CANADIAN COMMUNITY AS PARTNER

THEORY & MULTIDISCIPLINARY PRACTICE

Ardene Robinson Vollman, PhD, RN, CCHN(C)

Interim Scientific Director
Primary Health Care Strategic Clinical Network
Alberta Health Services
Adjunct Associate Professor
Department of Community Health Sciences
Cumming School of Medicine
University of Calgary
Calgary, Alberta
Chair, Canadian Public Health Association (2015–2016)

Elizabeth T. Anderson, DrPH, RN, FAAN

Professor Emerita
School of Nursing
The University of Texas Medical Branch
Galveston, Texas

Judith McFarlane, DrPH, RN, FAAN

Parry Chair in Health Promotion and Disease Prevention
College of Nursing
Texas Woman's University
Houston, Texas

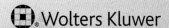 Wolters Kluwer

Philadelphia • Baltimore • New York • London
Buenos Aires • Hong Kong • Sydney • Tokyo

Art Director: Jennifer Clements
Acquisitions Editor: Christina Burns
Director of Product Development: Jennifer K. Forestieri
Supervising Development Editor: Heather Rybacki
Development Editor: Elizabeth Connolly
Editorial Assistant: Cassie Berube
Production Project Manager: Marian Bellus
Design Coordinator: Stephen Druding
Manufacturing Coordinator: Karin Duffield
Prepress Vendor: Aptara, Inc.

4th edition

Copyright © 2017 Wolters Kluwer.

Copyright © 2012 by Wolters Kluwer Health | Lippincott Williams & Wilkins.Copyright © 2008 by Wolters Kluwer Health | Lippincott Williams & Wilkins. Copyright © 2004 by Lippincott Williams & Wilkins. All rights reserved. This book is protected by copyright. No part of this book may be reproduced or transmitted in any form or by any means, including as photocopies or scanned-in or other electronic copies, or utilized by any information storage and retrieval system without written permission from the copyright owner, except for brief quotations embodied in critical articles and reviews. Materials appearing in this book prepared by individuals as part of their official duties as U.S. government employees are not covered by the above-mentioned copyright. To request permission, please contact Wolters Kluwer Health at Two Commerce Square, 2001 Market Street, Philadelphia, PA 19103, via email at permissions@lww.com, or via our website at lww.com (products and services).

9 8 7 6 5 4 3 2 1

Printed in China

Library of Congress Cataloging-in-Publication Data

Names: Vollman, Ardene Robinson, editor. | Anderson, Elizabeth T., editor. | McFarlane, Judith M., editor.
Title: Canadian community as partner : theory & multidisciplinary practice / [edited by] Ardene Robinson Vollman, Elizabeth T. Anderson, Judith McFarlane.
Description: Edition 4. | Philadelphia : Wolters Kluwer, [2017] | Includes bibliographical references and index.
Identifiers: LCCN 2016019632 | ISBN 9781496339980 (paperback)
Subjects: | MESH: Community Health Nursing–methods | Community Health Planning–methods | Consumer Participation | Health Promotion–methods | Models, Nursing | Canada | Case Reports
Classification: LCC RT98 | NLM WY 106 | DDC 610.73/430971–dc23 LC record available at https://lccn.loc.gov/2016019632

Care has been taken to confirm the accuracy of the information presented and to describe generally accepted practices. However, the authors, editors, and publisher are not responsible for errors or omissions or for any consequences from application of the information in this book and make no warranty, expressed or implied, with respect to the currency, completeness, or accuracy of the contents of the publication. Application of this information in a particular situation remains the professional responsibility of the practitioner; the clinical treatments described and recommended may not be considered absolute and universal recommendations.

The authors, editors, and publisher have exerted every effort to ensure that drug selection and dosage set forth in this text are in accordance with the current recommendations and practice at the time of publication. However, in view of ongoing research, changes in government regulations, and the constant flow of information relating to drug therapy and drug reactions, the reader is urged to check the package insert for each drug for any change in indications and dosage and for added warnings and precautions. This is particularly important when the recommended agent is a new or infrequently employed drug.

Some drugs and medical devices presented in this publication have Food and Drug Administration (FDA) clearance for limited use in restricted research settings. It is the responsibility of the health care provider to ascertain the FDA status of each drug or device planned for use in his or her clinical practice.

RRS1605

Dedication

For my family—my husband Ken, sons Rob and Mike, daughter-in-law Joanna,
our wonderful grandchildren Dylan and Sydney, and our angel Allyson.
You are the wind beneath my wings!
—ARV

Contributors

Gracia Adam, BSc en nutrition
Chargée de projet
Centre communautaire Jean-Guy Drolet
Québec, Québec

Robert C. Annis, PhD
Research Affiliate
Rural Development Institute
Brandon University
Cobble Hill, British Columbia

Annette Bailey, PhD, RN
Assistant Professor
Daphne Cockwell School of Nursing
Ryerson University
Toronto, Ontario

Ananya Tina Banerjee, PhD, R.Kin
Registered Kinesiologist
Women's Cardiovascular Health Initiative
Women's College Hospital
Toronto, Ontario

Shirley Bassett, BSc(Dent)
Honorary Colleague
Dental Program
School of Health and Human Services
Camosun College
Victoria, British Columbia

Kathy L. Belton, MEd, PhD(c)
Associate Director
Injury Prevention Centre
School of Public Health
University of Alberta
Edmonton, Alberta

Claire Betker, MN, PhD(c), RN, CCHN(C)
Director
Population Health and Health Equity
Public Health Branch
Manitoba Health, Healthy Living and Seniors
Winnipeg, Manitoba

Simon Carroll, PhD
Assistant Teaching Professor
Department of Sociology
University of Victoria
Victoria, British Columbia

Yvonne Chiu, BSc, PhD(Hon)
Executive Director
Multicultural Health Brokers Co-operative
Edmonton, Alberta

Alexandria Crowe, MN, NP Acute, RN(EC)
Nurse Practitioner
St. Joseph's Healthcare
Hamilton, Ontario

Cheryl Cusack, PhD, RN
Clinical Nurse Specialist
Winnipeg Regional Health Authority
Winnipeg, Manitoba

Mahdieh Dastjerdi, PhD, RN
Associate Professor
School of Nursing
Faculty of Health
York University
Toronto, Ontario

Gayleen Dimond, BN, RN
Public Health Nurse
Winnipeg Regional Health Authority
Winnipeg, Manitoba

Sophie Dupéré, PhD en santé communautaire
Professeure adjointe
Faculté des sciences infirmières
Université Laval
Québec, Québec

Daniel J. Dutton, PhD
Postdoctoral Fellow
The Prentice Institute for Global Population
  and Economy
University of Lethbridge
Lethbridge, Alberta

Dana S. Edge, PhD, RN
Associate Professor
School of Nursing
Faculty of Health Sciences
Queen's University
Kingston, Ontario

Laurie Fownes, BSW, MSc
Community Health Consultant
Calgary, Alberta

Ryan Gibson, PhD
Assistant Professor
Department of Geography and Environmental
  Studies
Saint Mary's University
Halifax, Nova Scotia

Kate Hall, MSc, PI
Community Planning Consultant
Minden, Ontario

Gwen K. Healey, PhD
Executive and Scientific Director
Qaujigiartiit Health Research Centre
Iqaluit, Nunavut

Rita Isabel Henderson, PhD
Postdoctoral Fellow
Department of Family Medicine
Cumming School of Medicine
University of Calgary
Calgary, Alberta

Marcia Hills, PhD, RN, FAAN
Professor
School of Nursing
Faculty of Human and Social Development
University of Victoria
Victoria, British Columbia

Cheryl Houtekamer, MPH
Program Supervisor
Youth Addiction Services
Addiction and Mental Health
Alberta Health Services
Calgary, Alberta

Anna Kirova, PhD
Professor of Early Childhood Education
Department of Elementary Education
Faculty of Education
University of Alberta
Edmonton, Alberta

Brigette Krieg, PhD
Associate Professor
Faculty of Social Work (Saskatoon Campus)
University of Regina
Saskatoon, Saskatchewan

Jennifer Langille, BN, RN
Nursing Instructor
Faculty of Nursing
University of Calgary
Calgary, Alberta

Candace Lind, PhD, RN
Associate Professor
Faculty of Nursing
University of Calgary
Calgary, Alberta

Melanie Lind-Kosten, MEd, RN
Nursing Instructor
Faculty of Nursing
University of Calgary
Calgary, Alberta

Wendi Lokanc-Diluzio, PhD, RN
Sexual and Reproductive Health Specialist
Alberta Health Services
Calgary, Alberta

Gail L. MacKean, MPA, PhD
Adjunct Assistant Professor
Department of Community Health Sciences
Cumming School of Medicine
University of Calgary
Calgary, Alberta

Sharon Mackinnon, BScN, BPHE, RN
Public Health Nurse
City of Hamilton, Public Health Services
Hamilton, Ontario

Bretta Maloff, MEd, RD
Alberta Health Services (retired)
Calgary, Alberta

K. Ashlee McGuire, PhD
Senior Planner
Alberta Health Services
Calgary, Alberta

Nancy C. McPherson, MSc, RN
Assistant Professor
Department of Nursing
Faculty of Health Studies
Brandon University
Brandon, Manitoba

Lynn M. Meadows, PhD
Adjunct Associate Professor
Department of Community Health Sciences
Cumming School of Medicine
University of Calgary
Calgary, Alberta

Melody Mendonça, MHSc
Research Coordinator
Centre for Studies in Food Security
Ryerson University
Toronto, Ontario

Pertice Moffitt, PhD, RN
Manager/Instructor
Health Research Programs
Aurora Research Institute, Aurora College
Yellowknife, Northwest Territories

Christina Murray, PhD, RN
Assistant Professor
School of Nursing
University of Prince Edward Island
Charlottetown, Prince Edward Island

Richard Musto, MD, FRCPC
Lead Medical Officer of Health
Calgary Zone
Alberta Health Services
Clinical Professor
Department of Community Health Sciences
Cumming School of Medicine
University of Calgary
Calgary, Alberta

Cameron D. Norman, MDes, PhD, CE
Principal
CENSE Research + Design
Toronto, Ontario

Nelly D. Oelke, PhD, RN
Assistant Professor
School of Nursing
Faculty of Health and Social Development
University of British Columbia, Okanagan
   Campus
Kelowna, British Columbia

Linda Ogilvie, PhD, RN
Professor Emeritus
Faculty of Nursing
University of Alberta
Edmonton, Alberta

Joyce M. O'Mahony, PhD, RN
Assistant Professor
School of Nursing
Thompson Rivers University
Kamloops, British Columbia

Katherine S. Pachkowski, MSc, RPN
Assistant Professor
Faculty of Health Studies
Brandon University
Brandon, Manitoba

André-Anne Parent, PhD
Professeure adjointe
École de sociale, Faculté des arts et des sciences
Université de Montréal
Montréal, Québec

J. David Patterson, BN, RN
Nursing Instructor
Faculty of Nursing
University of Calgary
Calgary, Alberta

Jennifer A.D. Price, PhD, RN, CCN(C)
Advance Practice Nurse
Women's Cardiovascular Health Initiative/
  Cardiology
Women's College Hospital
Toronto, Ontario

Frances E. Racher, PhD, RN
Professor
Faculty of Health Studies
Brandon University
Brandon, Manitoba

Sandra M. Reilly, EdD, RN
Associate Professor
Faculty of Nursing
University of Calgary
Calgary, Alberta

J. Renée Robinson, PhD, RPN
Professor
Department of Psychiatric Nursing
Faculty of Health Studies
Brandon University
Brandon, Manitoba

Cecilia Rocha, PhD
Director and Professor
School of Nutrition
Faculty of Community Services
Ryerson University
Toronto, Ontario

Manon Roy, BSc en travail social
Organisateur communautaire
Centre intégré universitaire de santé et service
  sociaux de la Capitale-Nationale
Québec, Québec

Gayle Rutherford, PhD, RN
Associate Professor
Faculty of Nursing
University of Calgary
Calgary, Alberta

Laura Ryan, MSW
Community Developer
Social Planning and Research Council
  of Hamilton
Hamilton, Ontario

Melissa Schaefer, Dip. D.T., Dip. D.H., MEd
Instructor
Dental Hygiene Program
School of Health and Human Services
Camosun College
Victoria, British Columbia

Catherine M. Scott, PhD
Chief Operating Officer and Lead
Policy Research
Alberta Centre for Child, Family and
  Community Research
Calgary, Alberta

Fran E. Scott, MSc, MD, CCFP, FRCPC
Associate Professor
Department of Clinical Epidemiology and
  Biostatistics
Faculty of Health Sciences
McMaster University
Hamilton, Ontario

Zahra Shajani, MPH, RN, CCHN(C)
Nursing Instructor
Faculty of Nursing
University of Calgary
Calgary, Alberta

Sue Shikaze, BSc, BEd
Health Promoter
Haliburton, Kawartha, Pine Ridge District
  Health Unit
Haliburton, Ontario

Malcolm Shookner, MA
Government of Nova Scotia (retired)
Halifax, Nova Scotia

Cynthia Smith, DrPH
Dean
School of Health and Human Services
Camosun College
Victoria, British Columbia

Sky Starr, MDiv, BRE, RMFT, CPC
Executive Director
Out Of Bounds (Grief Support)
Toronto, Ontario

Wilfreda E. Thurston, PhD
Professor
Department of Community Health Sciences
Cumming School of Medicine
University of Calgary
Calgary, Alberta

Brianne Timpson, MN, RN
Manager
Quality and Risk Assurance
Stanton Territorial Health Authority
Yellowknife, Northwest Territories

Christine Vandenberghe, MEd
Research Scientist (Evaluation)
Alberta Centre for Child, Family and
    Community Research
Calgary, Alberta

Gaynor Watson-Creed, MSc, MD, CCFP, FRCPC
Medical Officer of Health
Nova Scotia Health Authority
Dartmouth, Nova Scotia
Adjunct Professor
Department of Community Health and
    Epidemiology
Faculty of Medicine
Dalhousie University
Halifax, Nova Scotia

Sasha Wiens, BN, RN
Manager
Calgary Adult Bariatric Specialty Clinic
Alberta Health Services
Calgary, Alberta

Lewis Williams, Dip. S.W., MPH, PhD
Adjunct Associate Professor
School of Environmental Studies
Faculty of Social Sciences
University of Victoria
Victoria, British Columbia

Justine Zidona, BN, RN, IBCLC
Public Health Nurse
Winnipeg Regional Health Authority
Winnipeg, Manitoba

Reviewers

Carrie L. Allen, MN, RN
Undergraduate Adjunct Professor
Department of Nursing
University of Regina
Regina, Saskatchewan

Sherry Arvidson, MN, EdD, RN
Faculty of Nursing
University of Regina
Regina, Saskatchewan

Christine Balfour, MA, RN
Instructor of Nursing
University of British Columbia, Okanagan
    Campus
Kelowna, British Columbia

Nancy Barnes, MN, RN
Faculty Lecturer
Department of Nursing
University of Alberta
Edmonton, Alberta

Elizabeth Burgess-Pinto, PhD, RN
Assistant Professor
Bachelor of Science in Nursing Program
MacEwan University
Edmonton, Alberta

Sally Dampier, DNP, MMedSc(N), RN
Professor of Nursing
Confederation College
Thunder Bay, Ontario

Patricia Gregory, PhD, RN
Research and Scholarship Coordinator
Department of Nursing
Nursing Instructor
Red River College
Winnipeg, Manitoba

Deena Honan, MSN, RN
Instructor of Nursing
Grande Prairie Regional College
Grande Prairie, Alberta

Tracy Hoot, MSN, DHEd(c), RN
Instructor of Nursing
Thompson Rivers University
Kamloops, British Columbia

Frances Legault, PhD, RN
Lecturer
School of Nursing
University of Ottawa
Ottawa, Ontario

Marian MacLellan, MN, RN
Assistant Professor
Department of Nursing
Saint Francis Xavier University
Antigonish, Nova Scotia

Cheyenne Mary, BScK, BScN, MPH, RN
Senior Nursing Instructor
Faculty of Nursing
University of New Brunswick
Moncton, New Brunswick

Stephanie Montesanti, PhD
Assistant Professor
School of Public Health
University of Alberta
Edmonton, Alberta

Christina Murray, PhD, RN
Assistant Professor
School of Nursing
University of Prince Edward Island
Charlottetown, Prince Edward Island

Aroha Page, PhD, RN, FRCNA
Associate Professor of Nursing
Nipissing University
North Bay, Ontario

Mariann Rich, MSc, RN
Assistant Professor
Centre for Nursing & Health Studies
Athabasca University
Edmonton, Alberta

Ruth Schofield, BScN, MSc(T)
Assistant Professor
Faculty of Health Sciences
McMaster University
Hamilton, Ontario

Gail Sheppard, MSN
Faculty of Health
Kwantlen Polytechnic University
Langley, British Columbia

Laralea Stalkie, MSN, RN
Faculty of Nursing
St. Lawrence College/Laurentian University
    Collaborative
Kingston, Ontario

Shannon Vandenberg, MScN, RN, CCHN(C)
Nursing Instructor
Faculty of Health Sciences
University of Lethbridge
Lethbridge, Alberta

Cindy Versteeg, MScN, RN
Professor
Bachelor of Science in Nursing Program
Algonquin College
Ottawa, Ontario

Foreword

In writing this book, I have been faced with the challenge of aligning the concepts of population and public health with community development and health so that the Canadian community-as-partner (CCAP) process is meaningful for population and community assessment, action, and evaluation.

According to the Public Health Agency of Canada, *population health* is an approach that aims to improve the health of the entire population and to reduce health inequities among population groups.[1] To reach these objectives, population and public health professionals plan and carry out interventions that act upon the broad range of factors and conditions (determinants) that have a strong influence on people's health. *Community health* is defined by Baisch (2009)[2] as being grounded in the philosophical beliefs of social justice and empowerment. It is dynamic and contextual and is achieved through participatory community development processes that are based on ecologic models designed to address broad determinants of health. In both cases, an interdisciplinary approach is taken, but in the community health approach, partnership, public participation, engagement, and empowerment are core values. In Canada, using a population health approach incorporates many aspects of both population health and community health approaches while appreciating the science of epidemiology and social demography. Both perspectives value the promotion of health, both focus on the collective, and both recognize the determinants of health as foundational concepts and targets for action.

A paradigm shift regarding population and community health is advancing—interventions are less about professional control and more about community involvement, leadership, and empowerment. The CCAP model proposes an iterative and sequential process that demands creativity and courage to trust in people and the process. Community members have important and valuable "gifts" to offer—lived experiences and insider knowledge. Community health workers complement these "gifts" in the form of professional training, knowledge, and access to resources. By working together in respectful collaborations, positive change can be achieved.

In this book I have used a social planning perspective (which is admittedly traditional) combined with community development and social action examples. I have taken this approach because in many instances community work is initiated by health or social agencies of one sort or another in response to population or community concerns. Respect for the population and the community leads to the engagement of community members and the development of partnerships to build capacity for action to achieve health equity. Public participation is essential to facilitate fair and just decision making, even in contexts where wide disparities in wealth and health exist.

---

[1]Public Health Agency of Canada. URL=http://www.phac-aspc.gc.ca/ph-sp/approach-approche/index-eng.php#What
[2]Baisch, M. J. (2009). Community health: An evolutionary concept analysis. *Journal of Advanced Nursing, 65*(11), 2464–2476. doi:10.1111/j.1365-2648.2009.05068.x

The key message in this book is that a healthy community provides capacity and resources for a healthy population. The factors that determine the health of Canadians are complex and interrelated. To promote health and prevent disease and injury and reduce harm, an upstream approach is mandatory, taking into consideration the best evidence, putting into place clear accountability structures and processes, and using multiple action strategies, in multiple settings, across multiple sectors and systems. Hierarchical approaches are no longer acceptable in community work; horizontal partnerships and collaborations have demonstrated effectiveness in the creation of sustainable change, community health, and healthy people.

Aligning the concepts of population health and community development is necessary to clarify and illuminate the goals and objectives of community work, ensure open and clear communication among and between members of various disciplines and community partners, build community capacity, and facilitate change. Ultimately, if community partnerships are effective, the health of our communities will be sustained, health disparities between population groups will be reduced, and Canadians will have more equitable access to health.

Preface

Since the first edition of *Canadian Community as Partner: Theory & Multidisciplinary Practice* was published, I have had the pleasure of meeting many public health and community practitioners and students who have used the book to learn and to inform their practice. I have also learned that community groups have used the book to guide their own projects, and that the Catholic University of Health and Allied Sciences in Bugando, Tanzania has adopted the book for its Masters in Public Health Program. The book was originally written to provide a "made-in-Canada" resource for exactly these purposes: education, practice, and community development.

Canada continues to be a leader on the international stage in public health and health promotion, thanks in large part to the leadership exhibited by the Public Health Agency of Canada, the Canadian Public Health Association and other nongovernmental organizations, and provincial/territorial institutions. However, we have not often recognized the importance of the grassroots approach to community practice; in this book we tell the stories of projects that use the CCAP process and principles of primary health care to improve the health status of their communities and populations.

The book is organized in three sections: a *theoretical* section that sets the foundation for how and why we work as partners with the communities we serve; a *process* section that details the activities of the CCAP model in action; and a section of *stories* from a variety of contributors that tell the tales of working in and with communities from sea to sea to sea (and overseas).

Section 1: Theoretical Foundations

In this section of *Canadian Community as Partner,* the reader is invited to understand the fundamental principles of community practice. It uses the Ottawa Charter (1986) as its primary framework, incorporating the Charter actions, determinants of health, epidemiologic principles, the appreciation of ethics and culture, social justice, prevention and harm reduction, mental health promotion, and the expanding role of social media in public health. Fundamental to community practice is the interdisciplinary nature of teamwork; hence, there are no references to the wide variety of professions that comprise the community/public health workforce. We refer instead to the generic "community health worker," and anticipate that readers will adapt this to their respective professions, roles, and settings.

Section 2: The Process of Community as Partner

This section begins with the CCAP model that guides the process of working in and with communities. In subsequent chapters, each step of the process is detailed with specific examples. All of the steps in the CCAP process emphasize the importance of social justice, equity, public participation/engagement, and the determinants of health. The CCAP process is presented sequentially—however, in practice it is not linear; it is iterative and creative and contextual.

Section 3: Canadian Community-as-Partner in Practice: Case Stories

The chapters in this section tell the stories of field-based community workers in population/community health promotion from several disciplinary viewpoints. All action strategies of the Ottawa Charter are illustrated, along with stories that touch many populations across the country and internationally. The projects included took place in several different settings, illustrating how community health workers partner across sectors to achieve health outcomes that affect people and the communities in which they live. The stories are all new to this edition, and provide support for the successful application of the CCAP process in population and community health action.

Readers will note that not all issues challenging community health workers are addressed—that would be an impossible task! However, the CCAP process is transferable to multiple settings for action by a variety of players. As you will note in the case stories, data were collected to define and bound the issues of concern, literature was reviewed to examine options for action, and people were consulted in various ways to plan, carry out, and evaluate interventions. Readers can use the CCAP process to think about and plan actions to address issues they are facing that are not included in this book—youth homelessness, refugee and immigrant health, vaccine hesitancy, Aboriginal health, to name but a few topics that continue to challenge the health of Canadians.

The stories told in this book are but a minuscule sample of the extraordinary community work that is happening across Canada. I encourage all readers to share their own stories with others. It is through communication that knowledge is developed, exchanged, and translated into action. Provided throughout this book are internet sites and resources that can afford insights into the work of others. The book is also supported by a website—thePoint (http://thepoint.lww.com/Vollman4e). I encourage you to use the resources we have provided and find others, and to share what you learn with your colleagues.

This book would not be as valuable to readers without the stories and experiences shared by our many contributors. If you have a story you would like to share in the next edition of *Canadian Community as Partner,* or comments about any aspect of the book, please contact me (avollman@shaw.ca).

Ardene Robinson Vollman, PhD, RN, CCHN(C)

Acknowledgements

Without the efforts of Judith McFarlane and Elizabeth (Bets) Anderson over two decades and seven editions of their original book, *Community as Partner*, the first Canadian edition would never have been written.

Without the support of my family, I might not have embarked on the publishing journey that brings me to this fourth edition of *Canadian Community as Partner: Theory & Multi-disciplinary Practice*.

Throughout my career in public health and health promotion in Canada, I have met many people—educators, researchers, practitioners, students, and community members; all have inspired me and have been the motivation behind this book. Several have contributed their work to this book, and I am very grateful for their efforts.

I am particularly grateful to my colleague Kathy Dirk who has been a valuable assistant in the preparation of this edition of the book. Thanks also to the editorial team, led by Elizabeth Connolly, for their efforts throughout the publication process.

Contents

SECTION

2   The Process of Community as Partner   201

SECTION 3

Community as Partner in Practice   303

Common Acronyms Used in This Book

APHA	American Public Health Association
CBPAR	Community-Based Participatory Action Research
CCAP	Canadian Community-as-Partner
CCHS	Canadian Community Health Survey
CDC	Centers for Disease Control and Prevention
CIHI	Canadian Institute for Health Information
CIHR	Canadian Institutes of Health Research
CNA	Canadian Nurses Association
COPD	Chronic Obstructive Pulmonary Disease
CPHA	Canadian Public Health Association
CSDH	Commission on Social Determinants of Health
ESDC	Employment and Social Development Canada
HCC	Health Council of Canada
HIV	Human Immunodeficiency Virus
IMR	Infant Mortality Rate
LGBTIQ	Lesbian, Gay, Bisexual, Transgendered, Intersexed, and Queer/Questioning
LGBTQ	Lesbian, Gay, Bisexual, Transgendered, and Questioning (Two-Spirited)
LICO	Low-Income Cut-Off
MHCC	Mental Health Commission of Canada
NCCAH	National Collaborating Centre for Aboriginal Health
NCCDH	National Collaborating Centre for Determinants of Health
NCCEH	National Collaborating Centre for Environmental Health
NCCHPP	National Collaborating Centre for Healthy Public Policy
NCCID	National Collaborating Centre for Infectious Diseases
NCCMT	National Collaborating Centre for Methods and Tools
NCCPH	National Collaborating Centres for Public Health
NGO	Nongovernmental Organization
NHS	National Household Survey
PAHO	Pan American Health Organization
PAR	Participatory Action Research
PHAC	Public Health Agency of Canada
PHN	Public Health Nurse
PPD	Postpartum Depression
PTSD	Posttraumatic Stress Disorder

RN	Registered Nurse
SARS	Severe Acute Respiratory Syndrome
SES	Socioeconomic Status
STBBI	Sexually Transmitted and Blood Borne Infections
TB	Tuberculosis
UN	United Nations
WHO	World Health Organization

Note to Readers:

In this book, the term "Aboriginal" is used broadly as an umbrella term for the Indigenous peoples of Canada, including First Nations (status and nonstatus), Métis, and Inuit. While a broad definition has been adopted for the purpose of this book, it is important to recognize and appreciate the diversity among and within these groups.

Theoretical Foundations

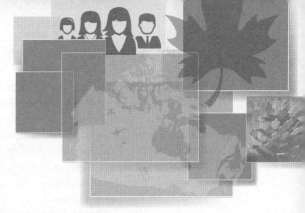

CHAPTER 1

Population Health Promotion: Essentials and Essence of Practice

Ardene Robinson Vollman

LEARNING OBJECTIVES

After studying this chapter, you should be able to:

1. Describe the philosophical foundations of population health promotion

2. List the five principles and eight essentials of primary health care

3. Outline the challenges, mechanisms, and strategies of the Canadian Framework for Health Promotion

4. Detail the prerequisites for health and the action strategies for health promotion as described in the Ottawa Charter for Health Promotion

5. List the factors that determine health

6. Describe population health and the population health approach

7. Understand the evolution of population health promotion

Introduction

In the 20th century, many gains in health status among the people of the developed world were achieved. Much was accomplished through four means: (1) advances in knowledge about the causes of disease, (2) development of new technologies and pharmaceuticals to treat and cure many diseases, (3) creation of vaccines and environmental solutions to prevent disease transmission and acquisition, and (4) innovations in surveillance techniques to measure health status. However, it has become increasingly accepted that health is more than the absence of disease—it is a broad manifestation of wellness of body, mind, and environment and is viewed as an essential resource for everyday living. This chapter chronicles the history and the evolution of thought around the concept of health as it relates to individuals, families, groups, and communities. Many of the principles and concepts presented in this chapter are discussed in more detail in other parts of the book.

In this text, the generic term "community health worker" or "community health team" is used to connote the multidisciplinary and intersectoral approach that underlies successful community practice. This book is intended to be useful to community social workers, dental health providers, nutritionists, health educators, community health nurses, community medicine physicians, pharmacists, health promoters, and community groups. It also recognizes that community health teams should have members of the public involved in all levels of activities to ensure that the foundational principles of community practice are implemented.

As you will see as you progress through this book and learn the processes of community and population assessment, planning, and evaluation, it will become evident that no single person or agency is capable of addressing the many and complex health problems of communities and populations. Because health is determined by a complex mix of factors, maintaining and creating health requires ongoing action from multiple partners whose mandates support similar goals. Hence, community health workers rely on cooperation with other workers, collaboration among agencies involved in similar work, and partnerships with people, communities, public and private sectors, and business to effect change that has a positive impact on the health of people.

Partnerships may be formed across *sectors* (i.e., broad fields of activity, such as education, health, justice) and at different *levels.* Levels may be defined by geography, scope of mandate (e.g., municipal, provincial), or vertical level within organizations (e.g., senior management, front line). Action is more effective when it includes vertical as well as horizontal partnerships and collaboration. Horizontal links are created when partnerships are formed at the same level. For instance, to deal with an outbreak of infection in a day care centre, the health district's environmental health officer and community nurse, the school board's preschool education specialist, and the social worker from children's services may be involved in the follow-up action. As an illustration of vertical collaboration, to set health policy regarding tobacco, a health region will work with the federal health department, the provincial health ministry, and the municipality, all of whom have different jurisdictions in policy development and enforcement. Horizontally, each partner may also need to work with justice counterparts (e.g., Royal Canadian Mounted Police, provincial police, local bylaw enforcement) and other departments to effect change in tobacco policy.

Key to all community practice is the principle of "doing with," not "to" or "for," the people served. This theme is pervasive in all the documents that form the foundation of community practice. The title of this book is *Canadian Community as Partner,* meaning that community workers partner not only with professional colleagues to serve the people in communities but also with members of those communities and groups.

FOUNDATIONS OF COMMUNITY PRACTICE

Whatever discipline in which community workers are trained, several documents published in the last quarter of the 20th century have been instrumental in the development of guiding principles for health promotion practice (Table 1.1).

TABLE 1.1   Seminal Documents in the Development of Health Promotion Practice

Title	Author/Year	URL
A New Perspective on the Health of Canadians	Lalonde, 1974	www.phac-aspc.gc.ca/ph-sp/pdf/perspect-eng.pdf
Declaration of Alma-Ata	WHO, 1978	www.who.int/publications/almaata_declaration_en.pdf
Achieving Health for All: A Framework for Health Promotion in Canada	Epp, 1986	www.hc-sc.gc.ca/hcs-sss/pubs/system-regime/1986-frame-plan-promotion/index-eng.php
Ottawa Charter for Health Promotion	WHO, 1986	www.who.int/healthpromotion/conferences/previous/ottawa/en/
Action Statement for Health Promotion in Canada	CPHA, 1996	www.cpha.ca/en/programs/policy/action.aspx

Two documents preceded the widespread acceptance of health promotion globally: the Lalonde report (1974) in Canada, and the WHO's Declaration of Alma-Ata (1978) on the international stage. These documents are discussed in the next section as they are foundational to understanding the impetus of the health promotion movement initiated in Canada by the Ottawa Charter.

The Lalonde Report

The publication of the report *A New Perspective on the Health of Canadians* heralded a change in the definition of health from having a focus on the absence of disease to emphasizing well-being in a larger context (Lalonde, 1974). The Lalonde report argues that health is not achievable from health care services alone but from the interaction of health services with human biology, lifestyle, and the environment in which we live (i.e., the four fields). This report suggested that health is tied to overall conditions of living, particularly the environment and the behaviours chosen by people. Lalonde's approach was directed primarily toward the individual and toward individuals taking responsibility for their health. Proponents of the approach tended to focus on behaviours, and when illness or injury resulted, people felt "blamed" for not carrying out the recommended health behaviours or not doing them "enough." Interventions focused on telling people what the healthy behaviour was, but did not address the social conditions that militated against its adoption. The emphasis on lifestyle captured the attention of governments, and the social-environmental elements were consequently downplayed in health policy and funding until the next decade when it became evident that the health education and social marketing approaches were insufficient to create the reduction in health expenditures envisioned by politicians and health planners.

Although the Lalonde report had obvious limitations, it did stimulate thought in a new direction and led to other important outcomes, not the least of which was the attention sparked across sectors such as economics, education, social welfare, and justice regarding the environmental imperatives of creating healthy people in healthy nations. As a result, the Lalonde report received international attention, and in response to the growing concern about the disparities in health status between developed and undeveloped countries and between people with many resources and those with few, the World Health Organization (WHO) convened a meeting of member countries.

Declaration of Alma-Ata

The WHO member states met in Alma-Ata, Kazakhstan in 1978 to develop an action plan to achieve the goal of "Health for All by Year 2000," proposed as the vision by the 30th World Health Assembly. From this conference came the *Declaration of Alma-Ata* (WHO, 1978) on primary health care, viewed as the bridge between the Lalonde perspective and the influence of postmodern thinkers and critical social theorists who critiqued social structures to better understand and transform the dominant social order. As historical, cultural, and gendered social constructions were questioned, new ways of working with people emerged so that the people themselves (not the politicians or the experts) could shape the world in which they live.

The Declaration of Alma-Ata (Box 1.1) became the philosophy of community action for health. Its emphasis on the principles of social justice, equity, public participation, appropriate technology, and intersectoral collaboration focused action on the needs of the population and the root causes of ill health, challenging the system to move beyond the traditional biomedical model (disease) to a framework that promoted health. Influenced by the work of critical social theorists, the Declaration of Alma-Ata called for health providers to work *with* people to assist them in making decisions about their health and how to meet health challenges in ways that are affordable, acceptable, and sustainable in the long term.

> **Box 1.1   Declaration of Alma-Ata: Primary Health Care**
>
> Primary health care is essential health care based on practical, scientifically sound, and socially acceptable methods and technology made universally accessible to individuals and families in the community through their full participation and at a cost that the community and country can afford to maintain at every stage of their development in the spirit of self-reliance and self-determination. It forms an integral part both of the country's health system, of which it is the central function and main focus, and of the overall social and economic development of the community. It is the first level of contact of individuals, the family, and community with the national health system bringing health care as close as possible to where people live and work and constitutes the first element of a continuing health care process. (Article VI)

Primary health care is more than the first point of contact with the health system. It implies the application of the primary health care philosophy that ensures public participation at all levels of the system, social justice and equity, and a system that balances prevention and promotion with the demands for care, cure, and rehabilitation. Primary health care also extends beyond the health system to the other societal systems that create conditions where health can flourish. We can see primary health care in action in participatory research, in emancipatory political action, in empowerment education in schools, and in other social movements where social justice, equity, and participation are valued.

A Framework for Health Promotion in Canada

In recognition of the social aspects of health promotion and as a signatory to the Declaration of Alma-Ata, the Canadian government published the discussion paper *Achieving Health for All: A framework for Health Promotion* (Epp, 1986) in preparation for the WHO First International Health Promotion Conference in Ottawa held in 1986 (Fig. 1.1).

The mid-1980s were characterized by rapid social change due to shifting family structures, an aging population, and wider participation in the workforce by women. These conditions exacerbate certain health problems, create pressure for new kinds of social support, and force community workers to seek new approaches to deal effectively with the impact of these social forces on the future health of Canadians.

The Epp framework defines health as a part of everyday living, an essential dimension of the quality of our lives. In this context, quality of life "implies the opportunities to make choices and gain satisfaction from living." Health is a state that individuals and communities alike strive to achieve, maintain, or regain and is influenced by circumstances, beliefs, culture, and socioeconomic and physical environments. This document reaffirmed the WHO (1986) definition of health promotion as "the process of enabling people to increase control over, and to improve, their health."

The **aim** of health promotion is the achievement of health for all. Although the prospects for the health of Canadians had improved over recent decades, three major issues remained that were not being adequately addressed by current health policies and practices:

- Disadvantaged groups had significantly lower life expectancy, poorer health, and a higher prevalence of disability than the average Canadian.
- Various forms of preventable disease and injuries continued to undermine the health and quality of life of many Canadians.
- Many thousands of Canadians suffered from chronic disease, disability, or various forms of emotional stress and lacked adequate community support to help them cope and live meaningful, productive, and dignified lives (Epp, 1986, p. 1).

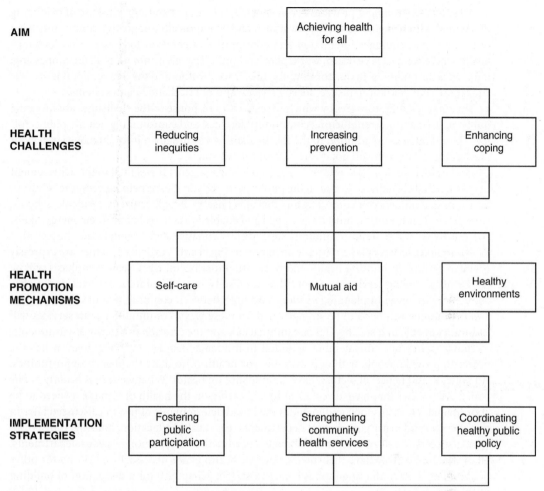

FIGURE 1.1   A Framework for Health Promotion in Canada.

To achieve the goal of "health for all," three *challenges* were articulated: reduce inequities in health status between Canadians with low and high incomes; increase the prevention effort and find new and more effective means to prevent injuries, illness, chronic conditions, and disabilities; and find ways to enhance people's ability to manage and cope with chronic conditions, disabilities, and mental health problems.

Three *mechanisms* intrinsic to health promotion are self-care, or the decisions and actions individuals take in the interest of their own health; mutual aid, or the actions people take to help each other; and healthy environments, or the creation of conditions and surroundings conducive to health.

Self-care refers to the decisions made and the behaviours practised by an individual specifically for the preservation of health; encouraging self-care means encouraging healthy choices. Beliefs, access to appropriate information, and being in surroundings that are supportive are factors that play important roles in making healthy choices.

Mutual aid refers to people's efforts to work together to deal with concerns; it implies people helping each other, supporting each other emotionally, and sharing ideas, information, and experiences. Frequently referred to as social support, mutual aid may arise in the context of the family, the community, a voluntary organization, a self-help group, informal networks, or a special interest association.

A *healthy environment* provides social support, the understanding and sense of belonging that comes with being in a socially, physically, and economically supportive community built in a way that encourages interaction and community integration to preserve and enhance health where we live, love, learn, work, play, and pray. The environment is all encompassing; it includes the buildings in our community, the air we breathe, and the jobs we do. It is also the education, transportation, justice, social services, and political and health systems.

The three leading *strategies* by which we can act in response to the challenges are fostering public participation, strengthening community services, and coordinating healthy public policy. These strategies, in addition to the mechanisms, are mutually reinforcing; one strategy or mechanism on its own will not create significant outcomes.

Public participation (also referred to as public engagement) is essential to the achievement of health for all Canadians. Encouraging public participation means helping people take part in decisions that influence or control factors that affect health. People (citizens, residents, schools, workplaces, communities) must be equipped and enabled to act; to channel their energy, skills, and creativity; and to build community capacity and enhance social capital (see Chapter 5).

Community services play a critical role in preserving health, particularly if they are expressly oriented toward promoting health and preventing disease/injury. Greater emphasis will be placed on providing services to groups that are disadvantaged, communities will need to become more involved in planning services, and links between communities and their services and institutions will need to be strengthened. In these ways, community health services will assume a key role in fostering self-care, mutual aid, and the creation of healthy environments.

Public policy has considerable potential to influence people's everyday lives; it has the power to provide people with opportunities for health or to deny them such opportunities. All policies, and hence all sectors, have an influence on health. What we seek is *healthy public policy*. All policies that have direct or indirect bearing on the health of Canadians need to be coordinated. The list is long and includes the broad determinants of health (discussed later in this chapter) and many government departments (e.g., health, education, housing, transportation, justice). It is not an easy undertaking to coordinate policies among various departments, all of which obviously have their own priorities; health is not necessarily a priority for other departments and conflicting interests may exist. (See Chapter 9 for a discussion of building healthy public policy.)

GLOBAL CONFERENCES ON HEALTH PROMOTION

In 1986, the WHO convened the First International Conference on Health Promotion, which resulted in the publication of the Ottawa Charter for Health Promotion (WHO, 1986) (Fig. 1.2). This conference originated as a result of the Declaration of Alma-Ata (WHO, 1978) and was dedicated to creating health for people in countries around the globe.

Seven International Health Promotion Conferences have followed since 1986 (Table 1.2). At each conference, participants reaffirmed commitment to the Ottawa Charter and extended the discourse by focusing research and discussion on a single Ottawa Charter strategy and making recommendations for action. Other WHO initiatives over the ensuing decades have been spawned by the Ottawa Charter (Box 1.2).

Canadian influence on global health promotion on the international scene is very strong; Canadian researchers, policy makers, educators, and practitioners have contributed significantly to each of the WHO global health promotion conferences. The Healthy Cities movement began in Canada and has become a dominant force in European countries. The conceptualization of population health has grown in prominence in Canada with the expansion of Lalonde's four-field concept to a more complete understanding of the determinants of health (Box 1.3).

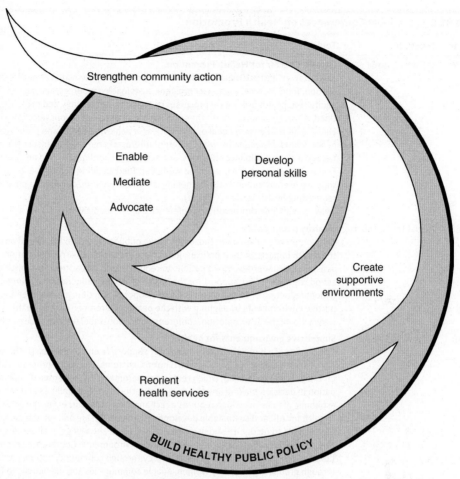

FIGURE 1.2   Ottawa Charter for Health Promotion. (Note: For an explanation of the logo, see http://www. who.int/healthpromotion/conferences/previous/ottawa/en/index4.html)

POPULATION HEALTH

Population health focuses on the health status of populations, which are conceptualized as coherent entities that are not simply the sum of individuals. Population health interventions address health inequities and a broad range of factors that impact health at the population level, such as environment, social structure, and resource distribution, as well as understanding these determinants in relation to biologic factors.

Box 1.2   Other WHO Initiatives for Health Promotion

The Global Conferences on Health Promotion have been influenced also by other WHO global initiatives such as conferences on sustainable development (e.g., Rio+20: The future we want [https://sustainabledevelopment.un.org/futurewewant.html]), UN General Assembly actions, and the WHO Commission on the Social Determinants of Health: Closing the gap in a genera-tion (www.who.int/social_determinants/thecommission/finalreport), among other national and international meetings.

TABLE 1.2 Global Conferences on Health Promotion

Year	Location	Topic
1986	Ottawa, Canada	**Ottawa Charter for Health Promotion** The Ottawa Charter explicitly identified the *prerequisites for health* as peace, shelter, education, food, income, a stable ecosystem, sustainable resources, and social justice and equity. The health promotion processes of enabling, advocating, and mediating were identified. *Advocacy* aims to create the social environmental conditions necessary for health. *Enabling* aims to ensure equal opportunities for achieving health and reducing inequities in health status. *Mediation* between different interests is required to ensure the collaboration needed among disciplines, agencies, and sectors to coordinate action and policy efforts. Five *strategies* for health promotion were identified: building healthy public policy, creating supportive environments, strengthening community action, developing personal skills, and reorienting health services (Fig. 1.2). www.who.int/healthpromotion/conferences/previous/ottawa/en/
1988	Adelaide, Australia	**Healthy public policy** This conference called upon those who make public policy to examine and be responsive to the health impacts of their policies. Pleas were made for industrialized nations to provide assistance to underdeveloped nations to reduce health disparities. Four priority areas for action were identified: support for the health of women; elimination of hunger and malnutrition; reduction of tobacco growing and alcohol production; and the creation of more supportive environments by aligning with the peace, environmental, and health movements. www.who.int/healthpromotion/conferences/previous/adelaide/en/index1.html
1991	Sundsvall, Sweden	**Supportive environments for health** This conference highlighted four aspects of supportive environments: (1) the social dimension, which includes the ways in which norms, customs, and social processes affect health; (2) the political dimension, which requires governments to guarantee democratic participation in decision making and the decentralization of responsibilities and resources; (3) the economic dimension, which requires a rechanneling of resources for the achievement of "Health for All" and sustainable development, including safe and reliable technology; and (4) the need to recognize and use women's skills and knowledge in all sectors to develop a more positive infrastructure for supportive environments. Conference recommendations for action were to strengthen advocacy through community action, particularly through groups organized by women; enable communities and individuals to take control of their health and environment through education and empowerment; build alliances to strengthen cooperation between health and environment campaigns; and mediate between conflicting interests in society to ensure equitable access to a supportive environment for health. www.who.int/healthpromotion/conferences/previous/sundsvall
1997	Jakarta, Indonesia	**Leading health promotion into the 21st century** The conditions (prerequisites) for health were expanded to include social security, social relations, empowerment of women, sustainable resource use, and respect for human rights. "Above all, poverty is the greatest threat to health." The statement noted the need for comprehensive approaches that work on several levels, within various settings, and effective partnerships among all levels of government, nongovernmental organizations (NGOs), and private and public sectors. Five priorities were set: (1) promote social responsibility for health, (2) increase investments for health development, (3) consolidate and expand partnerships for health, (4) increase community capacity and empower the individual, and (5) secure an infrastructure for health promotion. www.who.int/healthpromotion/conferences/previous/jakarta/declaration
1999	Mexico City, Mexico	**Bridging the equity gap** The theme of this conference was on strengthening the "art and science" (evidence base) of health promotion as well as strengthening political skills and actions for health promotion to ensure healthy public policy that reduces health inequity. Processes suggested were solidarity among practitioners and activists through networks, alliances, and partnerships; mobilization of resources; development of community capacity; development of human resources; and the creation of networks and associations of practitioners for mutual support and personal development. www.who.int/healthpromotion/conferences/previous/mexico

Year	Location	Topic
2005	Bangkok, Thailand	**Policy and partnership for action: Addressing the determinants of health** The Bangkok Charter for Health Promotion in a Globalized World identifies major challenges, actions, and commitments needed to address the determinants of health. It calls for all sectors and settings to advocate for health based on human rights and solidarity; invest in sustainable policies, actions, and infrastructure to address the determinants of health; build capacity for policy development, leadership, health promotion practice, knowledge transfer, research, and health literacy; regulate and legislate to ensure a high level of protection from harm and enable equal opportunity for health and well-being for all people; partner and build alliances with public, private, nongovernmental, and international organizations and civil society to create sustainable actions; and make the promotion of health a requirement for good corporate practice. www.who.int/healthpromotion/conferences/6gchp
2009	Nairobi, Kenya	**Promoting health and development: Closing the implementation gap** This conference identified key strategies and commitments urgently required to close the implementation gap in health and development through health promotion. Implementation gaps include gaps in health programs, in policy-making and intersectoral partnerships, and in health systems. Five strategies to combat such gaps were described: community empowerment, health literacy and health behaviour, strengthening health systems, partnerships and intersectoral action, and building capacity for health promotion. www.who.int/healthpromotion/conferences/7gchp
2013	Helsinki, Finland	**Health in all policies** This conference described an approach to public policy across sectors that systematically considers the health implications of policies, seeks partnerships, and forestalls negative health impacts in order to improve population health and health equity. This approach improves accountability for policy decisions while acknowledging that governments have a range of priorities in which health and equity do not automatically gain precedence over other policy objectives. www.who.int/healthpromotion/conferences/8gchp/statement_2013

Health Canada and the Public Health Agency of Canada (PHAC) have adopted the *population health approach* by which action is focused toward improved health outcomes, a sustainable and integrated health system, increased national growth and productivity, and strengthened social cohesion. The key elements of this approach are:

- Address the determinants of health, recognizing that they are complex and interrelated
- Focus on the health of populations
- Invest upstream
- Base decisions on evidence

Box 1.3 Principles and Essentials of Primary Health Care

According to the Declaration of Alma-Ata (WHO, 1978), primary health care refers to the five principles on which action on "health for all" must be based: equitable access to health and health services, public participation, appropriate technology, intersectoral collaboration, and reorientation of the health system to promotion of health and prevention of disease and injury. The Declaration further details eight essentials—services that nations must have in place to create positive conditions for health: education concerning prevailing health problems and the methods of preventing and controlling them; promotion of food supply and proper nutrition; an adequate supply of safe water and basic sanitation; maternal and child health care, including family planning; immunization against the major infectious diseases; prevention and control of locally endemic diseases; appropriate treatment of common diseases and injuries; and provision of essential drugs. (Article VII)

- Apply multiple strategies to act on the determinants of health
- Collaborate across levels and sectors
- Use mechanisms to engage citizens
- Increase accountability for health outcomes

A population health approach focuses on improving the health status of the population (PHAC, 2013). Action is directed at the health of an entire population, or subpopulation, rather than at individuals. Focusing on the health of populations also necessitates the reduction in inequalities in health status between population groups. An underlying assumption of a population health approach is that reductions in health inequities require reductions in material and social inequities. The outcomes or benefits of a population health approach, therefore, extend beyond improved population health outcomes to include a sustainable and integrated health system, increased national growth and productivity, and strengthened social cohesion and citizen engagement.

A population health approach reflects the evidence that factors outside the health care system or sector significantly affect health. Commonly referred to as the "determinants of health," the PHAC (2011) list (Table 1.3) is complemented by ongoing investigation by other researchers that adds to the current knowledge and understanding of what influences Canadians' health (Mikkonen & Raphael, 2010).

Take Note

Population health considers the entire range of individual and collective factors and conditions—and their interactions—that have been shown to be correlated with health.

Our knowledge of the determinants of health will continue to further develop, evolve, and be refined as interventions are implemented and successes chronicled. *Investing upstream* means directing attention at the root causes of illness and injury, rather than at the symptoms that are evident. In this way, interventions can be placed earlier in the causal stream and provide greater gains in population health. Traditional and new sources of qualitative and quantitative research and evaluation *evidence* are used to set priorities and identify best practices for influencing health; this is called evidence-based decision making. A *variety of strategies* applied in a variety of settings are required to create joint action among health and other sectors to effectively influence the factors that affect health and improve the health of Canadians. *Collaboration* and horizontal management strategies will require agreement on common goals, coordinated planning, development of related policies, and implementation of integrated programs and services. To do this means that citizens must be engaged in all aspects of health and social service priority setting, the determination of appropriate interventions, and the review of outcomes. (Chapter 5 discusses *public participation* and engagement in detail.) *Accountability* requires that process, impact, and outcome evaluations be undertaken to assess changes in health status and that the results of evaluations be reported widely not only to the scientific community but also to the public.

The population health approach has been proposed as a unifying force for the entire spectrum of health system interventions—from prevention, promotion, and protection to diagnosis, treatment, care, and rehabilitation—that integrates and balances actions among them. As an approach, population health targets factors that influence the health of Canadians across the life span, identifies variations in patterns of health, and uses the resulting knowledge to plan and implement interventions and policies to improve the nation's health status. Even though health and social services are funded by the provinces and territories, Health Canada and the PHAC exercise strong leadership roles in setting direction and standards in efforts to improve Canadians' health.

TABLE 1.3 Determinants of Health

Income and social status	Health status improves at each step up the income and social hierarchy. Higher income levels affect living conditions such as safe housing and the ability to buy sufficient and healthy food.
Social support networks	Support from families, friends, and communities is associated with better health. The health effect of the support of family and friends who provide a caring and supportive relationship may be as important as risk factors such as smoking, physical activity, obesity, and high blood pressure.
Education	Health status improves with level of education. Education increases opportunities for income and job security and gives people a sense of control over their lives—key factors that influence health.
Employment and working conditions	Unemployment, underemployment, and stressful work are associated with poorer health. Those with more control over their work and fewer stress-related demands on the job are healthier.
Social environments	The values and norms of a society affect the health and well-being of individuals and populations. Social stability, recognition of diversity, safety, good relationships, and cohesive communities provide a supportive society, which reduces or removes many risks to good health.
Physical environments	Physical factors in the natural environment (e.g., air and water quality) are key influences on health. Factors in the human-built environment, such as housing, workplace safety, and community and road design are also important influences.
Personal health practices and coping skills	Social environments that enable and support healthy choices and lifestyles, as well as people's knowledge, behaviours, and coping skills for dealing with life in healthy ways, are key influences on health.
Healthy child development	The effect of prenatal and early childhood experiences on subsequent health, well-being, coping skills, and competence is very powerful. For example, a low weight at birth links with health and social problems throughout life.
Culture	Culture comes from both personal history and wider situational, social, political, geographic, and economic factors. Multicultural health issues demonstrate how necessary it is to consider the interrelationships of physical, mental, spiritual, social, and economic well-being.
Gender	Gender refers to the many different roles, personality traits, attitudes, behaviours, values, relative powers, and influences that society assigns to the two sexes. Each sex has specific health issues or may be affected in different ways by the same issues.
Biology and genetic endowment	Physical characteristics we inherit play a part in deciding how long we live, how healthy we will be, and how likely we are to get certain illnesses.
Health services	It benefits people's health when they have access to services that prevent disease as well as maintain and promote health.

More detail on this approach is available from the PHAC website at http://www.phac-aspc.gc.ca/ph-sp/approach-approche/appr-eng.php

Target Populations

By incorporating the determinants, health services and health promotion activities have become targeted to specific groups within the population that had "needs" or deficits that could be addressed to improve health status. This approach rests on the foundation of risk factor assessment; that is, if people will reduce or eliminate risk-taking behaviours, and if risky environments can be fixed, then population health will improve. Therefore, individuals, groups, or aggregates of individuals, families, communities, and society itself became targets for action and intervention.

Many programs are directed toward individuals and aggregates—developing personal skills for healthy behaviours through health education and social marketing. The "BreakFree" campaign for youth tobacco reduction is an example of how program planners further categorize the target population through demographics. Youth were surveyed and then described in terms of subpopulations of youth, and messages were targeted accordingly, on the assumption that rural and urban youth, athletes, and honours students would respond differently to different marketing strategies to reduce tobacco use.

Other programs are directed to creating more supportive family environments for health; for instance, families living in poverty are provided opportunities in such programs as Head Start that prepares children for school entry, Nobody's Perfect that enhances parenting skills, and Canadian Prenatal Nutrition Program that supports early childhood development through family nutrition and prenatal support.

At the same time as Canadians' attitudes toward health and wellness are changing, social conventions are being altered so that behaviours such as tobacco use, substance use, intimate partner violence, and drinking and driving have become increasingly socially unacceptable. In addition, the move toward self-determination through public participation in policy decision making has become an imperative rather than a luxury. Canadians now expect to be consulted on matters that relate to health, and health is defined more broadly than the absence of disease.

Settings

As the targets for health interventions have expanded from the individual level, so too have settings for health service provision and health promotion expanded—from health settings (e.g., hospitals, clinics) to settings where people live, love, learn, work, play, and pray. The Healthy Cities, Health-Promoting Schools, and Healthy Workplace programs are attempts to develop strong communities and build social capacity and human capital that will enhance and strengthen the ability of communities, schools, and workplaces to influence the health and well-being of their residents, students and teachers, and employees.

The environment or context provided by various settings also contributes to health. As settings began to change and adapt in response to the needs and preferences of society, so too did environmental change affect people. That people behave or respond differently in different situations, contexts, and settings has led program planners to view settings or places as predisposing, enabling, and reinforcing factors for individual and collective behaviour (Green et al., 2000). Green and Kreuter (2005) state that the effectiveness of a health strategy depends on its fit with the target population, the health issue involved, and the environment in which it is applied. A multilevel, multicultural, multisectoral intervention runs the risk of being expensive and perhaps essentially meaningless, as well as not evaluable, because of the breadth of its target, lack of focus, and inability to specify indicators for assessing effectiveness. Using the setting as a focus fosters outcomes that are adaptable and sensitive to particular traditions, cultures, and circumstances.

POPULATION HEALTH PROMOTION

In response to the growing debate among health promotion practitioners and population health scientists, Hamilton and Bhatti (1996) offered for discussion a model they termed *Population Health Promotion* (Fig. 1.3). This model has been adapted over time to embrace levels of action, determinants of health, action strategies, and the foundations for practice in health promotion (Flynn, 1999).

In this model, the central concepts and action strategies of the Ottawa Charter, 12 determinants of health, and targets and/or settings are integrated with evidence-based decision making to ensure that policies and programs focus on the right issues, take effective action, and

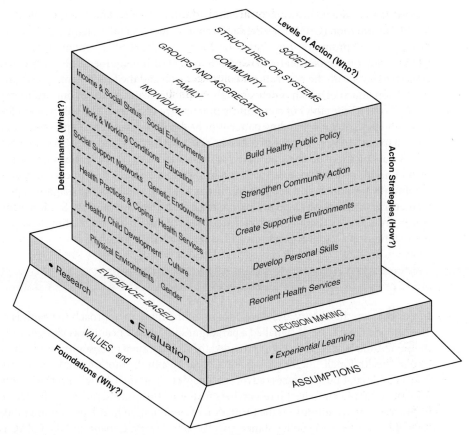

FIGURE 1.3   Population health promotion model. (Flynn, 1999)

produce sound results. Evidence is derived from three principal sources: research, experience, and evaluation studies.

A distinction is made between risk factors and risk conditions. *Risk factors* are behaviour patterns that tend to dispose people to poorer health and are modifiable through strategies that create individual behaviour change. *Risk conditions,* on the other hand, are general circumstances over which people have little or no control that are known to affect health status. Risk conditions are usually a result of public policy and are modified through collective action and social reform.

The population health promotion model allows for the integration of new knowledge from research, experience, and evaluation. It offers an analytic tool to assess situations that put people at risk, to assess populations at risk, and to move away from a victim-blaming approach to a more comprehensive determination of factors that contribute to ill health and injury.

IMPLICATIONS OF POPULATION HEALTH PROMOTION FOR "COMMUNITY AS PARTNER"

In 1986, the WHO took the lead in providing the scope, definition, and a framework for action to create "Health for All" as mandated by the Declaration of Alma-Ata (WHO, 1978). The Ottawa Charter serves to this day as the foundation of health promotion, and as health promotion action has taken place, the evidence generated by evaluation and research to support its value has expanded. Health Canada has sponsored several population health surveys, created the Canadian Institutes of Health Research (CIHR) and the Canadian Institute for Health Information (CIHI) to gather and report evidence, and realigned its own organization to support and promote a population health approach. Health promotion is a key means of taking action on population health and reducing health inequities. This book is written to be consistent both with the population health approach and the fundamental principles of health promotion, much of which is delivered by the public health sector of our health system.

In Chapter 3 the ethics of community practice are discussed. The basics of epidemiology as the foundation of understanding patterns of health in populations are presented in Chapter 4, and Chapters 5 to 9 present the five strategies of the Ottawa Charter. Section 1 ends with chapters discussing social justice and equity, culture and diversity, prevention and harm reduction, mental health promotion, and social media. Section 2 details the process of partnering with community for population and community assessment, analysis and diagnosis, planning, implementing interventions, and evaluating their outcomes and impacts. Section 3 contains case stories from across Canada that offer examples of successful population health promotion interventions in a variety of settings with a range of target groups.

Summary

In this chapter, the history and development of the modern approach to health is chronicled. The Lalonde report (1974) signalled a paradigm shift in how health was viewed, and the Declaration of Alma-Ata (WHO, 1978) provided the foundational philosophy by which to attain the goal of "health for all." Eight subsequent Global Health Promotion Conferences extended the understanding of the processes (advocacy, enabling, and mediating) and five action strategies for practice. Population health researchers furthered the understanding of the determinants of health, creating conditions for the formation of a population health promotion model (Hamilton & Bhatti, 1996). The policy stance now taken by Health Canada and the PHAC is based on its population health approach to policy and programming. Thus, the stage is set for readers to further investigate key concepts and develop a process for partnering with communities to enhance health and well-being.

REFERENCES

Flynn, L. (1999). *An adaptation of the Hamilton and Bhatti (1996) population health promotion model.* Manitoba and Saskatchewan Region: Health Canada.

Green, L. W., & Kreuter, M. W. (2005). *Health program planning: An educational and ecological approach* (4th ed.). New York, NY: McGraw-Hill Higher Education.

Green, L. W., Poland, B., & Rootman, I. (2000). The settings approach to health promotion. In B. Poland, L. W. Green, & I. Rootman (Eds.), *Settings for health promotion: Linking theory and practice* (pp. 1–43). Thousand Oaks, CA: Sage.

Hamilton, N., & Bhatti, T. (1996). *Population health promotion: An integrated model of population health and health promotion.* Ottawa: Health Canada.

Mikkonen, J., & Raphael, D. (2010). *Social determinants of health: The Canadian facts.* Toronto: York University School of Health Policy and Management. URL=http://www.thecanadianfacts.org

Public Health Agency of Canada (PHAC). (2011). What determines health? URL=http://www.phac-aspc.gc.ca/ph-sp/determinants/index-eng.php

Public Health Agency of Canada (PHAC). (2013). What is the population health approach? URL=http://www.phac-aspc.gc.ca/ph-sp/approach-approche/appr-eng.php

ONLINE RESOURCES

Please visit thePoint. at http://thepoint.lww.com/Vollman4e for up-to-date Internet resources and additional learning materials on this topic.

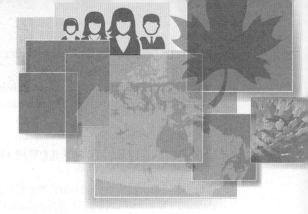

CHAPTER 2

Public Health in Canada

Ardene Robinson Vollman, Richard Musto, and Fran E. Scott

LEARNING OBJECTIVES

After studying this chapter, you should be able to:

1. Describe the history of public health and some of the achievements that have contributed to the health of Canadians

2. Discuss the functions of the public health system

3. Describe the organization and financing of Canada's public health system

4. List the principal disciplines that contribute to public health

Introduction

Public health has been an important part of the health system since the beginning of contemporary Canadian history. Public health is "the science and art of promoting health, preventing disease, prolonging life and improving quality of life through the organized efforts of society" (Last, 2001, p. 145). The mission of the public health system is to help society to create the conditions in which *all* people can be healthy. Public health focuses on the whole population, or on large sub-populations such as youth and new families, distinguishing it from medical and clinical services that focus on individual patients. Public health focuses on reducing health inequities between groups of people as a major strategy for improving overall population health.

Matters such as clean drinking water, clean air, waste management, safe food, and work safety concern everyone; individual action cannot achieve them—they are best addressed on a population or community basis.

Public health is grounded in the health and behavioural sciences, including epidemiology and biostatistics, leading to interprofessional and intersectoral action on the determinants of health of populations. Public health is committed to social justice: the concept of a society that gives individuals and groups fair treatment and an equitable (fair) share of the benefits of society. In the context of public health, social justice is based on the concepts of human rights and equity, maintaining that all groups and individuals are entitled equally to important rights such as health protection and minimum standards of income (see Chapter 10). The goal of public health—to minimize health disparity and preventable death and disability for all Canadians—is integral to social justice. Using a social justice perspective for public health interventions means ensuring that those in greatest need of public health services, or those most vulnerable or at-risk, receive more attention.

HISTORY OF PUBLIC HEALTH IN CANADA

For its centennial anniversary, the Canadian Public Health Association (CPHA) commissioned a history of public health in Canada, which was authored by Rutty and Sullivan (2010); the following text is based on this report. The CPHA has several historical documents on its website; readers interested in more detail are encouraged to visit that site.

The North American continent was home to Aboriginal people for thousands of years. Beginning in the 1600s, their health, economy, and social conditions were negatively affected by European immigration. The fur trade brought with it smallpox, measles, tuberculosis, and influenza that destroyed many Aboriginal lives and in some cases wiped out entire villages. Typhus was brought to Canada on ships coming from Europe, with many passengers arriving in the throes of disease. In 1710, efforts to inspect and quarantine ships became organized as fears grew that the black plague would also come to Canada. By the late 1790s, smallpox was less of a threat than epidemic cholera, typhus, tuberculosis, measles, and scarlet fever, which prompted sanitary reforms. In 1816, a physician was appointed as Health Officer in Lower Canada (Québec) and Quarantine Acts were legislated. Even though a quarantine station was established near Québec City, immigrants that appeared healthy but were in fact infected with cholera had entered Lower Canada in the 1830s. The disease spread, and by the time the epidemic was over, cholera had killed about 2,300 people (10% of the population) in Québec City and 4,000 (15% of the population) in Montreal. As cholera spread to Upper Canada, local boards of health were established and medical officers appointed to handle the epidemic; streets were cleaned of filth, pools of stagnant water were drained, and blocked sewers were cleared, particularly where poor immigrants lived in crowded housing conditions. Still, typhus and cholera continued to plague immigrants arriving on ships from Europe for the next two decades.

By the early 1860s, vaccination against smallpox became available and mandatory vaccination was introduced in the colonies. In the West, the Hudson's Bay Company provided vaccinations in an effort to protect Aboriginal communities. The Gold Rush in British Columbia, however, imported smallpox that devastated the coastal people.

Early in the 1900s, a social movement known as the *sanitary idea* took hold. Sanitary reformers undertook collective action to purify drinking water and manage sewage and garbage, leading to the development of the role of municipal government in health and creating the foundation for public health in Canada. After Confederation, and led by Ontario, health boards were formed and public health efforts expanded, including a larger role in public health for the federal government. However, the onset of World War I saw an increase in cases of typhoid, venereal disease, and the influenza pandemic known as the Spanish flu. After a period of growth in public health in the 1920s, the Great Depression occurred and public health interest and activity declined in the wake of the economic downturn. World War II brought an expansion in public health efforts, and the discovery of penicillin and widespread mandatory immunization programs began to have an impact on the spread and treatment of infectious disease. However, a poliomyelitis epidemic in the 1950s created havoc among the population until a vaccine was introduced. Many surviving children were left paralyzed as a result of polio. The 1960s saw a transformation in the social fabric of the country, led by Saskatchewan, with the introduction of universal health insurance and other social programs. In 1974, the Lalonde report brought new thinking to the understanding of health and in 1986 Canada led the way in health promotion action with the Ottawa Charter and the Epp framework (see Chapter 1). But new infections emerged in the form of HIV/AIDS, and the incidence of other viral infections (e.g., hepatitis C) grew along with the increasing injectable substance use in the country. Today, much as in the early days of Canada, we remain concerned about immigrant health, Aboriginal health, and the health of people living in poverty. While much of our history is linked to infectious diseases (Brunham, 2009), current and future challenges relate to chronic disease, mental health, and the determinants of health.

PUBLIC HEALTH ACHIEVEMENTS IN THE PAST CENTURY

Many of the major improvements in the health of Canadians have been brought about by the public health system. For example, the average life span of Canadians has increased by more than 30 years since the early 1900s, and 25 of those years can be attributed to advances in public health. Table 2.1 documents several public health achievements that led to this remarkable advancement in the health of Canadians (CPHA,2010).

TABLE 2.1   Twelve Canadian Public Health Achievements in the 20th Century

Achievement	Description
Acting on the social determinants of health	Recognition that health is influenced by many factors outside the health care system has strengthened public health's commitment and leadership in activities that address the broad determinants of health, such as income, education, early childhood development, and social connections.
Control of infectious diseases	There are many different infectious diseases—from anthrax to West Nile virus—and controlling their spread has been a fundamental goal since the beginning of public health in Canada.
Decline in deaths from coronary heart disease and stroke	Cardiovascular disease death rates have been declining steadily in Canada since the mid-1960s. The 1997 death rates were almost half those of 1969, and between 1994 and 2004 the death rate fell by 30%.
Family planning	Women have long been attempting to control when to have children through birth control and other techniques. Waiting until the mother is at least 18 years old before trying to have a child improves maternal and child health and it is healthier to wait at least two years after a previous birth before conceiving the next child. In 1969, all forms of contraception were legalized in Canada.
Healthier environments	Canadian environmental policies have helped to increase the community's health and dramatically reduce toxic emissions such as lead and mercury. Air and water quality have improved in some areas, despite population and economic growth. Fluoridation has improved children's oral health.
Healthier mothers and babies	In the early 1900s, many major health threats were associated with poor maternal and infant health. Today, the health of mothers and children in Canada is among the best in the world.
Motor-vehicle safety	In 1998, Canada's road fatality rate was ranked ninth among the 29 member countries of the Organization for Economic Co-operation and Development (OECD). Alcohol-related collisions decreased substantially and seatbelt use increased, resulting in many lives saved and injuries prevented.
Recognition of tobacco use as a health hazard	Canada has made more progress in tobacco control in recent years than most other countries in the world and has seen a dramatic decline in tobacco consumption, along with a pervasive shift in attitudes.
Safer and healthier foods	Canada is well known worldwide for its safe and high-quality food. Public health professionals have been working for 100 years to ensure Canadians have access to safer and healthier foods. Safer food, water, and milk were one of the earliest goals. Understanding the links between nutrition and health has increased dramatically over the past 100 years. Today, we continue to strive for healthy, affordable food for everyone in Canada.
Safer workplaces	Well into the 1900s, many diseases or injuries were associated with unsafe workplaces or hazardous occupations. The rate of work-related injury has been steadily declining since 1988—from 40 injuries among every 1,000 workers in 1988 to 20 per 1,000 in 2006.
Universal policies	The term "universal" generally applies to benefits that are awarded solely on the basis of age, residence, or citizenship, without reference to the recipient's income or assets. Universal programs for income maintenance, social welfare services, and health care services have helped Canadians maintain a high standard of living and of health.
Vaccination	One hundred years ago, infectious diseases were the leading cause of death worldwide. In Canada, they now cause less than 5% of all deaths—thanks to immunization programs. Immunization has probably saved more lives in Canada in the last 50 years than any other health intervention.

CPHA (2010).

TABLE 2.2   Essential Functions of a Public Health System

Function	Description
Population and community health assessment	• Describing and understanding people, factors that determine health, and the distribution of wealth, health, and risk factors across geographic areas and population segments • Outcomes: better targeted services, healthy public policies
Surveillance	• The ongoing systematic use of routinely collected health data • Purpose: tracking and forecasting health events, risks, and trends, prompting public health intervention • Outcomes: reports, program support, anticipatory program planning, program quality improvement
Injury and disease prevention	• Investigation, contact tracing, and preventive measures to reduce the risk of infectious disease emergence and outbreaks • Outcomes: activities to promote safe environments and healthy lifestyles to reduce preventable illness and injury

Health promotion	• Enabling people to make healthy choices through:
	  • Strengthening community action
	  • Creating supportive environments
	  • Developing personal skills
	  • Building healthy public policy
	  • Reorienting health services

Health protection	• Actions that ensure water, air, and food are safe • Based upon regulatory frameworks such as Public Health Acts and Regulations • Outcomes: control of infectious diseases, protection from environmental hazards and threats
Emergency and disaster preparedness	• Planning for natural and man-made disasters • Purpose: to minimize serious illness, death, and social disruption • Requires intensive intersectoral collaboration • Outcomes: organized responses to population/community emergencies

FUNCTIONS OF PUBLIC HEALTH

The programs, services, and institutions within Canada's public health system are focused on prevention and promotion, and consideration of the health status and needs of the whole population. Both the health care system (e.g., hospitals, medical clinics, community health centres, long-term care facilities) and the public health system share the same goal: maximizing the health of Canadians. Therefore, it is just as critical to have a well-functioning public health system as it is to have a strong health care system. Furthermore, both systems must work well together in responding to threats to the public's health. Table 2.2 describes the essential functions of Canada's public health system.

EMERGING THREATS TO THE HEALTH OF CANADIANS

While Canadians today are healthier than ever and have a longer life expectancy than previously (Decady & Greenburg, 2014), the risks to health have changed over the past decades. Compared with the first part of the 20th century, when infectious diseases were the most common cause of morbidity and mortality, now the leading causes of disability and death for all ages are injuries and chronic diseases. Today the health system battles obesity, tobacco, diabetes, mental illness, falls in the elderly, and childhood injuries. The challenge of infectious diseases remains, however, as old foes re-emerge (e.g., syphilis, tuberculosis, community waterborne disease, influenza) and new ones appear (e.g., West

---

Box 2.1 Definitions: Inequality and Inequity

Inequalities or disparities in health status between individuals and populations are inevitable consequences of genetic differences and various social and economic conditions, or a result of personal lifestyle choices (e.g., sexual activity, tobacco use).

Equity means fairness. Inequities occur as a consequence of unfair or modifiable conditions that create disadvantage in opportunity for health, access to health services, and to the necessities of a healthy life (e.g., food, housing).

From http://www.phac-aspc.gc.ca/php-psp/ccph-cesp/glos-eng.php

---

Nile virus, Middle Eastern respiratory syndrome [MERS], ebola, Zika virus, bioterrorism). Of special concern are the inequalities in life circumstances that lead certain population groups to have poorer health status than those with more advantages—this is termed as *health disparity* (see Box 2.1).

ORGANIZATION AND FINANCING OF CANADA'S PUBLIC HEALTH SYSTEM

Although health services are under provincial/territorial jurisdiction (Constitution Acts, 1867 to 1982, s92–7; Butler & Tiedemann, 2013), public health has become a shared responsibility among all levels of government (i.e., federal, provincial, territorial, and municipal). Each province/territory has its own public health legislation, the content of which varies considerably in scope, and comprehensiveness (National Collaborating Centre for Healthy Public Policy [NCCHPP], 2015). All provinces but Ontario have integrated all components of the health system—public health, acute care, and long-term care. The three territories are organized in various ways.

The public health system provides and supports a wide range of program and policy interventions including the development of health status reports; disease surveillance and responses to outbreaks; health promotion to advocate for and facilitate healthier public policies, improve skills, and support individual and community-level behaviour change; immunization programs; and inspection of restaurants and child-care facilities. Other programs include outreach to vulnerable populations, support for early child development, and provision of school health programs. How these programs "look" differs by province/territory based on identified population health needs (NCCHPP, 2015).

How much of Canada's health expenditures are dedicated to the public health system? The Canadian Institute for Health Information (CIHI) reported that health expenditures in 2010 accounted for about 11.6% of Canada's gross domestic product, and while there was a dip in percent of GDP to 11%, costs rose to $214.9 billion in 2014—an all-time high. Health spending per person varies among provinces but it translates to an average of over $6,000 per person. After rising at an average of 7% for a decade, the rate of growth is slowing (to 2.1% in 2014) and has not kept pace with inflation and population growth for the first time in 15 years. In contrast to the costs of hospitals (30%), health care professionals (25.6%), and pharmaceuticals (16%), spending on public health remained a small part of health expenditures over the recent decade—from 5.2% of total expenditures in 1998, 6.6% in 2008, and 5.3% in 2014 (CIHI, 2014, p. 42). In all provinces/territories but Ontario, public health services are funded by the province/territory. In Ontario, public health services are cost-shared with municipalities.

Box 2.2   Mandate of the PHAC

The role of the Public Health Agency of Canada is to:

- Promote health;
- Prevent and control chronic diseases and injuries;
- Prevent and control infectious diseases;
- Prepare for and respond to public health emergencies;
- Serve as a central point for sharing Canada's expertise with the rest of the world;
- Apply international research and development to Canada's public health programs; and
- Strengthen intergovernmental collaboration on public health and facilitate national approaches to public health policy and planning.

From http://www.phac-aspc.gc.ca/about_apropos/what-eng.php

KEY PLAYERS IN PUBLIC HEALTH IN CANADA

Following Canada's Severe Acute Respiratory Syndrome (SARS) outbreak in 2002, there were a number of reports with recommendations to improve public health capacity (Health Canada, 2003). In 2004, Canada created the Public Health Agency of Canada (PHAC) separate from Health Canada and named the nation's first Chief Public Health Officer. The PHAC leads public health activities at the federal level. The PHAC's mission is "to promote and protect the health of Canadians through leadership, partnership, innovation, and action in public health." (See Box 2.2 for the organization's mandate.) The PHAC collaborates with provinces/territories, NGOs, other countries, and international organizations (e.g., WHO) to share knowledge, expertise, and experiences.

The PHAC administers national laboratories in Winnipeg and Guelph and regional offices across the country. It includes the Centres for Chronic Disease Prevention and Control, Infectious Disease Prevention and Control, Emergency Preparedness and Response, Surveillance Coordination, Healthy Human Development, and the Office of Public Health Practice. Health Canada and other federal agencies also deal with a variety of public health concerns, including food safety and the regulation of drugs. The federal government also has jurisdiction over issues related to national borders and international concerns.

Other Public Health Agencies

In addition to formal public health agencies at the federal, provincial, territorial, and local levels there are a number of key organizations relevant to the public health system (Table 2.3). While public health services occur normally within the formal structure of government-funded services, this work is supported and complemented by the efforts of organizations and individuals within the voluntary (e.g., NGOs, interest groups) and private sectors (e.g., commercial vaccine laboratories).

Public Health Professional Disciplines

In 2008, after extensive consultation with the public health community across Canada, the PHAC released a document outlining the core competencies for public health workers in Canada (PHAC, 2008). Core competencies are the essential knowledge, skills, and attitudes necessary for the practice of public health. Core competencies can improve the practice of public health by providing a foundation for enhanced education and professional development. Their common language and values support collaboration and partnership development. They also provide an opportunity to improve recognition and understanding of public health. There are 36 core competencies in seven categories: public health sciences; assessment and analysis;

TABLE 2.3 Key Public Health Agencies in Canada

Agency	Description
National Advisory Committee on Immunization (NACI) (http://www.phac-aspc.gc.ca/naci-ccni/)	NACI is a pan-Canadian advisory committee of experts that makes recommendations for the use of vaccines currently or newly approved for use in humans in Canada, including the identification of groups at risk for vaccine-preventable diseases for whom vaccination should be targeted.
Canadian Task Force on Preventive Health Care (CTFPHC) (http://canadiantaskforce.ca)	Develops clinical practice guidelines that support primary care providers in delivering preventive health care.
Canadian Institutes of Health Research (CIHR) (http://cihr-irsc.gc.ca)	Institute of Population and Public Health leads research in this area; a number of the other institutes focus on determinants of health and upstream interventions.
Canadian Institute for Health Information (CIHI) (https://www.cihi.ca)	Provides health system reports including factors influencing health.
Canadian Food Inspection Agency (CFIA) (http://www.inspection.gc.ca/eng/1297964599443/1297965645317)	CFIA's mission is: "Dedicated to safeguarding food, animals and plants, which enhances the health and well-being of Canada's people, environment and economy." As such it is primarily a regulatory agency with minimal focus on health promotion.
Canadian Public Health Association (CPHA) (http://www.cpha.ca)	CPHA is the national, independent, not-for-profit, voluntary association representing public health in Canada. CPHA's members believe in universal and equitable access to the basic conditions that are necessary to achieve health for all Canadians. Most provinces/territories have corresponding associations.
National Collaborating Centres for Public Health (http://www.nccph.ca)	Of the six NCCs four have a strong health promotion focus (Determinants of Health, Methods and Tools, Aboriginal Health, and Healthy Public Policy) and two have a stronger focus on health protection (Infectious Diseases and Environmental Health).
Provincial agencies, such as the British Columbia Centre for Disease Control (BCCDC) (http://www.bccdc.ca), the Institut national de santé publique du Québec (INSPQ) (https://www.inspq.qc.ca), and Public Health Ontario (PHO) (http://www.publichealthontario.ca)	Provide scientific and technical knowledge creation and exchange on public health content relevant to decision makers and practitioners. Each of these agencies has some focus on health promotion, for example: a sexual health program at BCCDC, focus on expertise in individual and community development at INSPQ, and a health promotion chronic disease and injury prevention department at PHO.

policy and program planning, implementation and evaluation; partnerships, collaboration, and advocacy; diversity and inclusiveness; communication; and leadership. Discipline-specific competencies have been developed in consultation with seven public health disciplines and leadership competencies for public health practice were released in 2015 (Table 2.4). The PHAC has initiated a process through CPHA to investigate the feasibility of a general public health certification program in Canada after reviewing similar offerings in the United States.

There are many other valued professionals in public health departments, including those with expertise in information management and technology, social marketing, speech-language pathology, lactation, and health education, among others. In addition, many public health agencies hire others (e.g., data analysts, social workers, toxicologists, program evaluators, librarians, and research coordinators) who have specific public health expertise in addition to their discipline knowledge. The roles of some professionals are described in Table 2.5.

THE INTERSECTION OF PUBLIC HEALTH AND PRIMARY CARE

Just as there was a "rediscovery" in the early part of this century of the importance of public health with the experience of SARS, waterborne disease outbreaks, and the emergence of West Nile Virus, there has also been a realization of the foundational importance of a strong primary care system. Characterized by Starfield et al. (2005) as being the first point of access,

TABLE 2.4 Competency Statements for Public Health Disciplines in Canada

Discipline	URL
Core Competencies	http://www.phac-aspc.gc.ca/php-psp/ccph-cesp/about_cc-apropos_ce-eng.php
Medical Officer	http://nsscm.ca/Resources/Documents/Minimum%20MOH%20Competencies%20-%20FINAL%20-%20Clean-%20post-v5.pdf
Public Health Nursing	https://www.chnc.ca/documents/CHNC-PublicHealthNursingDisciplineSpecificCompetencies/index.html
Home Health Nursing	https://www.chnc.ca/documents/CHNC-HomeHealthNursingCompetencies/index.html
Dental Health	https://www.caphd.ca/sites/default/files/pdf/DisciplineCompetenciesVersion4_March31.pdf
Nutrition	http://www.dietitians.ca/publichealthnutrition
Inspection	http://www.ciphi.ca/pdf/dsc.pdf
Epidemiology and Biostatistics	http://journal.cpha.ca/index.php/cjph/article/viewFile/1645/1829
Health Promotion	http://www.healthpromotercanada.com/hp-competencies
Leadership	http://chnc.ca/documents/LCPHPC-EN/

person-focused, comprehensive, and coordinated, often with a family and community orientation, a robust primary care system is being advanced as the key to managing demand on hospital and other facility-based care. In Table 2.6, there are some examples, organized by the core public health functions, of how the two services, public health and primary care, complement one another. Two key general characteristics of the public health contributions are provision of the systems or programmatic elements, and response to unmet service needs, while for primary care it is the direct and continuing contact with patients.

Even greater benefit will be achieved with thoughtful collaboration between these two health system components. Valaitis (2012) found evidence of benefit across a number of areas including maternal-child programs, communicable disease prevention and control, health

TABLE 2.5 Roles of Seven Most Common Public Health Professionals

Public Health Professional	Description
Public/Community Health Nurse	Public health nurses (PHN) are the largest group of employees in public health; PHN work is diverse and carried out in a variety of settings (e.g., workplaces, schools, vaccination clinics), or on particular issues (e.g., communicable disease control, injury prevention, sexual health). PHNs also work with specific populations (e.g., young families, seniors, youth).
Environmental Public Health Professional/ Inspector	Public health inspectors do a variety of jobs to protect the public from environmental hazards and enforce provincial/territorial Public Health Acts and Regulations (e.g., inspection of food establishments, toxic waste sites, water treatments).
Epidemiologist	One of the responsibilities of epidemiologists and biostatisticians is surveillance, which involves collecting and analyzing health data that is used to plan and implement various programs and services.
Medical Officer of Health (MOH)	MOHs are physicians who specialize in working with communities and the population, rather than with individual clients. MOHs provide expertise, direction, leadership, and consultation in all of the public health functions.
Health Promoter	Health promoters come from a variety of disciplines and work to enable people and communities to increase control over and improve their health, with an emphasis on the social determinants of health. Health promoters have many roles that allow them to facilitate change in people's health behaviours within the context of social, institutional, and community development.
Public Health Dentist and Dental Hygienist	Together with public health dental hygienists, public health dentists are concerned with the diagnosis, prevention and control of dental diseases, and the promotion of oral health through organized community efforts.
Public Health Nutritionist/ Community Dietitian	Community dietitians are specialists in human nutrition. Public health nutritionists work both in primary care clinics and community-based programs. They also advocate for breast-feeding and food policies that increase access to healthy foods for disadvantaged people.

TABLE 2.6 The Intersection of Public Health and Primary Care

Function	Public Health	Primary Care
Population and community health assessment	• Regularly conduct and report an assessment of the health status of whole communities (often grouped as in a Zone or Region), or specific sub-groups of interest • Provide support and consultation to both regional health authorities and primary care groups, particularly with respect to primary data collection methods and interpretation of multiple data sources	• At minimum, regularly assess the practice population with a view to identifying health issues for attention in practice development • In the context of primary care groups, engage residents of communities in the geographic catchment area to define needs and priorities for the business plan
Surveillance	• Collect, collate, analyze, and report on key health indicators, identifying emerging issues or trends requiring health system response	• At minimum, report notifiable diseases • Particularly when the practices have an electronic medical record, monitor key indicators to assist with performance management
Health promotion	• Coordinate internally and partner with external stakeholders in a comprehensive plan to reduce key health threats such as tobacco use, including advocacy for policy and legislative measures. In support of primary care this may include the development of patient education tools, professional development, and community support services like a Smokers' Quit Line. • Develop and distribute resources and deliver prenatal classes • Develop and distribute resources, and provide early childhood care complementary to that done by primary care practitioners • Participate in community partnerships in the development and delivery of targeted programs for at-risk groups, with a focus on policy advocacy and enabling collaboration	• Counsel or refer patients and prescribe nicotine replacement therapy as required; participate in local advocacy • Provide prenatal care and manage emerging issues • Provide regular developmental assessment of infants and children, anticipatory guidance, and early intervention as required • Participate in community partnerships in the development and delivery of targeted programs for at-risk groups, with a focus on clinical expertise and patient care
Disease and injury prevention	• Advocate for appropriate legislation and enforcement of traffic safety • Participate in social marketing strategies and advocacy for a healthy food supply; participate in research and advocacy for food security • Manage cancer, neonatal metabolic, and other screening programs, including guideline development, mechanisms for encouraging client participation, and quality assurance	• Counsel patients on safe driving practices (e.g., use of seat belts and child passenger restraints); manage acute injuries and their rehabilitation • Assess and counsel patients on healthy diet, particularly in the presence of chronic health conditions such as diabetes and hypertension • Maximize participation of patients in screening programs, conduct testing as appropriate, and follow up with diagnostic workup when required
Health protection • Environmental Health • Communicable Disease Control	• Conduct regular inspections as per Public Health Act regulations (e.g., food operators, rental housing) • Manage the provincially funded vaccine program, including protocol development, professional education, and vaccine storage, distribution and administration; conduct surveillance of vaccine associated adverse events • Support the management and control of notifiable diseases through consultation, contact tracing, and provision of postexposure prophylaxis (PEP) when indicated • Manage the Tuberculosis and Sexually Transmitted Infection (STI) programs	• Report cases of enteric illness to PH when a food outlet is suspected as the source • Actively promote routine immunization; provide annual influenza vaccine; report vaccine associated adverse events • Diagnose, manage, and report notifiable diseases; assist with the prescription of postexposure prophylaxis • Manage STIs as per guidelines, referring to PH for contact tracing as appropriate; assist PH where appropriate in TB case management
Emergency and disaster management	• Maintain a current risk assessment; develop and exercise management plans • Engage community stakeholders, including primary care practitioners in both the planning and response to emergencies and disasters	• Maintain a practice-specific emergency response plan • Participate in the planning and response to community emergencies and disasters

promotion and health protection, chronic disease prevention and management, youth health, women's health, and working with vulnerable populations. Primary care and public health collaboration is an emerging area of research that should bear fruit in terms of improvements in overall health system efficiency and health equity.

Summary

The public health system in Canada has a long and valued history, and its many achievements have allowed Canadians to live healthier and longer lives. Seven principal disciplines, along with other professionals, contribute to the functions of public health: assessment, surveillance, health promotion, prevention, protection, and emergency preparedness. While the infectious disease challenges of the past have largely been conquered, new issues test the system today—health inequities, chronic diseases, and mental health promotion. The public health system must work collaboratively with all levels of government, across sectors, with NGOs, and with those who provide primary care to keep Canadians healthy at all stages of life, and to reduce inequities in life circumstances that lead to unfair disparities in health status for some groups of Canadians.

Acknowledgement

The authors wish to thank Anila Romaliu for her contribution to the discussion on the intersection of public health and primary care.

REFERENCES

Brunham, R. C. (2009). Infectious disease prevention and control: Remembering 1908 and imagining 2108. *Canadian Journal of Public Health, 100*(1), 5–6.

Butler, M., & Tiedemann, M. (2013). *The federal role in health and health care.* Ottawa: Library of Parliament. URL=http://www.parl.gc.ca/Content/LOP/ResearchPublications/2011–91-e.htm

Canadian Institute for Health Information (CIHI). (2014). *National health expenditure trends, 1975 to 2014.* Ottawa: Author. URL=https://www.cihi.ca/en/nhex_2014_report_en.pdf

Canadian Public Health Association (CPHA). (2010). *12 great achievements.* URL=www.cpha.ca/en/programs/history/achievements.aspx

Constitution Acts (1867 to 1982). Retrieved from the Government of Canada Justice Laws website: http://laws-lois.justice.gc.ca/eng/const/index.html

Decady, Y., & Greenburg, L. (2014). Ninety years of change in life expectancy. *Health at a glance,* July, 1–8. Ottawa: Statistics Canada. URL=http://www.statcan.gc.ca/pub/82–624-x/2014001/article/14009-eng.htm

Health Canada. (2003). *Learning from SARS: Renewal of public health in Canada.* A report of the National Advisory Committee on SARS and Public Health. Ottawa: Author.

Last, J. M. (2001). *A dictionary of epidemiology* (4th ed.). New York, NY: Oxford University Press.

National Collaborating Centre for Healthy Public Policy (NCCHPP). (2015). *Structural profile of public health in Canada.* URL=http://www.ccnpps.ca/en/structuralprofile.aspx

Public Health Agency of Canada (PHAC). (2008). *Core competencies for public health in Canada. Release 1.0.* Ottawa: Author. URL=http://www.phac-aspc.gc.ca/php-psp/ccph-cesp/about_cc-apropos_ce-eng.php

Rutty, C., & Sullivan, S. C. (2010). *This is public health: A Canadian history.* Ottawa: Canadian Public Health Association. URL=http://www.cpha.ca/uploads/history/book/history-book-print_all_e.pdf

Starfield, B., Shi, L., & Macinko, J. (2005). Contribution of primary care to health systems and health. *The Milbank Quarterly, 83*(3), 457–502. doi:10.1111/j.1468–0009.2005.00409.x

Valaitis, R. (2012). *Strengthening primary health care through primary care and public health collaboration.* Ottawa: Canadian Foundation for Healthcare Improvement. URL=http://www.cfhi-fcass.ca/Publications AndResources/ResearchReports/ArticleView/12–12–14/5a626084-a6e6–4c75-a421-feb115ccead5.aspx

ONLINE RESOURCES

Please visit thePoint at http://thepoint.lww.com/Vollman4e for up-to-date Internet resources and additional learning materials on this topic.

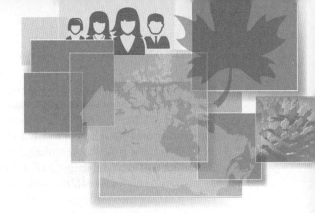

CHAPTER 3

Ethical Practice in Community Health

Katherine S. Pachkowski and Frances E. Racher

LEARNING OBJECTIVES

After studying this chapter, you should be able to:

1. Define the key concepts in ethical practice

2. Outline the differences between ethical pluralism and ethical relativism

3. Discuss the major features of deontologic, consequentialist, virtue, and feminist ethics

4. Describe the ethical foundations of public health and community practice

5. Discuss evolving ethical movements that are relevant to community practice

6. Identify ethical challenges in community practice and apply ethical principles, foundations, and strategies for their resolution

Introduction

Ethics is a crucial element of effective, just human services and health care. Community health professionals in various settings intervene in and influence the health and lives of individuals, groups, and communities. This influence places a moral responsibility on community health workers to understand the impacts of their actions, and a requirement for them to engage in ethical decision making and practice. To meet these obligations, community health professionals should strive to learn ethical theory, engage in critical thinking about the values held by themselves and others, and incorporate ethics into all aspects of practice. This chapter contains an overview of ethical theory, values related to community practice, and implications for community health professionals as they engage in ethical processes with the members of their communities.

The field of health care ethics was born out of a necessity to protect individuals. Rules and laws that were developed in response to the experimental atrocities committed upon unwilling prisoners in World War II were expanded to protect all medical research subjects. Over time, the principles protecting research subjects were applied to patients of health care services. While massive strides have been made toward protecting and upholding the rights and well-being of the individuals who are the focus of health care interventions, traditionally, limited focus has been placed on the rights and well-being of the collective. Defining the community as partner and engaging in activities with a broad health impact on and within the community requires different foci and different ethical approaches.

Health care professionals regularly face ethical challenges in their work. Learning to identify the elements of such challenges, to examine the relevant information, and to find reasoned and collaborative solutions requires critical thinking and openness. Solutions may be informed by understanding the rich history of ethics and contributions from philosophy, bioethics, and applied ethics. Community health professionals should consider relationships, environments, and dialogues with and among health professionals and members of the communities in which they work. Action should be based on respect for all people and their inclusion, diversity, participation, and empowerment.

HISTORICAL PERSPECTIVES AND KEY CONCEPTS

Ethics is the philosophical study of morality and the discipline that deals with the rightness or wrongness of actions. Ethics is a term that can describe the ways in which we understand and examine moral life (Beauchamp & Childress, 2013). The term *morality* refers to widely shared norms of right and wrong conduct (Beauchamp & Childress, 2013). Originally the domain of philosophers, ethics is now commonly identified as a core competency of many disciplines and professional groups.

Take Note

In its core competencies for public health in Canada, the Public Health Agency of Canada (PHAC) includes ethics in the category of Leadership, stating: "A public health practitioner is able to utilize public health ethics to manage self, others, information and resources" (PHAC, 2008, item 7.3).

Normative ethics is concerned with establishing standards of correctness by identifying and prescribing rules and principles of conduct, and developing theories justifying the norms (Johnstone, 2009). These theories are intended to guide action. This approach differentiates normative ethics from *descriptive ethics,* the study and description of ethical beliefs and practices, and *metaethics,* the study of the nature of ethics and ethical reasoning.

Applied ethics involves the use of ethical theories and methods of analysis to examine moral problems, practices, and policies. Applied ethics are used to lead health workers to reasoned decisions on ethical dilemmas.

Professional ethics are ethical theories that articulate the formalized, public, universal sets of values of a professional group (Johnstone, 2009). Most professional organizations have *codes of ethics* that articulate the ethical values of the profession and outline the norms and expectations for members' ethical conduct.

Bioethics is the systematic study of the moral dimensions of the life sciences and health care and involves the use of ethical methodologies in an interdisciplinary setting (Johnstone, 2009). A relatively new field of study, bioethics arose in response to rapid developments in these areas and concerns over ways that new technologies and procedures ought to be applied in society and to humans in medicine and research.

Values may refer to standards or qualities that are esteemed, desirable, or worthy of merit (Canadian Nurses Association [CNA], 2008), or to the ideals of importance to individuals, groups, communities, or societies. For example, the *Canadian Charter of Rights and Freedoms* contains the

---

Box 3.1 What Are Your Personal and Professional Values?

An important feature for any individual who seeks to serve the public is self-awareness and self-assessment. Community health professionals working with a community should ask themselves:

- What are my personal ethical values?
- What "rules" do I believe should never be broken? What rules are flexible?
- What are my professional values? Are they consistent with my personal values?
- What do I believe about individual freedom versus the public good?
- What are the cultural norms and values of the community in which I am working? Can I identify any conflicts with the values of the community and my personal or professional values? How do I approach ethical dilemmas in general? In community?
- How do I respond when a client or community holds different values than I do?

These questions facilitate the opportunity for the community health worker to reflect on practice and should be revisited on a regular basis. A focus on self-awareness may also help to mitigate moral distress, which emerges when a person is unable to act in a manner consistent with her/his personal and professional values.

---

societal values of individual freedom, health, fairness, honesty, and integrity (Canadian Charter of Rights and Freedoms, 1982). See Box 3.1 to reflect further on your personal and professional values.

ETHICAL DIVERSITY AND ETHICAL PRACTICE

Diversity or pluralism of moral values and beliefs is the characteristic of multicultural countries such as Canada. Those countries that abide by principles of *ethical pluralism* or *moral diversity* maintain the position that culturally diverse societies display multiple moral standards. These standards may lead to conflicting moral realities. However, divergence in values and differences in moral standards that exist across cultural boundaries are valued and considered to be resources that have historically led to the evolution of moral thinking (Volbrecht, 2002).

Ethical pluralism is an alternative view to *ethical relativism*. Relativism is the position that moral judgments can be viewed as right or wrong relative to the norms or standard patterns of behaviour of a particular culture or society. Different societies have different cultural norms and thus different moral codes (Card, 2004). Relativism allows that morality is therefore a function of cultural norms and should only be assessed within the context of that system of norms.

The use of ethical relativism does not provide direction in situations when cultures conflict, neither is guidance afforded when individuals belong to multiple cultures with differing perspectives. For example, an individual may belong to various groups that may include ethnic, religious, professional, and organizational cultures. Ethical pluralism emphasizes understanding difference rather than striving for uniformity to ensure that moral systems are responsive to the lived realities and experiences of all human beings, not just the select few who hold positions of power (Johnstone, 2009). Moral diversity ensures that no one point of view dominates. Diversity of values and beliefs is crucial to the continued evolution of morality, as it prompts critical reflection, inviting revision, and creative refinement.

THEORETICAL FOUNDATIONS

Community health professionals should understand a variety of ethical theories to guide ethical reasoning and support ethical decision making. While few ethicists endorse one theory as generally superior to others, each theory has particular strengths and limitations. Understanding different theories will give the community health worker different perspectives for examining an ethical issue and considering the implications of taking an action on the issue. The study of various forms of ethical theories can strengthen the ethical capacities of individuals, give them reason to critically reflect on a variety of issues that they may face, improve ethical critical thinking skills, and provide tools to evaluate the ethical dimensions of situations. Therefore, health care ethicists tend to study a broad range of ethical theories and endorse different theories for different types of situations.

In this chapter, we address two broad theories of ethics, deontology and consequentialism, as well as theories of principlism, virtue ethics, and feminist ethics. Each of these theories has had a major impact on the evolution of bioethics, health care ethics, and professional ethics.

Deontologic Ethics

Deontologic ethics encompasses those theories that centre on the duty of ethical agents to behave in a particular way. The phrase "deontology" is derived from Greek, and means "the study (or science) of duty" (Alexander & Moore, 2015). Deontologists believe that individuals can study morality and through reason come to an understanding of right or good. The most prominent deontologist was Immanuel Kant (1724–1804), whose theory of ethics remains highly influential. Deontologic theories provide guidance about the actions that are right or appropriate in a given situation. Because of this focus on action, deontology is often referred to as "rule ethics." The rightness or wrongness exists within the action taken, or the rule followed, regardless of the consequences of the action. Individuals are called upon to do their duty or abide by a certain prescribed set of rules, without any analysis of potential consequences of abiding by the rule. This approach is in contrast to other ethical schools that may focus on the consequences of actions (consequentialism) or the characteristics of individuals (virtue ethics).

Kantian Ethics

While "Kantian ethics" or "Kantianism" refers to the ethical theory of Immanuel Kant, the phrases also refer to other theories that derive from Kant's work (O'Neill, 1993). Kant emphasized the relationship between reason and morality. His theory of ethics is based on human autonomy and moral law from human reason (Alexander & Moore, 2015). This theory is focused on the question "What ought I do?" (O'Neill, 1993) and on *maxims* or principles of action that a person ought to adopt. These maxims are formulated in terms of *universal laws,* which must apply in all circumstances. For example, if one ought not to lie, one must never lie, under all circumstances, regardless of the potential consequences.

The concept of respect for persons is also central to Kant's ethics. His *Categorical Imperative* is to "treat humanity in your own person or in the person of any other never simply as a means but always at the same time as an end" (O'Neill, 1993). This ethical principle is a higher order constraint on any other maxim. This maxim requires that people always treat others with respect and dignity.

Criticisms of Deontologic Ethics

The ethical structure of deontology is based on action, while disregarding the consequences of the actions. In complex environments, sustaining a commitment to one particular maxim may be very difficult. Critics argue that duty-based ethics neglect or exclude important aspects of the moral experience of health care professionals, including moral judgements, the significance of emotions and experience, and the relational nature of professional practice. Deontologic ethics also generally reflect historically masculine values of autonomy, rationality, and independence of the moral subject, in contrast to an ethic of care that reflects characteristics of responsiveness to relational responsibilities, emotional connectedness, and contextuality (Volbrecht, 2002).

Consequentialist Ethics

Consequentialism, or *teleologic ethics,* is focused on the benefit or harm caused by actions. Morality is assessed based on the outcomes of a course of action, not on the action itself. Those actions that produce the greatest benefit with the least harm are considered to be the most moral actions (Sinnott-Armstrong, 2014). Consequentialism and deontology are often considered to be in opposition to one another.

Utilitarianism

Utilitarianism, the exemplar form of consequentialism (Sinnott-Armstrong, 2014), is a moral theory based on the goal of achieving the greatest good for the greatest number of people. Weighing consequences, benefits, or detriments that result from one's actions are instrumental in determining moral conduct and course of action. Utilitarianism is not concerned directly with a person's intentions but only with the outcome of the action. In contrast with deontology, the end justifies the means (Card, 2004).

Utilitarianism is split into two general categories, *act and rule utilitarianism* (Emmons, 1973). Act utilitarianism is focused on the consequences of individual actions. Rule utilitarianism, by contrast, is concerned with *classes* or types of acts. In rule utilitarianism, if people decide that the consequences of certain types of acts are morally good, it can be assumed that similar acts will also lead to morally good outcomes. This forms the basis of a rule that may be assumed and followed.

Criticisms of Consequentialism

Consequentialism has been accused of benefiting the elite, privileged social classes. The use of consequentialist theories may fail to provide clarity of central issues. Ethicists must consider the following questions: what consequences should be of concern?; who do the consequences affect?; how should these consequences be weighted?; what is good?; and how does one define a "good" outcome? (Sinnott-Armstrong, 2014).

Principlism

Principlism is based on the application of ethical principles (standards of moral behaviour) to situations. These principles have been developed from multiple ethical theories, to be used in concrete applications for decision making and problem solving. A principle is considered *prima facie* (on first pass) to be equal relative to other principles. In any given situation, principles must be assessed to determine which might take priority given the particular circumstances of the situation. Some individuals may consider particular principles to take priority or be more important in all contexts. Rules may be derived from these principles.

Beauchamp and Childress (2013) documented four key ethical principles: autonomy, beneficence, nonmaleficence, and justice. The strength of these four principles is their compatibility with various ethical theories. In recent literature there are three additional agreed-upon principles: fidelity, veracity, and respect for persons. Together, these seven ethical principles form the basis of ethics currently applied in community practice.

The principle of **autonomy** is focused on the right to self-determination, independence, and individual freedom. People should be free to make choices and entitled to act on their decisions, provided that their actions do not violate or impinge on the moral interests of others (Johnstone, 2009). In health care, autonomy involves respect for clients' rights to make decisions about and for themselves and their care. Informed consent is based on the principle of autonomy and a person's right to the information required to make informed decisions about one's care. Health care providers act to support the autonomy of clients by providing information that they can use in their decision making.

Limitations may be placed on autonomy in situations where individual choices interfere with the rights or well-being of others. As is often the case in community practice, personal choice or autonomy may be restricted by concern for the well-being of the community. For example, clients generally have the autonomous right to refuse treatment. However, if a contagious disease that has implications for the community or society, such as tuberculosis, is diagnosed, clients can be required to take prescribed medication and may be isolated or quarantined for a time to prevent the spread of the infectious disease to others.

Beneficence is an entreaty to "do good." Health care providers are expected to act for the benefit of others, be knowledgeable and technically competent, and ensure that their provision of care does good and benefits clients and their well-being. Beneficence requires that potential benefits to individuals and society be maximized and potential harms minimized, while promotion of the common good and protection of individuals are considered.

The principles of beneficence and autonomy may be at odds in community practice. For example, a community health initiative such as immunization, undertaken on a community-wide basis, may conflict with the autonomy of people whose religious beliefs do not support this practice. Such initiatives may cause a conflict due to the diversity of values and priorities among community members.

The principle of **nonmaleficence** requires that no harm be committed and health care professionals protect from harm those who cannot protect themselves—children, people living in poverty, people with disability, or people living on the margins of society. The principle of nonmaleficence is distinctly different from the principle of beneficence, and obligations to nonmaleficence may override obligations to beneficence. For example, allocation of resources to the benefit of one group is not morally defensible if the action takes resources from meeting the more basic needs of others (e.g., necessities such as food and shelter). In such situations, doing no harm to one group might take precedence over doing good for another group. The practice of community health requires advocacy for the benefit, well-being, and protection from harm for people in general and in particular for populations and groups who are vulnerable.

Community conflict arises when the benefits identified as the priority for one group conflict with harm identified as the priority for another group. For example, a group of rural residents may support the development of intensive livestock operations to provide anticipated employment and economic benefit to their community, while other community groups may be more concerned about the anticipated negative environmental impact on their community.

 Critical Thinking Exercise 3.1

Ethical Theories and Ethical Foundations

Consider that your community is struggling with a decision about how to approach the issue of homelessness experienced by some residents. Some community members want to divert resources to the building of a new homeless shelter in the core area. Others argue that the resources should instead be used toward employment and skill-building programs. Compare and contrast how decisions would be made using deontologic ethics, consequentialist ethics, virtue ethics, and feminist ethics, each in isolation of the other theories. What could each theory offer to a process and an outcome, if all three theories were considered concurrently for their potential contributions? How should the decision be made? What are the relevant considerations? What ethical foundations should be applied? What processes could be used to facilitate consideration of these ethical foundations?

The principle of **justice** is based on obligations of fairness regarding treatment of individuals and groups within society, the distribution of potential benefits and potential burdens (distributive justice), and the ways that those who have been unfairly burdened or harmed are compensated (compensatory justice). John Rawls articulated an influential view of justice based on social contracts. Rawls believed that each person should have equal basic rights and liberties, and inequalities should be attached to positions open to all and arranged to benefit the least advantaged (Wenar, 2013). These principles reflect a concern with *equity* (fairness of distribution, rather than equality of distribution). Rawls' theory of justice forms a framework for legitimate use of power, and preserving equity and fairness in the use of power by social institutions (Wenar, 2013).

Community practice is traditionally based on utilitarianism, adheres to the axiom "the greatest good for the greatest number," and supports the position that maximizing benefits to socially disadvantaged groups ultimately benefits society as a whole. Community health professionals advocate for distribution of health promotion and chronic disease prevention resources in ways that are fair and equitable to benefit the most people. They also focus on the needs of vulnerable populations and advocate for the distribution of resources to compensate for shortfalls or build individual capacity to address the challenges that members of these groups may be experiencing. At times, these two perspectives come into conflict, creating ethical dilemmas for community health workers and communities.

Respect for persons is based on the belief that human beings have worth and moral dignity. Persons are worthy moral agents and should be treated as ends in themselves, not merely as means to ends. Persons who are respected and have moral dignity can rightfully determine their own destiny, make choices, and take action. Respect for persons ensures their right to privacy and confidentiality. Sometimes in public health, the individual right to privacy is usurped by the public benefit of disclosure. For example, regulations were changed to allow the use of large health databases for epidemiologic research to benefit society without the informed consent of those people whose information was held in the database (Bayer & Fairchild, 2004). In community health and development, respect for persons is extended to respect for the experience and knowledge of community members, and supports the inclusion of members in community endeavours.

The principle of the sanctity of life is directly related to the respect for persons and may conflict with the principle of autonomy. For example, when persons with terminal illnesses are living in extreme pain they may consider assisted suicide as the preferred option. In Canada, the right for an individual to choose physician-assisted suicide has been upheld in a recent Supreme Court decision (Burki, 2015), striking down the previous ban on the practice. The ethical implications of this ruling are being debated intensely with some critics citing the principle of beneficence and a physician's mandate to heal as being in direct conflict with assisted suicide (Boudreau & Somerville, 2014).

The principle of **fidelity** is about faithfulness and focuses on maintaining loyalty, keeping promises, and being faithful in relationships. Being faithful entails meeting the client's reasonable expectations of the health care provider, including respect, competency, honesty, promise-keeping, and adherence to policies and laws (Purtilo & Doherty, 2011). Whether working with individuals or communities, health professionals must be careful in making promises and steadfast in keeping them.

The principle of **veracity** is the duty to tell the truth and be honest. As this principle is specific in directing behaviour, some consider it to be a second-level principle to guide behaviour and support the intent to be benevolent or to maintain fidelity (Purtilo & Doherty, 2011). Kant gave veracity a central role and considered truthfulness to be an absolute duty to be upheld without exception.

Veracity is essential in building and maintaining trust in relationships with individuals, groups, and communities. Health care providers working in and with communities must be truthful and transparent in the work they undertake and the relationships they establish. Health professionals have a responsibility to be clear and truthful about who they are, what roles they play, and what they bring to the community.

Criticisms of Principlism

Various issues arise when trying to apply the principles in practice: deciding which principle(s) apply in a given situation; interpreting the imperatives or required actions of the principle(s) in a given situation; deciding the relative weights of given principles; balancing the demands of different principles in situations where equally weighted demands might conflict; deciding whether ethical principles apply at all; and resolving disagreements in prioritizing ethical principles in a given situation (Johnstone, 2009). Principles may also be criticized as being culturally specific.

Virtue Ethics

Virtues are defining traits, strengths of character, and standards for noble conduct that predispose the possessor to consistent excellence of intent and performance. Instead of duties, consequences, or principles, virtue ethics focuses on characteristics of the moral agent. Aristotle conceived of ethics in this manner. While virtue ethics had fallen out of favour, it has seen a recent resurgence, particularly among health professions, and as a basis for some codes of ethics (Johnstone, 2009).

The main criteria of virtue ethics involve the type of person one should strive to be and the sort of life one ought to live. An action is deemed morally acceptable if an ideally virtuous agent would perform the same action under the same circumstances. Virtues are good, independent of any desire or ethical situation; every action depends on the person. Virtue connotes the moral excellence of intent and behaviour. For example, Volbrecht (2002) identified compassion, fidelity to trust, moral courage, justice, mediation, self-confidence, resilience, practical reasoning, and integrity as nursing virtues.

Criticisms of Virtue Ethics

The major criticism of virtue ethics is that virtues are not always compatible, and no process is offered to resolve this type of conflict (Glannon, 2005). The virtues often come into conflict in practice. Some argue that virtue ethics entails a justification of circularity whereby the virtuous person does what is good, and what is good is what the virtuous person does; the inability to explain its force or power as a moral guide in the absence of obligations, maxims, or principles; and unrealistic and unattainable expectations imposed on people to be excellent (Johnstone, 2009). Proponents respond by questioning the need to justify virtuous actions, rejecting the expectation that virtue ethics can be reduced to a set of ethical rules, and spurning the belief that expecting moral excellence is an unrealistic prospect.

Feminist Ethics and Ethics of Care

Feminist ethics has emerged as a response to other ethical theories and frameworks in the late 20th century, and is a relative newcomer to the field. It is centred on the value of relationships and the unique contributions of women to moral reasoning. Ethics of care has emerged from feminist ethics. The care focus is used to acknowledge the unique ethical perspective of women as separate from the dominant, male-oriented perspectives. Nursing ethics, though still in relative infancy, has evolved from feminist ethics and ethics of care.

Feminist Ethics

Feminist ethics is viewed by some as an extension of virtue ethics, as feminist ethics emphasizes an ethic of care that involves human connectedness and the importance of interpersonal relationships (Glannon, 2005). Feminist ethics initially was used to address the imbalance of power between men and women, and its use has expanded in some ways to a broader focus on equality and power dynamics. Feminist ethics are used first to account for women's moral experience and second to achieve social change with respect to women's oppression (Brennan, 1999). Feminist ethics draws attention to the distinguishing characteristics of relationships and the power within those relationships at individual, group, community, and societal levels. Feminist ethics is committed to the constructive process of designing alternative ways to restructure relationships, social practices, and institutions, with the ultimate goal of social transformation. By the late 1970s, feminists were questioning the ability of traditional ethical theories to address "women's issues"; others were recognizing the difficulties associated with using traditional ethical theories to address issues in a complex, multicultural world. Still others were identifying the contributions that feminist ethics could make to address these concerns and additional ethical issues.

Feminist ethics remains a vital and evolving field in its own right (Brennan, 1999). It has formed the foundation of other emerging theories and frameworks of ethics that focus on equity, disadvantage, and oppression (e.g., environmental ethics).

Ethics of Care

The work of Gilligan (1982) revolutionized discussions in moral theory and feminism, as she argued that women speak with a different voice than men and espoused a feminine ethic of care that considers responsibility to care and relationships between people as opposed to a masculine ethic of justice that considers ethical principles, conflicting duties, and consequences. Gilligan's work formed the foundation of ethics of care, which has been widely adopted (Tong & Williams, 2014). In essence, ethics of care is based on the moral frame of reference in which women "weave" their interests together with the interests of others (Tong & Williams, 2014). Moral decisions are made within the context of caring and empathetic relationships with others.

Criticisms of Feminist Ethics and Ethics of Care

The primary criticism of feminist ethics comes from those people who believe in the application of ethical principles in a rational manner, without complication of emotions or concern for relationships. Proponents of feminist ethics cover a continuum from recognizing this approach as a complement that extends rule ethics and virtue ethics, to advocating for the application of feminist ethics in new and evolving ways.

ETHICAL FOUNDATIONS OF PUBLIC HEALTH AND COMMUNITY PRACTICE

Seven concepts are foundational in public health and community practice: inclusion, diversity, participation, empowerment, social justice, advocacy, and interdependence. Of particular importance are the interrelationships among these concepts that weave a strong web upon which to base community practice.

Inclusion, the act of being included, means being accepted and able to participate fully within the family, the community, and the society within which one lives (Guildford, 2000). People who are excluded, whether because of poverty, ill health, sex, gender, race, or lack of education, do not have the opportunity for full participation in the social and economic bene-fits of the community or the society. *An Inclusion Lens* offers tools for analyzing practices, pro-grams, policies, and legislation to determine their ability to promote the social and economic inclusions of individuals, families, and communities (Shookner, 2002). Values that underpin this work are social justice and diversity. The goal is to provide a new way to encourage change that will transform organizations, communities, and society as a whole.

Diversity is the condition of being diverse, differing from one another, or composed of dis-tinct or unlike elements or qualities. Earlier in the chapter, diversity was discussed in relation to moral diversity and ethical pluralism. The value of diversity among people is key in ethical pluralism and required for the evolution of moral thought. Valuing diversity requires "recog-nition and respect for the diversity of cultures, races, ethnicity, languages, religions, abilities, age, and sexual orientation; valuing all contributions of both men and women to the social, economic, and cultural vitality of society" (Shookner, 2002, p. 2).

Engaging people in determining the ways a society guides its actions, makes decisions on public policy, and delivers programs and services is called public **participation**, or citizen en-gagement. The desired outcome of participation in decision making is greater social cohesion, evidenced by the creation of shared values, the reduction of health and wealth disparities, and the building of community spirit and capacity for action.

Increasingly, community and public health agencies are generating opportunities to involve and engage citizens in processes of service planning and program evaluation. Public engage-ment strategies must be designed and planned in collaboration with stakeholders to facilitate informed and meaningful public participation (see Chapter 5).

Empowerment is both a process and an outcome. As a process, empowerment is the de-velopment of knowledge and skills that increase one's mastery over decisions that affect one's life. As an outcome, empowerment is the achievement of mastery. To gain mastery or be empowered people must be able to predict, control, and participate in their environments. At the community or population level empowerment has been described as community competence. Community empowerment is exhibited as citizens actively participate and pro-mote inclusion, communicate with respect and in ways that accommodate and manage con-flict, demonstrate commitment to collectively determined goals, foster and share leadership and decision making, create supportive environments, strive for social justice, and nurture intercommunity relationships.

Social justice is the just distribution of resources and opportunity within a society. The concept is ideologically neutral and open to people of all political and religious affiliations, all socioeconomic brackets, all cultures and ethnic groups, both sexes, all genders, and all ages. The field of activity may be literary, scientific, religious, political, economic, cultural, athletic or other across the spectrum of human social activities. The virtue of social justice allows for people of good will to reach different, even opposing, practical judgments about the material content of the common good (ends) and ways to get there (means). Social justice is based on the application of equity, rights, access, and participation (see Chapter 10).

Social justice counters oppression and powerlessness. The role of community health work-ers is to support inclusion and empowerment of people living on the margin of society so that they may freely participate on footings of respect. Empowerment is the guarantor of equity and justice, and freedom is the result—freedom to fully participate in public decisions.

Advocacy can be defined as the act of disseminating information to influence opinion, con-duct, public policy, or legislation. Advocacy is the pursuit of influencing outcomes, including public policy and resource allocation decisions within political, economic, and social systems and institutions that directly affect people's lives. Advocacy consists of organized efforts and actions to highlight critical issues that have been ignored and submerged, to influence public attitudes, and to enact and implement laws and public policies so that visions of a just and decent society become reality. The goal of advocacy is to promote social justice and equity.

Human rights—political, economic, and social—are the overarching framework for this vision. Community health workers, as advocates, represent the interests of citizens, intervene to investigate problems and resolve conflicts, assist in capacity building within the community to advocate on its own behalf, review and comment on public policy, and disseminate information to the community and across communities.

A central concept in public health and community practice is the recognition of the **interdependence** of the people that underlies the most fulfilling aspects of community (Thomas et al., 2002). Public health strives for the health of entire communities and recognizes that the health of individuals is tied to the life of the community. Interdependence relates to the interdependence among human beings and also the interdependence of people with the world in which they live—their social, economic, and physical environments.

CONSIDERATIONS FOR COMMUNITY PRACTICE

Ethical theories have primarily focused on the rights of the individual. However, population health and public health have come to the foreground as a result of reminders posed by infectious diseases (e.g., human immunodeficiency virus [HIV], severe acute respiratory syndrome [SARS], tuberculosis [TB], Ebola virus). Public health efforts to manage infectious diseases have raised ethical questions related to the principle of autonomy and individual choice, which are often found in conflict with the collective good in public or population health. Ethical issues related to the determinants of health and access to employment, education, health services, and healthy environments have added to the ethical challenges presented by population health. Recent developments in which increasing numbers of families are choosing not to vaccinate their children against infectious illnesses have re-ignited the public debate around individual rights and the public good. Public health issues related to epidemiologic research and the use of large population databases without expressed consent of members of the population, surveillance related to HIV/AIDS, confinement related to SARS and TB, and restrictions related to tobacco consumption have generated ethical issues calling for a unique theory of public health ethics (Bayer & Fairchild, 2004).

In Canada, and indeed globally, ethics in public health remains largely guided by existing theoretical frameworks developed from a medical perspective, primarily from the four principles of Beauchamp and Childress (MacDonald, 2015). Many believe that this lack of a unique and distinct ethical framework incorporating the values of public health is problematic. The next step is the development of such a framework. While various public health crises have driven dialogue, this framework must not be reactive. A framework that is focused solely on pandemic planning, resource distribution, or justifications of autonomy and individual freedoms will not be adequate (MacDonald, 2015). Kenny et al. (2010) and MacDonald (2015) argue that the first step toward devising a public health ethic is the identification of the values that are at the heart of public health practice. These values should provide the core elements of any theoretical framework. However, these distinct values are yet to be clearly articulated.

A unique theoretical framework for public health is necessary and inevitable, and should reflect the core values of public health and community practice. Such a framework will articulate the ethical values of the field and provide a consistent guide for action and assessment, as well as for codes of ethics for professional groups working within public health or community settings. Some such codes already exist, as an attempt to communicate to the public the unique values of certain professional organizations and to provide guidance to the people within the organization. The American Public Health Association (APHA), for example, has developed a *Public Health Code of Ethics,* directed toward those in public health practice (Thomas et al., 2002). The APHA developed the code recognizing that, in contrast to medical ethics, public health is concerned more with populations than with individuals, more with prevention than with cure, and a key concept underlying public health is the interdependence of the people in a community (Thomas et al., 2002).

Ethics as Communal Dialogue

Ethics or morality exists on individual, group, community, and societal levels. Ethics, as communal dialogue, is a dynamic, ongoing conversation among members of a community about values and principles needed to make society and people's lives as civilized and fruitful as possible (Volbrecht, 2002). Ethics is a process of reflecting consciously on moral beliefs and consists of an ongoing dialogue about community values and community actions that should be taken in light of those values. Ethical pluralism promotes ongoing dialogue among community members facilitating the development and identification of a community's shared moral understandings and expectations of its members and the community as a whole (Volbrecht, 2002). Ethics is a continually evolving field, offering community health workers new challenges to consider. Research on ethical issues and health advances knowledge of ethics for community practice.

 Critical Thinking Exercise 3.2

Environmental Ethics

Traditional Western thinking and practice have been largely anthropocentric, focused on human considerations. With the growing understanding of the negative impact human practices have on the environment comes a moral obligation to attend to and mitigate the damage that human actions cause.

Consider for a moment a hospital environment. With a focus on the health of the patients within the hospital, vast amounts of resources are used on a daily basis. How can health care policy makers balance the environmental impact of these activities against the identified needs for hygiene, effectiveness, and efficiency? Should they?

Many health centres are seeing changes to policies with the intent of reducing the amount of hazardous waste that is flushed into local water supplies. For example, many health centres no longer allow unused medications to be washed down the sink. Once a common practice, it is increasingly clear that this activity contributes to the presence of pharmaceutical substances in waterways, including in potable water supplies.

Ethical Challenges in Community Practice

The various ethical theories emerged from vastly different philosophical positions. Using one particular theory over another to guide action can result in very different courses of action. Generally, community health workers should familiarize themselves with a number of theories to apply to different scenarios as appropriate.

While many community health workers are bound by professional codes of ethics, often these codes provide little practical guidance in the face of an ethical dilemma or crisis. An ethical dilemma is generally understood to be an issue in which two or more moral imperatives are in conflict. In practice decisions need to be made, individually or collaboratively, around thorny ethical issues. How does one parlay knowledge of philosophical ethical theories into action? Community health workers are concerned with *praxis,* the process by which the theory is realized in decisions and actions. Community health workers and those they serve benefit through the use of formalized decision-making processes when engaging in particularly

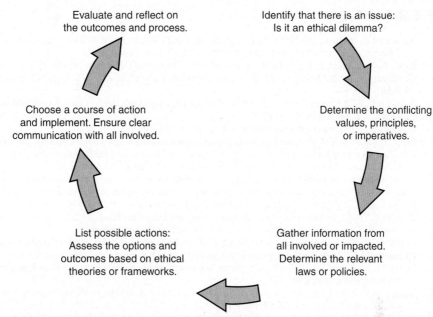

FIGURE 3.1   Framework for an ethical decision-making process.

challenging ethical dilemmas. The process is basic and has the potential to become intuitive to those who work in the field of health care services. A model of ethical decision making involves identifying the issue, collecting data, analyzing the issue from various ethical theoretical perspectives, and reaching a collaborative decision. Evaluation of the decision and reflection on issues are important components of the process. See Figure 3.1 for an ethical decision-making framework or tool to ensure accountability and thoroughness throughout the decision-making process. Many similar frameworks exist; their value lies in the process to ensure careful deliberation, rather than in providing an "answer" to a dilemma.

Health care workers are increasingly subject to moral or ethical distress, a phenomenon by which a care provider is unable to act in a manner that is consistent with her or his personal and professional values (CNA, 2008). Moral distress is linked to burnout of health care workers. Attention to ethical values and decision-making processes can help mitigate this risk.

Summary

The application of ethical theories in community practice offers ways to address ethical dilemmas and resolve ethical conflict. Feminist ethics have made way for the inclusion of responsiveness to relational responsibilities, emotional connectedness, and contextuality in discussions of ethical practice and may form the basis for a unique framework for public health ethics. Inclusion, diversity, participation, empowerment, social justice, advocacy, interdependence, and their interrelationships create a foundation to effectively underpin and support ethical community practice. The genesis of a public health code of ethics and identification of ethical challenges in community practice extend the dialogue. The interdependence, relationships, and collaboration among community health workers and members of the organizations, communities, and societies in which they practice, will facilitate the further development of moral thought and continue the evolution of ethical theory that underpins ethical community health practice.

REFERENCES

Alexander, L., & Moore, M. (2015). Deontological ethics. In E. N. Zalta (Ed.), *The Stanford encyclopedia of philosophy*. URL=http://plato.stanford.edu/archives/spr2015/entries/ethics-deontological/

Bayer, R., & Fairchild, A. L. (2004). The genesis of public health ethics. *Bioethics, 18*, 473–492.

Beauchamp, T., & Childress, J. (2013). *Principles of biomedical ethics* (7th ed.). New York, NY: Oxford University Press.

Boudreau, J. D., & Somerville, M. A. (2014). Euthanasia and assisted suicide: A physician's and ethicist's perspectives. *Medicolegal and Bioethics, 4*, 1–12.

Brennan, S. (1999). Recent work in feminist ethics. *Ethics, 109*, 858–893.

Burki, T. K. (2015). Canada removes ban on physician-assisted suicide. *The Lancet Oncology, 16*(3):e110.

Canadian Charter of Rights and Freedoms, Part I of the Constitution Act (1982). Retrieved from the Government of Canada Justice Laws website: http://lois.justice.gc.ca/eng/Const/page-15.html#h-39

Canadian Nurses Association (CNA). (2008). *Code of ethics for registered nurses*. Ottawa: Author.

Card, R. (2004). *Critically thinking about medical ethics*. Upper Saddle River, NJ: Pearson Prentice Hall.

Emmons, D. C. (1973). Act vs. rule-utilitarianism. *Mind, 82*(326), 226–233.

Gilligan, C. (1982). *In a different voice*. Cambridge: Harvard University Press.

Glannon, W. (2005). *Biomedical ethics*. New York, NY: Oxford University Press.

Guildford, J. (2000). *Making the case for social and economic inclusion*. Halifax: Health Canada, Atlantic Region.

Johnstone, M-J. (2009). *Bioethics: A nursing perspective* (5th ed.). Sydney: Churchill Livingstone.

Kenny, N. P., Sherwin, S. B., & Baylis, F. E. (2010). Re-visioning public health ethics: A relational perspective. *Canadian Journal of Public Health, 101*, 9–11.

MacDonald, M. (2015). *Introduction to public health ethics 3: Frameworks for public health ethics*. Montréal: National Collaborating Centre for Health Public Policy.

O'Neill, O. (1993). Kantian ethics. In P. Singer (Ed.), *A companion to ethics* (pp. 175–185). Oxford: Blackwell Publishing.

Public Health Agency of Canada (PHAC). (2008). *Core competencies for public health in Canada*. Release 1.0. Ottawa: Author. URL=http://www.phac-aspc.gc.ca/php-psp/ccph-cesp/about_cc-apropos_ce-eng.php

Purtilo, R., & Doherty, R. (2011). *Ethical dimensions in the health professions* (5th ed.). Philadelphia, PA: Elsevier Saunders.

Shookner, M. (2002). *An inclusion lens: Workbook for looking at social and economic exclusion and inclusion*. Halifax: Health Canada, Population and Public Health Branch.

Sinnott-Armstrong, W. (2014). Consequentialism. In E. N. Zalta (Ed.), *The Stanford encyclopedia of philosophy*. URL=http://plato.stanford.edu/archives/spr2014/entries/consequentialism/

Thomas, J. C., Sage, M., Dillenberg, J., & Guillory, V. J. (2002). A code of ethics for public health. *American Journal of Public Health, 92*, 1057–1059.

Tong, R., & Williams, N. (2014). Feminist ethics. In E. N. Zalta (Ed.), *The Stanford encyclopedia of philosophy*. URL=http://plato.stanford.edu/archives/fall2014/entries/feminism-ethics/

Volbrecht, R. (2002). *Nursing ethics: Communities in dialogue*. Upper Saddle River, NJ: Prentice Hall.

Wenar, L. (2013). John Rawls. In E. N. Zalta (Ed.), *The Stanford encyclopedia of philosophy*. URL=http://plato.stanford.edu/archives/win2013/entries/rawls/

ONLINE RESOURCES

Please visit the Point at http://thepoint.lww.com/Vollman4e for up-to-date Internet resources and additional learning materials on this topic.

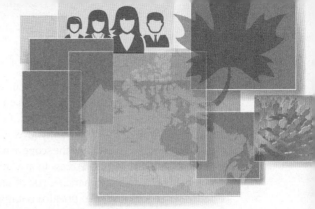

CHAPTER 4

Patterns of Health and Disease: The Role of Epidemiology in Population Health

Dana S. Edge

LEARNING OBJECTIVES

To assess community health needs and to plan, implement, and evaluate programs to meet those needs in conjunction with their community partners, community health professionals must understand basic concepts in epidemiology.

After studying this chapter, you should be able to:

1. Interpret and use basic epidemiologic and statistical measures of community health

2. Apply principles of epidemiology to your community practice

Introduction

Scrutiny of disease patterns, health conditions, and lifestyle behaviours in a population can provide valuable insights into disease etiology, the effects of health services, and the impact of health promotion strategies. To assess these patterns, epidemiology is used for studying the health of populations. Community health professionals integrate and apply concepts from epidemiology to promote, maintain, and restore the health of populations. In this chapter, we explore the meaning and usefulness of these concepts.

When program planners partner with communities, they contribute their expertise supported by the relevant science; in other words, they come armed with the statistics and models that explain health and disease patterns in populations. This information might include the current health status of the community according to a number of accepted indicators, allowing local data to be compared with data from other jurisdictions regionally, nationally, and internationally. By being able to see trends and patterns, strengths and risk factors can be identified and, working together, residents and community health workers can develop plans and set priorities to address concerns and build on community assets.

Epidemiologic and sociodemographic data have traditionally formed the scientific foundation of population health practice so that comparative and comprehensive evidence is available to inform decision making. Regardless of what epidemiologic information reveals, *how* decision making unfolds at the community level is essential to population health practice. Community members' perspectives define the scope of a health problem and influence the solution, in addition to the required resources. Access to available resources without fear of retribution or a threat to well-being is a defining characteristic of social justice (Kenny & Hage, 2009); the importance of addressing social justice in practice is emphasized in epidemiology and nursing (Carter-Pokras et al., 2012; Cohen & Gregory, 2009). Principles of primary health care—in particular, public participation and intersectoral collaboration—must be honoured at the local level if efforts to improve the health of Canadians are to be affordable and sustainable over time (Hutchinson et al., 2011). Therefore, being able to effectively communicate to a variety of stakeholders with standard measures of health and wellness is critical to accurately frame and understand health problems.

Take Note

The degree of equality in opportunities for health, regardless of different positions within a social hierarchy, forms the principle of social justice. Epidemiology is a tool used to assess equality and to highlight inequalities.

EPIDEMIOLOGY

Epidemiology ("the study of what is upon the people," from the Greek *logos* [study], *demos* [people], and *epi* [upon]) is the science of population health and is characterized by the study of the distribution and the determinants of health-related states (Centers for Disease Control and Prevention [CDC], 2012). Epidemiologic studies may take on the intrigue of detective stories as investigators track the factors associated with illness (morbidity) and death (mortality).

Epidemics, defined as outbreaks of illnesses greater than expected levels in a population, were a major focus of early epidemiologic work. In 1854, Dr. John Snow, a British anaesthesiologist, and William Farr, a statistician, conducted what is now considered to be a classic epidemiologic study; their collaboration capitalized on a naturally occurring phenomenon during a cholera epidemic in the SoHo district of London (Stanwell-Smith, 2013). At that time, the mode of transmission of cholera was unknown, although Snow suspected it was spread through contaminated water. In the area of London most affected, households randomly received their water supply from either the Lambeth Company or the Southwark & Vauxhall Company. Early in the outbreak, Snow went door-to-door to determine the name of the household water supplier. By mapping the cholera outbreak cases, using group comparisons, and applying epidemiologic principles, Snow and Farr determined that death rates from cholera were eight to nine times greater in households served by the Southwark & Vauxhall Company. The water supplied by Southwark & Vauxhall came from portions of the Thames River into which London sewage was discharged. Thus, this early epidemiologic work established the waterborne mode of transmission of cholera (Snow, 1936). Near the end of the epidemic, to make a political statement and prevent further transmission of cholera, Dr. Snow removed the handle of the Broad Street pump, eliminating the source of the cholera outbreak.

CONTEMPORARY COMMUNITY HEALTH PRACTICE

Today, advanced epidemiologic research methods are used not only to study outbreaks such as *Escherichia coli* food poisoning, Ebola, and severe acute respiratory syndrome (SARS) but also to investigate environmental conditions, lifestyles, health promotion strategies, and other factors that influence health. Epidemiology is extensively used in health surveillance, including monitoring the health status of disadvantaged populations, in the preparation of policy briefs, and in the evaluation of prevention programs. This chapter provides an introduction to epidemiologic and demographic concepts that are useful for community practice. Additional reading and in-depth discussion can be found in numerous textbooks (Gordis, 2013; Rothman, 2012).

EPIDEMIOLOGIC APPROACHES TO COMMUNITY HEALTH RESEARCH

In studying the determinants of population health, investigators are guided by epidemiologic models. A key understanding in epidemiology is the identification and definition of the population at-risk. To be part of the at-risk population, an individual must be susceptible to the condition or disease; for example, women would not be at risk for prostate cancer. This section describes three models and explains how each might guide the approach to the same problem.

The problem to be considered is an increase in the infant mortality rate (IMR) in a hypothetical community. The IMR is a particularly important health index that should be understood even by health professionals whose main concern is not maternal or child health. Because infant mortality is influenced by a variety of biologic and environmental factors affecting infants and mothers, the IMR is both a direct measure of infant health and an indirect measure of community health as a whole. IMRs, as well as the mortality of children under the age of 5 years, are used by the World Health Organization (WHO, 2012) as basic benchmarks of a nation's health status.

The Epidemiologic Triad

The epidemiologic triad or agent–host–environment model is a traditional view of health and disease, developed when epidemiology was concerned chiefly with communicable disease. As you will see, however, the model is applicable to other conditions as well. In the model, the *agent* is an organism capable of causing disease. The *host* is the population at risk for developing the disease. The *environment* is a combination of physical, biologic, economic, and social factors that surround and influence both the agent and the host. According to this model, by examining the characteristics of, changes in, and interactions among the agent, host, and environment, health (and illness) can be more holistically understood.

In Figure 4.1 the triad in its normal state of equilibrium is illustrated. Equilibrium does not signify optimum health but simply the usual pattern of illness and health in a population. Any change in one of the sides (agent, host, or environment) will result in disequilibrium—in other words, a change in the usual pattern.

How would this model guide the investigation of an increased IMR? To understand this, let us consider the three facets of the model.

At first glance, it might be concluded that any investigation should focus on types of infections as **agents** that cause infant deaths. However, the top five causes of infant mortality in Canada during 2011 were immaturity, congenital anomalies, asphyxia, infection, and sudden infant death syndrome (SIDS) (PHAC, 2013). In Figure 4.2 the leading causes (agent) of infant mortality in Canada during 2011 compared with 2004 are illustrated. Note that both the proportion of deaths from immaturity and congenital anomalies has dropped, whereas the cause of deaths from infection and SIDS has increased over the seven-year time period.

Investigators will also want to know the characteristics of the **host**—in this case, the infant population. This involves examining infant birth and death patterns in terms of age, ethnicity,

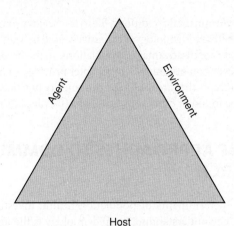

FIGURE 4.1   The epidemiologic triangle in the traditional view, showing health and disease as a composite state of three variables.

sex, and birth weight. These characteristics have been shown to be important risk factors for infant mortality. By studying these factors, it may be possible to identify groups of infants who are at particularly increased risk of dying.

Finally, the **environment** must be assessed. The mother is a significant part of an infant's pre-natal and postnatal environment. Therefore, investigators will analyze birth and infant mortality patterns according to factors such as maternal age, ethnicity, parity (number of previous live births), prenatal care, education, and socioeconomic status (SES). Analysis of these factors, which are also related to infant mortality, will help provide further identification of at-risk groups. Other conditions in the environment also need to be considered. For instance, has migration into the community from other geographic areas increased? Has adult morbidity or mortality, particularly among pregnant women, increased? Have there been changes in health services, medical practice, policies, personnel, funding, or other factors that could affect infant health?

The analysis of these three areas—the agent, host, and environment—should provide infor-mation regarding groups at risk for increased infant mortality and may point the way toward a program aimed at reducing that risk. Thus, the epidemiologic triad, although it was designed with a communicable disease orientation, can provide a useful guide for studying the multi-faceted problem of infant mortality as well as other health problems.

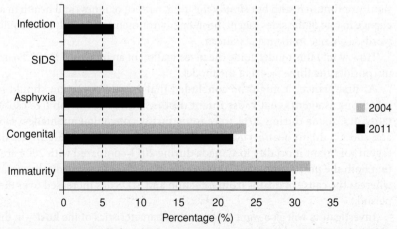

FIGURE 4.2   Leading causes of infant death, 2004 & 2011, Canada. (*Source:* PHAC, 2008 [p. 281], 2013 [p. 73].)

Box 4.1   Example of Research Using the Person–Place–Time Model

In the early 1980s, members of an Arctic Inuit community became very concerned about the number of suicides occurring in their region. Despite the community's alarm, no descriptive data were readily available to define who was at risk, at what time, or where. With permission of the local remote hospital, a community health nurse manually compiled information from the hospital emergency room (ER) logbook. From this review, sex, age, attempts, methods, location, and time of year were highlighted. Interestingly, it was noted that peaks in suicides and suicide attempts occurred in Spring and Fall—two seasons referred to as "break-up" and "freeze-up," respectively. During these seasonal variations, community members were restricted in travel, unable to traverse the ocean or rivers on snowmobiles. These data, when presented during the community town hall meeting, influenced community decisions about how to act.

The Person–Place–Time Model

An approach similar to the epidemiologic triangle is one that guides the investigators to consider the health problem in terms of person, place, and time (Gordis, 2013). The investigators examine characteristics of the persons affected (the host in the triangle model), the place (environment) or location, and the time period involved (which could relate to the agent, host, or environment). In studying infant mortality according to the person–place–time model, for example, infant and maternal factors are considered traits of "person." Aspects of "place" are such factors as whether the community is rural or urban, affluent or poor. "Time" characteristics might include seasonal variation, age-specific patterns, or trends in mortality. See Box 4.1.

The Web of Causation

Using the web of causation model, a health condition is viewed not as the result of individual factors but of complex interactions among multiple factors. One factor may lead to others, which, in turn, lead to others, all of which may interact with one another to produce the health condition. Factors can be at the *macro* (multisystem, societal) level, *meso* (familial, local) level, or *micro* (individual) level.

Central to this model is the concept of synergism, wherein the whole is more than the sum of its separate parts. For example, the effects of a *Shigella* infection on an infant, combined with the effects of poverty, youth, and low educational level of the mother, are more deleterious to infant health than the sum of the effects of the individual risk factors.

Use of the web of causation may result in a more expansive study of infant mortality than one guided by other models. Ideally, investigators using this model first identify all factors related to infant mortality. Next, secondary components that are related to each of the initial factors are identified. These two comprehensive steps provide the outline for the web of causation for infant mortality. Finally, investigators examine the relationships among all the identified components of the web and attempt to determine the most feasible point of intervention to improve infant mortality in the community. In Figure 4.3 a web of causation for infant mortality is depicted. Other webs are proposed in literature related to specific issues (e.g., myocardial infarction, lead poisoning, adolescent pregnancy, tobacco addiction).

This multifaceted approach addresses the concept of causation in a manner consistent with current knowledge of human health. Using a web of causation model can serve as a starting point to examine a facet of the web, acknowledging that other relationships exist. Thorough examination of one portion of the web may provide sufficient information for initiation of useful actions to improve community health.

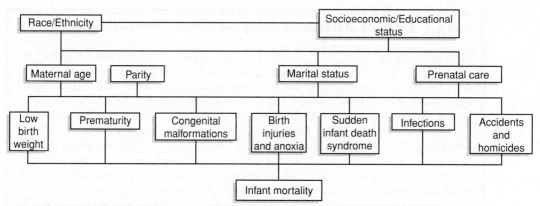

FIGURE 4.3   A web of causation for infant mortality based on information available from birth and death certificates.

The Haddon Matrix: Application of the Epidemiologic Triad

In the field of injury control, Haddon developed a matrix in the early 1970s to guide the development of public health strategies to prevent automobile crashes (Haddon, 1999). Using the epidemiologic triad of host–agent–environment (columns) and the concepts of pre-event, event, and post-event as prevention time points (rows), a matrix is formed and potential risk and protective factors can be filled in.

The Haddon Matrix has been instrumental in providing insights into injury causation and prevention for the past 40 years and continues to guide analysis (Baker & Li, 2012). Recently, researchers in Thunder Bay used the Haddon Matrix to identify trends from 20 studies that examined in motor vehicle crashes sustained by Canadian Aboriginal people (Short et al., 2013). Encapsulated in this three-dimensional unified model are the rows and columns of the Haddon Matrix, as well as four components of the public health approach: surveillance, risk factor definition, intervention/evaluation, and program implementation. This unified framework has the potential to foster comprehensive application and action plans when dealing with public health issues. The Haddon Matrix is described in greater detail in Chapter 12.

In this section, we showed how each of the three models provide a slightly different approach to a community issue and how frameworks can be used to identify preventive approaches. Community issues can be related to "problems" or "wellness," and in future chapters, you will see how the models can apply to both situations. There is no one "correct" model; as you gain experience, you will be able to choose or adapt those that are most appropriate to the community health issue at hand.

LEVELS OF PREVENTION IN COMMUNITY PRACTICE

The concept of prevention is a key component of modern community health. In popular terminology, prevention means intervening before an event occurs. In community health, four levels of prevention are practised: primordial, primary, secondary, and tertiary. For a more complete discussion of prevention refer to Chapter 12.

Take Note

Of prime importance to epidemiology is the prevention and control of disease in contrast to the secondary and tertiary curative approaches found in traditional clinical medicine.

DESCRIPTIVE MEASURES OF HEALTH

To plan appropriate methods of prevention, the community health worker must first assess the health of the community. This section covers some basic measures used in community health assessment.

Demographic Measures

Certain human characteristics, or *demographics,* may be associated with wellness or illness. Age, sex, ethnicity, income, and educational levels are important demographics that may affect health outcomes. For example, men are more likely than women to be diagnosed with cancer (PHAC, 2014), First Nations peoples are three to five times more likely to have diabetes than other Canadians (PHAC, 2011), and women between ages 35 to 40 are more likely to exclusively breastfeed their infants compared to younger women (PHAC, 2013). To plan interventions for population health, the community health worker must be familiar with the demographic characteristics of the community and with the health problems associated with those characteristics.

Morbidity and Mortality

Although epidemiology encompasses wellness as well as illness, wellness is difficult to measure. Therefore, many measures of "health" are expressed in terms of *morbidity* (illness) and *mortality* (death). Most Canadian indices of health are published by Statistics Canada and the PHAC, and include reports on communicable diseases and chronic diseases as well as other important topics and links to other relevant sites. An excellent source of US morbidity and mortality data is *Morbidity and Mortality Weekly Report* from the CDC.

Incidence

The *incidence* of a disease or health condition refers to the number of individuals in a population who develop the condition during a specified period of time (normally, a calendar year). The calculation of an incidence rate, therefore, generally requires that a population be followed over a period of time in what is called a prospective (forward-looking) study.

Prevalence

The *prevalence* of a disease or condition refers to the total number of individuals in the population who have the condition at a particular time. Thus, prevalence may be calculated in a "one-shot" cross-sectional ("slice of time") or retrospective (backward-looking) study, and is typically expressed as a proportion or percentage; when there is a known population at risk for a specific time period, the prevalence also may be expressed as a rate.

Take Note

Prevalence and incidence can be visualized by thinking of an open vessel, like a bottle. At any one time, there are new people being diagnosed with disease and entering the vessel (incidence); likewise, there are individuals with disease who die and leave the vessel (mortality). The number of people at any one time in the vessel represents the prevalence of the disease (Gordis, 2013).

Interpretation of Incidence and Prevalence

Measures of incidence and prevalence provide different information with various implications. For example, an increase in the prevalence of cancer means that there are more persons with cancer in the population. This may be because there are more new cases (in other words, increased incidence) or because persons with cancer are living longer. In either case, the community may need to direct resources toward cancer. However, if knowledge of incidence is lacking, it will be difficult to decide whether to target the resources toward primary prevention of cancer or toward secondary prevention (diagnosis and treatment) and tertiary prevention (rehabilitation) services.

Rates

Incidence is usually expressed as a mathematical measure, called a rate. Because epidemiology is the study of population health, these measures must relate the occurrence of a health condition to the population base. Rates do exactly this. They express a mathematical relationship in which the numerator is the number of persons experiencing the condition and the denominator is the population at risk, or the total number of persons who have the possibility of experiencing the condition over a period of time.

Rates must not be confused with other proportions that do not use the population at risk as the denominator. For example, the death rate from cancer is not the same as the proportion of deaths from cancer. In each, the numerator is the number of deaths from cancer. However, the denominators differ. In the death rate, the denominator includes all persons at risk of dying from cancer during a particular time frame. Therefore, the cancer death rate is an expression of the risk of dying from cancer. In the proportion of deaths, also called proportionate mortality, the denominator is the total number of deaths from all causes. Therefore, the proportionate cancer mortality simply describes the proportion of deaths attributable to cancer.

Calculation of Rates

Rates are calculated in this general format:

$$\text{Rate} = \frac{\text{number of people experiencing condition}}{\text{population at risk for experiencing condition}} \times K$$

K is a constant (usually 1,000, 10,000, or 100,000) that allows the ratio, which may be a very small number, to be expressed in a meaningful way. Let us apply this formula to the calculation of the IMR, which estimates an infant's risk of dying during the first year of life.

Example of a Rate: The Infant Mortality Rate

The IMR is usually calculated on a calendar-year basis: the number of infant deaths (deaths before the age of 1 year) in one year is divided by the number of live births (infants born alive) during that year. The numerator represents the number of infants experiencing the "condition" of dying in the first year of life, and the denominator represents the population of infants at risk for dying in the year.

In 2011, there was an average of 4.9 infant deaths for every 1,000 live births in Canada. In Saskatchewan, from 2005 to 2009, there were 65,481 live births and 432 infant deaths reported (Statistics Canada, 2013). To compare the IMR with the Canadian average, we calculate a rate. Applying the formula for a rate, we divide 432 by 65,481 and find that 0.0066 of an infant died during the first year of life. Because it is difficult to relate to 0.0066 of an infant, we multiply by a constant (K), in this case 1,000, and find that 6.6 infants per 1,000 live births died during the first year of life, that is, the IMR was 6.6 infant deaths per 1,000 live births in 2011. In comparison to the most recent national data available, we can say that Saskatchewan has a higher IMR than the national average. How does this compare with other provinces and territories?

TABLE 4.1 Infant Mortality (Rate per 1,000 Live Births) in Canada, 2000–2011[a]

Year	Infant Mortality Rate
2000	5.3
2001	5.2
2002	5.4
2003	5.3
2004	5.3
2005	5.4
2006	5.0
2007	5.1
2008	5.1
2009	4.9
2010	5.0
2011	4.8

[a]Includes stillbirths of unknown gestational period. Newfoundland, New Brunswick, and Québec do not report fetal death of less than 500 g.

By comparing rates rather than raw numbers, we can then rank parts of the country by IMR to determine areas of greatest need for intervention. In 2009, Prince Edward Island and Nova Scotia had the lowest IMRs at 3.4 infant deaths per 1,000 live births, whereas the Northwest Territories had the highest rate at 15.5 per 1,000 (Statistics Canada, 2013). Regional variations also occur within provinces. Each province and local region may have a very different actual number of births, but by comparing rates, health program planners are able to determine where need is greatest for programming to improve birth outcomes.

Additionally, trends can become apparent by tracking rates longitudinally over time. In Table 4.1, we can see that the trend in the national IMR decreased for the first 2 years and has stabilized over the 10-year period.

Interpretation of Rates

Rates enable researchers and practitioners to compare different populations in terms of health problems or conditions. To assess whether the population in a specific community is at greater or lesser risk for the problems or conditions, the rates for the community should be compared with rates from similar communities, from the province or territory, or from Canada as a whole. Estimates of preventable infant mortality enable us to better understand the nature of the disparities between population subgroups and the factors that may be responsible and help to direct interventions toward areas where improvement is possible.

Some caution must be taken in interpreting rates. Like most statistical measures, rates are less reliable when based on small numbers. This must be kept in mind when assessing relatively infrequent events or conditions or communities with small populations.

Many rates are based on data from a calendar year, which may also present some difficulties. When calculating an IMR for a particular year, such as 2011, be aware that some of the infants who die during the 2011 calendar year were actually born in 2010 and thus were not part of the 2011 population at risk (denominator), and some of the infants who were born in 2010 might die in 2011 (numerator) and not be reflected in the 2010 IMR. Also, populations may increase or decrease during a calendar year. In such cases, the midyear population estimate (June 30) is generally used because the population at risk cannot be determined exactly. A study that follows a cohort, or specified group, prospectively can help overcome the limitations of the conventionally calculated calendar-year rate.

Box 4.2 presents more information regarding causes of infant death.

Box 4.2 Example of Research Using the Person–Place–Time Model

- **Person:** Late fetal, neonatal, and postneonatal deaths among babies weighing less than 1,500 g may be largely attributable to factors affecting maternal health. Late fetal deaths among babies weighing ≥1,500 g may result from suboptimal maternal care. For example, regions characterized by relatively high rates of late fetal death among babies with normal birth weight may benefit from better access to caesarean delivery.
- **Place:** Suboptimal newborn care or lack of access to neonatal intensive care is likely to contribute to early neonatal (0–6 days of age) deaths among babies with birth weight ≥1,500 g and late neonatal deaths among babies with intermediate birth weight, between 1,500 and 2,499 g.
- **Time:** Infant deaths during the late neonatal (7–27 days) period for birth weight ≥2,500 g and postneonatal (28–364 days) deaths for birth weight ≥1,500 g may be largely attributable to factors in the infant environment (e.g., access to immunization, injury prevention, and control).

From Canadian Perinatal Health Report. (2008). URL=http://www.phac-aspc.gc.ca/publicat/2008/cphr-rspc/index-eng.php

---

Commonly Used Rates

Table 4.2 summarizes a number of important rates. Note that the measures of natality and mortality are, in essence, measures of incidence of the conditions of "being born" and "dying." Note also the various ways in which the denominator, or population at risk, is determined in different rates.

Crude, Specific, and Adjusted Rates

Rates that are computed for a population as a whole are called *crude rates.* Subgroups of a population may have differences that are not revealed by the crude rates. Rates that are calculated for subgroups are referred to as *specific rates.* Specific rates help identify groups at increased risk within the population and also facilitate comparisons between populations that have different demographic compositions. Most frequently, specific rates are computed according to demographic factors such as age, ethnicity, or sex.

In comparing populations with different distributions of a factor that is known to affect the health condition being studied, the use of *adjusted rates* may be advisable. An adjusted rate is a summary measure that statistically removes the effect of the difference in the distributions of that characteristic. In essence, adjustment produces an estimate of what the crude rate would be if the populations were identical in respect to the factor for which adjustment is made. A rate can be adjusted for age, ethnicity, sex, or any factor or combination of factors suspected of affecting the rate. Adjusted rates are helpful in making community comparisons, but they are hypothetical as the numerical value of an adjusted rate depends on the standard population used in the standardization calculations (Gordis, 2013). Therefore, adjusted rates must be interpreted with care. See Box 4.3.

Box 4.3 Example of Epidemiologic Research Using Rates

Using autopsy reports in Manitoba between 1989 and 2010, Herath et al. (2014) examined traumatic and nonnatural deaths of children in the province, which represented 22% of all childhood deaths during the 21-year study period. Rural and northern parts of the province had higher traumatic injury mortality rates, and most children died at the scene or shortly thereafter. In 2010, the mortality rate for all traumatic and nonnatural deaths was 2.3/100,000 children, which was markedly lower than the 4.8/100,000 mortality rate in 1999.

TABLE 4.2 Commonly Used Rates

Measures of Natality

$$\text{Crude birth rate} = \frac{\text{Number of live births during time interval}}{\text{Estimated midinterval population}} \times 1{,}000$$

$$\text{Fertility rate} = \frac{\text{Number of live births during time interval}}{\text{Number of women aged 15–44 at midinterval}} \times 1{,}000$$

Measures of Morbidity and Mortality

$$\text{Incidence rate} = \frac{\text{Number of new cases specified health conditions during the time interval}}{\text{Estimated midinterval population at risk}} \times 1{,}000$$

$$\text{Prevalence rate} = \frac{\text{Number of current cases of specified health condition at a given point of time}}{\text{Estimated population at risk at same point of time}} \times 1{,}000$$

$$\text{Crude death rate} = \frac{\text{Number of deaths during time interval}}{\text{Estimated midinterval population}} \times 1{,}000$$

$$\text{Specific death rate} = \frac{\text{Number of deaths in a subgroup during time interval}}{\text{Estimated midinterval population of subgroup}} \times 1{,}000$$

$$\text{Cause-specific death rate} = \frac{\text{Number of deaths from specified cause during time interval}}{\text{Estimated midinterval population}} \times 1{,}000$$

$$\text{Infant mortality rate} = \frac{\text{Number of deaths of infants aged <1 year during time interval}}{\text{Total live births during time interval}} \times 1{,}000$$

$$\text{Neonatal mortality rate} = \frac{\text{Number of deaths of infants aged <28 days during time interval}}{\text{Total live births during time interval}} \times 1{,}000$$

$$\text{Postneonatal mortality rate} = \frac{\text{Number of deaths of infants aged} \geq 28 \text{ days but <1 year during time interval}}{\text{Total live births during time interval}} \times 1{,}000$$

ANALYTIC MEASURES OF HEALTH

As you have learned, rates are used to describe and compare the risks of dying, becoming ill, or developing other health conditions. It is also desirable to determine if health conditions are associated with, or related to, other factors. The related factors, also known as risk factors, may point the way to preventive actions (e.g., the linking of air pollution to health problems has led to environmental controls). To investigate potential relationships between health conditions and other factors, analytic measures of community health are required. In this section, three analytic measures are discussed: relative risk, odds ratio, and attributable risk.

Relative Risk

To determine if a relationship or association exists between a health condition and a suspected factor, it is necessary to compare the risk of developing the health condition for the population exposed to the factor with the risk for the population not exposed to the factor. The *relative risk* (RR) *ratio* does exactly this by expressing the ratio of the incidence rate of those exposed and those not exposed to the suspected factor:

$$RR = \frac{\text{incidence rate among those exposed}}{\text{incidence rate among those not exposed}}$$

The RR tells us whether the rate in the exposed population is higher than the rate in the nonexposed population and, if so, how many times higher it is. A high RR in the exposed population suggests that the factor is a *risk factor* in the development of the health condition.

Internal and External Risk Factors

The concept of RR is understood readily when one group of people is clearly exposed and another is not exposed to an external agent such as a virus, cigarette smoke, or an industrial pollutant. However, it may be confusing to see RR applied to internal factors such as age, race, or sex. Nevertheless, as can be seen in the next example, persons are also "exposed" to intrinsic factors that may carry as much risk as extrinsic ones.

Example of Relative Risk: Diabetes

Type 2 diabetes mellitus is complicated by conditions such as ischemic heart disease, peripheral vascular disease, cerebral vascular disease, retinopathy, renal vascular disease, and peripheral neuropathy. Complications of diabetes lead to a poorer quality of life and premature death.

There is general agreement that type 2 diabetes has a genetic basis but that environmental factors, the most important of which is obesity, are also involved in the disease onset. It appears that nongenetic factors may be subject to intervention, and studies of controlling obesity are needed, especially by diet and exercise. Participation in a community-based exercise program can successfully facilitate weight loss in a group of individuals with type 2 diabetes. Exercise decreases fasting blood glucose values and decreases the need for insulin or oral hypoglycaemic agents, or both.

Diabetes and the First Nations

From the 2009–2010, Canadian Community Health Survey (CCHS), the age-standardized, self-reported prevalence of diabetes among the non-Aboriginal Canadian population ages 12 and older was 5%, whereas for off-reserve First Nations peoples, the self-reported prevalence was 10.3% (PHAC, 2011). With this information, we can calculate a relative risk. Among off-reserve First Nations peoples, the prevalence rate was 10.3/100, and among non-Aboriginal Canadians, the rate was 5.0/100. Thus, the RR of diabetes for First Nations peoples living off-reserve compared with Canadians in general can be calculated as follows:

$$RR = \frac{10.3 \text{ per } 100}{5.0 \text{ per } 100} = 2.60$$

In other words, the risk of diabetes is nearly three times greater for off-reserve First Nations peoples than for non-Aboriginal Canadians. Clearly, First Nations ancestry is a risk factor. The risk factor itself cannot be altered, but the information provided by this analysis can be used to plan protective services for the population at greatest risk. We must be cautious in making generalizations, as further analysis indicates that diabetes rates differ among Aboriginal groups. In a report of off-reserve First Nations, Métis, and Inuit peoples, diabetes was reported among 9.3% of First Nations peoples compared to 7.5% of Métis, and 4.9% of Inuit (Garner et al., 2010).

Odds Ratio

Calculation of the RR is straightforward when incidence rates are available. Unfortunately, not all studies can be carried out prospectively as is required for the computation of incidence rates. In a retrospective study, the RR must be approximated by the *odds ratio* (OR).

As shown in Table 4.3, the OR is a simple mathematical ratio of the odds in favour of having a specific health condition when the suspected factor is present and the odds in favour of having

TABLE 4.3   Cross Tabulation for Calculation of Odds Ratio

	Health Condition		
	Present	Absent	Total
Exposed to factor	a	b	a + b
Not exposed to factor	c	d	c + d
Total	a + c	b + d	a + b + c + d

the condition when the factor is absent. The odds of having the condition when the suspected factor is present is represented by *a* divided by *b* in the table (*a*/*b*). The chance of having the condition when the factor is absent is represented by *c* divided by *d* (*c*/*d*). The odds ratio is thus

$$\frac{a/b}{c/d} = \frac{ad}{bc}$$

An example may help. Groundwater contamination from bacteria is a serious public health concern because the spread of antibiotic-resistant organisms can transfer through water to humans and animals. A group of Canadian researchers used water samples submitted for testing to public health laboratories between 2005 and 2006 in Ontario and Alberta to determine the proportion of water samples that were contaminated with *Escherichia coli (E. coli)* from private wells and to identify factors related to the contamination (Coleman et al., 2013). One of the factors examined was whether livestock on the property affected the well water, and the sample included farming and nonfarming properties with livestock. Let us use the *E. coli* data in Table 4.4 to calculate the OR for properties with livestock.

$$OR = \frac{ad}{bc} = \frac{100(310)}{114(133)} = 2.41$$

From the OR calculation, we can state that private wells on properties with livestock were nearly two and a half times more likely to test positive for antibiotic-resistant *E. coli* than were properties without livestock.

Relative Risk and Odds Ratio: Caution in Interpretation

A word of caution: Regard a high RR or OR with appropriate concern, but do not allow the finding to obscure the potential involvement of other factors. Refer to Table 4.4 again and note that 133 private wells on properties without livestock in the sample had multiclass-resistant organisms in the well water. In other words, livestock was not the sole cause of *E. coli* contaminated well water.

In addition to assessing the strength of the association based on either the OR or RR, the confidence interval (CI) surrounding the estimate must be evaluated. Since RR and OR are ratios,

TABLE 4.4   *E. coli* Contaminated Private Wells by Presence of Livestock

	Multiclass-Resistant *E. coli*		
	Present	Absent	Total
Properties with Livestock	100	114	214
Properties without Livestock	133	310	443
Total	233	424	657

Data from Coleman et al. (2013). Table 4, p. 3032.

Box 4.4   Use of the Odds Ratio in Epidemiologic Research

Czoli, et al. (2014) reported on the prevalence of e-cigarette use among
Canadian youth and young adults, ages 16 to 30. Of the 1,188 participants, 16% reported trying
e-cigarettes. The authors reported that compared to nonsmokers, former and current smokers
were four times (OR = 4.25, 95% CI, 2.11–8.56) and nearly 10 times (OR = 9.84, 95% CI, 6.52–
14.86), respectively, more likely to have tried e-cigarettes than nonsmokers.

---

an estimate of 1.0 indicates that there is no difference between the variables being compared. Therefore, if the confidence interval includes the integer "1," then the estimate is considered statistically "nonsignificant." For example, if a reported odds ratio is 1.8, with an accompanying 95% confidence interval of 0.6–2.3 (e.g., OR = 1.8, 95% CI = 0.6–2.3), the integer 1 is included in the confidence interval, thus rendering the finding as statistically nonsignificant. See Box 4.4.

Attributable Risk and Attributable Risk Percent

Another measure of risk is *attributable risk* (AR), or the risk difference between the incidence rates for those exposed and those not exposed to the risk factor. This measure estimates the excess risk attributable to the factor being studied. It shows the potential reduction in the overall incidence rate if the factor could be eliminated.

AR = incidence rate in exposed group *minus* incidence rate in nonexposed group. AR is usually further quantified into attributable risk percent:

$$\frac{\text{Attributable risk}}{\text{Incidence rate in exposed group}} \times 100$$

This provides an estimate of the percentage of occurrences of the health condition that could be prevented if the risk factor were eliminated. For example, a study examining lung cancer risk in Ontario estimated that the percent of AR associated with radon gas in homes was 13.6% (Peterson et al., 2013). The authors estimated that removing radon in homes to background levels would prevent 91 lung cancers per year.

Cause and Association

Ultimately, community health workers hope to determine causes of health conditions so that steps can be taken to improve health. In view of the complexity of the human body and human behaviour, establishing causality is difficult. Therefore, investigations of population health generally examine relationships or *associations* between variables. The variables are the characteristics or phenomena (such as age, occupation, or physical exercise) and the health conditions (such as heart disease) being studied. A disease that is perceived to be dramatically increasing in a community frequently results in residents searching for a cause, and emotions can run high. When explaining "risk," it is important to remember that increased risk determined from a statistically significant association does not connote "causation."

Variables and Constants

An important requirement in any study is that the factors studied must have the potential to vary from person to person. If a factor cannot vary, it is not a variable but a constant. It is impossible to establish an association between a constant and a variable because the constant, by definition, cannot change when the variable changes. Thus, a study that looks only at men cannot establish an association between sex and, for example, heart disease; the study has made sex a constant. A study that looks only at persons with heart disease cannot establish an association between heart disease and any other variable; heart disease has become a constant in the study.

Control or Comparison Groups

To ensure that associations between variables can be examined, *control groups* or *comparison groups* may be needed. A study of heart disease might compare persons with the disease with a control group of persons without the disease. An investigation of a new treatment would study persons who receive the treatment and a control group of persons who do not receive the treatment.

Independent and Dependent Variables

Frequently, variables are referred to as *dependent* or *independent*. The dependent variable is the outcome or result that the investigator is studying. It is a characteristic that conceivably could be altered (e.g., health status, knowledge, or behaviour). The independent variable is the presumed "cause" of or contributor to variation in the dependent variable. For example, in the radon gas study cited earlier (Petersen et al., 2013), radon gas, the independent variable, is seen to contribute to lung cancer risk, the dependent variable. An independent variable may be a naturally occurring event or phenomenon such as level of usual physical activity, exposure to ultraviolet radiation, or type of employment, or it might be a planned intervention such as an exercise regimen, a medical treatment, or an educational program. An independent variable might also be an intrinsic quality such as age, ethnicity, or sex. Note that these intrinsic qualities, although they cannot vary within an individual, can vary from person to person; thus, they can be studied as independent variables.

Confounding Variables

When an association is identified between variables, it is tempting—but incorrect—to assume that one variable causes the other. If, for example, a study found that communities with lower salaries for public health workers had higher crime rates, we could not conclude that low public health salaries led to high crime rates. Common sense suggests that economic conditions might influence both salaries and crime, that is, economic conditions intervene in the study and confound the results. Any factor that is associated with both the independent (exposure) and dependent (disease) variables is considered a confounding variable.

Criteria for Determining Causation

If an association is found between variables, it means that variables tend to occur or change together, but it does not prove that one variable causes the other. Because of the possibility of confounded results, guidelines for determining causation have been identified. An association must be evaluated against these criteria; the more criteria that are met, the more likely it is that the association is causal. However, an association may meet all the criteria for causation and later be shown to be spurious because of factors that were not known at the time the study was done. For this reason, investigators must interpret their results with great caution; rarely can results be shown to be causal. Nine widely used guidelines for evaluating causation, first established by Bradford Hill in 1965, are listed below (Gordis, 2013). Of these, time sequence, strength of association, and consistency with existing knowledge are considered to be the most critical.

1. The association is strong. The strength of the relationship may be evaluated statistically by a variety of measures. For example, the higher the RR or OR with a narrow CI, the stronger the association.

2. Consistency with other knowledge. An association that contradicts current scientific views must be evaluated very carefully. However, associations may be inconsistent with current knowledge simply because current knowledge is not as advanced as a new discovery.

3. The association is temporally correct. The hypothesized cause of the health condition must occur before the onset of the condition.

4. Dose–response relationship. A strong argument can be made for a causal relationship if the risk of disease or condition increases with increased exposure. However, absence of a dose–response relationship does not necessarily rule out a causal relationship.

5. Consideration of other alternative explanations. Not all potential intervening variables can be explored, of course, but alternate explanation for the association, including the possibility of confounding, must be examined carefully before considering an association to be causal.

6. The association is biologically plausible. Consistency with existing biologic knowledge is sought; however, there have been instances where the epidemiologic identification of a syndrome or disease has preceded the biologic understanding of a disease (e.g., human immunodeficiency virus [HIV]/acquired immune deficiency syndrome [AIDS]).

7. Replication of findings. The same association must be found repeatedly in other studies, in other settings, and with other methods.

8. Cessation of exposure. If a causal exposure or factor for a condition is removed, it is expected that the incidence of the disease would also decrease. While this is normally the case, there are instances where the pathologic progression of a disease is irreversible by the time the exposure is removed, and the occurrence of the condition may not fall accordingly.

9. The association is specific. The hypothesized cause should be associated with relatively few health conditions. For example, speaking English may be associated with many health conditions, but it is a cause for none. This criterion must be tempered by the knowledge that certain factors or behaviours, such as cigarette smoking, have been shown to have multiple effects.

The usefulness of information to a community depends on its accuracy, completeness, and reliability. If data are to provide a realistic profile of a community, identify issues placing people at risk, and assess areas of strength on which to build programs, then planners must have confidence in the information they gather and in the interpretations made by residents and community workers. Hence, data must be from credible sources, collected by ethical and valid methods, appropriate to the issues involved, and detailed enough to allow quality interventions to be developed. In the next section, common sources of data are identified and, when combined with assessment strategies presented in Chapter 16, can form a solid foundation for community action.

SOURCES OF COMMUNITY HEALTH DATA

To be an effective community health worker, you will also need to interpret and use data from various sources. In this section, we present the use of several important sources of data.

Census

The census is the most comprehensive source of population data for Canada. Every 5 years since 1951, under the Statistics Act, the government of Canada enumerates the population and surveys it for basic demographics such as age, sex, marital status, and mother tongue as well as numerous other factors such as employment, ethnicity, housing, income, migration, and education.

Although census data are comprehensive, bias does occur. For example, people may answer personal questions dishonestly. Perhaps more significant, the census is believed to underrepresent low-income residents, residents of First Nations reserves, and transients. These people are more difficult to locate and enumerate and tend to be less likely to respond to census surveys. However, efforts are made to capture information on as many people as possible; forms are available in more than 50 languages, in Braille, and in large print. Forms are also available in electronic formats, and a census representative is available to collect the data in person if necessary. To find out more about the Canadian census, go to the Statistics Canada website at http://www12.statcan.ca/census-recensement/index-eng.cfm

Vital Statistics

Vital statistics are the data on legally registered events (e.g., births, deaths, marriages, and divorces) collected on an ongoing basis by government agencies. Provincial health departments usually publish vital statistics annually. The Canadian Institute for Health Information (CIHI) gathers data from the provinces and publishes annual volumes as well as periodic reports on specific topics. Vital statistics for provinces and territories can be found online.

Beginning researchers tend to consider vital statistics "hallowed" because they are, after all, legal data. However, legality does not guarantee validity. For example, the manner in which cause of death is recorded on death certificates is inconsistent. The numbers of unmarried but cohabiting couples also demonstrate that marriage and divorce records are also not completely valid measures of reality. Despite their limitations, vital statistics are often the best available data, and much useful information can be gained from them.

Notifiable Disease Reports

The PHAC reports data collected by provincial and local health departments on legally reportable diseases and also periodically requests voluntary reporting of nonnotifiable health conditions of special interest. Canada Communicable Disease Report (CCDR), other reports on chronic diseases, and reports on special topics are available from the PHAC.

Even legally mandated disease reports may not be representative of all cases of the disease. Thus, they may not provide valid description of a disease as it exists in the community. In practice, health care providers may fail to report diseases that should be reported; for instance, chickenpox (varicella) is consistently underreported.

Medical and Hospital Records

Medical and hospital records are used extensively in community health research. These records, however, do not provide a completely representative or valid picture of community health. In the first place, not all persons with health problems receive medical attention, so medical records are obviously biased. Second, medical documentation is not always complete. Finally, hospitalized patients are also more likely to have another illness along with the one being studied. This phenomenon, called Berkson bias, creates the likelihood of finding a false association between the two illnesses (Porta, 2014).

Social Welfare Reports

Statistics Canada as well as Employment and Social Development Canada (HESDC) publish regular reports on current issues about the social situations experienced by Canadians. A survey of the websites of these organizations can offer the community professional insight into social conditions such as homelessness, poverty, education, and the economy. Other national Internet sites offer opinion and analysis of social and economic conditions. There are also regional "think tanks" that offer comment on issues specific to people in groups of provinces.

Various national and provincial professional associations also offer publications on issues relevant to their disciplines. As with any site, you must be cautious in interpreting the opinions and analysis because they will come from a particular perspective and are trying to make an argument that supports their specific viewpoint. Seeking information from several sites will provide the community health professional with a broad perspective on issues.

SCREENING FOR HEALTH CONDITIONS

Thus far, we have focused on methods for studying community health problems and assessing health risks for populations. Screening, a method of secondary prevention, is an effort to detect unrecognized or preclinical illness among individuals. Screening tests are not intended to be diagnostic. Their purpose is to rapidly and economically identify persons who have a high probability of having (or developing) a particular illness so that they can be referred for definitive diagnosis and treatment.

Considerations in Deciding to Screen

Screening goes further than identifying groups at risk for illness; it identifies individuals who may actually have an illness. Screening carries an ethical commitment to continue working with these individuals and provide them access to diagnostic and treatment services. In general, screening should be conducted only if:

- Early diagnosis and treatment can favourably alter the course of the illness.
- Definitive diagnosis and treatment facilities are available, either through the screening agency or through referral.
- A group being screened is at risk for the illness (in other words, the group is likely to have a high prevalence of the illness).
- Screening procedures are reliable and valid.

Ideally, a screening test should be simple to perform, cause minimal distress to patients, and be of low cost. Acceptability by the public and clinicians is also crucial for the adoption and implementation of any screening test (Fletcher et al., 2012).

Screening Test Reliability and Validity

Reliability refers to the consistency or repeatability of test results; *validity* refers to the ability of the test to measure what it is supposed to measure.

A reliable screening test yields the same result even when administered by different screeners. Training for all screening personnel in use of the test is essential. Lack of reliability may suggest that the screeners are administering the test in an inconsistent manner or that a chemical reagent is unstable.

To be valid, a screening test must distinguish correctly between those individuals who have the condition and those who do not. This is measured by the test's sensitivity and specificity, as shown in Table 4.5. *Sensitivity* is the ability to correctly identify individuals who have the disease—that is, to identify a true positive. A test with high sensitivity will have few false negatives. *Specificity* is the ability to correctly identify individuals who do not have the disease or to call a true negative "negative." A test with high specificity has few false positives.

Ideally, a screening test's sensitivity and specificity should be 100%; in practice, however, screening tests vary in this regard. As shown in Table 4.5, sensitivity, or the true-positive rate, is the complement of the false-negative rate, and specificity, or the true-negative rate, is the complement of the false-positive rate. Thus, as sensitivity increases, specificity decreases, and vice versa. Therefore, decisions regarding screening test validity may require uncomfortable compromises, as you will see from the following examples.

TABLE 4.5 Sensitivity and Specificity of a Screening Test

Screening Test Results	Reality	
	Diseased	**Not Diseased**
Positive	True positive	False positive
Negative	False negative	True negative
Total	Total diseased	Total not diseased

$$\text{Sensitivity (true-positive rate)} = \frac{\text{True positives}}{\text{Total diseased}}$$

$$\text{Specificity (true-negative rate)} = \frac{\text{True negatives}}{\text{Total not diseased}}$$

$$\text{False-negative rate} = \frac{\text{False negatives}}{\text{Total diseased}} \quad or \quad 1 - \text{Sensitivity}$$

$$\text{False-positive rate} = \frac{\text{False negatives}}{\text{Total not diseased}} \quad or \quad 1 - \text{Sensitivity}$$

DECISION MAKING IN SCREENING: PRACTICAL AND ETHICAL CONSIDERATIONS

Suppose you are screening for a deadly disease that is curable only if detected early, and you have a choice between a test with high sensitivity and low specificity or one with high specificity and low sensitivity. To save the most lives, you need high sensitivity, that is, a low rate of false negatives (people who *have* the disease but are not detected by the screening test). However, if you select the test with high sensitivity, its low specificity means that you will have a high number of people who do *not* have the disease but whom the test identifies as having it (false positives). Using such a test will alarm many people needlessly and will cause unnecessary expenses by over-referring them for nonexistent disease. Which test would you choose?

Now, suppose you are screening for the same disease, but the diagnostic and treatment facilities in the community are already overloaded, and further budget cuts are projected. To minimize unnecessary referrals of false positives, you would want the test with high specificity. However, because of the low sensitivity of this test, you will have to weigh the benefits of a low false-positive rate against the ethics of a high false-negative rate. Is it justifiable to lull the undetected diseased persons into a false—and potentially fatal—sense of security? Which test would you choose now?

Decisions regarding screening involve seeking the most favourable balance of sensitivity and specificity. Sometimes, sensitivity and specificity can be improved by adjusting the screening process (e.g., adding another test or changing the level at which the test is considered positive). At other times, evaluating sensitivity and specificity may result in a decision not to conduct a screening program because the economic costs of over-referral or the ethical considerations of under-referral outweigh the usefulness of screening. An understanding of the principles discussed in this section will help you make informed decisions regarding community screening.

OUTBREAK MANAGEMENT

The emergence of newly identified infectious diseases in the past 30 years (e.g., HIV, Ebola virus, SARS, Zika) highlights the importance of preparedness of the public health system as well as an organized, logical approach to the investigation of outbreaks. Critical with any report of an outbreak is early verification of the diagnosis, plus the establishment of an epidemic. Key to diagnosis verification is ascertaining what constitutes a "case" and that laboratory and clinical assessments are accurate; simultaneously, potential missing cases are searched for. If previous records exist about the prevalence of a disease, it is important to compare the current findings with historical data. Once the existence of an epidemic has been established, identification of "when" (time), "where" (place), and "who" (person) occurs. Plotting the occurrences on a map and the cases on a time line assists in describing the nature of the epidemic. Determination as to whether the epidemic has a common source versus whether it is propagated aids in identifying potential control measures. Finally, it is important to analyze the findings and develop and test hypotheses. Appropriate public health agencies are notified once an epidemic is verified and it has been determined who is at risk. This is not always easily accomplished, particularly when dealing with a new condition or disease not previously known.

A case in point was the 2003 SARS outbreak in Toronto, Ontario, as there was no diagnostic test, no treatment, and very little information on the characteristics of the viral agent (Basrur et al., 2004). A total of 224 SARS cases were documented among Toronto residents, and of 23,300 people identified as contacts, 13,374 were placed in quarantine (Basrur et al., 2004). The strain on the public health system was enormous, particularly given the clinical uncertainty of the disease; lessons from the experience continue to inform preparedness efforts today (Ferguson-Paré, 2014). The need for comprehensive disease control strategies with strong communication linkages among health agencies was one of the most salient lessons learned from the experience. For more information about accessing the Canadian Notifiable Diseases On-Line, go to the PHAC website at http://dsol-smed.phac-aspc.gc.ca/dsol-smed/ndis/index-eng.php

Summary

In this chapter, you have been introduced to epidemiology, the specific science of population health. Examples have been offered as to how epidemiology can be used to accurately assess a community's health status in order to appropriately intervene as a community health professional. Answers to many health questions can be obtained by examining existing data and by remaining inquisitive. Our practice is better informed through applying epidemiologic principles to community health problems.

 ## Critical Thinking Exercise 4.1

Demographic Analysis and Population Risk Factors

- The life expectancy in 2007/2009 for Canadian men was 78.8 years of age and among women, 83.3 years. In the same year, men in the Territories had a life expectancy of 72.5 years, the lowest in the country, whereas men in British Columbia had the highest at 79.5 years. What factors could explain the differences in life expectancy?
- Can you identify health conditions that would have a stable incidence rate, but a growing prevalence rate? How are incidence and prevalence connected? Are there disease conditions where the incidence is higher than the prevalence?

REFERENCES

Baker, S. P., & Li, G. (2012). Epidemiologic approaches to injury and violence. *Epidemiologic Reviews, 34*, 1–3.

Basrur, S., Yaffe, B., & Henry, B. (2004). SARS: A local public health perspective. *Canadian Journal of Public Health, 95*, 22–24.

Carter-Pokras, O. D., Offutt-Powell, T. N., Kaufman, J. S., Giles, W. H., & Mays, V. M. (2012). Epidemiology, policy, and racial/ethnic minority health disparities. *Annuals of Epidemiology, 22*, 446–455.

Centers for Disease Control and Prevention (CDC). (2012). Section 1: Definition of epidemiology. In *Principles of epidemiology in public health practice* (3rd ed.) [Self-study course]. URL=http://www.cdc.gov/ophss/csels/dsepd/ss1978/lesson1/section1.html

Cohen, B. E., & Gregory, D. (2009). Community health clinical education in Canada: Part 2—Developing competencies to address social justice, equity, and the social determinants of health. *International Journal of Nursing Education Scholarship, 6*, 1–15.

Coleman, B. L., Louie, M., Salvadori, M. I., McEwan, S. A., Neumann, N., Sibley, K., et al. (2013). Contamination of Canadian private drinking water sources with antimicrobial resistant Escherichia coli. *Water Research, 47*, 3026–3036.

Czoli, C. D., Hammond, D., & White, C. M. (2014). Electronic cigarettes in Canada: Prevalence of use and perceptions among youth and young adults. *Canadian Journal of Public Health, 105*, e97–e102.

Ferguson-Paré, M. (2014). The SARS experience. *Canadian Nurse, 111*(9), 27.

Fletcher, R. H., Fletcher, S. W., & Fletcher, G. S. (2012). *Clinical epidemiology: The essentials* (5th ed.). Philadelphia, PA: Lippincott Williams & Wilkins.

Garner, R., Carrière, G., Sanmartin, C., & the Longitudinal Health and Administrative Data Research Team. (2010). *The health of First Nations living off-reserve, Inuit and Métis adults in Canada: The impact of socio-economic status on inequalities in health.* Ottawa: Statistics Canada, Health Information and Research Division. URL=http://www.statcan.gc.ca/pub/82–622-x/82–622-x2010004-eng.htm

Gordis, L. (2013). *Epidemiology* (5th ed.). Philadelphia, PA: Elsevier Saunders.

Haddon, W., Jr. (1999). The changing approach to the epidemiology, prevention and amelioration of trauma: The transition to approaches etiologically rather than descriptively based. *Injury Prevention, 5*, 231–236.

Herath, J. C., Kalikias, S., Phillips, S. M., & Del Bigio, M. R. (2014). Traumatic and other non-natural childhood deaths in Manitoba, Canada: A retrospective autopsy analysis (1989–2010). *Canadian Journal of Public Health, 105*, e103–e108.

Hutchinson, B., Levesque, J-F., Stumpf, E., & Coyle, N. (2011). Primary health care in Canada: Systems in motion. *The Milbank Quarterly, 89*, 256–288.

Kenny, M. E., & Hage, S. M. (2009). The next frontier: Prevention as an instrument of social justice. *Journal of Primary Prevention, 30*, 1–10.

Petersen, E., Aher, A., Kim, J., Li, Y., Brand, K., & Copes, R. (2013). Lung cancer risk from radon in Ontario, Canada: How many lung cancers can we prevent? *Cancer, Cause and Control, 24*, 2013–2020.

Porta, M. (2014). *Dictionary of epidemiology* (5th ed.) . Oxford: Oxford University Press, Oxford Reference.

Public Health Agency of Canada (PHAC). (2008). *Canadian perinatal health report: 2008 edition.* URL=http://www.phac-aspc.gc.ca/publicat/2008/cphr-rspc/index-eng.php

Public Health Agency of Canada (PHAC). (2011). *Diabetes in Canada: Facts and figures from a public health perspective.* URL=http://www.phac-aspc.gc.ca/cd-mc/publications/diabetes-diabete/facts-figures-faits-chiffres-2011/index-eng.php

Public Health Agency of Canada (PHAC). (2013). *Perinatal health indicators for Canada 2013: A report from the Canadian Perinatal Surveillance System.* URL=http://www.phac-aspc.gc.ca/rhs-ssg/phi-isp-2013-eng.php

Public Health Agency of Canada (PHAC). (2014). *Chronic disease and injury indicator framework, Quick Stats, Fall 2014 edition.* Ottawa: Centre for Chronic Disease Prevention, PHAC. URL=http://infobase.phac-aspc.gc.ca/cdif/Publications/Quick-Stats_2014_EN-FINAL.pdf

Rothman, K. J. (2012). *Epidemiology: An introduction* (2nd ed.). Toronto: Oxford University Press.

Short, M. M., Mushquash, C. J., & Bedard, M. (2013). Motor vehicle crashes among Canadian Aboriginal people: A review of the literature. *Canadian Journal of Rural Medicine, 18*, 86–98.

Snow, J. (1936). *Snow on cholera, being a reprint of two papers by John Snow, M.D., together with a biographical memoir by B. W. Richardson and an introduction by W. H. Frost.* New York, NY: Commonwealth Fund.

Stanwell-Smith, R. (2013). The remarkable Dr. John Snow. *Perspectives in Public Health, 133*, 237.

Statistics Canada. (2013). *Infant mortality rates, by province and territory (both sexes)* [table]. URL=http://www.statcan.gc.ca/tables-tableaux/sum-som/l01/cst01/health21a-eng.htm

World Health Organization (WHO). (2012). *Newborns: Reducing mortality (Fact Sheet No. 333).* URL=http://www.who.int/mediacentre/factsheets/fs333/en/

ONLINE RESOURCES

Please visit the Point at http://thepoint.lww.com/Vollman4e for up-to-date Internet resources and additional learning materials on this topic.

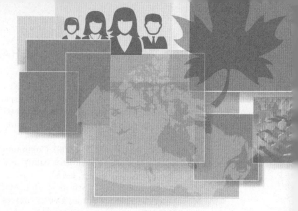

CHAPTER 5

Strengthening Community Action: Public Engagement for Social Innovation and Collective Impact

Catherine M. Scott, Gail L. MacKean, Bretta Maloff, Cheryl Houtekamer, and Christine Vandenberghe

> *Health promotion works through concrete and effective community action in setting priorities, making decisions, planning strategies and implementing them to achieve better health. At the heart of this process is the empowerment of communities—their ownership and control of their own endeavours and destinies.*
>
> *Community development draws on existing human and material resources in the community to enhance self-help and social support, and to develop flexible systems for strengthening public participation in and direction of health matters. This requires full and continuous access to information, learning opportunities for health, as well as funding support.*
>
> —Ottawa Charter (1986)

LEARNING OBJECTIVES

After studying this chapter, you should be able to:

1. Describe links between strengthening community action, community development, and public engagement

2. Describe elements of community development methods and processes

3. Discuss the role of public engagement in health

4. Understand the roles of partnerships in population health promotion

5. Describe links among the concepts of collaboration, partnerships, social innovation, and collective impact. How are they similar? How do they differ?

6. Discuss how these key concepts relate to current discussions regarding to social innovation and collective impact

Introduction

The opening quote from the Ottawa Charter is timeless—in essence it encapsulates the foundation of population health promotion. The principles of engagement, ownership, and control reflect a commitment to democratization of knowledge that remains salient in guiding all that we do in health and human services. Over the past several decades, population health interventions have met with varying levels of success. Increasingly, health professionals, researchers, policymakers, and the public have acknowledged that meaningful engagement of stakeholders in conceptualizing, developing, and implementing health interventions is vital to the success of such initiatives. Over the past four decades, population health promotion policies and programs have placed high priority on active public engagement in activities that affect health and human services. Comprehensive action strategies to improve health are embedded within the population health promotion model; strengthening community action (SCA) is one of its cornerstones (see Chapter 1, Fig. 1.3).

Seminal health promotion documents from the 1970s and 1980s (see Chapter 1, Table 1.1) outlined the principles of public engagement and the potential impact engagement could have on social innovation. Despite this foundation, we have only recently seen a dramatic shift in rhetoric to action; from the need to generate and "translate" research evidence for practice to a greater focus on using diverse sources of evidence, taking risks (i.e., the risk of failure) associated with rapid innovation cycles, and engaging those who will use the evidence. The shift has been slow and speaks to the complexity of social innovation. Approaches and bodies of literature remain segmented (e.g., developing separate strategies for public, patient, clinician, and community engagement in health systems planning). In this chapter, we will draw together these diverse discourses.

SCA combines community development processes with the goal of stimulating social action for health. Engaging the public in a social innovation agenda, however, raises a host of questions. For example:

- How is *community* defined and by whom?
- Whose agenda(s) is(are) being addressed?
- In what areas can public engagement have meaningful impact (i.e., rather than being token involvement)?
- How do individuals, communities, and organizations work with health systems to meaningfully address joint goals?

In this chapter, we begin to address these questions. We introduce values and principles that are common to public engagement, community development, and collaboration. We follow with an overview of theory that informs the process of community development. We then discuss how the public can be engaged in individual level care, health systems decision making, and population health promotion with particular focus on the development of interdisciplinary and intersectoral partnerships to address health. We argue that developing in-depth understanding of community development processes, public engagement, and collaboration is fundamental to SCA and ultimately to achieving population health goals.

VALUES AND PRINCIPLES

Two key underlying core values of SCA are that:

1. People who are affected by a decision or a series of decisions have a right to participate in the planning and decision-making processes (IAP2, 2015).[1]

---

[1] The terms public engagement and public participation have become interchangeable over time. For example, the public participation frameworks developed by the International Association for Public Participation (IAP2) are used as the foundation for engagement approaches across health systems. We will use the term *public engagement* throughout this chapter.

2. Better decisions will be made if we recognize the value of diverse perspectives, and actively use different sources of evidence (i.e., evidence generated from research, evaluation, and experience) (Scott et al., 2009).

In addition, the following principles have been identified as contributing to effectiveness and sustainability of engagement, community development, and collaboration (American Institutes for Research [AIR], 2014; Government of British Columbia, 2011; International Association for Public Participation [IAP2], 2015; Scott et al., 2012; Scott & Thurston, 2004).

- Jointly established and agreed-upon goals, objectives, and principles
- Respect for diversity
- Commitment to relationship development based on mutual respect and trust
- Commitment to learning and improvement
- Sensitivity to inherent power differences
- Power-sharing strategies explicitly embedded in planning and implementation
- Open, honest, and clear communication
- Flexible structures and processes to accommodate changing needs
- Capacity building to sustain innovations

COMMUNITY DEVELOPMENT

When people think about *community,* it is often in terms of geographic or demographic boundaries. While such definitions may be useful in some circumstances, they can be of limited value when it comes to community organizing. People often attach themselves to, and are active in, communities that stretch beyond their place of residence (e.g., school and work communities). Thinking of communities as collectives of people who share common values and concerns provides a broader definition that more accurately reflects the way that people think about and organize their social relationships.

There are many definitions for *community development* in part because *community development* is both a process and a product. Commonalities in defining community development include: improving health outcomes, supporting both capacity development and empowerment, mobilizing multiple stakeholders, strengthening communities and, addressing common needs and goals (Winnipeg Regional Health Authority [WRHA], 2014).

It involves building collective commitment, knowledge, resources, and skills that can be deployed for purposive community change and social innovation, building on community strengths to address community needs. It means that members of a community work together to develop their capacity and competencies, identify and meet their needs, and participate more fully in society. Community development is central to many of the core concepts developed in this and other chapters (i.e., creating supportive environments for health [see Chapter 7], reorienting health services [see Chapter 8], and building healthy public policy [see Chapter 9]).

Community development is therefore concerned with people working together to create opportunities for learning through experience and collective effort to inform and influence decisions that affect them (Abelson et al., 2004; O'Doherty et al., 2012). Thus, individual involvement and collective activity go hand-in-hand; the aim is for people in a community to join together with others to address community needs in such a way that all who take part, professionals and non-professionals alike, develop their own potential as members of society (Box 5.1).

> ### Box 5.1 Developing Communities: Where Do We Start?
>
> Start where people are, because it reflects a respect for the rights of individuals and communities to affirm their own values and ways of living. Second, one should recognize and build on community strengths instead of only assessing community needs. Third, while we need to work closely with communities, to respect their capacities and rights to self-determination, we must at the same time strive to live up to our own ethical standards and those of our professions in not letting blind faith in the community prevent us from seeing and acting on the paramount need for social justice. Fourth, high-level community participation must be fostered. Fifth, one should not forget sense of humour in their work. Sixth, the role of political analysis and activism in health education must be recognized. Health problems and their solutions need to be re-framed in terms of their political, economic, and social contexts. Think globally, act locally, foster individual and community empowerment, and finally, work for social justice (Minkler, 1994).

Take Note

Beware romanticization of communities. "Community, as implied in the landmark Ottawa Charter (WHO, 1986) and some more recent documents, can do no wrong.... Although it is important to accept community self-determination in principle, it is also vital to recognize that what communities do for their own health may be inimical to a broader public health.... [The idea of community] becomes romanticized in a way that can obscure very real and important power inequities between different communities that may subtly imperil the health and well-being of less powerful groups, for example the community of urban land developers versus the community of the homeless" (Labonté, 2012, pp. 97–98).

Community Development Drivers

What stimulates community development is often a result of citizens' perceived lack of government responsiveness or unfairness or inequity within a community. Often inequity in housing, employment, or education as a result of poverty, race, or gender motivates action on the part of communities. Inequity is not an isolated event or unique to one part of the world. The recent report on global risks (World Economic Forum [WEF], 2015) outlines five areas that threaten societies: economic, environmental, geopolitical, societal, and technological, which, interestingly, parallel the social determinants of health (see Chapter 1, Table 1.3). The impact on health is strongly influenced by public policy decisions across these broad domains (Mikkonen & Raphael, 2010).

As communities increase their understanding of the complexity of these issues, and recognize that scarce resources are being outstripped by community needs, they are becoming increasingly concerned about how they can effect change in their localities to address these issues through either novel approaches or policy change. Some recent Canadian examples are: the development of a palliative care network in Ontario (Bainbridge et al., 2011); childhood intervention programs in Canada (Shan et al., 2014); improving patient safety (Baum et al., 2012); community health workers in immigrant and refugee populations (Torres et al., 2013); and capacity building among immigrant communities (Narushima et al., 2014).

Critical Thinking Exercise 5.1

Evidence indicates that when local community members are committed to investing in their community, they can successfully develop and mobilize their assets, capacities, and abilities to construct a new social reality. A community development approach that is focused on community assets and opportunities rather than on needs and deficiencies builds on opportunity, competence, and empowerment. Think of a community issue that is important to you. What are the community assets that could be mobilized to address this issue? What are the benefits of taking an assets-based approach rather than focusing on deficits?

Whatever the impetus, people come together to take action. It is in these initial gatherings that community development begins, gains momentum, creates leaders, and focuses efforts. There are several steps in the community development process (Table 5.1).

Community Development Practice

Although there are no prescribed methods to community development because each community will have unique challenges and assets, the following action list extends the values and principles outlined earlier and are fundamental to all community development initiatives.

- Promote active and representative engagement toward enabling all community members to meaningfully influence the decisions that affect their lives
- Engage community members in learning about and understanding community issues, and the economic, social, environmental, political, psychological, and other impacts associated with alternative courses of action
- Incorporate the diverse interests and cultures of the community in the community development process; and disengage from support of any effort that is likely to adversely affect the disadvantaged members of a community
- Work actively to enhance the leadership capacity of community members, leaders, and groups within the community

TABLE 5.1 Steps in the Community Development Process

Step	Description
Defining the issue	Articulate the issue; what is known about it, and who is affected.
Initiating the process	Research the veracity of the issue and perspectives, identify the full range of stakeholders, and gather people together to create commitment for action.
Planning community conversations	Invite all stakeholders to participate; develop both informal and formal processes of consultation that allow all viewpoints to be properly aired.
Talking, discovering, and connecting	Prepare handouts that outline the issue and why you are gathering information and mobilizing the community; connect with key people and community members; share information and garner support.
Creating an asset map	Develop lists as you talk to people and initiate relationships, communicate regularly and widely; attract resources.
Mobilizing the community	Bring people together in central locations to discuss options, share experiences, create a common vision, and plan activities.
Taking action	Involve and educate community members, help to shape opinion, and galvanize commitment.
Planning and implementing	Have a vision in mind of what must change so that community-driven initiatives improve the situation, organize people and work, and sustain efforts.

- Be open to using the full range of action strategies to work toward the long-term sustainability and well-being of the community (Community Development Society [CDS], 2015)

External champions in the form of local politicians or professional service providers (e.g., health care providers and community workers) are helpful to the community development process, but such supporters must take care to allow community control over directions, agendas, and processes and not highjack the process for their professional purposes. This is particularly important when undertaking community-based research.

The community development process involves commitment, resources, and skills. Each community has its unique starting point. For instance, some communities know exactly what they want but either do not know how to get there or need support. Other communities rarely get decisions made because of deep-rooted conflicts or historical divisions among groups of people who stubbornly refuse to cooperate. Some communities have experienced too much change too quickly, and old-timers and newcomers have not yet formed a common bond. Other communities have given up trying to do anything because too many people have moved away and the energy of those remaining has been sapped, resulting in general apathy.

Whatever the starting point, and no matter what the community is facing, some key lessons learned over time must be kept in mind: have patience; be flexible; be organized; communicate often; embrace challenges and novel approaches; build networks; encourage others; and appreciate that champions/leaders exist in all communities (Community Tool Box, 2015; Scott et al., 2012).

 Critical Thinking Exercise 5.2

Striking the Balance

Community development initiatives focus on empowering community members to take action to address community issues. Within health systems across Canada, there is increasing emphasis on encouraging community and individual responsibility for health. For example, some policy discussions emphasize empowering families to provide care for patients. Using this policy example, answer the following questions:

- Empowerment for whom? Is increasing family responsibility for care in the best interest of patients and their families?

In addition, Hage and Kenny (2009, p. 77) pose the following critical questions for consideration prior to engaging in social innovation initiatives:

- "For whose benefit are we intervening?
- Whose values are we espousing?
- Are we simply replacing one set of values for another?
- Are middle class values being superimposed on the working class?"

With your colleagues, discuss how consideration of these questions will influence your engagement in community development initiatives.

AN OVERVIEW OF PUBLIC ENGAGEMENT IN HEALTH

As community health workers, and as public health organizations, are there strategies in addition to community development that can be used to engage individuals, groups, and communities in decisions that affect their health and their health care? In what kinds of health and health care decision making can the public effectively be involved; how? Can the public engage in health services planning and development decisions? Can patients and families participate more actively in decisions around their own health and health care?

In this next section, we address some of these questions by providing an overview of what is known about public engagement in health.

History

Public engagement is central to the WHO's definition of *health promotion* (refer to Chapter 1). Fostering public participation is one of the three strategies for enabling people to have more influence in areas that affect their health, outlined in the Epp framework (1986). The underlying rationale for strengthening community action is that involving the public and communities in their health has benefits for the health of individuals and the population.

Over the past twenty-five years, there has been increasing attention paid to involving the public in decisions that affect their health and well-being. A number of social trends have influenced this movement. Democratization of knowledge means that people have access to an increasing amount of information to inform their thoughts and actions. As people become more knowledgeable, they also are less likely to turn to or automatically trust authority figures and experts. Part of health care culture is the expert model. Traditionally, members of the public—including patients and families—have believed that health care and human service professionals know best; that is, they know what the best therapy or treatment or service is for them as individuals, and/or the best way to design and deliver services for a particular population. There has been a long history of engaging the public in community and children's health and health care. More recently public engagement is gaining credibility in adult health and health care.

As you will note throughout this chapter, the theory of public engagement, community development, and collaboration has been well established. The major advances in knowledge about effective public engagement and partnership over the past decade have come from the implementation of established approaches, as people in a variety of practice contexts actively explore different ways of engaging people, communities, and community-based organizations in collective endeavours. In the health and human service sectors, over this same period of time, we have also seen increasing integration among the concepts of community development, public engagement, and partnership. Our understanding of community has broadened, and increasingly people who require services and their families are being recognized as the "public" that needs to be engaged in the design of services if they are to meet the needs of people.

Central to the conceptualization of public engagement is the concept of a spectrum or continuum that builds on the understanding that there is a range of ways in which the public can be engaged in decisions that affect health. This conceptualization of public engagement as a spectrum is generally attributed to Arnstein (1969), whose ladder of public participation has been widely adopted and continually evolved by researchers and practitioners and is now fundamental to discussions of public engagement in health, health care, and human services (IAP2, 2015).

The degree of public involvement increases as one moves across the spectrum from "inform" to "empower." More public involvement is not necessarily better than less public involvement; rather, it depends on the context of the public engagement. This spectrum is illustrated in Figure 5.1.

Building Capacity for Public Engagement

The public as individuals, groups of people, organizations, and entire communities are engaged in a variety of activities that ultimately have an impact on health. This participation can be envisioned as taking place at three broad levels—micro, meso, and macro (Table 5.2).

→ **Increasing Public Involvement** →

	Inform	Input	Engage	Collaborate	Empower
Description	Information out— Information goes from a health organization to the public	Information in— input comes from the public to a health organization	A health organization and the public talk and understand each other	A health organization and the public work together over a period of time	A health organization works with the public to build capacity
Purpose	Creating awareness, public education	Getting citizen and/or stakeholder input, advice, and feedback	In-depth exploration of views, perspectives, and interests, with emphasis on listening and achieving mutual understanding	To make decisions and/or develop policy on an issue	To enable the public to make decisions and take action in areas that affect health
Public participation scenarios	A social marketing campaign is used to increase public awareness about active living strategies	A broad community survey is used to obtain public input on playground safety	A structured public consultation day is held to explore a geographic community's perspectives on the determinants of health	A health organization works collaboratively with community partners on issues (e.g., comprehensive school health, smoke-free municipalities)	Communities make decisions in areas that impact health through community development and social action

FIGURE 5.1 Spectrum of public engagement (IAP2, 2014; Smith, 2003).

COLLABORATION AND PARTNERSHIPS FOR INNOVATION AND COLLECTIVE IMPACT

Addressing complex health and social issues requires that people work together to explore their differing perspectives and develop strategies to move forward. Increasingly, community health workers are encouraged to act in collaboration and develop partnerships with the public in order to more effectively address health and health service issues (Scott et al., 2012). This type of engagement is more formal and involves shared decision making for collective impact (Kania & Kramer, 2011) but may range from short-term (e.g., deliberative dialogues) (O'Doherty et al., 2012) to long-term commitments (e.g., partnership agreements). In this section, we provide a brief overview of the concepts of collaboration and partnerships and introduce strategies for more effectively engaging the public in decisions related to population health promotion, health systems decision making, and individual care.

TABLE 5.2 Public Participation at Micro, Meso, and Macro Levels

Level of Participation	Examples of Types of Activities
Micro (individual)	Individuals engaged in decision making with frontline providers, about their own service and care needs.
Meso (community, organization)	Groups engaged at an operational level in designing health and human services (e.g., new parents participating in the development of pre- and post-natal services; community members participating in the planning and design of a new hospital)
Macro (provincial, national health and health care policy)	Citizens are engaged in a deliberative dialogue to shape government health care policies and/or healthy public policies. Deliberative processes allow a group of people to obtain and exchange information, explore an issue, and arrive at an agreement that informs decision making (NCCHPP, 2015; O'Doherty et al., 2012).

Terminology and Meaning

Collaboration and partnerships are terms that are frequently used synonymously. Although they are closely linked, they have distinct meanings. *Collaboration* is an umbrella term often used for a range of strategies for building relationships to address health and social issues. Collaboration may be motivated by a need to resolve conflict or to advance a shared vision (Gray, 1996). *Partnership* is a type of collaboration that occurs when the purpose is to advance a shared vision of a need and the expected outcome is the development and implementation of a joint agreement to address the need and bring the shared vision into reality. As a result, formal structures such as committees or backbone organizations are usually created to manage agreements (Berger, 2013; Doll et al., 2012; Kania & Kramer, 2011; Scott & Thurston, 2004).

Collective impact is a state achieved when partnerships achieve their goal of directing their varied resources toward remedying an identified social problem and develop a backbone organization to coordinate efforts. The concept of collective impact arose out of efforts to develop shared approaches for performance, outcome, and impact measurement across multiple non-profit organizations in order to inform innovation in practice (Kania & Kramer, 2011).

Over the past 10 years, there has not been a great deal added to the research literature on the topics of collaboration and partnership but practice approaches continue to evolve. Partnership theory, frameworks, and models derived in the 1990s and 2000s clearly provide the foundation for recent thinking related to collective impact (Box 5.2).

Collaboration is not a static process; it is generally described as flexible and iterative, having characteristics in common with the community development process described earlier. Development of partnerships usually commences with a few potential partners exploring issues of common interest, articulating a common vision, and developing a preliminary strategy before approaching other potential partners. Before commitment to proceed is achieved, many relationship-building activities are required. Achieving "collaborative advantage" and moving through "collaborative inertia" (Huxham & Vangen, 2005) is dependent on remaining responsive to changes (Box 5.3).

Changes in membership and context require ongoing negotiation of purpose, strategies to build and maintain trust among members, accepting accountability, attention to the role of power, identifying resources, developing and adapting action plans, agreeing on communication

---

Box 5.2 Sources of Influence of Backbone Organizations

Characteristics of partnerships are embedded in the Turner et al.'s (2013) description of six sources of influence that backbone organizations (i.e., formal collaborative structures created to manage agreements) should have to assist in guiding collective impact efforts:

1. Competence: Backbone organizations should be competent in terms of their knowledge of the issue, problem solving, leadership, and interpersonal skills.
2. Commitment: The backbone organization should have a successful history of working on the issue being addressed through the collective impact effort.
3. Objectivity: Organizations serving in this role should be seen by others as being objective, and should create a safe space for others to interact.
4. Data and information: Backbone organizations should have access to data, research, and information on the problem as well as means to disseminate that information.
5. Network: Backbone organizations should have a large network of connections with cross-sectoral organizations which would in term allow them to broker relationships at the individual and group levels.
6. Visibility: The community must be aware of the backbone organization and have a good opinion of the organization, as well as an awareness of the collective impact effort.

Box 5.3 Collaborative Advantage and Inertia

Collaborative advantage: Something is achieved that could not have been achieved by any one individual, group, or organization working alone (Huxham & Vangen, 2005).

Collaborative inertia: A situation that arises when the apparent rate of work output from a collaboration is slowed considerably compared to what a casual observer might expect to be able to achieve (Huxham & Vangen, 2005).

---

strategies, and adopting a broad understanding of leadership (Huxham & Vangen, 2005; Kania & Kramer, 2011; Scott et al., 2012) (Box 5.4).

A Partnership Framework

The partnership framework (Table 5.3) described in this chapter comprises five categories: extra-local relations, domain, partner characteristics, partnership characteristics, and communication.

Extra-Local Relations

Extra-local relations are those institutional influences exerted by the social, political, and economic systems among which the partnership is situated. Institution influences occur at the macro, meso, and micro levels. Although extra-local relations may not play a predominant role in a partnership, they must always be considered. Organizations, communities, and individuals not directly involved in the partnership are potential sources of extra-local influence.

Domain

The domain is the area of interest that is the focus of partnership activities (e.g., human immunodeficiency virus [HIV]/AIDS prevention; primary health care reform; housing and homelessness). Partners may represent interests in several different domains; however, at the partnership level, success is more likely if differing interests are focused in an attempt to address one particular recognized and supported domain.

Partner Characteristics

Partner characteristics are those factors that distinguish the partners. The distinctive characteristics each partner brings to the partnership will directly and indirectly influence its development. These characteristics include:

- The structure and processes of the partner agency
- The resources that the partner and the partner representative are able to contribute

---

Box 5.4 What Does Leadership Mean?

In collaborative contexts, leadership is NOT about a single formal leader influencing members to achieve goals. Three leadership media—structures, processes, and participants—influence whether or not collaborative advantage is achieved. Leadership is about balancing the facilitative roles (i.e., embracing, empowering, involving, mobilizing the structures, processes, and participants) with directive roles (i.e., manipulating the collaborative agenda and playing politics) (Huxham & Vangen, 2005).

TABLE 5.3 Partnership Framework

Categories	Properties	Partnerships		
		Dimensions		
Extra-local factors	Administrative	Organizational		
	Service provision	Individual		
		Community		
Domain	Recognition	Funders		
	Support	Community		
		Vulnerable group		
		Partners		
		Personnel		
Partnership characteristics	Groundwork	Research	Activities	
	Organizational structure	Administrative		
		Operational		
	Resources	Funding	Space	
		Personnel	Time	
		Material		
	Representation	Areas	Characteristics	
	Reputation	Positive	Negative	
Partner characteristics	Organizational structure	Administrative		
		Operational		
	Resources	Commitment	Funding	
		Knowledge	Time	
		Skills		
	Representation	Areas	Characteristics	
	Reputation	Partners		
		Personnel		
		Vulnerable group		
Communication	Type	Formal	Informal	
	Area	Service recipient		
		Personnel		
		Partnership		
		Partner		
		Community		
Operations	Type	Administrative		
		Service provision		
	Area	Service recipient		
		Personnel		
		Partnership		
		Partner		
		Community		

Adapted from Scott-Taplin (1993, p. 107).

- Representation of the target group in the partner agency
- The reputation of the partner, of the personnel working for the partner, and of the group(s) served by the partner agency

Representation of the target group within partnering agencies will need to be discussed, as this representation will vary from partner to partner. For example, the target group might be involved at the board or management committee level, or through more indirect means (e.g., surveys, public forum). It is important that partners accept the legitimacy of a range of representation strategies.

Partnership Characteristics

Each partnership initiative is unique. This uniqueness is a function of the way in which a partnership is established between the individuals and organizations that participate. The characteristics that distinguish a partnership include:

- The groundwork completed before the initiation of the partnership
- The structure and processes of the partnership
- The resources available to the initiative
- The representation of the target group within the partnership
- The reputation of the partnership

Partnerships that are effective develop strategies to break down professional territorial barriers (Scott & Hofmeyer, 2007). These strategies include the implementation of communication mechanisms and professional development opportunities that encourage collaboration (Scott & Thurston, 1997).

Communication

Communication and sharing lessons learned throughout the life of the partnership are vital to the success of a partnership, as it will directly or indirectly affect all of the categories discussed previously. Ongoing evaluation of both formal and informal communication strategies will facilitate the determination of which strategies are appropriate for the partnership at a given time.

Partnership Configuration

The configuration of categories, properties, and dimensions must be unique to the specific requirements of the partnership. It is recommended that all categories and their associated properties and dimensions be appraised and adapted to meet the specific needs of individual partnership initiatives.

Categories within the framework must never be considered in isolation. Each category interacts with each of the other categories. Changes in one area may directly, or indirectly, influence changes in all other categories. Just as the cogs within a toy must all work together to propel the toy, within this framework all of the categories and their properties and dimensions must be considered and configured to advance the partnership toward a common vision.

The configuration will vary from partnership to partnership with some categories taking precedence in some partnerships and other categories taking precedence in others. Failure to assess each of the elements in the framework to determine its appropriateness for a specific partnership model may result in some essential elements being neglected, some nonessential elements being implemented, or some essential elements being implemented improperly. In any of these situations, the result may be that increased work will be required to ensure the success of the partnership or the partnership may fail to achieve its vision.

Partnership Organization

The model of partnership organization (Fig. 5.2) extends the description of partnerships. This model portrays the categories of the partnership framework enmeshed in the partnership culture. All of the categories are displayed in a relationship of mutual dependency. The linkages (direct and indirect) between each of the categories will vary from partnership to partnership.

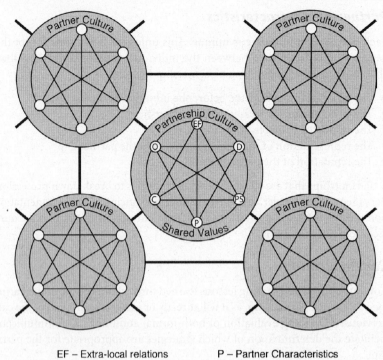

EF – Extra-local relations   P – Partner Characteristics
D – Domain   C – Communications
PS – Partnership Characteristics   O – Operations

FIGURE 5.2   Failure to include essential elements in the partnership. In this example, the partnership has failed to address the issue of representation of the partners. As a result, the partnership is not as successful as it otherwise would have been. (Redrawn from Scott-Taplin, 1993.)

The organizational culture of individual partners may overlap with, or be distinct from, the partnership culture. The similarity between the partnership culture and that of the individual partners should be considered carefully when forming a partnership. If the partnership and partners' cultures are in conflict, decisions will have to be made about whether the partnership is appropriate or whether the inclusion of those partners is important enough to warrant extra resources being devoted to support their participation. For example, some additional strategies may be required to make a successful partnership between a government organization based on hierarchical structures and a non-profit organization based on principles of equity and consensus decision making. Partners may also develop relationships with one another that are external to the partnership. Consideration should be given to how external relationships may influence the partnership (Berger, 2013; Doll et al., 2012; Scott & Thurston, 1997).

A Process Model of Partnership Development

It is one thing to recognize that specific elements in the partnership framework are essential or nonessential for the development of a partnership; it is another to determine when to implement these elements. The process model describes some phases of partnership development (Fig. 5.3).

As described earlier, partnership development is an iterative process. Although elements of the process are arranged in a circle, after the partnership has been initiated, the order in which these activities occur will vary. As the partnership evolves, some elements of the process may need to be revisited.

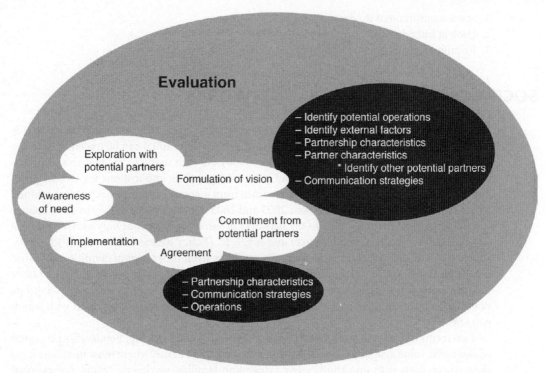

FIGURE 5.3   A process model for partnership development. (Redrawn from Scott-Taplin, 1993.)

The process begins with the awareness of a need. It is important to discuss the formation of the partnership with potential partners early in the process. This informal group will formulate a vision for the collaborative initiative. When the vision has been formulated, this group will be able to:

● Identify potential actions that will support attaining the vision
● Identify extra-local relations that may affect the partnership
● Identify essential partnership characteristics
● Identify other potential partners
● Contact the partners that are identified
● Identify communication strategies
● Identify aligned activities (Huxham & Vangen, 2005)
● Identify opportunities for shared measurement (Kania & Kramer, 2011)

The next stage of the process involves going to the identified partner agencies to discuss their potential commitment to the project. Before proceeding, it is recommended that potential partners achieve agreement on issues relating to partnership characteristics and communication strategies. Once these factors have been established, the partnership initiative can be implemented.

Many process descriptions of collaboration and collective impact emphasize the importance of evaluation strategies throughout (Scott et al., 2012). Evaluation procedures are an integral part of the entire partnership development process. Cabaj (2014) shares five rules for evaluating collective impact efforts:

1. Use evaluation to enable strategic learning
2. Use different designs for different users

3. Share measurement if necessary
4. Look at intended and unintended outcomes
5. Examine contribution not attribution to community changes

SOCIAL CAPITAL AND SOCIAL NETWORKS

The term *social capital* has come into increasing prominence over the past 20 years and is linked to building community capacity. The origins of social capital can be traced back to the 19th century classics of sociology (Woolcock, 1998). As with many terms that rise to prominence, there are differing opinions about its meaning and its implications for the design of interventions. The definition that we use comes from a social capital project commissioned by the Government of Canada between 2003 and 2005 that uses social networks as its central component: "*Social capital refers to the networks of social relations that may provide individuals and groups with access to resources and supports*" (Policy Research Initiative [PRI], 2005; Shookner et al., 2012). Social capital definitions differ from other *capital* definitions because they relate to the quality and quantity of social processes and what flows from the links, rather than the common measures of individual well-being and success (e.g., income levels). For example, human capital is about *what* you know, and social capital is concerned with *whom* you know.

Two forms of the concept of social capital are bonding and bridging. *Bonding* social capital relates to the value assigned to social networks that are quite dense, where most members have close connections with one another (e.g., close-knit families, workplace teams, professional groups). *Bridging* social capital is the value generated from social networks that cut across groups, creating connections that have the potential to bring in resources that a group does not currently have or to share information between groups. While bonding social capital is frequently described in terms of its negative potential (i.e., for excluding others or creating an insular environment), the appropriate balance of these two forms of social capital is dependent on the setting or context (Shookner et al., 2012).

 Critical Thinking Exercise 5.3

Defining Social Capital

Consider the two differing definitions of social capital: What are the key distinctions? What would be the strengths and limitations of applying each of these in your practice? Propose an alternate definition that builds on the strengths of each.

The community development approaches we describe in this chapter are about building social capital (as well as other forms of capital, such as economic and cultural). Tapping into and possibly strengthening social networks has the potential to facilitate the achievement of common goals. Social networks have the potential to bring many benefits (e.g., goods and services, connections to jobs and funding sources, emotional support) and to enable or constrain behaviours (e.g., family and friends may influence choices related to diet and exercise); they also have the potential to exclude people and break apart communities. There is much debate about the potential for using social capital to create more supportive environments; some people argue that it may be possible to facilitate the development of bridging social capital but not bonding. Whatever strategies are used, it is important to remember that the value of different forms of social capital is dependent on the context (Shookner et al., 2012).

Critical Thinking Exercise 5.4

Putting It All Together

Imagine that you are a community health worker at a junior high school (grades 7–9), and that you have been asked by your manager to develop an "active living" program with the school. Using "Strengthening Community Action," think about how you would go about working collaboratively with the school to develop and implement an active living program. Some of the questions that you might want to ask yourself as you go through this exercise include:

- What is currently going on in the school that contributes to active living? How high a priority is it for the school?
- Are there teachers, other staff, students, and/or parents who are potential active living champions that you can approach to be involved in and help lead this work?
- What are you and your organization bringing to this collaboration that will contribute in a meaningful way to where the school community wants to go?
- What type of mechanisms can you help to create where everyone's voice can be heard, and where people feel that their ideas are contributing to the development of the program?
- What other ways can you think of to initially engage the school community in this work?
- If you conceptualize the school community (i.e., teachers, administrative and other school staff, students, parents) as a type of "public," think about where you are on the public engagement spectrum (i.e., inform to empower) and where you want to be.
- How might you sustain the commitment to the program over time?
- How can you tell when it is time for your involvement in the collaboration to end, and how might you withdraw?

Summary

In this chapter, we described links between community development, public engagement, collaboration, and partnerships. We have argued that developing in-depth understanding of these concepts is fundamental to SCA and ultimately to achieving population health goals. The positive effects of healthy communities become evident as citizens participate in making choices and decisions that affect the quality of community life.

REFERENCES

Abelson, J., Forest, P. G., Eyles, J., Casebeer, A., & MacKean, G. (2004). Will it make a difference if I show up and share? A citizens' perspective on improving public involvement processes for health system decision making. *Journal of Health Sciences and Policy Research, 9*, 205–212.

American Institutes for Research (AIR). (2014). *A roadmap for patient + family engagement in healthcare: Practice and research.* URL=http://patientfamilyengagement.org/

Arnstein, S. R. (1969). A ladder of participation. *American Institute of Planners Journal, 35*, 216–224.

Bainbridge, D., Brazil, K., Krueger, P., Ploeg, J., Taniguchi, A., & Damay, J. (2011). Evaluating program integration and the rise of collaboration: Case study of a palliative care network. *Journal of Palliative Care, 27*, 270–278.

Baum, F., Freeman, T., Lawless, A., & Jolley, G. (2012). Community development: Improving patient safety by enhancing the use of health services. *Australian Family Physician, 41*, 424–428.

Berger, S. (2013). *Harvesting the wisdom of coalitions.* Edmonton: Government of Alberta and Early Child Development Mapping Project, University of Alberta.

Cabaj, M. (2014). Evaluating collective impact: Five simple rules. *The Philanthropist, 26*, 109–124.

Community Development Society (CDS). (2015). *Principles of good practice.* URL=http://www.comm-dev.org/about-us/item/86-principles-of-good-practice

Community Tool Box. (2015). *Section 8: Some lessons learned on community organization and change.* Lawrence: Work Group for Community Health and Development, University of Kansas. URL=http://ctb.ku.edu/en/table-of-contents/overview/model-for-community-change-and-improvement/lessons-learned/main

Doll, M., Harper, G. W., Robles-Schrader, G., Johnson, J., Bangi, A. K., Velagaleti, S., et al. (2012). Perspectives of community partners and researchers about factors impacting coalition functioning over time. *Journal of Prevention and Intervention in the Community, 40*, 87–102.

Epp, J. (1986). *Achieving health for all: A framework for health promotion.* Ottawa: Health and Welfare Canada.

Government of British Columbia. (2011). *Integrated primary and community care patient and public engagement framework.* URL=https://www.patientsaspartners.ca/sites/default/files/attachments/ipcc_ppe_framework.pdf

Gray, B. (1996). Cross-sectoral partners: Collaborative alliances among business, government and communities. In C. Huxham (Ed.), *Creating collaborative advantage* (pp. 57–79). Thousand Oaks, CA: Sage Publications.

Hage, S. M., & Kenny, M. E. (2009). Promoting a social justice approach to prevention: Future directions for training, practice, and research. *Journal of Primary Prevention, 30*, 75–87.

Huxham, C., & Vangen, S. (2005). *Managing to collaborate: The theory and practice of collaborative advantage.* London: Routledge.

International Association for Public Participation (IAP2). (2014). *IAP2's public participation spectrum.* URL=http://c.ymcdn.com/sites/www.iap2.org/resource/resmgr/Foundations_Course/IAP2_P2_Spectrum.pdf

International Association for Public Participation (IAP2). (2015). *Core values.* URL=http://www.iap2.org/?page=A4

Kania, J., & Kramer, M. (2011). Collective impact. *Stanford Social Innovation Review, 94*(Winter), 36–41. URL=http://www.ssireview.org/articles/entry/collective_impact

Labonté, R. (2012). Community, community development and the forming of authentic partnerships: Some critical reflections. In M. Minkler (Ed.), *Community organizing and community building for health* (3rd ed., pp. 95–109). New Brunswick, NJ: Rutgers University Press.

Mikkonen, J., & Raphael, D. (2010). *Social determinants of health: The Canadian facts.* Toronto: York University School of Health Policy and Management. URL=http://www.thecanadianfacts.org/

Minkler, M. (1994). Challenges for health promotion in the 1990s: Social inequities, empowerment, negative consequences, and the common good. *American Journal of Health Promotion, 8*, 403–413.

Narushima, M., Wong, J. P., Li, A., & Sutdhibhasilp, N. (2014). Sustainable capacity building among immigrant communities: The raising sexually healthy children program in Canada. *Health Promotion International, 29*, 26–37.

National Collaborating Centre for Healthy Public Policy (NCCHPP). (2015). *Deliberative processes.* URL=http://www.ncchpp.ca/57/Deliberative_Processes.ccnpps

O'Doherty, K. C., Gauvin, F. P., Grogan, C., & Friedman, W. (2012). Implementing a public deliberative forum. *Hastings Center Report, 42*(2), 20–23.

Policy Research Initiative (PRI). (2005). *Social capital as a public policy tool: Project report.* Ottawa: Author.

Scott, C., & Hofmeyer A. (2007). Networks and social capital: A relational approach to primary healthcare reform. *Health Research Policy and Systems, 5*(9).

Scott, C. M., MacKean, G. L, & Maloff, B. (2012). Strengthening community action: Public participation and partnerships for health. In A. R. Vollman, E. T. Anderson, & J. McFarlane (Eds.), *Canadian community as partner: Theory & multidisciplinary practice* (3rd ed., pp. 103–124). Philadelphia, PA: Wolters Kluwer Health.

Scott, C. M., Seidel, J., Bowen, S., & Gall, N. (2009). Integrated health systems and integrated knowledge: Creating space for putting knowledge into action. *Healthcare Quarterly, 13*(Special Issue), 30–36.

Scott, C. M., & Thurston W. E. (1997). A framework for the development of community health agency partnerships. *Canadian Journal of Public Health, 88*, 416–420.

Scott, C. M., & Thurston, W. E. (2004). The influence of social context on partnerships in Canadian health systems. *Gender, Work and Organization, 11*, 481–505.

Scott-Taplin, C. M. (1993). *The development of partnerships among community agencies working with vulnerable groups.* Unpublished master's thesis, University of Calgary, Calgary, Canada.

Shan, H., Muhajarine, N., Loptson, K., & Jeffery, B. (2014). Building social capital as a pathway to success: Community development practices of an early childhood intervention program in Canada. *Health Promotion International, 29*, 244–255.

Shookner, M., Scott, C. M., Vollman, A. R., & Hofmeyer, A. (2012). Creating supportive environments for health: The role of social networks. In A. R. Vollman, E. T. Anderson, & J. McFarlane (Eds.), *Canadian community as partner: Theory & multidisciplinary practice* (3rd ed., pp. 71–86). Philadelphia, PA: Wolters Kluwer Health.

Smith, B. L. (2003). *Public policy and public participation: Engaging citizens and community in the development of public policy.* Prepared for Population and Public Health Branch, Atlantic Regional Office, Health Canada. URL=http://www.phac-aspc.gc.ca/canada/regions/atlantic/assets/pdf/public_policy2003_e.pdf

Torres, S., Spitzer, L., Labonté, R., Amaratunga, C., & Andrew, C. (2013). Community health workers in Canada: Innovative approaches to health promotion outreach and community development among immigrant and refugee populations. *Journal of Ambulatory Care Manager, 36*, 305–318.

Turner, S., Errecart, K., & Bhatt, A. (2013). Exerting influence without formal authority [Web log post]. URL=http://www.ssireview.org/blog/entry/exerting_influence_without_formal_authority

Winnipeg Regional Health Authority (WRHA). (2014). *Community development framework.* URL=http://www.wrha.mb.ca/community/commdev/files/CommDev-Framework.pdf

Woolcock, M. (1998). Social capital and economic development: Towards a theoretical synthesis and policy framework. *Theory and Society, 27,* 151–208.

World Economic Forum (WEF). (2015). *Global Risks 2015* (10th ed.). Genera: Author. URL=http://www3.weforum.org/docs/WEF_Global_Risks_2015_Report15.pdf

World Health Organization (WHO). (1986). *The Ottawa Charter for Health Promotion.* Geneva: Author.

ONLINE RESOURCES

Please visit the Point. at http://thepoint.lww.com/Vollman4e for up-to-date Internet resources and additional learning materials on this topic.

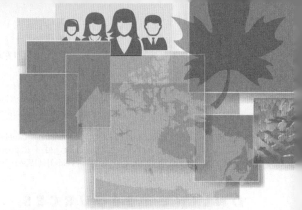

CHAPTER 6

Developing Individual Skills: Building Capacity for Individual, Collective, and Sociopolitical Empowerment

Lewis Williams and Lynn M. Meadows

> *Health promotion supports personal and social development through providing information, education for health, and enhancing life skills. By so doing, it increases the options available to people to exercise more control over their own health and over their environments, and to make choices conducive to health.*
>
> *Enabling people to learn, throughout life, to prepare themselves for all of its stages and to cope with chronic illness and injuries is essential. This has to be facilitated in school, home, work, and community settings. Action is required through educational, professional, commercial and voluntary bodies, and within the institutions themselves.*
>
> —Ottawa Charter (1986)

LEARNING OBJECTIVES

After studying this chapter, you should be able to:

1. Understand how the development of individual capacities is closely related to and contingent on collective and sociopolitical forms of empowerment

2. Understand how health and empowerment are culturally contingent constructs

3. Understand how empowerment is mediated by power-culture dynamics and the relevance of critical and postmodern theories in explaining these processes

Introduction

The development of personal skills[1] is one of the five action areas of the Ottawa Charter for Health Promotion (World Health Organization [WHO], 1986). At the heart of this action is individual empowerment—the development of individual capacities and the mobilization of these toward health promoting behaviours and increased control over health. In the years since the Ottawa Charter many people throughout Canada and other parts of the world still struggle for the basic prerequisites for health—peace, shelter, education, food, and income—and at a larger level, organizations concerned with the governance and regulation of our societies continue to fall short of providing the conditions conducive to a stable and sustainable ecosystem, social justice, and equity among people. The Charter represented a huge leap forward in approaches to health, at least in Western biomedically driven health system contexts; it clearly went beyond the lifestyle approach to health to make the links to the influence of ecologic factors. However, the Charter was drafted when health promotion theory was in its infancy. Since 1986, significant shifts have occurred in terms of the contextual factors that shape individual empowerment, understanding of what individual empowerment means, and how it is actualized.

Various forms of globalization have increasingly influenced these contextual factors. Contemporary globalization describes an accelerated constellation of processes by which nations, businesses, and people are becoming more interconnected and interdependent. Two forms of globalization are relevant. Economic globalization refers to the increasing flow of capital, labour, and goods across national boundaries. At local levels, it is characterized by flatter tax rates, decreased state regulation and assistance to those in need, and the concentration of wealth and employment opportunities in urban centres. Cultural globalization refers to the globalization of perception and consciousness, the transmission of cultural symbols and systems (including knowledge systems), and the actual movement of people across and within national borders. Both processes are closely linked, as the ability to produce and disseminate culture on a large scale is closely tied to economic power.

The globalization of economy and culture influence the ways people think and how they see and feel about themselves (self-identity) and others, and more generally shape the power relations within which opportunities for individual empowerment are embedded. Globalization continues to contribute to the increased wealth, power, and health inequities between people. In the newly created Canada Social Report (Tweddle et al., 2014) it is reported that compared to average after-tax incomes of Canadians, "welfare incomes for the four illustrative households[2] generally ranged between 20 and 40 percent of after-tax average incomes. Only in one case did they exceed 50 percent of after-tax average incomes—i.e., 55.4 percent for single parents in Newfoundland and Labrador" (p. 61). Paradoxically, population health promotion approaches to well-being recognize that literacy and culture are increasingly recognized as shaping access to other health determinants including individual health practices and coping skills (Ronsman & Rootman, 2009).

Meanings of individual empowerment on the whole have been shaped within neo-colonial contexts that privilege Western identities and biomedically oriented beliefs and knowledge systems over others, including those of Aboriginal peoples. Such meanings tend to view the individual as being a discrete entity and development of individual skills and capacities (e.g., empowerment) part of but separate from the environment. Aboriginal conceptualizations of individual empowerment, on the other hand, are more anchored to ideas of having a secure cultural identity and are relational with respect to extended family, land, and metaphysical

---

[1]Personal skills are hereafter referred to as individual capacities. The term "individual capacities" refers to the broad array of attributes that can be ascribed to the individual—for example, self-identity, knowledge, life skills, literacy, biological characteristics, and the like.
[2]Four categories are: individual considered employable; single person with a disability; single parent, one child; and couple, two children (Tweddle et al., 2014, p. 3).

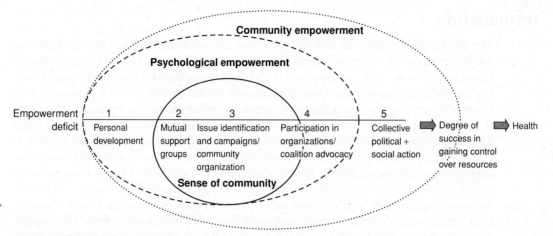

FIGURE 6.1 Community empowerment components and process.

realities. Therefore, while individual empowerment continues to serve as an important public health construct and tool, it continues to warrant some cultural critique.

Actualizing individual empowerment and the understanding of how and why this occurs generally remains a much under-theorized area. Some of the most significant Western-based theoretical work rightfully makes the interconnections between individuals and social structures. For example, empowerment has been conceived as a multi-levelled construct involving intra-individual, inter-individual, and sociopolitical elements (Wallerstein, 2006) and as a process progressing along a dynamic continuum of action from individual and small group development to community organization, partnerships, and advocacy/political action (Rissel, 1994) (see Fig. 6.1). In this sense, individual empowerment is contingent on collective empowerment and the creation of supportive environments, and the latter two are equally contingent on individual empowerment. However, empowerment theory has generally stopped short of theorizing the forms of power inherent in these processes. Neither has it given much consideration to the identity and power-culture relations that mediate these processes. In this chapter, you are encouraged to think critically about the concept of individual empowerment and its application within public health through making linkages between individual, collective, and sociopolitical empowerment; critiquing and extending meanings of well-being and individual empowerment to include Aboriginal peoples; demonstrating the relevance of power-culture dynamics to empowerment processes, both as they mediate access and influence people's experiences; and considering empowerment terrain and critical postmodern theory in empowerment conceptualization.

INDIVIDUAL EMPOWERMENT IN CONTEXT

Within public health contexts, individual empowerment is often taken to mean development of individual skills via activities aimed at health education, life-skills enhancement, and individual and social development. The underlying rationale and intent of public health programs is that they will reduce risk behaviours for specific diseases through interventions focused on individual determinants of behaviour affecting diet, physical activity, stress management, and tobacco use. However, rates of recidivism from individualized behaviour change interventions can be very high as individuals slip back into their normal (less healthy) behaviour patterns in nonsupportive environments. Evidence abounds that an individual's health promoting behaviours and practices are undoubtedly strongly influenced by socioecologic influences such as income, housing quality, location, and social capital (Mikkonen & Raphael, 2010; Raphael, 2008). Even if we know the power of regular physical activity with respect to physical and mental health benefits, formidable barriers may reside in our work, family, neighbourhood, and cultural circumstances. Comfort measures such as food, alcohol, or tobacco may be hard to resist if people lack social sources that comfort; people who feel depressed, socially isolated, or trapped may sense a lack of individual control over their circumstances. In itself, individual empowerment is not enough to achieve healthier communities. Sustained changes in health promoting behaviours require the transformation of risk environments to those that support healthy behaviours. Earlier research tended to emphasize empowerment as an individual construct and emphasized its psychological components. However, Wallerstein (2006) describes empowerment as "a complex strategy that sits within complex environments. Effective empowerment strategies may depend as much on the agency and leadership of the people involved, as the overall context in which they take place" (p. 15). This conceptualization makes the link among the five action strategies of the Ottawa Charter and clearly articulates the need to address risk environments as well as risk behaviours. The development of individual capacities and their successful mobilization toward increased control over health is inseparable from other forms of empowerment.

Williams (2005) defines empowerment as "a process of enabling individuals and communities to express consciously constructed (cultural) identities and aspirations through access to capacities such as land, language, housing, economic resources, and decision making institutions in ways that are mutually empowering" (p. 2).

This definition of empowerment recognizes that health, as self-defined by communities, and empowerment, as the means to health, are both culturally contingent. The importance of countering the influence of culturally dominant discourses and practices over groups at the margins, including the concept of authentic expression through consciously constructed identities, is also recognized. Authentic expression refers to chosen forms of expression that are self-defined as being congruent with people's sense of self and identity. The material expression of a community's aspirations, worldviews, and cultural systems must be sufficiently supported by access to economic resources, social structures, and decision-making institutions (environmental supports) for authentic expression. Where life circumstances do not support the expression of people's identities and cultural systems, the development and mobilization of individual and community capacities and alignment of health systems and policy organizations with community needs and realities are key means through which desired changes may be made. For example, community health promotion is defined as "a participatory empowering equity focused process—one that regards community participation as being essential to every stage of health promoting actions as well as one that leverages community assets and knowledge to create the necessary conditions for health" (Nishtar, 2007, p. 61).

Maton (2008) suggests three pathways through which empowering community settings influence individuals, the surrounding community, and the larger society: increased numbers of individually empowered citizens; the radiating influence of empowered citizens; and external organizational activities. Maton also proposes a set of six characteristics of empowering community settings: the group-based belief system; core activities of the setting; the relational environment; opportunity role structure; leadership (and staff); and setting maintenance and change.

While the need for empowerment initiatives to deal comprehensively with community differences is acknowledged, various aspects of identity and culture are still often compartmentalized, as are discussions regarding the impact of ethnic cultures on development, or literature drawing the connections between gender identities and women's health (Pederson et al., 2010). Furthermore, our limited understanding of how social identities and cultural systems mediate empowerment processes has tended to be confined to either individual or community levels of empowerment.

HEALTH AND EMPOWERMENT

Health in itself is culturally constructed, contingent on worldview. Worldviews are embedded in deeply held values and cultural beliefs, influencing how we experience our world and explain these experiences. They incorporate our perceptions about the nature of life, how human beings interact with each other, and the natural world. Aboriginal approaches to health are distinct from current dominant Western constructions, placing emphasis on wholeness, connection, balance, harmony, and growth. "For First Nations people the development of the individual is interwoven with the well-being of the community and of the nation. Moreover, an individual's identity, status, and place in the world are tied not only to the [extended] family…, but also to one's ancestors and community" (Aboriginal Healing Foundation, 2006, p. 24).

Approaches have been developed to specifically advance the health status of Aboriginal peoples in response to the dominant Western paradigm. Aboriginal models are holistic and culturally connected; they contextualize well-being within culturally specific frameworks and are about empowerment in a broader sense, including connections between health status and access to determinants of health. While Western conceptualizations of empowerment are now making the connections between individual and collective forms of empowerment, these remain distinct from Aboriginal approaches. For Aboriginal peoples, empowerment is generally much more a collective phenomenon within which the individual is metaphysically indistinct from extended family, ancestors, land, and historical tribal context.

A report by the Advisory Group on Suicide Prevention (2000–2003) reported that cultural continuity (self-government, land claims, education, health service, cultural facilities, and police and fire services) was protective for youth suicide. Indeed, communities with three or more of these factors in place reported substantially fewer suicides than those with no protective factors. Compared to those without cultural continuity (where youth suicide rates were 138 per 100,000), communities where all six factors were present had youth suicide rates of 2 per 100,000 (p. 28). Research by Kirmayer et al. (2011) supports this holistic idea of empowerment, articulating Canadian Aboriginal notions of resilience within an ecological framework that results from interactions among individuals, communities, and larger regional, national, and global settings. Sources of resilience include the importance of collective history, the richness of Aboriginal languages and traditions, and the historical continuity with traditional lands. For Aboriginal peoples, the development of individual capacities, including a secure sense of cultural identity and the means to express these—empowerment in its fullest sense—is actually a project of decolonization, including claiming back Aboriginal meanings of health and empowerment.

LITERACY AND HEALTH FOR ALL

Forms of literacy include conversation, reading and writing, linguistic, cultural, spiritual, and technological. Literacy is a tool or the means by which people negotiate their environments to achieve full health and human potential. Literacy is central to the development of individual capacities and empowerment and thus an important determinant of health. Low literacy affects health directly; people without functional reading ability tend to make ineffective use of the health care system, manage chronic diseases poorly, experience difficulty using medication, and exercise fewer safety precautions in the workplace. Low literacy also has indirect effects on health related to difficulty obtaining and retaining employment, low income, low self-esteem, social isolation, and the abuse of alcohol and tobacco. Indeed, the impact of these indirect effects may have a more pervasive influence on health than the direct effects (Hauser & Edwards, 2006; Ronsman & Rootman, 2009). Furthermore, it is suggested that literacy is clearly linked to or associated with other health determinants such as income and social status, culture, gender, quality of living and working conditions, individual health practices and coping skills, and healthy child development (Pederson et al., 2010; Ronsman & Rootman, 2009).

Canada has significant problems with low levels of literacy. The International Adult Literacy and Skills Survey (IALSS) provides a comprehensive picture of literacy in Canada (Statistics Canada, 2007). Forty-eight percent of the adult population—some 12 million Canadians— performed below a level of literacy that is considered desirable for coping with the demands of our knowledge- and information-based society (Hauser & Edwards, 2006). The PHAC (2015) reports that approximately 60% of Canadians and 88% of seniors are not health literate. Literacy in Canada is profoundly influenced by culture and language. Aboriginal, francophone, and immigrant peoples have lower literacy scores relative to the rest of the population. Literacy studies have drawn attention to the importance of first language acquisition to literacy, and Aboriginal practitioners have found Native language studies to be an important precursor or complement to literacy studies in English or French. Conceivably, when one feels more grounded in one's own culture, language, and traditions, literacy will improve (Ronsman & Rootman, 2009).

Approaches to defining and measuring literacy are based on worldview. Western conceptualizations that primarily assess literacy through prose and document literacy, numeracy, and problem solving have predominated in Canada. Non-Western peoples have considerably different conceptualizations. The rainbow approach to literacy proposes that there are several forms of Aboriginal literacy, each of which can be characterized by a colour. For example, red is mother tongue literacy, while green is English and/or French literacy, yellow is the literacy of symbolism and blue the literacy of technology, indigo is spiritual literacy, and violet is holistic literacy—an appreciation of the interconnections between mind, body, spirit, and family for a healthy life. "When viewed in these terms literacy is not [just] a skill to be learned but an approach to life that includes healthy relationships, healthy nutrition, language instruction, ceremonial practices and family literacy" (Hauser & Edwards, 2006, p. 25). Literacy is increasingly thought of as an active phenomenon deeply linked to individual and cultural identity and self-determination (Chinn, 2011). Literacy is strongly linked to the ability to think critically about discourses and belief systems (spoken language, written text, and practices) and the ways in which one is positioned by self and others within these, undoubtedly influencing our sense of self and capacity to act for health. Literacy, whether perceived as the ability to read and write or as a multiple phenomenon and active tool for shaping one's own life, is closely linked to health and empowerment (Chinn, 2011).

 Take Note

Next time you are in a pharmacy examine the literature on display through the lens of health literacy.

POWER-CULTURE, EMPOWERMENT, AND HEALTH

In this section we take a critical postmodern approach to explaining how power-culture relations influence health for different groups, particularly those at the economic and cultural margins of societies. We introduce the concepts of material and relative disparities and, using the example of mental well-being, demonstrate how dynamics of power and culture structure environments. Power-culture is defined in Box 6.1.

> **Box 6.1 Definition of Power-Culture**
>
> *Power-culture* refers to the interplay of dynamics of power and culture that are operative in any context and influence all stages of self-determination or empowerment, including the development and mobilization of individual skills. Different levels of power (such as individual, group, or institutional) are brought into dynamic interaction with different cultural systems (such as ethnicity, gender, sexual identity, or class), resulting in various forms of empowerment relations (Williams & Labonté, 2007).

There is overwhelming evidence that, for individuals, higher socioeconomic position is associated with better health (Pickett & Wilkinson, 2015). Both material and relative deprivations have significant implications for health and empowerment. *Material deprivation* refers to lack of access to environmental capacities conducive to health, including the alignment of communities' realities and cultural values with the rules, norms, and conventions on which institutions and public policies are based. *Relative deprivation,* or relative access to environmental capacities, is significant with respect to both health and empowerment. The nature and context of work can also contribute to health inequalities. Paralleling trends in research on the social determinants of health, a number of industrial relations researchers have argued that the study of injustice or inequality should occupy a pivotal place in the study of employment relations. Employment relations refer to the "individual and collective power relations aspects at work" (Benach et al., 2010, p. 196). Using the lens of power-culture provides another way of thinking how material and relative deprivation structure health. Different levels of power (individual, group, and institutional) are brought into dynamic interaction with different cultural systems (such as ethnicity, gender, class, and sexuality), differentially shaping health contexts and opportunities for empowerment. The effects of material and relative disadvantage on the health of groups are particularly evident with respect to mental well-being.

Among those displaying symptoms of poorer mental health relative to other populations are Aboriginal people, immigrants, rural communities, youth, low-income groups, LGBTIQ people, people with disabilities, and seniors. Such experiences of mental health are also gendered, strongly influenced by social power, roles, and identity (Williams, 2005). Overall, mental health status of Aboriginal peoples is significantly worse than that of non-Aboriginal peoples by almost every measure—suicide rates for Aboriginal youth in Canada, for example, are roughly five to six times higher than for non-Aboriginal youth (Government of Canada, 2006). Research largely demonstrates that the mental health of immigrants, particularly those with low income and education, tends to erode over time in response to pressures of racism, poverty, and social exclusion and to lesser degrees the vulnerability of immigrants to stress by the disruption of social and cultural networks (Hansson et al., 2010). Members of sexual minority groups also bear excessive burdens of mental disease; lesbians have rates of depression, anxiety disorders, and suicidal ideation that are two to three times higher than women in the general population (Robinson, 2012). The experiences of these groups are by no means homogeneous. For example, the experience of immigrant people will vary, contingent on ethnic, class, and gender identities; associated social status; and access to social and structural forms of power. However, research also reveals clear patterns across groups even when other factors are controlled.

Access to environmental supports (structural forms of power) for mental well-being is clearly mediated by sociocultural identities and status, with groups at the economic and cultural margins having consistently less access than others. Many examples across these groups in Canada are evident—relative to national averages, Aboriginal people live in substandard housing conditions (Adelson, 2005), immigrants (particularly recent immigrants) have lower rates of labour force participation (Yssaad, 2012), and women and people with disabilities have lower income levels (Statistics Canada, 2013).

Experiences of relative deprivation have significant implications for health, including the ways by which marginalized groups are discriminated against or negatively positioned with respect to self-identity by members of dominant groups. The ability to produce and disseminate culture on a large scale is closely tied to economic or material forms of power. Members of economically and culturally dominant groups (e.g., Caucasian, male, middle class) tend to control major sources of media and therefore hold the power to construct beliefs.

Take Note

Examine a local or national newspaper for examples of the ways in which people and newspaper media depict Aboriginal people, women, people with disabilities, people living in poverty, and members of LGBTIQ communities.

The effects of relative deprivation are enormous. Studies demonstrate that Aboriginal people, visible minorities, and immigrants are particularly vulnerable to unemployment, underemployment, lower incomes, and social segregation (Department of Canadian Heritage, 2005). Studies have found racism to be a determinant of mental well-being, either through institutionalized forms or via the disempowering ways in which individuals and groups are positioned by more economically and culturally dominant groups (Nestel, 2012). Paradies (2006) undertook a review of 138 empirical qualitative, population-based studies on racism and health (which included a direct measure of self-reported racism and a direct measure of a health-related factor as an outcome) and found that nearly half of the studies related primarily to mental health. Homosexual and bisexual men and women are consistently discriminated against across a number of categories (Robinson, 2012). For example, they are more likely to be fired from a job, denied a promotion, forced out of the neighbourhood by neighbours, and given inferior medical care than their heterosexual counterparts.

Same-sex–attracted young people have higher rates of homelessness and cannot necessarily rely on support and protection of their families of origin. Lesbian, gay, and bisexual youth are more likely than heterosexual young people to engage in self-endangering behaviours, such as abusing alcohol and drugs, vomiting or taking laxatives to lose weight, and thinking about planning and attempting suicide (Robinson, 2013). The meanings people attribute to their experiences and the subsequent modes of subjectivity they adopt are key to individual identity, empowerment, and health. How people feel about themselves, their life chances, and their perceived and real ability to make changes is clearly linked to health outcomes. The development of individual capacities (skills) and their mobilization is closely related to people's self-identity and cultural identity and their ability to think critically. Further, access to mediating structures such as networks and institutions that reflect one's aspirations, cultural identity, and day-to-day realities depends on having individual capacity.

THE EMPOWERMENT TERRAIN

The empowerment terrain conceptualizes the interrelationships among social identities, cultural systems, and empowerment processes. Developed by Williams (2005), the *empowerment terrain* refers to the elements that exist both within and outside of individuals whose dynamic interaction constitute an individual's or community's capacity to exercise control over health and well-being. The *internal empowerment terrain* refers to the more subjective or psychological elements of empowerment—consciousness, identity, and culture. Culture refers to a system through which a social order is communicated and reproduced. The internal empowerment terrain is conceptualized as the individual capacities or the internal world that people carry from

TABLE 6.1 Key Elements of Internal and External Empowerment Terrains

Internal Empowerment Terrain	External Empowerment Terrain
Consciousness • Knowledge, critical thinking, spontaneity, and intuition	Colonization Economic globalization • Global movement of capital and goods
Identity • Sense of self and herstory/history • Self-esteem, sense of belonging	Cultural globalization • The globalization of culture via migration, electronic, and print media
Culture • Internalized systems of meaning • Worldviews and symbols shared by a collective	Economic and other physical resources • Housing, access to health care, and the like Dominant social structures (rules, norms, conventions) and institutions (democracy, neoliberalism, religion, professions) that transmit cultural systems Social and interorganizational networks

one locale to another. The ways in which these elements combine shapes the internal empowerment terrain and thus empowerment capacities of the individual.

The *external empowerment terrain* refers to physical and economic resources (e.g., housing and income), social structures, discourses, community social networks, and community cohesiveness (e.g., social connections) and strategic partnerships (e.g., employment, faith) to which one may have access. Globalization (including sociohistoric and contemporary processes of colonization) is also considered to be an important element that has very real effects on the lives of people. Empowerment is constrained or enabled by the elements that constitute both internal and external empowerment terrains (Table 6.1).

The external and internal empowerment terrains are each mediated by the other and are constituted by the flow of actions between actors. For example, discourses are articulated within print media and policies and are also internalized by people. Positions and self-identity are reconstituted via the mediating influences of internal empowerment terrain elements (e.g., consciousness, self-esteem, knowledge) on the external elements and vice versa. Access to public health services that are institutionally supportive of one's culture is more clearly external, while a strong sense of culture and identity is located internally. However, an interdependent relationship exists between the two. A strong sense of identity assists one in accessing culturally appropriate health services and, in turn, is nurtured by those same social structures. Some empowerment capabilities even more clearly span people's internal and external worlds, such as an alliance with another group, which may be both formalized (institutional aspects) and also have subjective elements (the felt relationship as in a sense of connection/belonging).

The empowerment capacity of individuals and communities to act and make changes of their choice is undermined by deprivations within any of the empowerment terrain elements. For example, unemployment undermines empowerment capacity through loss of income, self-reliance, self-confidence, and psychological and physical health. Such deprivations in empowerment capacities are often linked to health determinants such as income or housing conditions, to inequities within populations of wealth and power, and to health itself.

A CRITICAL POSTMODERN APPROACH TO EMPOWERMENT

According to postmodern philosophers, reality is socially and culturally constructed, and pluralism is a fact of life. Critical postmodernists are concerned with power, oppression, and inequality. Theoretically, this conceptualization of empowerment rests on postmodern thought wherein the ensuing power-culture dynamics are unstable and shifting, contingent on the relative natures of empowerment elements operative within particular locales. It also bases its account of empowerment relations on conceptualizations of power that suggest power is dispersed throughout the social system (empowerment terrain), is fluid and unpredictable (particularly at micro, inter-individual, and community levels), yet is also more deterministic in nature at macro levels (Williams & Labonté, 2007).

Power-culture dynamics shaping empowerment terrains are contingent on who is present and the context. Thus, power-culture dynamics and resulting relations of empowerment will vary from situation to situation. Community level power-culture dynamics will be influenced by access of individuals and communities to structural power, whereas at the macro, institutional level, the relationship becomes more deterministic. Large amounts of structural power are leveraged through the institutionalization of discourses and practices that reproduce particular cultural systems, representing the interests of those communities.

A HEALTH PROMOTION EXAMPLE

The mobilization of identities and cultural systems as capacities for individual and community empowerment within health-related initiatives is increasingly apparent within Canada and throughout the world.

For example, First Nations communities in Canada are increasingly asserting their rights to combine traditional and locally based approaches with Western models. Such projects often require activities that articulate and build awareness among community members about traditional and locally based approaches; strengthen connections to mediating structures, such as health advocacy groups; and advocate for public policy development to enable programs that better reflect community-defined and culturally based approaches to healing.

A pan-Canadian project explored local and cultural meanings of mental health and healing in five mental health programs across the country that represented a broad cross section of rural, remote, and urban regions, in- and out-patient services, and cultures (Waldram, 2008). While participants in the research did not experience residential schools, the residual effects, both intergenerational and intragenerational, were common. One important theme identified in the project was "the cultural, age, and gender heterogeneity of the client or patient base that [was] served by these programs" (p. 3). The report further notes "the importance of flexibility and eclecticism in the development of treatment models. There is no singular Aboriginal client, as there is no singular Aboriginal individual" (p. 4). Healing was found to be an active process done by an individual within the context of the various programs and their eclectic resources focused on the common goal of supporting healing through personal agency. Taken together, the processes and results of the five projects illustrate the need to explore, acknowledge, and work with the eclectic characteristics of individuals in Aboriginal communities (e.g., Western and heterogeneous Aboriginal beliefs and practices) in the development of personal skills to support healing and health.

Initiatives such as those actively work with cultural identities and systems (at individual, community, and organizational capacities) to address systematic power-culture inequities. Grounding research projects in the PHAC determinants of health does not provide an adequate base for culturally sensitive and appropriate research with Aboriginal communities. There is a need to incorporate the worldview encompassed in the Four Worlds 14 determinants of health, especially "strong families and healthy child development" (Nesdole et al., 2014, p. e211), in the context of individual skills.

Summary

The development of individual capacities is closely connected to collective and sociopolitical forms of empowerment as health promoting environments enable the translation of individual skills and knowledge into health promoting behaviours. The ways in which empowerment processes are strongly influenced by cultural identities, social status, and other forms of power are still not well understood; globalization has added to the complexity of these dynamics. Health is a culturally contingent construct, as is empowerment. Literacy is a key health determinant and a consideration for other health determinants such as income, housing, and occupation. It is closely connected to the development of individual capacities (including positive self-identity and critical thinking), cultural identity, and empowerment. Literacy in a broad sense, that is, multiple literacies, may be thought of as the means by which we negotiate our environments in the pursuit of health and human potential. It is therefore closely linked to empowerment processes.

Power-culture is a potentially useful framework for thinking about and analyzing how the dynamics produced between different forms of power and cultural systems influence access to material capacities, experiences of power (and powerlessness), and health outcomes. Developing individual skills is not just a matter of increasing capacities such as knowledge, life skills, and reading and writing but ultimately is closely linked to self-identities, beliefs, and worldviews of individuals and communities in ways that enable the diverse development and expression of human potential.

The Ottawa Charter remains an important health promotion guide. Our Canadian society is culturally heterogeneous; however, disparities in economic and cultural power continue to be perpetuated. Understanding and addressing power-culture inequities must be a key part of health promotion. Beginning points for this are thinking more critically about the ways in which the development of individual capacities are intricately linked to cultural identity, worldview, and social institutions, and building these considerations into health promotion initiatives.

REFERENCES

Aboriginal Healing Foundation. (2006). *Final report of the Aboriginal Healing Foundation: Vol. III. Promising healing practices in Aboriginal communities.* Ottawa: Author.

Adelson, N. (2005). The embodiment of inequity. Health disparities in Aboriginal Canada. *Canadian Journal of Public Health, 96*(Suppl 2), S45–S61.

Advisory Group on Suicide Prevention. (2000–2003). *Acting on what we know: Preventing youth suicide in First Nations.* URL=http://www.hc-sc.gc.ca/fniah-spnia/alt_formats/fnihb-dgspni/pdf/pubs/suicide/prev_youth-jeunes-eng.pdf

Benach, J., Muntaner, C., Solar, O., Santana, V., & Quinlan, M. (2010). Introduction to the WHO Commission on Social Determinants of Health Employment Conditions Network (EMCONET) study, with a glossary on employment relations. *International Journal of Health Services, 40*, 195–207.

Chinn, D. (2011). Critical health literacy: A review and critical analysis. *Social Science & Medicine, 73*, 60–67.

Department of Canadian Heritage. (2005). *A Canada for all: Canada's action plan against racism.* Gatineau: Multiculturalism National Office, Government of Canada. URL=http://publications.gc.ca/collections/Collection/CH34-7-2005E.pdf

Government of Canada. (2006). *The human face of mental health and mental illness in Canada 2006.* URL=http://www.phac-aspc.gc.ca/publicat/human-humain06/pdf/human_face_e.pdf

Hansson, E., Tuck, A., Lurie, S., & McKenzie, K, for the Task Group of the Services Systems Advisory Committee, Mental Health Commission of Canada. (2010). Improving mental health services for immigrant, refugee, ethno-cultural and racialized groups: Issues and options for service improvement. URL=https://www.mentalhealthcommission.ca/English/system/files/private/Diversity_Issues_Options_Report_ENG_0.pdf

Hauser, J., & Edwards, P. (2006). *Literacy, health literacy and health: A literature review.* Ottawa: Canadian Public Health Association, Expert Panel on Health Literacy.

Kirmayer, L., Dandeneau, S., Marshall, E., Phillips, M., & Williamson, K. (2011). Rethinking resilience from Indigenous perspectives. *Canadian Journal of Psychiatry, 56*, 84–91.

Maton, K. I. (2008). Empowering community settings: Agents of individual development, community betterment, and positive social change. *American Journal of Community Psychology, 41*, 4–21.

Mikkonen, J., & Raphael, D. (2010). *Social determinants of health: The Canadian facts.* Toronto: York University School of Health Policy and Management. URL=http://www.thecanadianfacts.org/

Nesdole, R., Voigts, D., Lepnurm, R., & Roberts, R. (2014). Reconceptualizing determinants of health: Barriers to improving the health status of First Nations peoples (commentary). *Canadian Journal of Public Health, 105*, e209–e213.

Nestel, S. (2012). *Colour coded health care: The impact of race and racism on Canadians' health.* Toronto: Wellesley Institute.

Nishtar, S. (2007). Community health promotion—a step further (editorial). *IUPHE Promotion and Education, 14*(2), 61–62.

Paradies, Y. (2006). A systematic review of empirical research on self-reported racism and health. *International Journal of Epidemiology, 35*, 888–901.

Pederson, A., Raphael, D., & Johnson, E. (2010). Gender, race, and health inequalities. In T. Bryant, D. Raphael, & M. Rioux (Eds.), *Staying alive: Critical perspectives on health, illness, and health care* (2nd ed., pp. 205–238). Toronto: Canadian Scholars' Press.

Picket, K. E., & Wilkinson, R. G. (2015). Income inequality and health: A causal review. *Social Science & Medicine, 128*, 316–326.

Public Health Agency of Canada (PHAC). (2015). *Health literacy.* URL=http://www.phac-aspc.gc.ca/cd-mc/hl-ls/index-eng.php

Raphael, D. (2008). *Social determinants of health: Canadian perspectives* (2nd ed.). Toronto: Canadian Scholars' Press.

Rissel, C. (1994). Empowerment: The holy grail of health promotion? *Health Promotion International, 9*, 39–47.

Robinson, M. (2012). *Fact sheet: LGBTQ mental health.* Toronto: Rainbow Health Ontario. URL=http://www.rainbowhealthontario.ca/wp-content/uploads/woocommerce_uploads/2011/06/RHO_FactSheet_LGBTQMEN-TALHEALTH_E.pdf

Robinson, M. (2013). Fact sheet: LGBTQ youth suicide. Toronto: Rainbow Health Ontario. URL=http://www.rainbowhealthontario.ca/wp-content/uploads/woocommerce_uploads/2013/08/RHO_FactSheet_LGBTYOUTH-SUICIDE_E.pdf

Ronsman, B., & Rootman, I. (2009). Literacy and health literacy: New understandings about their impact on health. In D. Raphael (Ed.), *Social determinants of health: Canadian perspectives* (2nd ed., pp. 170–187). Toronto: Canadian Scholars' Press.

Statistics Canada. (2007). *International adult literacy and skills survey (IALSS).* URL=http://www23.statcan.gc.ca/imdb/p2SV.pl?Function=getSurvey&SurvId=15029&InstaId=15034

Statistics Canada. (2013). *Disability in Canada: Initial findings from the Canadian survey on disability.* URL=http://www.statcan.gc.ca/pub/89-654-x/89-654-x2013002-eng.htm

Tweddle, A., Battle, K., & Torjman, S. (2014). *Canada social report: Welfare in Canada, 2013.* Ottawa: The Caledon Institute of Social Policy. URL=http://www.canadasocialreport.ca/WelfareInCanada/2013.pdf

Waldram, J. B. (2008). Models and metaphors of healing. In *Aboriginal healing in Canada: Studies in therapeutic meaning and practice* (pp. 1–8). Ottawa: Aboriginal Healing Foundation.

Wallerstein, N. (2006). *What is the evidence on effectiveness of empowerment to improve health? (Health Evidence Network report).* Copenhagen: WHO Regional Office for Europe. URL=http://www.euro.who.int/__data/assets/pdf_file/0010/74656/E88086.pdf

Williams, L. (2005). Taking a population health approach to mental well-being: Identity, power and culture. Opening keynote address presented at Summer School 2005, Prairie Region Health Promotion Research Centre, Saskatoon.

Williams, L., & Labonté, R. (2007). Empowerment for migrant communities: Paradoxes for practitioners. *Critical Public Health, 17*, 365–379.

World Health Organization (WHO). (1986). *The Ottawa charter for health promotion.* Geneva: Author.

Yssaad, L. (2012). *The immigrant labour force analysis series: The Canadian immigrant labour market, 2008–2011.* Ottawa: Statistics Canada, Labour Statistics Division. URL=http://www.statcan.gc.ca/pub/71-606-x/71-606-x2012006-eng.htm

ONLINE RESOURCES

Please visit the Point at http://thepoint.lww.com/Vollman4e for up-to-date Internet resources and additional learning materials on this topic.

CHAPTER *7*

Creating Supportive Environments for Health: Enabling Community Action

Malcolm Shookner and Catherine M. Scott

> *Our societies are complex and interrelated. Health cannot be separated from other goals. The inextricable links between people and their environment constitutes the basis for a socio-ecological approach to health. The overall guiding principle for the world, nations, regions and communities alike, is the need to encourage reciprocal maintenance—to take care of each other, our communities and our natural environment. The conservation of natural resources throughout the world should be emphasized as a global responsibility.*
>
> *Changing patterns of life, work and leisure have a significant impact on health. Work and leisure should be a source of health for people. The way society organizes work should help create a healthy society. Health promotion generates living and working conditions that are safe, stimulating, satisfying and enjoyable.*
>
> *Systematic assessment of the health impact of a rapidly changing environment— particularly in areas of technology, work, energy production and urbanization—is essential and must be followed by action to ensure positive benefit to the health of the public. The protection of the natural and built environments and the conservation of natural resources must be addressed in any health promotion strategy.*
>
> —Ottawa Charter (1986)

LEARNING OBJECTIVES

After studying this chapter, you should be able to:

1. Describe the links between creating supportive communities and an ecological perspective

2. Discuss the role of environments in health

3. Discuss the rationale for a settings approach to health interventions

4. Describe the role of civic engagement in strategies for creating supportive environments

Introduction

The quote at the beginning of this chapter is an extract from the Ottawa Charter, written in 1986. If we were to rewrite it today, we might be tempted to change a few words but, in essence, it has stood the test of time. On a day-to-day basis, people are influenced by, and influence, environments within which they live, learn, work, play, and worship. The population health promotion model introduced in Chapter 1 is based on an ecological perspective that acknowledges health as a product of interdependence between people and ecosystems. Based on this point of view, individuals are not solely responsible for their actions; environments influence the way people view the world and the choices they make.

Following the 1986 Global Health Promotion Conference held in Ottawa (World Health Organization [WHO], 1986), the Canadian effort to understand the relationship between health and the environment was extended when a commission recommended actions for Canada to move toward healthier environments for its citizens. Five components for action were identified: ending prejudice and oppression; creating a new vision of environmental choice; fostering technology for assessing our environment; accommodating diversity through participation; and becoming world experts in intersectoral action in the design of healthy environments (Small, 1990). Four strategies for action arise from a commitment to make healthy environments available to all Canadians: political vision and leadership in all five action components listed above; scientific and social research and industrial incentive to produce materials that are cleaner, less risky, and less damaging; public education about environmental effects on health; and legislative review and reexamination of policies to ensure that individuals control their environments.

POLICY FOUNDATIONS

Three documents, in addition to the Ottawa Charter, form the basis for current thinking on healthy, equitable, and supportive environments.

Sundsvall Conference and Statement

As highlighted in Chapter 1, there was tremendous policy momentum in the last three decades of the 20th century that clearly placed environment as a determinant of health and creating supportive environments as a strategy for action to address health for all. Between 1986 with the First International Conference on Health Promotion and 2013 with the eighth global conference in Helsinki, commitment to action on the environment was consistently strengthened. However, it was at the third international conference in Sundsvall, Sweden, with its focus on Supportive Environments for Health, that enduring policy foundations were created: "The way forward lies in making the environment—the physical environment, the social and economic environment, and the political environment—supportive to health rather than damaging to it" (Box 7.1) (WHO, 1991).

A supportive environment is of paramount importance for health; environment and health are interdependent and inseparable. Sundsvall participants noted significant health inequalities as reflected in the widening gap in health status both within nations and between rich and poor countries; millions of people live in extreme poverty and deprivation in an increasingly degraded environment; an alarming number of people suffer from the tragic consequences of armed conflicts; and rapid population growth is a major threat to sustainable development forcing people to survive without clean water and adequate food, shelter, or sanitation. Thus, action to create supportive environments must be coordinated at local, regional, national, and global levels to achieve solutions that are truly sustainable. The need for worldwide, cross-sectoral

---

Box 7.1 Dimensions of a Supportive Environment for Health

1. The *social* dimension, including ways in which norms, customs, and social processes affect health
2. The *political* dimension, including democratization, decentralization of power and resources, and commitment to human rights and social justice
3. The *economic* dimension, including sustainable development and reliable and safe technology
4. A positive *infrastructure,* which includes and values women's skills and knowledge

WHO, 1991.

---

collaboration to address pressing environmental issues was again reinforced at the Bangkok conference in 2005.

The Sundsvall Statement suggests that interventions to achieve health for all must reflect two basic principles: equity and public action. *Equity* is the priority in creating supportive environments for health. Any action and resource allocation should be based on clear priorities and a commitment to those marginalized by poverty, gender, race, or disability. *Public action* must recognize the interdependence of all living beings and manage all natural resources effectively, taking into account the needs of future generations and recognizing the importance of involving indigenous peoples in sustainable development activities.

There were four key action strategies identified at Sundsvall to create supportive environments at community level: *strengthen advocacy* through community action, particularly through groups organized by women; *enable communities* and individuals to take control over their health and environment through education and empowerment; *build alliances* for health and supportive environments in order to strengthen the cooperation between health and environmental campaigns and strategies; and *mediate* between conflicting interests in society in order to ensure equitable access to supportive environments and health.

Take Note

Four key action strategies from the Sundsvall Statement for creating supportive environments: strengthen advocacy, enable communities and individuals to take action, build alliances, and mediate conflicting interests.

The Future We Want—Rio+20

Twenty years after the ground breaking United Nations Conference on Environment and Development (informally called the Earth Summit, held in Rio de Janeiro, Brazil, 1992), the UN convened Rio+20, the latest in a series of conferences to follow up on the commitments made at the original conference. Its report, "The Future We Want," stated "Our Common Vision":

> *We recognize that poverty eradication, changing unsustainable and promoting sustainable patterns of consumption and production and protecting and managing the natural resource base of economic and social development are the overarching objectives of and essential requirements for sustainable development. We also reaffirm the need to achieve sustainable development by promoting sustained,*

inclusive and equitable economic growth, creating greater opportunities for all, reducing inequalities, raising basic standards of living, fostering equitable social development and inclusion, and promoting the integrated and sustainable management of natural resources and ecosystems that supports, inter alia, economic, social and human development while facilitating ecosystem conservation, regeneration and restoration and resilience in the face of new and emerging challenges (United Nations Conference on Sustainable Development [UNCSD], 2012, p. 2).

Health Equity—World Health Organization

The WHO Commission on Social Determinants of Health released its report, "Closing the gap in a generation: Health equity through action on the social determinants of health" in 2008. The first of its overarching recommendations was "Improve Daily Living Conditions."

The inequities in how society is organized mean that the freedom to lead a flourishing life and to enjoy good health is unequally distributed between and within societies. This inequity is seen in the conditions of early childhood and schooling, the nature of employment and working conditions, the physical form of the built environment, and the quality of the natural environment in which people reside. Depending on the nature of these environments, different groups will have different experiences of material conditions, psychosocial support, and behavioural options, which make them more or less vulnerable to poor health. Social stratification likewise determines differential access to and utilization of health care, with consequences for the inequitable promotion of health and well-being, disease prevention, and illness recovery and survival.

One has only to listen to the news on a regular basis to know that the topics of environment and health remain as pressing issues of our time. We know a great deal about the interconnectedness of global and local environmental challenges. There is, however, much work to be done to galvanize worldwide collaboration to tackle these challenges. In this chapter, we will focus on the roles that communities and neighbourhoods play to ensure access to basic goods that are socially cohesive, that are designed to promote good physical and psychological well-being, and that are protective of the natural environment and essential for health equity (CSDH, 2008, p. 4).

THE PHYSICAL ENVIRONMENT AND HUMAN HEALTH

In this section, the mechanisms by which contaminants enter human populations are presented. Airborne contaminants and other environmental toxins (e.g., tobacco smoke) affect people exposed to them. Some hazards can seem innocuous, but people are becoming increasingly sensitive to commonly occurring environmental conditions. Perfume is such an instance; hence, we are seeing more "scent-free" buildings, conferences, and meetings as people become aware of these situations. Following are summaries from the report "Health and the Environment—Partners for Life" (Health Canada, 1997) that remains relevant today. This seminal work aligns with recent updates from the Canadian Environmental Health Atlas (http://www.ehatlas.ca/about-atlas).

The Natural Environment

Over past decades, the environment has been used as a convenient biologic, radioactive, physical, and chemical waste disposal site. In some parts of Canada, the results of this environmental abuse have caused many Canadians, particularly those populations that live near manufacturing and processing plants, or in remote areas, to have detectable levels of contaminants (e.g., mercury and lead) in their blood, hair, and body tissues.

Air Quality

Air is the mixture of gases that surrounds the planet and makes up the atmosphere; it consists of 21% oxygen and 78% nitrogen by volume, plus traces of other gases and water vapour. However, its composition may vary from one location to another and between indoors and outdoors because of contamination with particulate matter or other gases. These airborne contaminants pose health risks either directly through inhalation or indirectly through their effects on the environment (e.g., pollution of the water supply or contamination of foods). When inhaled and depending on its physical properties, amount, the rate and depth of breathing, and the health of those exposed, air pollution can cause a variety of health effects.

Natural sources of outdoor contaminants include smoke from forest fires, wind-blown dust particles from soil and volcanoes, fungi, bacteria, plants, and animals. Pollutants are also released from motor vehicles, industrial processes, burning fuels, and the like. The level of contamination in outdoor air is influenced by population density, degree of industrialization, local pollution emission standards, season, climate, and daily weather conditions. Air pollutants may originate from local sources or from remote locations, travelling thousands of kilometres from one part of the world to another through the phenomenon called "long-range atmospheric transport."

Outside air quality can affect the quality of indoor air, but pollutants can also arise from poor ventilation that allows contaminants from building materials, furnishings, heating, cooking, consumer products (e.g., tobacco, perfumes), and the soil to build up indoors.

Ultraviolet (UV) radiation is one of the main causes of skin cancer in Canada. While some exposure to UV radiation is beneficial (because it helps produce vitamin D, although dietary sources are also available), UV rays pose a health hazard to anyone who is exposed for long periods of time. The increased incidence of skin cancer is attributed in part to sun tanning, but scientists are also concerned about the depletion of the earth's ozone layer, which acts to prevent UV radiation from penetrating the atmosphere.

Water Quality

Canada contains 15% of the earth's fresh water supply, but 60% of Canada's supply exists far from the heavily populated areas where it is needed for human use. The proportion that is accessible, although generally of high quality, often contains small amounts of environmental contaminants. Compared with other transmission media, such as food and air, drinking water is a minor source of most pollutants—although it is the principal source of exposure to some microorganisms and to water disinfection by-products.

About 87% of Canadians receive municipal tap water that is treated. Chlorine is a simple, effective, yet relatively inexpensive agent for destroying harmful microorganisms in tap water. With a few exceptions, the most serious contamination problems involve tap water from untreated sources, such as private wells. Recent outbreaks of water-borne disease have affected thousands of people and have been responsible for several deaths.

Water fluoridation helps prevent tooth decay in children without endangering their health. However, even at optimal levels in some children, fluoride may cause dental fluorosis, a generally mild condition involving tooth discoloration. Despite claims to the contrary, there is no evidence that fluoridated water causes heart disease, cancer, thyroid problems, birth defects, miscarriages, or hearing or vision problems.

Chemical and Biologic Hazards

Canadians are exposed to environmental contaminants primarily through food despite strict control by federal and provincial legislation and by voluntary actions taken by food producers, processors, and packagers. Contaminants can enter the food supply via a number of different routes and from different sources. Contamination may occur at the site of production, in the processing plant, at the distribution centre, in the retail outlet, in the refrigerator at home, or even on the kitchen counter. Exposure to food-borne contaminants is affected by many factors: food availability, the preparation method, the amount and type eaten, age, occupation, sex, health status, culture, religion, socioeconomic factors, geography, and the nature of the contaminant. People who have high intakes of wild game, birds, fish, and shellfish are exposed to higher levels of contamination because certain organic pesticides that are no longer registered in Canada may persist in soil or enter the environment through long-range atmospheric transport from countries where they are still in use. Some groups are more susceptible than the general population to the effects of food-borne contaminants (e.g., unborn foetuses, breast-fed infants, the elderly, people with weakened immune systems). However, proper food handling and cooking practices could prevent most adverse incidents.

The Built Environment

We are as much a part of our fabricated or built environment as we are part of our natural environment. The built environment encompasses all of the buildings, spaces, and products that are created or significantly modified by humans. It includes our homes, schools, workplaces, parks, business areas, and roads. It extends overhead in the form of electric transmission lines, underground in the form of waste disposal sites and subway trains, and across the country in the form of highways. The way communities are planned and built, including such aspects as the availability of affordable housing, public transportation, and bicycle paths, and the design of public spaces, can also affect health (McCormack & Shiell, 2011). For example, people are more likely to exercise when recreation and sport facilities are located near their homes. Commuting can have a negative impact on the psychological state of commuters and the quality of social life. Available parks and green spaces provide opportunities for reducing stress and meeting spiritual needs. Urban planners must keep in mind the needs of people with limited mobility, the proximity of required services to sustain a community (e.g., schools, community centres, shopping), the negative effects of overcrowding, and the need for safety and security.

ACTION PROCESS FOR CREATING SUPPORTIVE ENVIRONMENTS FOR HEALTH

A planning approach called the Action Process for Creating Supportive Environment for Health Action Plan (APCSEH), adapted from MacArthur (2002), suggests following concrete steps that begin with the preparatory stages of gaining commitment, forming partnerships, and creating the processes of working together; followed by assessment, analysis, public participation, and priority setting; and completed by the planning approval, launch, and evaluation stages (Fig. 7.1). More detail regarding approaches to collaboration and collective impact is discussed in Chapter 5.

As models of health promotion have evolved over the past four decades, the targets for health interventions have shifted from a preoccupation with individual-level behaviour change to an ecological approach that considers interactions among the target population, the health issue involved, and environmental influences. Many initiatives focus on creating supportive environments through particular settings (e.g., work, school, home) as a starting point to address the determinants of health (e.g., the WHO's Healthy Cities, Health Promoting Schools, and Healthy Workplaces).

Environments may predispose, enable, and reinforce individual and collective behaviour; they may also limit choices and behaviours. Many groups of Canadians are exposed to unhealthy environments. Devaluing or undervaluing groups of people (e.g., people who are homeless, women, immigrants, elderly, gays and lesbians, Aboriginal peoples, people who have disabilities) and

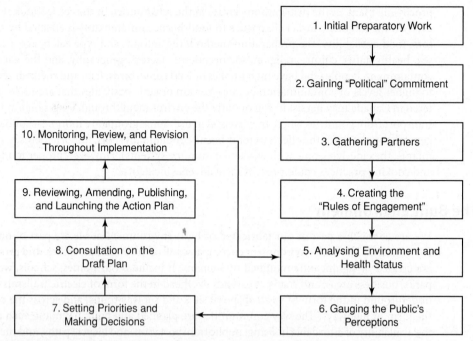

FIGURE 7.1   Action process for creating supportive environments for health.

environmental issues (e.g., climate change, pollution, affordable housing, workplace determinants, urban development) have generated tremendous disparities across the economic, sociocultural, and physical components of the environment with which people interact. Yet, ensuring that all citizens have access to supportive environments benefits society as a whole.

In the next part of this chapter, we will explore how local communities can take action to influence the environments that impact their lives. We describe the ecological perspective, using it as a starting point for describing overlapping environmental influences on health. We then briefly distinguish environments from settings, the latter being the focus of many health promotion interventions. The ecological perspective reflects complex interactions among determinants of health and as such implies that strategies for creating supportive environments adopt an interdisciplinary, multisectoral approach. The concepts of social capital and social networks are conceptually linked to the ecological perspective and are discussed in more detail in Chapter 5.

ECOLOGIC PERSPECTIVE: OVERLAPPING ENVIRONMENTAL INFLUENCES ON HEALTH

The WHO Commission on Social Determinants of Health (CSDH, 2008) and Rio+20 (UNCSD, 2012) both took ecological approaches to addressing health inequities, recognizing the importance of the environment and place.

Why Place Matters for Health Equity

The WHO emphasizes why place matters for health equity:

The disruption and depletion of natural environmental systems, including the climate system, and the task of reducing health inequities around the world go hand in hand. Ecological damage is affecting the lives of everyone in society but it has the greatest impact on the most vulnerable groups

(CSDH, 2008, p. 71). It is critical to ensure that economic and social policy responses to climate change and other environmental degradation take into account health equity (CSDH, 2008, p. 196).

The Rio+20 report also has this to say about population health and the environment:

We recognize that health is a precondition for and an outcome and indicator of all three dimensions of sustainable development. We understand the goals of sustainable development can only be achieved in the absence of a high prevalence of debilitating communicable and non-communicable diseases, and where populations can reach a state of physical, mental and social well-being. We are convinced that action on the social and environmental determinants of health, both for the poor and the vulnerable and for the entire population, is important to create inclusive, equitable, economically productive and healthy societies. We call for the full realization of the right to the enjoyment of the highest attainable standard of physical and mental health (UNCSD, 2012, p. 27).

The field of social ecology focuses on relationships between human populations and their environments. The word *environment* means different things to different people. For some, it is limited to a discussion of physical components of an environment—air, water, and soil quality. While threats to the physical components of an environment can have direct and immediate impacts on health, our discussion of human environments is somewhat broader. Using an ecological perspective means that we include the physical components as well as political, economic, sociocultural, and biologic environmental influences in our discussion (Fig. 7.2). By adopting this perspective, the proponents of population health promotion explicitly focus interventions toward *populations and their environments.* While such a broad perspective does more accurately reflect the influences on human health, it also complicates things. If health is determined by the complex interplay between people and the environment that surrounds them, then population health interventions must take this complexity into account, thus requiring cross-disciplinary and cross-sectoral collaboration to create supportive environments.

Environments and Settings

The broad definition of *environments* is helpful for thinking about the complex influences on human health, but it is not as helpful for thinking about how to implement strategies that focus

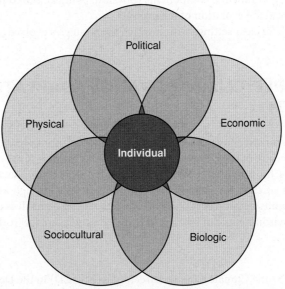

FIGURE 7.2   An ecological model of the influences on human environments.

TABLE 7.1 Stages in Community Project Implementation

Project Phase	Description and Key Considerations
Development of vision for project	A small group coming together based on a perceived need
Identification of other potential participants	Making sure that all who should be at the table are there
Understanding the context	Taking stock of the overlapping environmental influences and identifying appropriate settings
Developing the ground rules (structures and processes for project management)	Communication, decision making, dealing with conflict, dealing with power
Obtaining commitment to proceed	Explicit commitment from each participant to work within the ground rules
Implementation	Being prepared to change direction based on life circumstances, changing membership, new opportunities, etc.
Maintenance and sustainability	Paying ongoing attention to the needs of participants
Winding down	Recognizing when the time has come to move on

on creating supportive environments. It is perhaps more helpful to think in terms of specific settings in which people interact (e.g., workplaces, schools, communities) and to look at the environmental influences within that setting in order to develop strategies that are feasible, focused, evaluable, and effective. The Jakarta Declaration (WHO, 1997) states *"settings for health* offer practical opportunities for the implementation of comprehensive strategies" (p. 2).

A more focused settings-based approach means that interventions can be tailored to the characteristics of the setting. Environments that are created within a setting can predispose, enable, and reinforce individual and collective behaviour (Poland et al., 2000). For example, the sociocultural and political environmental influences in a particular setting may either enable people to interact with one another, to share resources and ideas, or they may constrain such behaviour because people behave differently in different settings. The success of health strategies therefore depends on their fit with the people involved, the health issue at hand, and the environmental characteristics of the setting (Table 7.1).

The following case example provides an example of an initiative that was designed to create supportive environments. We encourage you to think about the following questions as you read:

- What environmental components (physical, political, economic, sociocultural, biologic) influenced the evolution of the project?
- Were there clear settings within which the strategies evolved? How did this influence the project?

CASE EXAMPLE: CLIMATE CHANGE ADAPTATION AND HEALTH

This case example illustrates the complex relationships involved in addressing climate change through the use of the Ottawa Charter action of creating a supportive environment for health. In this case, the provincial government provided leadership, a social entrepreneur took knowledge from an expert workshop and put it into action through her work with municipalities, and the results became part of their local adaptation plans. It is a good example of how supportive environments can be created by people and agencies working together.

Context

The Nova Scotia Climate Change Directorate (NSCCD) in the Department of Environment is trying to better understand and assess how socioeconomic factors and socioeconomic change affect community vulnerability, adaptive capacity, and resilience to climate change. The Directorate has a mandate to support municipalities and provincial departments in the development of impact assessments and adaptation plans and to provide relevant climate and socioeconomic data to assist with these efforts (Government of Nova Scotia, 2014).

The Nova Scotia Government has acknowledged the essential leadership role that municipalities possess in response to climate change both in terms of mitigation and adaptation. In recognition of this important role, the province asked municipalities to prepare a Municipal Climate Change Action Plans (MCCAP). To aid in this undertaking, an MCCAP Guidebook was prepared (Service Nova Scotia and Municipal Relations and Canada-Nova Scotia Infrastructure Secretariat, 2011) that provided a six-step framework to assist in identifying priority areas for action central to mitigation and adaptation efforts, though the emphasis was on adaptation. The overall intent of the framework was to promote a screening process that would assist municipalities in gaining perspective on what natural hazards they should be protecting themselves from and be ready to respond to in the context of climate trends and projections. In essence, the MCCAP was a screening process to figure out what hazards municipalities needed to address to protect infrastructure, community well-being, and essential services. The MCCAP was about delineating the places or issues that warrant action.

There are many socioeconomic circumstances and patterns that affect community vulnerability to climate impacts that are not captured in climate change or economic scenarios. These circumstances and patterns underpin a community's current or plausible future state of adaptive capacity and resilience. Researchers have found that climate assessments that look only at climate scenarios (i.e., climate trends and projections) and do not consider relevant socioeconomic conditions, or assume that they will remain static, are less complete and useful as a basis for effective adaptation planning.

The NSCCD made use of a tool for measuring socio-economic status, the SES Rating Tool, developed by Nova Scotia Community Counts (a former unit, now closed, of the Nova Scotia Department of Finance). Selecting from a list of ten social and economic variables, the rating tool enables display and mapping of relative socioeconomic advantage and disadvantage in communities across Nova Scotia. NSCCD applied this tool to the communities with which they were working in a pilot project on community adaptation to climate change.

Local strategies for climate change adaptation require a holistic view of the environmental, social, and economic issues at play. The human element, the social and economic conditions that people live in, will make them more or less capable of taking up the challenge or being adversely affected by it.

Current Status

Following an Expert Workshop in 2013 to explore how to apply SES variables to climate change adaptation scenarios, there was no further action at the provincial level. However, one workshop participant took what had been discussed and applied it to her work with two municipalities in Nova Scotia as part of the climate change planning effort. In each place, municipal staff and council were guided through a process that revealed and discussed similarities and differences in perception of current socioeconomic circumstances. They then used a newfound collective awareness to more fully evaluate the severity of plausible consequences of climate change impacts on local populations and select where adaptation effort was warranted.

The importance of having trust for honest conversations about community vulnerabilities was recognized in the municipal discussions. It was also recognized by municipalities that the involvement of the public health sector was needed to best understand the magnitude and nature of local health circumstances that could exacerbate vulnerabilities to weather events. As well, public health's involvement highlighted opportunities for adaptation strategies to positively impact health.

What are the results to date?

- Municipalities have considered SES vulnerability to identified hazards and impacts.
- Optional adaptation actions have been identified, influenced in part by the SES conversation about what adaptive measures could help protect vulnerable populations.
- Municipal Climate Change Plans have been adopted by Councils.

This is still a work in progress. It is a municipal infrastructure planning project that places emphasis on SES and resonates with social determinants of health, giving it a holistic or ecological perspective. There are explicit references to the health of the population that resonate with the Ottawa Charter.

The central role of municipalities in community adaptation to climate change is reminiscent of the central role of municipalities in the Healthy Communities movement. The Healthy Communities approach offers community groups and local governments a process that helps everyone focus their efforts toward a common goal: to strengthen the social, environmental, and economic well-being of their community (Ontario Healthy Communities Coalition [OHCC], 2003).

Critical Thinking Exercise 7.1

The Role of Public Working with Municipalities

What is the role of the public health sector in working with municipalities on environmental issues that affect health, especially with vulnerable populations? Share your thoughts with colleagues to learn what other public health roles are considered to be important when addressing these issues.

Summary

Creating supportive environments for health is a complex undertaking. Recognizing that individuals are surrounded by overlapping environmental influences is fundamental to the ecological perspective underpinning population health promotion. Developing strategies that address only physical environmental influences without considering social, political, or economic contexts will be of limited value when attempting to address health issues.

At this point in time, this type of work is not "how we do business" in health systems. It requires time and commitment on the part of all involved and resources that are frequently in short supply. But that is not to say that we should avoid advocating for supportive environments at home, work, school, and play for ourselves and for others.

Critical Thinking Exercise 7.2

Mobilizing Knowledge for Creating Change in Your Environments

Describe one *ah ha* as you read about the relationship between environment and social action. What challenges do you perceive to addressing environmental issues in your work setting? How will you use what you have learned in this chapter to influence change related to creating supportive environments for health?

Acknowledgement

I would like to acknowledge the contribution to the case study made by Anne Warburton, Elemental Sustainability Consulting, who was a participant in the Expert Workshop. She took the initiative after the workshop to apply what she learned to her work with local municipalities in the preparation of their climate change adaptation plans. Her observations about how SES factors influenced these plans add to our understanding about the relationship between climate change adaptation and health equity.—MS

REFERENCES

Commission on Social Determinants of Health (CSDH). (2008). *Closing the gap in a generation: Health equity through action on the social determinants of health.* Geneva: World Health Organization. URL=http://www.who.int/social_determinants/thecommission/finalreport/en/

Government of Nova Scotia. (2014). *Climate Change Nova Scotia—Adapting to climate change.* URL=http://climatechange.novascotia.ca/adapting-to-climate-change

Health Canada. (1997). *Health and the environment: Partners for life.* Ottawa: Public Works and Government Services Canada. URL=http://publications.gc.ca/pub?id=9.695412&sl=0

MacArthur, I. D. (2002). *Local environmental health planning: Guidance for local and national authorities.* WHO Regional Publications, European Series, No. 95. Copenhagen: World Health Organization, Regional Office for Europe.

McCormack, G. R., & Shiell, A. (2011). In search of causality: A systematic review of the relationship between the built environment and physical activity among adults. *International Journal of Behavioral Nutrition and Physical Activity, 8,* 125.

Ontario Healthy Communities Coalition (OHCC). (2003). *Communities and local government: Working together – A resource manual* (2nd ed.). Toronto: Author. URL=http://www.ohcc-ccso.ca/en/webfm_send/185

Poland, B. D., Green, L. W., & Rootman, I. (Eds.). (2000). *Settings for health promotion: Linking theory and practice.* Thousand Oaks, CA: Sage.

Service Nova Scotia and Municipal Relations and Canada-Nova Scotia Infrastructure Secretariat. (2011). *Municipal climate change action plan guidebook: Canada-Nova Scotia agreement on the transfer of federal gas tax funds.* Halifax: Author. URL=http://www.fcm.ca/Documents/tools/PCP/municipal_climate_change_action_plan_guidebook_EN.pdf

Small, B. (1990). Healthy environments for Canadians: Making the vision a reality. *AEHA Quarterly, Winter.* URL=http://www.environmentalhealth.ca/w90vision.html

United Nations Conference on Sustainable Development (UNCSD). (2012). *The future we want.* A/RES/66/288, Resolution adopted by the General Assembly on 27 July 2012. URL=http://www.uncsd2012.org/thefuturewewant.html

World Health Organization (WHO). (1986). *The Ottawa charter for health promotion.* Geneva: Author.

World Health Organization (WHO). (1991). *Sundsvall Statement on Supportive Environments for Health.* Geneva: Author.

World Health Organization (WHO). (1997). *Jakarta Declaration on Leading Health Promotion into the 21st Century.* Geneva: Author.

ONLINE RESOURCES

Please visit the Point at http://thepoint.lww.com/Vollman4e for up-to-date Internet resources and additional learning materials on this topic.

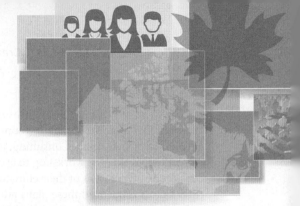

CHAPTER 8

Reorienting Health Services: New Directions for Health Promotion

Laurie Fownes and Rita Isabel Henderson

> *The responsibility for health promotion in health services is shared among individuals, community groups, health professionals, health service institutions and governments. They must work together towards a health care system that contributes to the pursuit of health.*
>
> *The role of the health sector must move increasingly in a health promotion direction, beyond its responsibility for providing clinical and curative services. Health services need to embrace an expanded mandate that is sensitive and respects cultural needs. This mandate should support the needs of individuals and communities for a healthier life, and open channels between the health sector and broader social, political, economic and physical environmental components.*
>
> *Reorienting health services also requires stronger attention to health research as well as changes in professional education and training. This must lead to a change of attitude and organization of health services [that] refocuses on the total needs of the individual as a whole person.*
>
> —Ottawa Charter (1986)

LEARNING OBJECTIVES

After studying this chapter, you should be able to:

1. List the principles of primary health care and discuss how they influence health reform

2. Understand the role of health promotion and prevention approaches in the traditional biomedical model and in a reoriented system

3. Discuss the healthy settings approach and the healthy communities movements

4. Identify the role of capacity building strategies in the reorientation of health services

5. Reflect on what an integrated model of health would contribute to the health system

Introduction

Despite efforts in recent decades to reform the Canadian health care delivery system so that it reflects changing understandings of health, there are challenges that limit the success of innovative and timely reforms. As such, a reorientation of health services is an ongoing and critical debate within the sector. This chapter focuses on the action strategy for health promotion, reorienting health services (World Health Organization [WHO], 1986). Health systems are defined "as comprising all the organizations, institutions and resources that are devoted to producing health actions" (WHO, 2000, p. xi). The reorientation of health services in Canada includes a call for action by provincial governments that are charged with delivering health services, the federal government that sets national health policy and delivers health services to Inuit and on-reserve First Nations peoples, as well as social and economic sectors, NGOs and voluntary organizations, local authorities, industry, and the media.

This chapter begins with a focus on primary health care then addresses shifts that have occurred within the Canadian health system in recent decades, including a transition away from the conventional biomedical model toward models aimed at health promotion and disease/injury prevention. This is followed by a review of the broader settings approach to health promotion, where emphasis is placed on the health promoting hospital, school health, and healthy community movements as well as on service innovations that have emerged from these. An exploration of an integrated model of health concludes the chapter.

PRIMARY HEALTH CARE

The 1974 Lalonde Report paved the way for recommendations on strengthening the primary health care system in Canada and globally. A few years later, the International Conference on Primary Health Care in Alma-Ata (WHO, 1978) catalyzed action on reorienting health care delivery systems to address health inequalities between people living in developed countries and those living in developing nations. These seminal documents, listed at the beginning of the book, frame a paradigm shift away from the biomedical model of health toward a social justice approach.

The WHO (2008) describes primary care as focusing on the provision of health services, whereas primary health care more broadly mobilizes forces within a society toward a transformed health systems agenda framed by social values such as equity, solidarity, and participation. While primary care has historically referred narrowly to family physician services, primary health care is a philosophy as much as a service framework and refers to principles on which "Health for All" action can be based. Population-level issues are addressed within primary health care, including: equitable access to health and health services; public participation; appropriate technology; intersectoral collaboration; and the reorientation of the health system toward health promotion, as well as disease and injury prevention. At the system level, there has been a shift toward a more encompassing perspective in order to address population-level inequities in a variety of areas, such as in oral health (Honkala, 2014) and nutrition (Bains et al., 2014). Using the primary health care philosophy, an integrated health system approach links acute and chronic health care needs, recognizing the importance of both preventive and curative health approaches. Recent primary health care transformations in Canada have seen the incremental, though relatively rapid, implementation of change through public and stakeholder engagement to address key components of an integrated system that includes team-based service provision, alternative funding models, and ongoing performance measurement.

Understanding of health service and system requirements has shifted over time. This shift followed demographic and technological changes, including growing incidence of chronic and preventable diseases, an aging population, and structural pressures related to the evolution of health technology (e.g., data management, e-health). Such shifts have influenced the context of policy making and health care delivery, as well as responsibilities of governments, requiring a process of redefining health sector objectives.

The Declaration of Alma-Ata (WHO, 1978) advocates for a basic level of health services essential to the health of populations (see Chapter 1, Box 1.1). Initially conceived of as both a health development strategy and a level of health service, the basic principles and values of primary health care promote access to health (not health care alone) based on equity, social justice, and participation.

National efforts to achieve the aims of Alma-Ata were accompanied by "dramatic changes in the pattern of disease, in demographic profiles, and in socioeconomic environment" (WHO, 2003b, p. 8). These efforts included changes in government roles and responsibilities, program delivery, and policy development and implementation. NGOs became increasingly recognized as important stakeholders in health. To overcome complex health inequities that communities encounter, governments were called upon to offer their populations "universal access and coverage on the basis of need; health equity as part of development oriented to social justice; community participation in defining and implementing health agendas; and intersectoral approaches to health" (WHO, 2003a, p. 103). These principles remain central to ongoing strategies.

Four strategic imperatives were recommended for integrating primary health care into WHO strategies: reduce excess mortality among marginalized populations[1]; reduce leading risk factors to health; develop sustainable health systems; and develop enabling policy and institutional environments. For the first strategy, interventions were expected to "directly impact on the major causes of mortality, morbidity and disability" (WHO, 2003b, p. 6) among marginalized populations. To address the second strategy, health promotion and prevention approaches were expected to address known risk factors. For the third, financially sustainable approaches supported by leaders and populations were expected to be sought. Finally, to integrate the fourth strategy, it was outlined that primary health care policy "must be integrated with other policy domains, and play its part in the pursuit of wider social, economic, environmental and development policy" (WHO, 2003b, p. 7).

Dr. Margaret Chan, former Director General of the WHO, argued that the principles underpinning primary health care were key to reaching the Millennium Development Goals, signed in 2000 by all 191 United Nations member states. The eight goals to reach by 2015 included eradicating poverty; achieving universal primary education; promoting gender equity; reducing child mortality; improving maternal health; combating HIV/AIDS, malaria, and other diseases; ensuring environmental sustainability; and making global partnerships for development (UN, 2014).

TOWARD AN INTEGRATED MODEL OF HEALTH

Reorientation implies moving from the *status quo* to something new; this something new being better in some way, ideally more effective or more efficient in meeting stated health goals motivated by a social justice framework (Baum et al., 2009). How we understand health has been largely influenced by the different models through which we have viewed health systems. The biomedical model has long dominated the health sector, narrowly defining health as the absence of disease (Burowy, 2014) and leading to a prominent public health focus on communicable disease instead of chronic disease prevention (Kirk et al., 2014). The Lalonde Report (1974) expanded our understanding by acknowledging that lifestyle factors influence

---

[1]"Marginalization occurs when people are systematically pushed away from economic, social, political, and cultural participation and power" (Sharma, 2014, p. 1). It is "a process of social location, [that] creates conditions contributing to vulnerabilities" (Lyman & Cowley, 2007, p. 138). In terms of health, scholars have observed that marginalized populations face greater discrimination, resource scarcity, chronic illness, environmental threats, limited access to health services, among other health risks (Lyman & Cowley, 2007).

health, while at the same time a broader definition of health that included mental and social well-being, not just physical health status, was being embraced. In recent years, health promotion has been entreated to move beyond "the immediate causes of disease … [to] focus on the causes of the causes" of illness (Commission on Social Determinants of Health [CSDH], 2008, p. 4).

Initially, these definitions fuelled debates about what health entailed and led to a reexamination of the way in which we define, measure, and understand health. Recently, attention has moved beyond describing approaches that define health, to highlighting new realities that were unforeseen when the Ottawa Charter and earlier initiatives were drafted. Today's realities include global capitalism, climate change, and responses to inequities that have tended to erode health and social protections for the most vulnerable (Labonté, 2011). As the understanding of health has grown to incorporate the multiple factors that influence people's day-to-day activities, "upstream" thinking about disease and injury prevention has focused attention on social justice issues related to distribution patterns of illness and injury in the context of the determinants of health (Baum et al., 2009), or the root causes of illness and injury.

Interestingly, studies of cost distribution for specific conditions indicate that the greatest proportion of health care funding still goes to treatment services (e.g., hospitals, physicians, pharmaceuticals) rather than to disease and injury prevention and health promotion services (Slomp et al., 2012). Meanwhile, some have argued that Canada's move toward an integrated approach to health service delivery has not embraced crucial health promotion questions of how and why people access health services when they do (Rosella et al., 2014). Others have noted that an increasingly business-minded approach in recent decades has flourished as limited funding is committed to implementation and meaningful accountability measures based on local knowledge, patient satisfaction measures, and cultural contexts (Smith, 2010). For critics, this "allowed health authorities to focus attention on the more pressing needs of acute care, while health promotion took a back seat" (Kirk et al., 2014, p. 19). The same authors argue that lack of funding for complex chronic health problems in favour of more seemingly urgent concerns is further exacerbated by lack of foundational training among health practitioners in the social determinants of health.

The Canadian health system has several components—acute care, rehabilitation and long-term care, mental health care, and community and public health care—which result in health service provision being organized around those functions. The system comprises multiple practitioners and specialists working within complex organizational structures that have been created around the needs of professional groups. As a consequence, patients have become increasingly dissatisfied with health services, costs have escalated, and many provinces are now attempting to reform their health sector by better integrating the various components of the health system. The growing emphasis on chronic disease prevention and management has provided much of the impetus for these reforms.

As indicated, building an integrated health service model has faced challenges related to competition from biomedical approaches, requiring professionals in health promotion to work toward broadening the definition of evidence-based practice as a means of strategically influencing decision making (Juneau et al., 2011). The ongoing nature of this challenge is highlighted in the limited investment by government in health promotion activities that address systemic inequities.

One challenge to health promotion is that, in principle, politicians and governments respond to the demands of their constituents. However, a dilemma emerges here for health promotion, as Canadians tend to focus their health policy concerns toward direct interactions with health systems, demanding more funding for hospital beds or reduced referral wait times over less tangible and longer-term outcomes of public spending on reoriented health services. This dilemma challenges health promotion proponents to have effective communication skills that help the public at large appreciate the complex causal links between social determinants of health (e.g., income, education, food security, safe housing) and population health status. In the process of reorienting health services in Canada, the turn toward community-based health care delivery models highlights questions of accessibility, affordability, acceptability, and appropriateness of services for the groups who use them. As such, community health workers increasingly recognize that health is created and sustained in places where people live, love, learn, work, play, and pray, requiring the meaningful involvement of community agencies and institutions in population health efforts.

Innovations in technology are fostering innovations for Canadians. For example, e-health technology offers a means of reaching rural and remote clientele for diagnosis and referrals, and social media tools (e.g., text messaging, mobile apps, Facebook, YouTube) appeal to distinct population groups, potentially enhancing the engagement of underserved populations in health promotion action (see Chapter 5).

THE SETTINGS APPROACH TO HEALTH

Building on the Ottawa Charter's principles, to optimize the influence of health care resources to tackle social determinants (Graham et al., 2014), the process of reorienting health services involves a reexamination of the role that institutions and professionals play in our communities. Focusing on external factors that impact people's health, the settings approach has arguably been a successful strategy emerging from the Ottawa Charter's call for action. As health services looked beyond the prevailing treatment- and cure-based efforts, promising settings included schools, communities, faith institutions, and workplaces. The traditional biomedical model in turn became recognized as one option among many. On a practical level, it involved moving "beyond the delivery of individually oriented lifestyle-focused health promotion *in* a setting, appreciating that the contexts in which people live their lives are themselves crucially important in determining health" (Dooris et al., 2014, p. 7). As such, a hospital is but one *setting* in which health promotion occurs.

The Health Promoting Hospital Movement

In response to the Ottawa Charter's call to action around reorienting health services, the WHO launched the Health Promoting Hospital (HPH) movement in 1988, which included the establishment of an International Network of HPHs in 1990. Between 1993 and 1997, WHO launched the European Pilot Hospital Project on the role of HPHs. Principles underlying the HPH movement are that "hospitals provide considerable opportunity to engage a broad section of the community through patients and their family members as well as their own staff and personnel" (Kar et al., 2012).

The HPH movement was designed to assist hospitals to steer toward the reorientation of service delivery by incorporating the principles of capacity building and organizational change in order to promote health within and outside the physical boundaries of hospitals. A key principle of the HPH approach is to "maximize the influence of healthcare resources (including social capital) on the foremost determinants of health: the social, economic, ecologic and built environments" (Graham et al., 2014). One effect of an HPH approach has been to reorient both local and higher level leadership toward playing supportive roles in disease and injury prevention through shared responsibility for system innovation (Carlfjord et al., 2011). The HPH movement now includes more than 700 hospitals in Europe and growing interest worldwide has resulted in the development of coherent direction, standards, and effectiveness measures. Five standards to assess quality of HPHs are outlined in Table 8.1 (WHO Europe, 2004).

TABLE 8.1 Standards for Health Promotion in Hospitals

Standard	Description
1: Management policy	The organization has a written policy for health promotion. The policy is implemented as part of the overall organizational quality improvement system, aiming at improving health outcomes. This policy is aimed at patients, relatives and staff.
2: Patient assessment	The organization ensures that health professionals, in partnership with patients, systematically assess needs for health promotion activities.
3: Information and intervention	The organization provides patients with information on significant factors concerning their disease or health condition, and health promotion interventions are established in all patient pathways.
4: Promoting a healthy workplace	The management establishes conditions for the development of the hospital as a healthy workplace.
5: Continuity and cooperation	The organization has a planned approach to collaboration with other health service levels, institutions, and sectors on an ongoing basis.

WHO Europe, 2004.

Groene and Jorgensen (2005) noted that HPHs can include interventions that are directed at "structures and processes, as well as interventions directed at individuals" (p. 7). As a physical setting, activities such as waste disposal, architectural design, and healthy policies (e.g., nonsmoking spaces) can be either destructive or health promoting. Participatory governance and strong policies against sexual, racial, and other forms of harassment are activities that foster a healthy social environment. As a workplace, there are empowerment measures and risk reduction measures (e.g., against stress and injury) that make a hospital a healthy work environment. Examples of integrating principles of health promotion into service provision include quality assurance measures; patient participation in service planning, delivery, and evaluation decisions; and reorienting in-service education so that personnel develop an appreciation of nonmedical factors (i.e., determinants of health) that affect health and well-being.

School Health Promotion

School health promotion is based on the premise that health is a prerequisite for learning. Healthy children in safe and health-promoting school environments are not only more likely to view school as a positive and safe place to be, but less likely to engage in risk behaviours (e.g., smoking, risky sexual activity, alcohol, drugs). Because of a focus on violence prevention, health promoting schools create a context wherein students are less prone to bullying or racism, and are less likely to endure serious injury or experience psychosomatic symptoms (Boyce et al., 2008). Schools are uniquely positioned to inspire action on many determinants of healthy child and adolescent development because they are situated in the community, have connections to health-related services and personnel (e.g., public health unit, social services, justice), and have a "captive" population (including parents).

The comprehensive school health model (Joint Consortium for School Health [JSCH], 2008) is based on the principle that administration, staff, faculty, and students must act on several fronts simultaneously to develop healthy young people: instruction, psychosocial environment, physical environment, and support services. To become responsible for their own health, students need age-appropriate instructions to develop lifelong positive personal health practices. These include media literacy, problem-solving, and communication skills. Social support can be informal (e.g., peers, teachers) or formal (e.g., rules, clubs), and is demonstrated by the respectful application of school policies in order to foster students' sense of belonging to the school community. For optimal growth and development, children need safe and violence-free physical environments. Clean air and water, ergonomic facilities, safe spaces to play, and reliable transportation to school are important aspects of the environment. The school can also be a convenient and economical access point for support services (e.g., early diagnosis and treatment) to help students and families who are experiencing difficulties.

A health promoting university approach is evolving across Canada and globally with conferences held every two years under the auspices of WHO and the Pan American Health Organization (PAHO). This movement promotes a comprehensive approach to the creation and maintenance of health promoting universities. The Edmonton Charter for Health Promoting Universities and Institutions of Higher Education (PAHO, 2005) was created at the second international conference held in Edmonton, Canada.

Healthy and Safe Communities

The reorientation of health services and systems includes models conducive to enhancing the capacity of communities to improve their health, embracing efforts that focus on building leadership not just within hospitals and schools, but within local organizations, businesses, and governments.

A reorientation of health services means embracing movements that are outside of the traditional health purview, such as programs developed to ensure that the built environment of cities, towns, and neighbourhoods in which we live are safe and healthy (Mowat, 2015) and that the role of nonhuman actors in public health, such as pets, are appreciated. Coalitions are key to bringing together municipal, provincial/territorial, and national organizations (private, public, and not-for-profit) with individual citizens to better understand and address priority health and quality of life issues. Collaborative action and efficient use of resources from multiple sectors are mobilized to produce positive community-focused long-term solutions and build foundations for healthier physical and social environments. Actions are built on an assets approach that promotes healthy public policy as well as structural and systemic change, resulting in quality of life improvements for the community as a whole. See Box 8.1 for specific examples of the settings approach.

Is your setting a health promoting setting? Johnson and Paton (2007) propose a typology to assess the level of commitment of a setting to health promotion (Table 8.2) on a continuum from 1 (mostly rhetoric) to 4 (reorientation and organizational reform). This typology allows people to assess whether (or not) their faith institutions (e.g., churches, parishes, mosques), neighbourhoods, sports teams, and professional associations are indeed health promoting settings.

TABLE 8.2   Typology to Assess Commitment to Health Promotion

Type 1	Type 2	Type 3	Type 4
"Do" a health promotion project	Delegate health promotion to a specific staff person or department to "do"	"Being" a health promoting setting	"Being" a health promoting setting and improving the health of the community
No attention to developing a program; ad hoc activities	Not integrated into the organization; limited attention to a program. Does not effectively use resources or challenge the whole setting to rethink its role in health	Commitment to developing a program of health promotion and infrastructure to support it; strategic direction. The direction is inward—getting its own house in order	Commitment to developing strategic responses to population health issues; outward-looking to the broader community; incorporates structural and organizational changes to support community action

> ## Box 8.1 Examples of the Settings Approach for Health Promotion
>
> ### YouThrive
> *http://youthrive.ca*
>
> *YouThrive* is a practical resource for leaders in communities and schools across Ontario who work with youth aged 12 to 19. It is designed for people who want to create communities in which young people can thrive and develop capacity to realize their own abilities, make a contribution to society, and learn how to take control of their own lives. It shows how using a health promotion approach supports positive mental health and prevents risk-taking behaviour among young people.
>
> ### Healthy Schools BC
> *www.healthyschoolsbc.ca*
>
> A healthy school is a place where students have many opportunities—in the classroom, and in every aspect of their school experience—to foster their healthy physical, mental, social, and intellectual development. Healthy schools—also known as health-promoting schools—work with partners from the health and education sectors, and with those from the broader community, to support students to develop healthy habits that will last a lifetime.
>
> ### Parachute Canada
> *http://www.parachutecanada.org/safecommunities*
>
> Safe Communities has joined with Safe Kids Canada, SMARTRISK, and ThinkFirst Canada to create Parachute, a national, charitable organization dedicated to preventing injury and saving lives. Parachute's injury prevention programming and advocacy efforts are designed to help Canadians reduce their risks of injury while enjoying long lives lived to the fullest.
>
> ### Alberta Health Services
> Twelve ways to make your community healthier, in Apple Magazine Spring 2011, pp. 42–43
>
> http://www.applemag-digital.com/applemag/spring_2011#article_id=448160
>
> This article builds on what we know about the determinants of health to offer suggestions about what actions individual citizens can take to create a healthier, safer, and more vibrant community.
>
> ### Community Campus Partnerships for Health
> *https://ccph.memberclicks.net*
>
> Established in 1997, Community Campus Partnerships for Health (CCPH) is a nonprofit membership organization that promotes health equity and social justice through partnerships between communities and academic institutions. By mobilizing knowledge, providing training and technical assistance, conducting research, building coalitions, and advocating for supportive policies, CCPH helps to ensure that the reality of community engagement and partnership matches the rhetoric.

CAPACITY BUILDING AND THE REORIENTATION OF HEALTH SERVICES

Community capacity building is a critical component to health promotion action and is commonly linked to an increased ability of communities to take action concerning health (Wong et al., 2010). Relevant and effective capacity building requires moving "beyond the popular discourses of 'cultural competence' and 'cultural sensitivity' to integrate the principles of social justice, access and equity into the research—policy—practice cycle to guide interventions at the grassroots" (p. 111). Although terms such as *community empowerment, competence,* and *readiness* are often used interchangeably, capacity refers to a broader construct. Community capacity building is an approach that focuses on understanding the obstacles that inhibit groups and communities from realizing their potential while enhancing people's knowledge, skills, and abilities that will allow their groups and communities to achieve the results they desire and overcome the causes of their exclusion and distress (e.g., inequity, violence, racism). Health promoters value community capacity building because they want to work *with* communities and to do so they need a reciprocal understanding of lived experience (from community members' perspective) and knowledge (from the health workers' experiences in community development).

HEALTH SECTOR REFORM

Reports in recent decades from several provinces call for the reorientation of services from institutions (e.g., hospitals) to the community (e.g., community-based services and home care). There is a common message in these reports: Canadians value their health system, but changes are needed to make health service delivery more efficient, effective, and affordable. To do this, sweeping changes are recommended regarding how services are organized, funded, and resourced. In most instances, keeping people well is a high priority, while competition, choice, and accountability are significant concerns about service delivery sustainability if Canada is to maintain health and care for those who need it. It is well understood today that the health system cannot be held solely responsible for the health of the nation's people; cooperation and collaboration are required with other sectors and governments to align services, policies, and programming.

Community involvement in making policy decisions around education, health, and social services is more apparent as agencies deal with lower levels of funding, high consumer expectations, increased competition for limited resources, and changing demographics. For this purpose, community-based health workers play an instrumental role in fostering community capacity for health promotion using the principles and processes of public participation and intersectoral collaboration.

Take Note

We should not assume that the locus of health promotion practice is a health service, a health professional, or linked closely to a formal health program. Increasingly, the community has become the centre for health promotion. Listening to the people, starting from their issues and perspectives, respecting their points of view and culture, and allowing community members to exercise leadership are important caveats for successful community work. Advocacy means using skills and resources to blend knowledge and politics to foster social justice and make the system work better for people with the fewest resources.

Summary

The process of reorienting health systems is adaptive to shifts that occur among individuals, communities, organizations, and populations on multiple levels. Since the origins of the primary health care approach in the Declaration of Alma-Ata, there have been rapid shifts in trends, demographics, priorities, and ways of working. No single approach to health service delivery is equipped to address the broad health experiences in our communities. The traditional biomedical model has historically played a critical role in the delivery of health services; however, today's reality requires that this model become more encompassing. The healthy community and healthy settings movements have informed the reorientation of health services and exacted measurable standards and demonstrable outcomes. Workplace health promotion, school health promotion, healthy communities programming, and community capacity building play integral roles in the implementation of strategies that are meaningful and relevant for the communities in which we live, love, learn, work, play, and pray.

REFERENCES

Bains, A., Pakseresht, M., Roache, C., Beck, L., Sheehy, T., et al. (2014). Healthy Foods North improves diet among Inuit and Inuvialuit women of childbearing age in Arctic Canada. *Journal of Human Nutrition & Dietetics, 27*(Suppl 2), 175–185.

Baum, F. E., Bégin, M., Houweling, T., & Taylor, S. (2009). Changes not for the fainthearted: Reorienting health care systems toward health equity through action on the social determinants of health. *American Journal of Public Health, 99*, 1967–1974.

Boyce, W., King, M., & Roche, J. (2008). *Healthy settings for young people in Canada.* Ottawa: Public Health Agency of Canada. URL=http://www.phac-aspc.gc.ca/hp-ps/dca-dea/publications/yjc/pdf/youth-jeunes-eng.pdf

Burowy, I. (2014). Shifting between biomedical and social medicine: International health organizations in the 20th century. *History Compass, 12*, 517–530.

Carlfjord, S., Kristenson, M., & Lindberg, M. (2011). Experiences of working with the tobacco issue in the context of health promoting hospitals and health services: A qualitative study. *International Journal of Environmental Research and Public Health, 8*, 498–513.

Commission on Social Determinants of Health (CSDH). (2008). *Achieving health equity: From root causes to fair outcomes.* Geneva: Author. URL=http://whqlibdoc.who.int/publications/2007/interim_statement_eng.pdf?ua=1

Dooris, M., Will, J., & Newton, J. (2014). Theorizing healthy settings: A critical discussion with reference to healthy universities. *Scandinavian Journal of Public Health, 42*(Suppl 15), 7–16.

Graham, R., Boyko, J., & Sibbald, S. (2014). Health promoting hospitals in Canada: A proud past, an uncertain future. *Clinical Health Promotion, 4*, 70–75.

Groene, O., & Jorgensen, S. J. (2005). Health promotion in hospitals—a strategy to improve quality in health care. *European Journal of Public Health, 15*, 6–8.

Honkala, E. (2014). Primary oral health care. *Medical Principles & Practice, 23*(Suppl 1), 17–23.

Johnson, A., & Paton, K. (2007). *Health promotion and health services: Management for change.* Sydney: Oxford University Press.

Joint Consortium for School Health (JSCH). (2008). *What is comprehensive school health?* URL=http://www.jcsh-cces.ca/upload/JCSH%20CSH%20Framework%20FINAL%20Nov%2008.pdf

Juneau, C-E., Jones, C. M., McQueen, D. V., & Potvin, L. (2011). Evidence-based health promotion: An emerging field. *Global Health Promotion, 18*(1), 79–89.

Kar, S., Roy, G., & Lakshminarayanan, S. (2012). Health promoting hospital: A noble concept. *National Journal of Community Medicine, 3*, 558–562.

Kirk, M., Tomm-Bonde, L., & Schreiber, R. (2014). Public health reform and health promotion in Canada. *Global Health Promotion, 21*(2), 15–22.

Labonté, R. (2011). Towards a post-charter health promotion. *Health Promotion International, 26*(Suppl 2), ii183–ii186.

Lalonde, M. (1974). *A new perspective on the health of Canadians.* Ottawa: Government of Canada.

Lyman, J., & Cowley, S. (2007). Understanding marginalization as a social determinant of health. *Critical Public Health, 17*, 137–149.

Mowat, D. (2015). Healthy Canada by design: Translating science into action and prevention. *Canadian Journal of Public Health, 106*(Suppl 1), eS3–eS4.

PAHO. (2005). Edmonton Charter for health promoting universities and institutions for higher education. Available at Pan American Health Organization, Health Promoting Universities documents, URL=http://www.paho.org/hq/index.php?option=com_content&view=article&id=10621&Itemid=41391&lang=en

Rosella, L., Fitzpatrick, T., Wodchis, W., Calzavara, A., Manson, H., & Goel, V. (2014). High-cost health care users in Ontario, Canada: Demographic, socio-economic, and health status characteristics. *BMC Health Services Research, 14*, 532.

Sharma, M. (2014). Developing an integrated curriculum on the health of marginalized populations: Successes, challenges, and next steps. *Journal of Health Care for the Poor and Underserved, 25*, 663–669.

Slomp, M., Jacobs, P., Ohinmaa, A., Bland, R., & Block, R. (2012). The distribution of mental health service costs for depression in the Alberta Population. *Canadian Journal of Psychiatry, 57*, 564–569.

Smith, N. (2010). Incorporating local knowledge(s) in health promotion. *Critical Public Health, 20*, 211–222.

United Nations (UN). (2014). *The millennium development goals report 2014.* New York, NY: Author. URL=http://www.un.org/millenniumgoals/2014%20MDG%20report/MDG%202014%20English%20web.pdf

Wong, Y.-L. R., Wong, J., & Fung, K. (2010). Mental health promotion through empowerment and community capacity building among East and Southeast Asian immigrant and refugee women. *Canadian Issues, Summer,* 108–113.

World Health Organization (WHO). (1978). *Declaration of Alma-Ata.* Geneva: Author.

World Health Organization (WHO). (1986). *The Ottawa charter for health promotion.* Geneva: Author.

World Health Organization (WHO). (2000). *The world health report 2000—Health systems: Improving performance.* Geneva: Author. URL=http://www.who.int/whr/2000/en/

World Health Organization (WHO). (2003a). Health systems: Principled integrated care. In *The world health report 2003—Shaping the future 3* (Chapter 7, pp. 103–131). Geneva: Author. URL=http://www.who.int/whr/2003/en/

World Health Organization (WHO). (2003b). *Primary health care: A framework for future strategic directions.* Geneva: Author.

World Health Organization (WHO). (2004). *Standards for health promotion in hospitals.* Copenhagen: WHO, Regional Office for Europe. URL=http://www.euro.who.int/__data/assets/pdf_file/0006/99762/e82490.pdf

World Health Organization (WHO). (2008). *The world health report 2008—Primary health care: Now more than ever.* Geneva: Author. URL= http://www.who.int/whr/2008/en/

ONLINE RESOURCES

Please visit thePoint at http://thepoint.lww.com/Vollman4e for up-to-date Internet resources and additional learning materials on this topic.

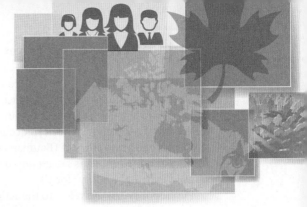

CHAPTER 9

Economic Thinking in Healthy Public Policy

Daniel J. Dutton and Wilfreda E. Thurston

Health promotion goes beyond health care. It puts health on the agenda of policy makers in all sectors and at all levels, directing them to be aware of the health consequences of their decisions and to accept their responsibilities for health.

Health promotion policy combines diverse but complementary approaches including legislation, fiscal measures, taxation and organizational change. It is coordinated action that leads to health, income and social policies that foster greater equity. Joint action contributes to ensuring safer and healthier goods and services, healthier public services, and cleaner, more enjoyable environments.

Health promotion policy requires the identification of obstacles to the adoption of healthy public policies in non-health sectors, and ways of removing them. The aim must be to make the healthier choice the easier choice for policy makers as well.

—Ottawa Charter (1986)

LEARNING OBJECTIVES

After studying this chapter, you should be able to:

1. Describe the cycle model of policy development
2. Identify the role economic thinking can play in policy development
3. Discuss the role of communities in policy development
4. Acknowledge the need for critical social analysis in developing healthy public policy

Introduction

Healthy public policy is an important strategy for health promotion, and economic analysis is one tool that can aid advocates as well as politicians in making decisions. Economics is a discipline that emphasizes mathematical modeling, however, political science reveals that healthy public policy is not just about common sense or the right data as the policy making process is complex. The central concern of economics is the study of the allocation of resources in the face of scarcity. Scarcity exists when people have unlimited wants in the face of limited resources. Healthy public policies are those that influence the health of populations; they can occur in all sectors, require collaboration, and depend on strong advocacy and support (Bauman et al., 2014). Since we are always operating in times of scarcity and the problems facing population health are always evolving, not all policies will succeed in being "healthy" for all.

Public policy "always refers to the actions of government and the intentions that determine those actions" (Cochrane et al., 2009, p. 1). Public policy, therefore, incorporates more than actual legislation, deals with public problems, and provides a framework for action, but it does not include the operations and structures that result from policy (or lack of policy). Governments have three categories of policy instruments: do nothing; act indirectly (e.g., educate); or act directly through state agencies, corporations, or in partnership with private or not-for-profit organizations (Pal, 2013). Thus, while public policy in a democracy is made by elected officials (Pal, 2013), there is interaction among various locations of public policy (e.g., federal, provincial, or municipal) and actual implementation.

THE POLICY CYCLE AND ECONOMIC ANALYSIS

Howlett (2009) presents a policy cycle that is iterative: agenda setting, policy formulation, decision making, policy implementation, and policy evaluation. Figure 9.1 is a representation of how the processes work together. The common idea of a rational decision-making model and

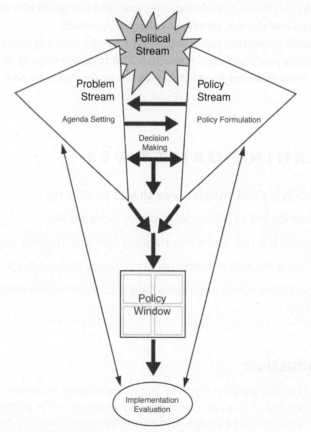

FIGURE 9.1   A nonlinear, nonrational policy process.

a linear process where problems and solutions are broken into discrete parts is rare in complex societies. Linear models are incompatible with much of healthy public policy because analysis inevitably reveals the complex nonlinear nature of most problems and solutions (Howlett, 2009). (See also "Figure 1 Stages in policy making: a turbulent flow" in Benoit, 2013, p. 2.)

Agenda Setting

Agenda setting is the process through which problems come to the attention of elected officials. The problem stream is the process whereby the lack of an ideal state becomes perceived as something they should address (Howlett et al., 2009). The relative strengths of various parts of the policy community (discussed later) clearly affect this feedback process. The way a problem is defined shapes the policy options available (Pal, 2013). In defining the problem, wants should not be confused with needs; we all *need* housing but some *want* a specific house or neighbourhood. Economists can help define a problem and identify trade-offs associated with policy choices, recommending a course of action that is closest to a stated policy objective without removing funds from other actions that may be equally valued.

A long-standing debate in health economics concerns how to define the social objective for a population and what is *best* at a given time. The regulation of risk-taking behaviour in society is important in health policy where debates over objectives are unavoidable. Is it best to regulate behaviour in the whole population in order to reduce risks to zero, presumably at a high cost, or is there a point where the risk is *low enough* even though there is a substantial risk facing some people? An everyday life example of this type of trade-off is policy around traffic laws. We could minimize traffic-related fatalities and injuries with strict enforcement of 30 kilometers per hour speed limit. If the objective is to minimize traffic-related fatalities and injuries, then the overall best interest of the population is served. If the objective is to maximize well-being, then the population may prefer to face some risk of fatalities and injuries in return for the benefits of reduced travel times and lower costs to businesses. Many of the public health problems that face community health workers, such as traffic injuries, HIV/AIDS, poverty, and chronic disease, are complex and described as "wicked problems" (Howlett, 2009, p. 160).

Take Note

In preparation for the Vancouver Winter Olympics in 2010, Dr. Bob McCormack, the medical officer for the Canadian Olympic Committee, said that the Canadian athletes should be among the first people vaccinated against H1N1 flu. Responding to claims his suggestion was unfair, Dr. McCormack said, "The example that will make most sense to Canadians is, what if the men's hockey team got swine flu and were unable to achieve their goal of a gold medal? Canadians would be very disappointed." Scarcity means that if the Olympians get their flu shots first, people in other high-risk groups, like the elderly or pregnant women, would go longer without their flu shot. In that case Canadian society would be implicitly valuing Olympic medals more than the lives of vulnerable individuals (Nguyen, 2009).

POLICY FORMULATION

The policy stream is the process whereby experts and analysts pose solutions to the problem and is consistent with the stage of policy formulation. When solutions become joined to problems, and a favourable political stream exists, a policy window opens (Howlett et al., 2009). The political stream refers to the societal context and sources of power. The policy window refers to a favourable opening for a public policy. Even if the work of the problem and policy streams goes well, if the political stream is not favourable (e.g., politicians fear vociferous opposition) then the policy window may never open. Public support can open a window. For example, when the issue of domestic violence was first raised in the House of Commons in 1982 some members made jokes and laughed. In general the public was outraged by that response and their reaction was reflected in the media, prompting a House of Commons report on domestic violence from the Standing Committee on Health. In 2015, many provinces have special offices, social services, and judicial responses to domestic violence.

The example also highlights the influential role of the media (Howlett et al., 2009) in both reflecting and shaping the political stream. Fraser (2010) discusses the concept of political space for those experiencing injustice and their frequent exclusion. She also argues that policy networks should often extend beyond state boundaries in our interconnected world. An important aspect of political space is its influence on the range of ideas that are circulating in the political stream. Observers of the political process will note that some actors in the policy game have more power than others to hinder or realize agenda setting and solution identification. Bureaucrats can filter the information that politicians receive, for instance, therefore the representative nature of bureaucracy (Bradbury & Kellough, 2011) can influence whether there is a political space for groups such as the poor, people of various sexual orientations, or Aboriginal peoples. Social media is now emerging as a tool for creating space for people to share ideas and to create action (Clay, 2011) (see Chapter 14).

Development of a policy decision related to interventions should build from considerations of efficacy, effectiveness, and safety. Efficacy, whether an intervention improves population health, is most directly assessed in one or more randomized controlled trails (RCTs). Economists also want to know if intervention A provides a greater improvement in health than intervention B, and if the new intervention is safe. Community health workers often cannot use RCTs because the costs would be enormous for population level interventions, so other evaluation methods must be employed. The effectiveness of an efficacious intervention outside of the research environment should also be considered, that is, whether people behave the same way in day-to-day life as they do under research conditions. There is little economics can add to the decision-making process when an intervention is no better than doing nothing, no better than the current standard intervention, does not work in nonresearch settings, or simply is not safe.

Even where an intervention is effective and safe, it may take resources that could have been used elsewhere. The application of economics to questions of population health amounts to considering how scarce resources can be directed to provide optimal outcomes. Examples of questions that health economics could address include:

- Is a health intervention worth doing compared to other things that could be done with the same resources?
- Are we generally satisfied with the way resources are presently spent and what we get for them? Are there better ways to improve health for the same amount of money?
- Are the service delivery systems sustainable?
- Who should pay for interventions?

Economists can help clarify policy options that are presented to government by clarifying trade-offs, opportunity costs, sunk and fixed costs, marginal benefits and costs, incentives, trading, markets, and market failures. Whenever we make choices, or decisions, it is because something is scarce and we face a **trade-off**. For example, funding a day care might mean those funds are no longer available for a long-term care facility. Doing nothing has a cost: time spent waiting. If a decision is deferred to a later date that means the value of time spent waiting is implicitly less than the cost of acting now.

The cost of something is what you give up, including trade-offs, to get it. The **opportunity cost** of any decision is the "next best alternative" that could have been chosen. This means that decision makers have to consider both the explicit and implicit costs of any decision. For example, what is the opportunity cost of tending to a frail elderly person in a bed in a full-service acute care hospital? It is whatever care is forgone in order to keep that person in the bed. In times where that bed would otherwise sit empty the opportunity cost is low. However, as the Canadian population grows and ages, the demand for acute care beds rises. If the number of acute care beds per capita does not grow on pace with demand, then the opportunity cost of occupying that bed with a frail elderly patient rises, since more pressing acute cases are not getting the bed. Emergency department wait times and wait lists for surgical procedures make this cost apparent: long-term care patients are using acute care beds necessary for higher numbers of patients needing short hospital stays.

A **sunk cost** is something that cannot be recovered no matter what decision is made and, as such, should not be considered in policy formulation. What distinguishes sunk costs from other costs is that at the time of the decision they are not *opportunity costs*. This is because the resources are already gone, there is no alternative use for the resources, or they are incurred no matter what decision or course of action is taken. Health education campaigns are sometimes justified by incorrectly invoking sunk costs. For example, suppose that the government spent $1 million on a smoking cessation education campaign that showed no impact on smoking behaviour one year later. A common argument for continuing with an ineffective program such as this one is the high level of resources previously expended. These sunk costs of the program should not affect the decision since they cannot be recovered.

A **fixed cost** is an upfront cost that must be incurred no matter which decision is made. An example would be a decision to reduce poverty by changing the income distribution of a population through redistributive taxes. If staff have to be employed to administer it whether the tax system changes or not, then the cost of the administration is fixed and should not be considered to be an economic cost associated with the decision. Extra training for those personnel in the event of a change in the tax structure, however, is not a fixed cost (see Box 9.1 for another consideration of costs).

Marginal thinking refers to considering only incremental units of benefits and costs when considering a course of action. A **marginal benefit** is the additional benefit gained per action; a **marginal cost** is the additional resources spent. A decision maker is considered "rational" in economic theory if the marginal benefit of an action exceeds the marginal cost of undertaking that action when fixed and sunk costs are properly ignored. In most situations, the marginal

---

Box 9.1 Fixed and Sunk Costs: The Value of Information

A closely related concept to fixed and sunk costs concerns the value of information. From an economic perspective, information is only of value for a decision maker if it has the potential to influence the decision. A population-wide nutrition intervention is one example. Vitamin D is a cheap supplement with some proven benefits from high-quality studies (e.g., skeletal health) and some inconsistent estimates of other health benefits from observational studies. Increasing the level of vitamin D in fortified foods might improve many health conditions for a low price for government. Production companies, however, may face high costs of changing equipment that are passed onto the consumer. If decision makers decide to keep fortification levels constant they are making the implicit decision that the costs of a population intervention (monetary and potential health risks) are too high. In other words, they are valuing more information on vitamin D benefits (i.e., a reduction in uncertainty regarding those benefits) more than the estimated impact. This line of thinking can explain why doing nothing could be a reasonable option for decision makers: they value certainty.

Box 9.2 Thinking on the Margin

In 2009, the Alberta government elected to change the schedule for pap smears for women from once per year to once every three years. The idea behind the switch was that when women are tested once a year there are many false positives, abnormal tests that do not end up being cancer but lead to expensive follow-ups. The amount of benefit for testing every year is lower and the costs are higher than if testing is done every three years, where abnormalities that are detected tend to be serious and not fluctuations that clear themselves up (Alberta Health Services, 2011). The government appears to have weighed the marginal costs and marginal benefits and decided the opportunity cost of doing these tests annually was too high.

---

cost increases and the marginal benefit decreases as the intensity of the action considered increases. For example, it would not make sense to vaccinate every single person in the country against meningitis since the marginal cost of vaccinating the last person is very expensive compared to the benefit of that vaccination, which could be almost zero in some low-risk groups after the rest of the population is vaccinated. An alternative consideration would be vaccinating every teenager in the country against meningitis, a higher-risk group, where the marginal benefits in terms of "disease avoided" are far higher (see Box 9.2 for another example).

Take Note

The economist's notion of "rational" refers to the logical consistency of a person's choices, such that an individual can identify his or her most preferred choice from a set of options. That is, at different times, facing the same circumstances, a rational person makes the same choice. If a person prefers cola to fruit juice, and fruit juice to water, then an economist's notion of rationality requires that this person prefers cola to water. People would be called "irrational" in an economic context if they were to make a decision in the presence of a better option while having full knowledge of what they were doing. People who are not economists tend to use the term rational to refer to someone who makes choices that are considered "reasonable." For example, it is common to view someone with an addiction as making unreasonable choices to use drugs or alcohol. That is, from a health perspective we would judge this choice to be a poor one. For economists, even those with an "unreasonable" objective can still be rational in their choices, as illustrated by the literature on "rational addiction" pioneered by economists Becker and Murphy (1988).

The ability to alter **incentives** is a powerful tool for policy makers. When costs or benefits change, so does behaviour; people respond to incentives. For example, to increase the country's birth rate, Australia introduced a baby bonus policy in 2004. The $3000 bonus for families that had a baby was to take effect on July 1, 2004, but it had been announced seven weeks beforehand. On that date there was an unusual large increase in the birth rate. Economists Gans and Leigh (2009) estimated that over 1000 births were delayed from June to July and that around 300 births were delayed by more than two weeks. Because a prolonged pregnancy is dangerous for both the mother and the infant, Gans and Leigh concluded that such an incentive should not have happened on a set day but could have been phased in gradually. The government claimed that "on the margin" there would be very little effect as families would only delay birth by one or two days at most, an assumption that proved wrong. One decision maker was quoted as saying advance notice was not wrong because "well if I thought that mothers would put their babies at risk, but I don't believe mothers would put them at risk" (Gans & Leigh, 2009, p. 247). So, even when decision makers believe they are thinking rationally (on the margin) they may create unintended negative consequences.

Through **trade** everyone is made better off by gains that can be realized from specialization in society. By specializing and then trading a good or service with others who are specializing in something else, a person will have a higher standard of living than they would otherwise. When people in society specialize at something they are good at, they can each individually purchase more than they could if they were forced to make or grow everything they needed themselves. Therefore, an economy with specialization is considered more efficient than one without. This idea can be used to consider more efficient ways of delivering health interventions. For example, in the Canadian health care system, physicians get reimbursed only for services that they provide personally. There is a view that many services provided by physicians can be supplied by other skilled health professionals. However, there is no incentive for physicians to delegate these services to others, so there is no realization of the possible gains to specialization. Compare this situation to dentists, who have organized their practices so they can earn an income by managing a team of dental hygienists. The success of physician lobbyists to disallow specialization by task in medical service delivery has a large opportunity cost since physicians could be employed doing things others are not trained to do.

In a market-based economy, households of consumers interact with entities known as firms that are attempting to maximize their profits. These two groups of economic agents operate as if they are guided by an "invisible hand" that leads the **market** to allocate resources efficiently. In general, in a competitive market, prices will summarize all the information needed for a decision to be made. For example, salaries will determine the opportunity cost of labour and prices for goods will capture their cost of production. Then consumers and producers will respond to the prices and guide the allocation of resources. In response to the actions of the agents, prices may in turn adjust. This means that people are going to be making decisions that are best for them individually but will result in an efficient allocation of goods and services. Efficient in this sense means that no one can be made better off without making another person worse off. Thus, the degree to which some people will be worse off is an important consideration.

To illustrate how market forces can operate in a health system context, consider the aging population of most of the Western world. With an older population there will be a higher demand for hip replacements. In Canada, patients currently pay nothing out-of-pocket for hip replacement surgery and the market does not dictate physicians' fees. The number of hip replacements per year is dictated by the provincial government's budget. This is a system where fees and prices do not reflect market demand. As a consequence, there are wait lists for these procedures. If Canada were to switch overnight to a market-based system of health care delivery, then the greater demand on orthopaedic surgeons would raise the fees they are able to charge for their services and people with the means to pay would not have to wait. As the salaries to orthopaedic surgeons rose, more doctors would enter the local market and increase the supply of services, which alleviates the pressure driving up rising salaries. In this scenario wait lists would disappear for two reasons: (1) at the higher price, more doctors would supply the surgery and enter the market; and (2) at the higher price, fewer patients would demand the service. From a healthy public policy perspective, therefore, inequities are created as people who *want* a hip replacement and could pay would get it before someone who might *need* it more but could not pay.

Markets, however lauded they are, are imperfect, and the reliance on markets to allocate resources is particularly problematic with regard to health. When a market, for some reason, does not supply the most efficient allocation of resources it is known as a **market failure**. *Externalities,* a form of market failure, occur when a consumer's decisions influence a third party without their buy-in. For example, second-hand exposure to tobacco smoke can increase risk for those who otherwise would not smoke. This is a market failure, since the second-hand smoke exposure imposes a cost on those who are not part of the smoker's decision to smoke. To limit this negative externality, governments have adopted some smoking bans. In another example, if vaccinations are voluntary and have some cost associated with them (e.g., standing in a queue, taking time off work), then consumers may decide to attempt to free-ride off of the protection they receive from others being vaccinated. In this case, there may not be enough people vaccinated to attain proper protection for the population, which means there is a market failure.

Information asymmetry between providers, patients, and payers is another form of market failure. Professionals are privileged in their interactions with service users in that they have specialized information that other people usually do not have. If presented with an incentive to do so, professionals might induce demand for their services by exploiting this information asymmetry. On the other hand, people may misrepresent their true need to get services. Both of these situations can result in inefficient allocation of resources to those that need them least.

Consumers may waste resources, or would have recovered from illness without the intervention of the health system or other alternative therapies, because they have *uncertainty with respect to the need and effectiveness of care.* Since they are uncertain, they will just consume a level of health service or alternatives that they perceive to be best for them, leading to inefficient outcomes in the pure market economy. Further, *an absence of competition* is a market failure. Doctors and nurses are organized as cartels that choose not to compete with each other based on price over the provision of health services. When there is a long wait list, those in need cannot penalize less efficient and effective services. When there is a *missing market,* as in the case of rare diseases, there may not be adequate opportunity for the private sector to profit in their treatment; therefore, in a pure market economy there may be a lack of service providers or companies willing to invest in research.

When a market fails to provide resources efficiently, the government can change the outcome through public policy. Examples of this in health policy practice are the regulation of monopolies to prevent price gouging and the establishment of government agencies in charge of enforcing safety standards in drugs or food. The government can also step in to correct information asymmetries by providing information or acting where markets are missing. Finally, the public often seeks government intervention when the market economy fails to produce an allocation of resources that is deemed equitable. To redistribute resources, the government can introduce a system of taxes and transfers. Canada's current health insurance coverage is a system of taxes being transferred to run health systems.

Decision Making

In the decision-making stage, policy makers select from among policy options developed in the formulation stage. Estimating both the costs and benefits, and if possible the direct and indirect costs and benefits, of a policy can form an important aspect of rationales for policies along with statistical, moral, and ethical arguments. Even at this stage, the policy-making process may cease when options that satisfy competing agendas (agendas other than solving that particular societal problem) or that are low cost and low risk are not evident. Politicians may "float" a policy idea to gauge public reaction, and a negative reaction, whether founded in evidence or not may mean that the policy never sees implementation even if it has the most marginal benefits over marginal costs.

Policy Implementation and Evaluation

Policy implementation is the process by which governments put solutions or policies into effect, and evaluation monitors the outcomes of policies. Evaluation can lead back to a fuller understanding of either the problem or potential solutions. For example, domestic violence rates do not appear to be going down according to studies of service use. There are several possible explanations for this, including: women may be more likely to report than in the past, and they may report earlier; record keeping may have improved so that more cases enter public statistics; or the policies enacted may not be addressing the root causes of domestic violence. Evaluations can help assess whether social change has occurred and how (Thurston & Potvin, 2003).

Economic evaluation has many metrics, tools, processes, and heuristics that have emerged to make it a discipline unto itself. A major part of economic evaluation is enumerating costs and benefits. Costs, whether fixed, sunk, or marginal, are normally wholly contained in one metric: money spent to achieve the action described. Costs not normally measured in dollars (e.g., time) are converted to dollars by employing assumptions. For example, if an individual had to perform some task for 10 hours, those 10 hours would be priced as the salary that individual could command doing their regular job (this would be the opportunity cost of the task for the individual).

Economic evaluation of health policies joins costs and outcomes, and therefore makes the values of the decision makers clear. An evaluation will therefore encourage understanding of the agenda setting, policy formulation, and decision-making phases of healthy public policy. Economic evaluation is more common in the acute care sector of health systems than in health promotion, including healthy public policies, but economic evaluation of population health promotion is emerging as a separate field (Edwards et al., 2013).

Benefits in health are less straightforward than costs but can be broadly divided into direct and indirect benefits in applied work. Direct benefits are those received by the individual or community with respect to the action under consideration. For example, a direct benefit of a program that increased physical activity could be the lower incidence of chronic disease later in life and higher community support. Indirect benefits are those received as a consequence of the action under consideration but not directly related to the action. Using the same example, an indirect benefit could be additional productivity of employees who are physically active. By employing assumptions these benefits can also be measured in dollars. Employing the language of costs and benefits necessitates defining the point to which these costs and benefits are being accrued. In Canada, with our public health care system, most of the benefits and costs accrue to the government, or more broadly to society. In relation to our example, society benefits directly from lower rates of chronic disease in the population, and indirectly from greater productivity in the workplace. The costs are relevant to society too if the intervention is publicly funded.

After enumerating all the costs and benefits, economic evaluators can define a cost–benefit ratio, which is literally the cost per unit of benefit. If the costs and benefits are both measured in dollars then we can think of the intervention as an investment that generates value, or return in the case of society accruing the benefits. A return-on-investment is the ratio of the net benefits and the costs. An intervention that generates \$3 of benefit for every \$1 of cost would have a return-on-investment of 2 ([\$3 benefit − \$1 cost]/\$1 cost); that means for every one dollar invested, the public receives an additional two dollars in return. Decision makers, by using this metric along with many other possible metrics, are able to compare different interventions that otherwise might not be comparable. For example, the health impact of drug education in children could be compared with expanding a current hospital or building more community playgrounds (see Box 9.3).

Box 9.3 Public Health: A Return on Investment

The CPHA, in cooperation with the Canadian Coalition for Public Health in the 21st Century and the Canadian Network of Public Health Associations produced a short video that illustrates return on investment in a variety of public health actions.

https://www.youtube.com/watch?v=TVZxtuZhN_M

One further point on economic evaluation is that time matters. Understanding the trade-off between future and present benefits is important for decision makers to take full advantage of the information contained in any economic evaluation. Benefits accrued today are inherently more valuable than benefits accrued in the future. This comes from the economic idea of "discounting," which is manifest in the concept of interest: in order to invest money most people expect a higher return in the future. In terms of health, this means that prevention, a future benefit, has no immediate return on investment in comparison to treatment. Often this means that evaluation of prevention requires a longer time period to track outcomes, evidence that may not occur during the career of sitting politicians.

POLICY COMMUNITIES, NETWORKS, AND COALITIONS

People who are concerned about a particular policy issue can be called a policy community (Fig. 9.2) or policy subsystem (Howlett et al., 2009). A policy community may include members of the general public, representatives of organizations, government employees, and elected or appointed officials. Within these communities, people share information, exchange views, and try to persuade others to take a position. Some members of the policy community interact on a regular basis and these form a policy network. Advocacy coalitions form yet another subset of the policy community comprising people with common knowledge and beliefs who participate together in urging action on a policy (Howlett et al., 2009). Bureaucrats, that is, those hired by government, have many mechanisms for influencing public policy; that many bureaucratic discussions are held in secret is one source of control. However, the heterogeneity within bureaucracies should not be underestimated (Howlett et al., 2009). Having an economist in a policy network may be a considered an advantage in formulating economic arguments.

Actors in a policy subsystem vary in knowledge and expertise and in ultimate goals. The arrows in Figure 9.1 point to the importance of a varied membership in a policy network and the role of advocacy coalitions and the broader policy community. In the early stages of the West African Ebola crisis, "top public health officials" from across Canada, a policy network, were reported to have held weekly teleconferences for several months (Grant, 2014, p. A9). Most

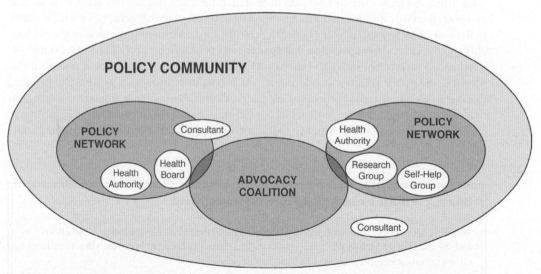

FIGURE 9.2   Policy subsystems: Policy communities, networks, and advocacy coalitions.

of the officials were likely public health physicians and the costs of examining this "low-risk" disease were high in terms of salary and other meeting costs. The problem and policy streams need accurate information to do their jobs well and rely on experts and analysts examining problems and proposing solutions. Economists may provide one source of expert advice.

Economic analysis can be used to advocate for a particular public policy. Given scarce resources, decision makers are often left choosing between competing interest groups, all of which can have compelling arguments. Following the example of the Ebola virus, health professionals may have the power to make the threat to health a public policy issue and divert policy maker attention from other issues, like poverty. In economic terms, doctors and nurses have professional skills that they can trade upon for attention, whereas people already marginalized in society must rely on other means of being heard. Understandings of power and how it circulates may therefore be important in analyzing a policy network.

Howlett et al. (2009) discuss policy regimes as a way of identifying how some policies and approaches to policy endure over time. A policy regime represents common ideas or principles underlying policies and a typical set of participants in the policy community. There may therefore be differences in policy regimes among issues in different sectors of the government. Discussion and analysis of power and equity within policy communities must therefore be a central focus in assessing inter-organizational arrangements, or participation in policy communities is more likely to be about social control than social change. It is the critical analysis that distinguishes social justice participation from social control participation (Fraser, 2010). One of the unintended consequences of ignoring power and equity is that participation of social elites can be strengthened at the expense of redistribution of power and resources (Carroll & Jarvis, 2015). The discussion of international markets and development by Caroll and Jarvis is also an example of analysis of policy regimes.

Healthy public policy strengthens communities (see Chapter 5), and a policy process built on participation strengthens the ability of communities to develop the ways and means to address its issues, to nurture the talent and leadership that enhance the quality of community life, to tackle problems that threaten the community, and to take advantage of opportunities that can help create conditions for people to mutually support and care for each other.

Interdependence among sectors that influence the health of populations has made intersectoral action critical to addressing the "wicked problems" of public health. Internationally, emphasis has been placed on the need for intersectoral action to effectively address the broad determinants of health (Blas et al., 2008), but as Adeleye and Ofili (2010) report about low and middle income countries, intersectoral action is not common in governments. Strengthening the impact of intersectoral policy requires detailed knowledge of collaborative planning and evaluation strategies. Scott et al. (Chapter 5) present an overview of collaboration literature and describe a partnership framework and process model that has been used effectively for planning and evaluation.

Summary

In this chapter we have provided a brief introduction to economic analysis and public policy in community health. Policy that is designed to effectively address population health must do so with a critical social lens to analyze all elements of the policy cycle from construction of the problem to evaluation of policy implementation. The area of cost and benefits is just one in which economists can play a crucial role. We have linked the purposes, processes, and outcomes of developing strong communities and strengthening social action to the policy development process. We have also noted that the borders for policy development are more flexible than in the past and we are wise to think how interrelated we are on this planet.

REFERENCES

Adeleye, O. A., & Ofili, A. N. (2010). Strengthening intersectoral collaboration for primary health care in developing countries: Can the health sector play broader roles? *Journal of Environmental and Public Health*, 2010, 272896.

Alberta Health Services. (2011). Everything about pap testing in Alberta just changed. In *Road to health living series*. URL=http://www.albertahealthservices.ca/hp/if-hp-tr-en-pap-testing.pdf

Bauman, A. E., King, L., & Nutbeam, D. (2014). Rethinking the evaluation and measurement of health in all policies. *Health Promotion International, 29*(Suppl 1), i143–i151.

Becker, G., & Murphy, K. M. (1988). A theory of rational addiction. *Journal of Political Economy, 96*, 675–700.

Benoit, F. (2013). *Public policy models and their usefulness in public health: The stages model.* Montréal: National Collaborating Centre for Healthy Public Policy. URL=http://www.ncchpp.ca/docs/ModeleEtapes PolPubliques_EN.pdf

Blas, E., Gilson, L., Kelly, M. P., Labonté, R., Lapitan, J., Muntaner, C., et al. (2008). Addressing social determinants of health inequities: What can the state and civil society do? *Lancet, 372*, 1684–1689.

Bradbury, M., & Kellough, J. E. (2011). Representative bureaucracy: Assessing the evidence on active representation. *American Review of Public Administration, 41*, 157–167.

Caroll, T., & Jarvis, D. S. L. (2015). The new politics of development: Citizens, civil society, and the evolution of neoliberal development policy. *Globalizations, 12*, 281–304.

Clay, S. (2011). The political power of social media: Technology, the public sphere, and political change. *Foreign Affairs, 90*(1), 28–41.

Cochrane, C. E., Meyer, L. C., Carr, T. R., & Cayer, N. J. (2009). *American public policy: An introduction* (9th ed.). Boston, MA: Wadsworth Cengage Learning.

Edwards, R. T., Charles, J. M., & Lloyd-Williams, H. (2013). Public health economics: A systematic review of guidance for the economic evaluation of public health interventions and discussion of key methodological issues. *BMC Public Health, 13*, 1001.

Fraser, N. (2010). *Scales of justice: Reimagining political space in a globalizing world.* New York, NY: Columbia University Press.

Gans, J., & Leigh, A. (2009). Born on the first of July: An (un)natural experiment in birth timing. *Journal of Public Economics, 93*, 246–263.

Grant, K. (2014, October 15). Nurses sound alarm about Ebola readiness. *The Globe and Mail*, pp. A1, A9.

Howlett, M. (2009). Policy analytic capacity and evidence-based policy-making: Lessons from Canada. *Canadian Public Administration, 52*, 153–175.

Howlett, M., Ramesh, M., & Perl, A. (2009). *Studying public policy: Policy cycles & policy subsystems* (3rd ed.). Don Mills, ON: Oxford University Press.

Nguyen, L. (2009, October 14). Athletes should get the first jab. *Calgary Herald*, p. A8.

Pal, L. A. (2013). *Beyond policy analysis: Public issue management in turbulent times* (5th ed.) Toronto: Nelson Education.

Thurston, W. E., & Potvin, L. (2003). Evaluability assessment: A tool for incorporating evaluation in social change programs. *Evaluation, 9*, 453–469.

World Health Organization (WHO). (1986). *The Ottawa charter for health promotion.* Geneva: Author.

ONLINE RESOURCES

Please visit the Point at http://thepoint.lww.com/Vollman4e for up-to-date Internet resources and additional learning materials on this topic.

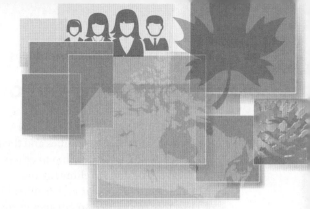

CHAPTER 10

Social Justice and Equity for Health Promotion

Candace Lind, Claire Betker, and Melanie Lind-Kosten

LEARNING OBJECTIVES

After studying this chapter, you should be able to:

1. Define the concepts of social justice and equity
2. Identify the links among social justice, equity, and population health
3. Outline steps to integrate social justice into practice and policies
4. Identify socially just language to describe populations

Introduction

Often credited as the birthplace of the health promotion movement, Canada has a rich background of involvement in its worldwide development, including partnering in the creation of the Ottawa Charter in 1986, the creation of the Population Health Promotion Model, and further development of the evidence base for the social determinants of health that arose from these foundational documents (see Chapter 1). Social justice and equity were identified as prerequisites for health in the Ottawa Charter, but social justice has a long history as a human rights issue. The links between social justice, equity, and health have become clearer in recent years and form part of discourses in practice, policy, research, and education. A growing body of literature shows a clear relationship between the root causes of health problems/concerns in communities or populations and issues of social justice and equity.

This chapter includes a summary of the history of social justice and equity. Social justice is discussed as a human rights issue, using Canadian exemplars of marginalized populations. Discussion points include issues related to the effects of ignoring social justice, a movement to shift away from a biomedical model of health care, a critique of language that may perpetuate the stigmatizing of particular populations, and issues related to enacting social justice and equity in practice. Policy development for socially just practices and examples of social justice in research and practice are shared. The chapter closes with strategies to improve action from a social justice approach and the necessity of treating all people with dignity and respect as a means of creating a socially just world.

DEFINITIONS AND HISTORY OF SOCIAL JUSTICE AND EQUITY

The Canadian Nurses Association (CNA, 2010) defines social justice as "the fair distribution of society's benefits, responsibilities and their consequences. It focuses on the relative position of one social group in relationship to others in society as well as on the root causes of disparities and what can be done to eliminate them" (p. 10). In this definition, social justice is much more than a means to an end; it is also an end in itself for which to strive. In 2002, the CNA Board of Directors committed to advancing social justice as an organizational priority, solidifying it as an important concept to guide nursing policy development, practice, research, and education. Community health nurses are leaders in service provision to vulnerable populations using a social justice approach and a determinant of health focus. The concepts of social justice and equity are not well integrated into other public health discipline-related competencies (National Collaborating Centre for Determinants of Health [NCCDH], 2015) and definitions from other disciplines are lacking, but change is happening. For example, the Dietitians of Canada identify food insecurity as a social justice issue, and the Public Health Physicians of Canada include equity and justice as components of ethical practice.

Social justice focuses on the health of populations and defines the determinants of health as societal in nature. The ten defining attributes of social justice are equity, human rights (including the right to health), democracy and civil rights, capacity building (of individuals or institutions), just institutions (fair institutional practices), enabling environments, poverty reduction, ethical practice, advocacy, and partnerships (between individuals and institutions: public, private, government, education, or communities) (CNA, 2010, p. 7). Societal outcomes from using a social justice approach to community health practice include positive social development, universal respect and dignity, and all individuals' needs met and potentials realized.

Equity in health refers to the absence of differences in health that are systematic and avoidable, and therefore unfair and unjust (Cohen et al., 2013). Health equity is based on a human rights perspective where everyone has the right to opportunities for health, the right to participate fully in society, and the right to nondiscrimination (Reutter & Kushner, 2010). Health equity implies that all groups in a population should have equal opportunities for health; it does not mean identical health outcomes for everyone (Cohen et al., 2013). The Canadian Association of Public Health Dentistry CAPHD, 2006 position statements include a dedication to work toward equity in oral health. The Canadian Institute of Public Health Inspectors' CIPHI, n.d. code of ethics includes a statement on the nondiscriminatory human right to health, and the Pan-Canadian Network for Health Promoter Competencies (2015) lists health equity as a practice competency (see Chapter 2).

Action to advance health equity is occurring in Canada and internationally. Members from 25 disciplines including nursing and medicine are represented in the CPHA, which is an "independent, not-for-profit, voluntary association representing public health in Canada with links to the international public health community" (Canadian Public Health Association [CPHA], 2013, p. 2). Policy development and advocacy to reduce health inequities is a core function of the organization. The CPHA advocates for universal and equitable access to the basic conditions that are necessary for all people to achieve health. One example of the scope of the CPHA's work was co-hosting the first International Conference on Health Promotion in 1986 (see Chapter 1) where a charter for action to achieve health for all the world's populations by the year 2000 and beyond was created. The Ottawa Charter is credited with sparking a worldwide movement for health promotion and an understanding that action on the social determinants of people's health is crucial if any meaningful impact on the health of the world's population is to occur. Social justice and equity are listed as prerequisites for health along with a stable ecosystem, sustainable resources, peace, shelter, education, income, and food.

Established in 2004, the mission of the Public Health Agency of Canada (PHAC) is to promote and protect the health of Canadians. Its roles include prevention and control of infectious and chronic diseases and injuries, and strengthening intergovernmental collaboration on public health. The PHAC funds public health activities by communities and voluntary and not-for-profit agencies that support government policies and priorities. One PHAC goal is the reduction of health disparities. The PHAC (2010) defines social justice as "the concept of a society that gives individuals and groups fair treatment and an equitable share of the benefits of society. In this context, social justice is based on the concepts of human rights and equity. Under social justice, all groups and individuals are entitled equally to important rights such as health protection and minimal standards of income. The goal of public health—to minimize preventable death and disability for all—is integral to social justice" ("S" section, para. 1).

Internationally, the World Health Organization (WHO) is the directing and coordinating authority for health within the United Nations, responsible for providing leadership on global health matters, engaging in partnerships for joint action, shaping the global research agenda, setting norms and standards, providing technical support to countries, and monitoring and assessing health trends. Health is a shared responsibility, involving equitable access to essential care. The WHO's work is focused on improving people's health outcomes and life expectancy, recognizing that action is necessary across a range of contextual factors and inequitable health outcomes.

The WHO holds an unequivocal position on social justice and its links to health, stating "social justice is a matter of life and death. It affects the way people live, their consequent chance of illness, and their risk of premature death" (Commission on Social Determinants of Health [CSDH], 2008, p. 3). In addition to fulfilling basic needs for healthy living, access to quality housing, clean water, and sanitation are global human rights issues. Health inequities are unjust when these differences in health are avoidable by reasonable action taken globally and within societies. Recently, the WHO completed an analysis of the changing political, economic, and institutional context in which it works. Social justice remains high on its agenda: "In a context of growing inequity, competition for scarce natural resources and a financial crisis threatening basic entitlements to health care, it would be hard to find a better expression of health as a fundamental right, as a prerequisite for peace and security, equity, social justice, popular participation and global solidarity" (WHO, 2014b, p. 9).

Nursing is recognized for having a long history of social justice advocates who have focused their political efforts on social and economic issues (CNA, 2010). Social justice advocacy work is well developed in public health dentistry and dental hygiene where inequities in oral health and access to care for marginalized populations have resulted in policy statements and lobbying efforts (CAPHD, 2006; NCCDH, 2015). In the acute-care setting, the primacy of the biomedical model and the focus on individuals have obscured the determinants of health and action on social justice advocacy. Nevertheless, Housing First policies ensure that people have safe and affordable shelter in place before being discharged from hospital (Employment and Social Development Canada [ESDC], 2014). Housing First is an evidence-based approach capable of reducing homelessness and decreasing pressure on health services.

OPPRESSION AND DISCRIMINATION

Oppression, a concept discussed in conjunction with social justice and equity, is an experience of repeated, widespread systemic injustice. Civilized oppression is used to refer to the everyday processes of oppression in life; it "refers to the vast and deep injustices some groups suffer as consequences of often unconscious assumptions and reactions of well-meaning people in ordinary interactions which are supported by the media and cultural stereotypes as well as by the structural features of bureaucratic hierarchies and market mechanisms" (Deutsch, as cited in Fine, 2008, p. 219). There are many examples of unjust practices in everyday life. Consider these two: a child standing in a store lineup is ignored by the clerk and the next adult is served instead, and a health professional directs initial questions to a family member instead of the older adult seeking care. The agist assumptions in both of these examples may be that the recipient is not competent or worthy of attention and inclusion. The message received by the child or the older adult is that they do not matter, leading them to feel invisible, devalued, and voiceless.

A cycle of oppression may be visible in practice settings and policy decision making. An example is health care access for social assistance recipients; starting with biased information and perceptions about recipients, practitioners develop a stereotype, such as the commonly held belief that people receiving assistance are lazy. On the contrary, the reasons for unemployment among social assistance recipients are multiple and complex. Stereotyped views of people lead to health care providers missing important contexts related to income, transportation, and access to employment and child care when they are working with people to develop care plans or when making referrals on their behalf. Stereotypes lead to prejudice and influence providers to think in a particular way. For example, the belief that people receiving social assistance are lazy leads us to think they do not want to work. When we act disrespectfully toward them based on that prejudice, we are participating in discrimination. In this way, we are contributing to lack of full access to competent and compassionate health care. When discriminatory actions are supported by systemic power within the health care system and substandard assessments are not challenged, oppression is the result (Pycroft & Bartollas, 2014).

Discrimination in health care settings is a barrier to receiving health care services (Gerlach et al., 2014). It is conveyed through opinions, attitudes, and behaviours of staff, with a significant impact on the mental and physical health of recipients (Skosireva et al., 2014). The most common complaint among people with mental illness accessing help through a physician or emergency department is lack of respectful treatment. Perceived discrimination and stigma has led to avoidance of help seeking and decreased access to care. Skosireva et al. (2014) found high unmet health needs despite good access to health care among people in Toronto who are homeless and experiencing mental illness, suggesting discrimination may be an important determinant of access for marginalized populations (see Chapter 13).

Barriers to service delivery can include professional attitudes and discriminatory behaviour based on ageism, racism, sexism, classism, or heterosexism. Access issues are also rooted in government and institutional policies (Reutter & Kushner, 2010). Economic growth is the common driver of government policies, creating significant challenges to mobilizing action to pursue ends that benefit everyone in a society, but profit no one (Burris & Anderson, 2010).

SOCIAL JUSTICE AND HUMAN RIGHTS

There are many international and Canadian examples of well-established links among social justice, equity, and human rights, as well as research on the effects of ignoring social justice issues. The human right to health was established by the WHO's constitution, which provided the first legal instrument to recognize health as a fundamental human right. "Human rights highlight the discrimination, inequality, powerlessness and accountability failures that lie at the root of poverty and deprivation" (WHO, 2008, p. 1). Evidence on the role of determinants of health has established the interconnectedness between health and the factors and conditions that support health, and "individuals' right to health cannot be realized without realizing their other rights, the violations of which are at the root of poverty, such as the rights to work, food, housing and education, and the principle of non-discrimination" (Office of the United Nations High Commissioner for Human Rights [OHCHR], 2008, p. 6). These are the roots of social justice issues. Two Canadian examples are explored to highlight these connections.

Social justice and equity issues are especially prevalent in Aboriginal populations. The Health Council of Canada (HCC, 2012) states: "It is well documented that many underlying factors negatively affect the health of Aboriginal people in Canada, including poverty and the inter-generational effects of colonization and residential schools.... many Aboriginal people don't trust—and therefore don't use—mainstream health care services because they don't feel safe from stereotyping and racism" (p. 1). The legacy of colonization that lives on today includes entrenched poverty, ongoing discrimination, and associated distress (Gerlach et al., 2014).

Life expectancy for Aboriginal Canadians is well below that of other Canadians, averaging approximately seven years less for men and five years less for women. Poor health outcomes experienced by Aboriginal populations are related to economic, political, and social disparities, resulting in a disproportionate burden of ill-health and overwhelming disparities in health and well-being. Health care service delivery has been experienced as paternalistic and even latently hostile (Adelson, 2005). Racism is a persistent human rights issue and must be addressed by employing culturally competent and safe practices developed in partnership with Aboriginal communities. A health care environment that is free of racism and where Aboriginal peoples are treated with respect and dignity is essential (HCC, 2012). Workplace policies and prac-tices that support cultural competency training are crucial. Solutions to reduce these injustices require political will and use of policy frameworks that acknowledge the relationship between inequity and ill-health (Adelson, 2005).

Another group that experiences disproportionate human rights violations and social injus-tice is the lesbian, gay, bisexual, transgendered, intersexed, and queer/questioning (LGBTIQ) youth population (Dysart-Gale, 2010). Feelings of isolation, exclusion, and fear persist despite legislative acceptance of the civil and human rights of "sexual minorities" in Canada as wide-spread social acceptance has not yet occurred. Determinants of health are jeopardized for these youth when they are forced from their homes (verbally or physically) when their sexuality is acknowledged. Heteronormative assumptions and assessments by health care practitioners in-adequately assess and further marginalize these populations, and worse, homophobic attitudes can lead to the neglect of professional duty to provide care (Dysart-Gale, 2010).

Elements central to human rights and health discourse acknowledge that human rights are an important social goal and include a focus on the dignity of individuals, nondiscrimination, and the importance of the engagement of individuals in issues affecting them. The notions of charity and helping others must be replaced with socially just language that does not situate people as "the problem," but rather as partners in decision making. Policies and programs that guide practice can inadvertently disadvantage already marginalized populations (Silva et al., 2013), so language is an essential area where close examination is required regarding how it may perpetuate assumptions (e.g., that everyone is heterosexual; homeless people are mentally ill).

One of the irreversible and tragic effects of ignoring social justice issues is suicide, which is overrepresented in marginalized and discriminated groups in society (WHO, 2014a). World-wide, more than 800,000 people die each year from suicide. Societal issues such as barriers to health care and the stigma associated with seeking help, and community issues such as discrimination, abuse, acculturation and dislocation, and sense of isolation and lack of social support are risk factors for suicide (WHO, 2014a).

POPULATION HEALTH PROMOTION AND INEQUITY

The WHO stated unequivocally: "Social injustice is killing people on a grand scale" (CSDH, 2008, p. 1). Action must be taken on the social determinants of health. The structure of a society and conditions of daily life are responsible for a large majority of the health inequities between and within countries. Through its mandate to promote population health, the public

---

Box 10.1 Health Effects of Social Inequality

A study of geographic-based health statistics in Montreal showed a 10-year difference in life expectancy between upper and lower SES neighbourhoods, demonstrating the health effects of social inequalities (Lessard & Raynault, 2009). Mobilized for change, the city of Montreal created the Direction de Santé Publique (DSP) to address poverty and public health. Its focus is on understanding the impact of social disparities on the most vulnerable citizens and working to reduce this impact. The Montreal DSP has been a driver of social change by publicly positioning itself as fostering the protection of the poorest people's health and taking on public policy issues that extend well beyond immediate health protection, the traditional purview of public health.

---

health sector is ideally situated to take action on health inequities and social justice (Cohen et al., 2013). A Canadian framework called the Population Health Promotion Model was developed to guide action (see Chapter 1).

Reducing health inequities is a priority direction to improve health in Canada (Reutter & Kushner, 2010). The cause of the health disparities that arise from inequities is rooted in societal structures, necessitating interprofessional and intersectoral collaboration to take action on the multiple social determinants of health. Additional factors that influence health include food security and housing. The most significant health disparities in Canada are related to socioeconomic status (SES), Aboriginal identity, gender, and geographic location. Poverty and social inequalities are the root causes of many poor health outcomes and stem from societal structures and government policy decisions (Reutter & Kushner, 2010) (see Box 10.1).

The WHO has taken the position that to close the health gap, equity must start with quality compulsory primary and secondary education for all children, regardless of families' abilities to pay. Post-secondary education in Canada is linked to the development of more sophisticated skills to self-evaluate one's own harmful or beneficial behaviours and more resources to attain healthier lifestyles.

THE OTTAWA CHARTER REVISITED

Recently, CPHA leaders stated there is a crisis of values in which Canadian society is becoming more unequal and less interested in achieving health and social equity, recognizing "now more than ever, public health needs a strong voice to advocate for social justice" (Paradis, 2012, p. 241). In an invited commentary on the centennial of public health in Canada, Lessard and Raynault (2009) stated, "Since we know that education and income are the most significant factors for improving health, and that for decades the poorest have had poor health from one generation to the next, public health needs to move beyond the comfort of the disease paradigm" (p. 248).

Despite progress in health promotion since the Ottawa Charter was written, the challenge of achieving greater equity in health remains. Hancock (2011) called the then 25-year-old Ottawa Charter an "unfulfilled promise," as the concept of inequity had been largely ignored on the global stage. In Canada, political reluctance to identify and address the root causes of ill-health and health inequity has been prevalent. Governments must shift to place ecosystems and human health at the centre of their decision making, rather than focusing their attention more narrowly on economic development.

One of the significant barriers to a focus on the determinants of health and health equity is the current illness care system. Until the focus shifts from illness care to an upstream focus on prevention and health promotion, little change is likely to occur. Hancock (2011) calls for "a revolutionary transformation in the political and healthcare leadership in Canada. So far, there has only been rhetoric" (p. ii266). A health-in-all-policies (HIAP) approach (as opposed to health just viewed as the responsibility of the health care sector) has yet to be realized in any meaningful way in Canada. This approach is key to tackling the social determinants of health and realizing equity and social justice.

In 2010, the WHO issued the guiding *Adelaide Statement on Health in All Policies,* described as a "new social contract between all sectors to advance human development, sustainability and equity, as well as to improve health outcomes" (p. 1). The statement is part of a global process that recognizes the causes of ill-health and well-being exist outside of the health sector, and accordingly governments must engage in cross-sector policy development and integration to advance human development and equity. To be effective, HIAP requires "joined-up leadership within governments, across all sectors and between levels of government" (WHO, 2010, p. 2). Successful strategies incorporate a clear mandate; accountability, transparency, and participatory processes; engagement with stakeholders outside of government; and practical, intersectoral initiatives that build trust and partnerships.

The public health sector has been described as ideally situated to take action on poverty, health, and social justice issues (Basch, 2014). However, the focus on individual change (vs. social change) can lead to situations where victims of circumstances are blamed for failing to rise out of those circumstances. Therefore, interventions that focus on changing the social and economic environments in which economically disadvantaged people live are needed if we are to reduce disparity and foster a socially just society (Basch, 2014). Burris and Anderson (2010) suggest that employing a social justice standpoint could help community health workers act more effectively to advance health. A significant public health contribution would not only include sharing reasons for the importance of using a social justice framework for practice, but would also include showing how social injustice kills people.

POLICY: FROM EVIDENCE TO ACTION

The relationship between social justice and public policy advocacy is complex as there are diverse views, values, and beliefs about how to promote health or prevent problems. While it may be agreed a situation is unjust and requires policy action, a clear path for action is often difficult to discern. Baum (2007) articulated a vision of policy action on health equity using the metaphor of a "nutcracker": action requires top-down political commitment combined with bottom-up pressure from communities and civil society groups. Adding horizontal pressure from those who witness the effects of health inequities every day in their professional practices would help strengthen action.

A literature review to identify barriers preventing health equity issues reaching government policy agendas found that while there is advocacy for healthy public policies, few policies have been adopted and health inequity continues to grow (Embrett & Randall, 2014). Challenges to the adoption of healthy policy include poor framing of issues, poor links between a problem and its solution, lack of public awareness of issues and their implications, little political will to address issues, and weak dissemination of information about equity issues. Embrett and Randall concluded that advocacy based on evidence is insufficient to move an equity issue onto a policy agenda, but employing policy analysis theory could help guide strategies to move an issue forward (see Chapter 9).

Cacari-Stone et al. (2014) explored how two community-based participatory action research projects influenced policy to address racial and ethnic health inequities. The interplay of civic engagement through a participatory research process coupled with political participation and evidence sharing influenced the policy-making process. Public testimonies in town hall meetings and the use of media advocacy helped alter public opinion and increase awareness of a problem that required action by politicians. Data were translated into principles and recommendations for action. Their findings suggested a participatory approach to engage communities most affected by health inequities had influenced policy change.

Silva et al. (2013) suggested the use of health equity impact assessments could help protect against public health policies or practices that disadvantage marginalized populations. A health impact assessment (HIA) offers a structured process to incorporate health into public policy and thereby influence the development of all policies. HIA can be effective as a health equity policy formulation instrument within the policy cycle; however, successful implementation requires a cross-government high-level mandate and support (Harris et al., 2014).

HIA uses a variety of qualitative and quantitative techniques and tools to evaluate the potential health effects of a policy, program, or project. Originating from the mid-1990s, HIAs can be applied to assess any policy proposal with potential for "impacts on the socio-economic and physical determinants of the health of the population" (St-Pierre, 2009, p. 1), and use a five-step process that includes screening, scoping, appraisal, reporting, and monitoring. Recently, an explicit focus on equity has been included in each step. HIA guides action to promote healthy public policy and combat inequities. HIA highlights the potential effects of a program or policy on vulnerable groups and thereby helps reduce health inequities by informing policy makers of probable negative or positive effects that must be considered (St-Pierre, 2010). The use of HIA has been repeatedly called for in light of the burgeoning evidence of the health impact of inequities.

PRACTICE IMPLICATIONS

The language used to describe populations frames how they are viewed, which in turn affects community health workers' assumptions, beliefs, and attitudes and how they work with people. Although using language such as "at risk," "high needs," or "vulnerable" helps community health workers realize pockets of greater need, and may garner public and political support resulting in the channeling of more resources to some populations, there is a risk attached to the use of such terms. Deficit-based language inadvertently stigmatizes and marginalizes populations. For example, using the label "vulnerable" may suggest a problem resides inside an individual (or a community) and requires intervention using outside (often paternalistic) solutions. Using language and terms that remove the focus from blaming an individual or community and directs the focus of attention to include examining potential societal causation is more inclusive and positive. Action developed in partnership with community members engages them in the change rather than limiting them to passive recipients of assistance (Frohlich & Abel, 2013). Interventions at larger systems or societal levels address the root causes of problems. Mindfulness to avoid language that holds the potential to further stigmatize a population creates a shift to using more socially just language.

Venkatapuram and Marmot (2009) suggest the individual-level framework of causation that is dominant in epidemiology excludes the important effects of social phenomena on individuals' impairments and mortality. A single-focused lifestyle approach to health holds a danger of potentially blaming people for their poor health status and limiting not only the resources and efforts of health workers, but also limiting the possibilities for partnering with individuals and communities in health promoting action for change that would enhance social justice and equity (see Box 10.2). To move away from the concept of individual behaviours, Frohlich and Abel (2013) suggest community health workers must also shift their inequity language to one of discussing unequal chances. There is an inequality of opportunity for people that limit some groups' abilities to engage in healthy behaviours. The biomedical lifestyle approach that has driven many public health practices has shown "the inability of public health to change individual behaviour on a large scale...despite expensive and labour-intensive

> ### Box 10.2 Harm Reduction to Address Inequities
>
> Harm reduction strategies (e.g., needle exchange programs and supervised injection sites) as a value-neutral approach that reduces the harms associated with substance use has been studied with homeless and substance-using populations that face multiple inequities in health. Harm reduction alone is insufficient to address the root causes of inequities and could possibly even further marginalize these groups. Institutional structures must be a focus of social justice initiatives to move past individual-focused harm reduction strategies, to address the root causes of problematic substance use and homelessness, and link with other actions on the determinants of health. In one study of the ethical practices of nursing in the context of homelessness, Pauly (2008) concluded: "An ethical commitment to social justice by nurses suggests that action which addresses the determinants of health inequities such as housing is needed.... [However] in this study, nurses did not take action to redress the broader social conditions that contribute to inequities in health and access to health care for those who are street involved" (p. 202). A social justice lens provides a broad framework for including those who use illegal substances in the development of policy and programs and in engaging in systemic change. More nurses must shift their focus from being solely on the context of providing care to individuals to engaging in this systemic change.

large-scale interventions... [and this] has given epidemiologists reason to pause with regard to how they view behaviour and its causes and their ability to modify it" (Frohlich & Abel, 2013, p. 200). It is time for change.

Using the community development process (see Chapter 5) helps support a social justice approach to practice. Relationship development skills facilitate community development as does employing a strengths-based partnership approach in which community members co-create solutions to their problems. Community development employing a social justice lens builds on the existing strengths of a community and requires a worker skill set in the awareness of inequalities, colour-blind racial attitudes, understanding differing multicultural and social identities, use of inclusive language and cultural sensitivity, engaging those who are underrepresented or underserved, communication and team development that promotes diverse identity and interest representation (Checkoway, 2013).

EDUCATIONAL IMPLICATIONS

Despite the inclusion of a social justice statement in some public health disciplines' codes of ethics, many do not see its relevance for their practice and have a limited understanding of social justice. The importance of embedding social justice and equity into the education of health professionals is becoming increasingly evident in curriculum innovations described in the literature. Rising student enrollments coupled with health care system downsizing and fewer community health practicum opportunities has led to students' immersion in nontraditional practicum placements where they may be exposed to poverty, inequities, and marginalization of populations. This poses an ideal opportunity for first-hand student learning about social justice and equity. Substantive theory in curricula regarding social justice, health disparities, and relations of power is needed. Creative methods of teaching about these concepts include innovations such as Mawji and Lind's (2013) development of a simulation mannequin dressed as a homeless, battered sex trade worker. This mannequin effectively teaches key community health concepts such as social justice and equity, advocacy and activism, community development, harm reduction, and social determinants of health.

> ### Box 10.3   Education Example: Harvest Supper
>
> Every October, two local businesses host a "five-star" three-course meal for the homeless population in Calgary. In an elegant banquet room, attendees are seated at tables set with white tablecloths, napkins, and cutlery for three courses. Waiters take individual orders and courteously serve each homeless guest their chef-prepared meal on fine china. Each course is modified to accommodate personal likes, dislikes, and food restrictions with the greatest respect—the entire staff go out of their way to ensure each guest is served a meal with which they are satisfied.
>
> In 2014, a group of eight community health practicum students were invited to attend the dinner, experiencing a first-hand opportunity to challenge their assumptions about homelessness, table manners, and respect and learn the value of treating every person with dignity regardless of social status.
>
> Prior to the meal, students assumed the homeless guests would have poor table manners and would not appreciate the fine meal. However their assumptions were overturned, and some students noted it was their own manners that were lacking by comparison! Afterward the students discussed how the experience challenged their assumptions; they understood that homeless people have come from families that are not all that different from their own, and from a societal level homelessness should not be an acceptable way of life, as it constitutes a poor solution to personal crises.

STEPS TOWARD CREATING A SOCIALLY JUST WORLD

Venkatapuram and Marmot (2009) identified a range of psychosocial determinants that affect people's health and provided beginning steps the community health team can use toward creating a socially just world. These determinants include the ethical concepts of autonomy, dignity, respect, trust, and reciprocity (see Chapter 3) (see Box 10.3). In the research of Perez-Arechaederra et al. (2010), exploration of perceived fairness in health services delivery by physicians helps clarify the concept of reciprocity. They suggest a physician must consider patients as colleagues and welcome patients' voices in decision making. The way that patients are treated by staff, along with the information exchange between patient and service provider, has a strong impact on justice perception. To feel they are treated fairly, people must feel their voices are heard, and they are treated with dignity and respect.

Interdisciplinary and cross-sectoral collaboration that extends well beyond individual-level practice to taking action on systems and societal levels is required. The consideration of health must infuse all government policies, not just health sector policies, and "multiple dimensions of health should matter for realizing social equity and justice.... [which] requires making changes to a range of basic social practices and institutions" (Venkatapuram & Marmot, 2009, p. 85). Ultimately, adopting a social justice standpoint could help advance health more effectively as social structures and power relations have a large impact on the level and distribution of a population's health (Burris & Anderson, 2010).

Efforts to promote equity and social justice are not confined to those at political or policy levels. Social justice is also fostered through day-to-day efforts and interactions with others. Our ways of being, knowing, and choosing are rooted in social justice. We witness social injustice in the community, where we also have the opportunity to advocate for and work toward achieving health equity (Falk-Rafael & Betker, 2012). The following suggestions are offered as starting points to help community health workers integrate social justice into their roles, within organizations, and at a societal level.

- As a community health worker:
  - Promote the urgency to address the social determinants of health and health inequities.
  - Arm yourself with facts. The seminal documents in Chapter 1 are essential reading. Additional resources are identified in many chapters.

- Nurture leadership in yourself and in others; when opportunity presents itself, ensure your voice is heard.
- Within your organization:
  - Support current and future community health workers' acquisition of competencies to meet practice and policy challenges.
  - Advocate for and initiate coordinated policy efforts—be part of the "nutcracker" pressure for action on the determinants of health.
  - Share historical and current accounts of how others are taking action on the determinants of health from a social justice perspective.
  - Engage in discussions about equality, equity, social justice, and advocacy using stories from your practice and your own community.
  - Promote equity in health policy and program planning. Universal and targeted services are needed to combat rising health inequities due to a faster uptake of programs by more socially advantaged populations. Consider tools designed to incorporate equity and social justice in health policy and program planning.
- At a system level:
  - Challenge societal beliefs that individuals are solely responsible for their health outcomes.
  - Act politically.
  - Seek opportunities to increase Canadians' awareness of the importance of action on the social determinants of health.
  - Use accessible videos and tools to engage in conversations about health, equity, and social justice.

Summary

This chapter offered an in-depth discussion about the concepts of social justice and equity and their impact on the health of populations. Social justice is a human rights issue. Poverty and social inequalities are the root causes of many poor health outcomes necessitating interprofessional and intersectoral collaboration with action taken on the multiple social determinants of health. For example, a practice focus when working with people who live with poverty must include interventions that move away from an individual-focused lifestyle orientation toward changing social and economic environments. Health equity action requires top-down political commitment, bottom-up pressure from communities, and horizontal pressure from practitioners. Social justice may be fostered through day-to-day practitioner efforts and interactions with others that incorporate dignity and respect, and that avoid potentially stigmatizing language such as "at-risk" or "vulnerable." Human rights are fostered by policies and practices that include a focus on the dignity of people, nondiscrimination, and the importance of the engagement of people in issues affecting them. The outcomes of using a social justice approach to community practice include positive social development, universal respect and dignity, and people's needs met and potential realized. A focus on the root causes of disparities in society provides guidance for policy development, practice, research, and education that align with social justice. However, much work remains to be done to incorporate social justice and equity into community health practices and government policies to effect meaningful societal health promoting change.

REFERENCES

Adelson, N. (2005). The embodiment of inequity: Health disparities in Aboriginal Canada. *Canadian Journal of Public Health, 96*(Suppl 2), S45–S61.

Basch, C. H. (2014). Poverty, health, and social justice: The importance of public health approaches. *International Journal of Health Promotion and Education, 52*, 181–187.

Baum, F. (2007). Cracking the nut of health equity: Top down and bottom up pressure for action on the social determinants of health. *IUHPE—Promotion & Education, 14*(2), 90–95.

Burris, S., & Anderson, E. D. (2010). A framework convention on global health: Social justice lite, or a light on social justice? *Journal of Law, Medicine & Ethics, 38,* 580–593.

Cacari-Stone, L., Wallerstein, N., Garcia, A. P., & Minkler, M. (2014). The promise of community-based participatory research for health equity: A conceptual model for bridging evidence with policy. *American Journal of Public Health, 104,* 1615–1623.

Canadian Association of Public Health Dentistry (CAPHD), Position Development Committee. (2006). *A brief analysis of position statements on oral health and access to care.* URL=http://www.caphd.ca/sites/default/files/pdf/caphd-access-position-statement.pdf

Canadian Institute of Public Health Inspectors' [CIPHI]. (n.d.). URL=http://www.ciphi.ca/pdf/ethics.pdf

Canadian Nurses Association (CNA). (2010). *Social justice…a means to an end, an end in itself* (2nd ed.). Ottawa: Author. URL=http://www.cna-aiic.ca/~/media/cna/page-content/pdf-en/social_justice_2010_e.pdf

Canadian Public Health Association (CPHA). (2013). *2013 annual report.* Ottawa: Author. URL=http://www.cpha.ca/uploads/annual-reports/2013_ar_e.pdf

Checkoway, B. (2013). Social justice approach to community development. *Journal of Community Practice, 21,* 472–486.

Cohen, B. E., Schultz, A., McGibbon, E., VanderPlaat, M., Bassett, R., GermAnn, K., et al. (2013). A conceptual framework of organizational capacity for public health equity action (OC-PHEA). *Canadian Journal of Public Health, 104,* e262–e266.

Commission on Social Determinants of Health (CSDH). (2008). *Closing the gap in a generation: Health equity through action on the social determinants of health.* Geneva: World Health Organization. URL=http://www.who.int/social_determinants/thecommission/finalreport/en/

Dysart-Gale, D. (2010). Social justice and social determinants of health: Lesbian, gay, bisexual, transgendered, intersexed, and queer youth in Canada. *Journal of Child and Adolescent Psychiatric Nursing, 23,* 23–28.

Embrett, M. G., & Randall, G. E. (2014). Social determinants of health and health equity policy research: Exploring the use, misuse, and nonuse of policy analysis theory. *Social Science & Medicine, 108,* 147–155.

Employment and Social Development Canada [ESDC]. (2014). Housing First. http://www.esdc.gc.ca/eng/communities/homelessness/housing_first/index.shtml

Falk-Rafael, A., & Betker, C. (2012). Witnessing social injustice downstream and advocating for health equity upstream: "The trombone slide" of nursing. *Advances in Nursing Science, 35,* 98–112.

Fine, M. (2008). An epilogue, of sorts. In J. Cammarota & M. Fine (Eds.), *Revolutionizing education: Youth participatory action research in motion* (pp. 213–234). New York, NY: Routledge.

Frohlich, K. L., & Abel, T. (2013). Environmental justice and health practices: Understanding how health inequities arise at the local level. *Sociology of Health & Illness, 36,* 199–212.

Gerlach, A., Sullivan, T., Valavaara, K., & McNeil, C. (2014). Turing the gaze inward: Relational practices with Aboriginal peoples informed by cultural safety. *Occupational Therapy Now, 16*(1), 20–21.

Hancock, T. (2011). Health promotion in Canada: 25 years of unfulfilled promise. *Health Promotion International, 26*(Suppl 2), ii263–ii267.

Harris, P., Sainsbury, P., & Kemp, L. (2014). The fit between health impact assessment and public policy: Practice meets theory. *Social Science & Medicine, 108,* 46–53.

Health Council of Canada (HCC). (2012). *Empathy, dignity, and respect: Creating cultural safety for Aboriginal people in urban health care.* Toronto: Author. URL=http://www.healthcouncilcanada.ca/rpt_det.php?id= 437#.php?mnu=2

Lessard, R., & Raynault, M-F. (2009). Public health and poverty. *Canadian Journal of Public Health, 100,* 247–248.

Mawji, A., & Lind, C. (2013). Imogene: A simulation innovation to teach community health nursing. *Clinical Simulation in Nursing, 9,* e513–e519.

National Collaborating Centre for Determinants of Health (NCCDH). (2015). *Do public health discipline-specific competencies provide guidance for equity-focused practice?* Antigonish, NS: NCCDH, St. Francis Xavier University.

Office of the United Nations High Commissioner for Human Rights (OHCHR), & World Health Organization. (2008). *The right to health.* (Fact sheet no. 31). Geneva: Author. URL=http://www.ohchr.org/Documents/Publications/Factsheet31.pdf

Pan-Canadian Network for Health Promoter Competencies. (2015). *Pan-Canadian network for health promoter competencies and glossary.* URL= http://www.healthpromotercanada.com

Paradis, G. (2012). Public health needs you! *Canadian Journal of Public Health, 103,* e241.

Pauly, B. (2008). Shifting moral values to enhance access to health care: Harm reduction as context for ethical nursing practice. *International Journal of Drug Policy, 19,* 195–204.

Perez-Arechaederra, D., Herrero, C., Lind, A., & Masip, J. (2010). Exploration of fairness in health services: A qualitative analysis. *Health Marketing Quarterly, 27,* 244–261.

Public Health Agency of Canada (PHAC). (2010). *Glossary of terms.* URL=http://www.phac-aspc.gc.ca/php-psp/ccph-cesp/glos-eng.php

Pycroft, A., & Bartollas, C. (Eds.). (2014). *Applying complexity theory: Whole systems approaches to criminal justice and social work.* Bristol, UK: Policy Press.

Reutter, L., & Kushner, K. E. (2010). Health equity through action on the social determinants of health: Taking up the challenge in nursing. *Nursing Inquiry, 17,* 269–280.

Silva, D. S., Smith, M. J., & Upshur, R. E. (2013). Disadvantaging the disadvantaged: When public health policies and practices negatively affect marginalized populations. *Canadian Journal of Public Health, 104,* e410–e412.

Skosireva, A., O'Campo, P., Zerger, S., Chambers, C., Gapka, S., & Stergiopoulos, V. (2014). Different faces of discrimination: Perceived discrimination among homeless adults with mental illness in healthcare settings. *BMC Health Services Research, 14,* 376.

St-Pierre, L. (2009). *Introduction to HIA.* Montréal: National Collaborating Centre for Healthy Public Policy. URL=http://www.ncchpp.ca/docs/Introduction_HIA_EN_.pdf

St-Pierre, L. (2010). *HIA and inequities.* Montréal: National Collaborating Centre for Healthy Public Policy. URL=http://www.ncchpp.ca/docs/HIA_Inequities_EN_March2010.pdf

Venkatapuram, S., & Marmot, M. (2009). Epidemiology and social justice in light of social determinants of health research. *Bioethics, 23,* 79–89.

World Health Organization (WHO). (2008). *Human rights, health and poverty reduction strategies.* Geneva: WHO and Office of the United Nations High Commissioner for Human Rights. URL=http://www.ohchr.org/Documents/Issues/ESCR/Health/HHR_PovertyReductionsStrategies_WHO.pdf

World Health Organization (WHO). (2010). *Adelaide statement on health in all policies: Moving towards a shared governance for health and well-being.* Geneva: Author. URL=http://www.who.int/social_determinants/hiap_statement_who_sa_final.pdf

World Health Organization (WHO). (2014a). *Preventing suicide: A global imperative.* Geneva: Author. URL=http://www.who.int/mental_health/suicide-prevention/world_report_2014

World Health Organization (WHO). (2014b). *Twelfth general programme of work: Not merely the absence of disease.* Geneva: Author. URL=www.who.int/about/resources_planning/twelfth-gpw

ONLINE RESOURCES

Please visit the Point at http://thepoint.lww.com/Vollman4e for up-to-date Internet resources and additional learning materials on this topic.

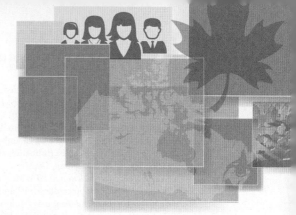

CHAPTER 11

Negotiating the Cultural Context of Community Care

Ryan Gibson, Frances E. Racher, and Robert C. Annis

LEARNING OBJECTIVES

After studying this chapter, you should be able to:

1. Describe the cultural composition of Canada

2. Define key concepts related to culture and ethnicity

3. Discuss multiculturalism in Canada, including the benefits

4. Outline barriers and facilitators related to multiculturalism in community practice

5. Develop cultural attunement and apply cultural humility in working with groups and organizations in the community

Introduction

Canada is a country of ethnic and cultural diversity. The Aboriginal peoples, the British and French founding peoples, and a wide variety of other ethnic groups create the cultural mosaic that is Canada. Health professionals work with individuals, families, groups, and communities whose lives are both enriched and challenged by the cultural diversity that exists across this country. In this book, the focus is "community as partner", which denotes work with groups, organizations, populations, and the community as a whole. Therefore, this chapter will diverge from the traditional health professional practice of working with individuals to discussions related to working with collectives and to community practice beyond individuals and families, beyond community as context. Health professionals are more frequently turning their attention and contributing their knowledge and skills to this focus of community as partner.

Culture is identified as one of the 12 determinants of health (see Table 3.1 in Chapter 1). These determinants do not act in isolation but are known to be complex and interrelated, creating an intricate web. For example, culture affects people's opportunities for education and occupation, which in turn has considerable consequences for income, knowledge of support structures, access to informal support in social networks, and personal coping skills.

The chapter begins with a description of the cultural landscape of Canada and the composition of the Canadian population. Key concepts, related to culture and ethnicity, are defined to set the stage for discussions of theory and the application of theory to practice. A dialogue on the history of multiculturalism in Canada and its benefits provides a context for community practice. Given the paucity of health care literature on matters of racism, marginalization, and inequities in health and health care (Kirkham, 2003), challenges to multiculturalism including prejudice, ethnocentrism, stereotyping, and racism are incorporated. Cultural competence, cultural attunement, and cultural humility are examined and thoughts about effective community practice in working with groups and organizations are shared.

THE CULTURAL LANDSCAPE OF CANADA

In 2011, some 32,852,325 people comprised the diverse cultural landscape of Canada (Statistics Canada, 2013a). Three particular influences contributed to that diversity, including (1) the various cultures of Aboriginal peoples, (2) the heritage of the British and French founding nations, and (3) the diverse cultures of immigrants to this country.

Aboriginal Peoples

According to the 2011 National Household Survey (NHS), the population of Canada included 1,400,685 Aboriginal people, or 4.3% of the total population (Table 11.1) (Statistics Canada, 2013b). These population figures may reflect increases in population and greater involvement in census participation by Aboriginal people.

In the 2011 NHS (Statistics Canada, 2013b), of the Aboriginal people reporting, 60.8% considered themselves to be First Nations, 32.3% Métis, and 4.2% Inuit. Over 85% of the population of Nunavut, 50% of the Northwest Territories, and 23% of the Yukon Territory were composed of Aboriginal peoples. The provinces of Manitoba and Saskatchewan were reported to have the highest proportions of Aboriginal residents, with 16.7% and 15.6% of their populations, respectively. Although proportions of the populations were lower for Ontario and British Columbia,

TABLE 11.1 Aboriginal Identity Population, 2011 Counts for Canada, Provinces, and Territories

	First Nations	Métis	Inuit	Aboriginal Population[a]	
	N	N	N	N	(%[b])
Canada	851,560	451,795	59,445	1,400,685	4.3
Newfoundland and Labrador	10,382	7,160	6,086	35,800	7.1
Prince Edward Island	1,048	379	45	2,230	1.6
Nova Scotia	14,894	8,801	677	33,850	3.7
New Brunswick	11,762	4,298	452	22,620	3.1
Quebec	62,443	35,479	12,772	141,915	1.8
Ontario	141,672	78,372	3,014	301,430	2.4
Manitoba	111,660	74,440	0	195,895	16.7
Saskatchewan	97,799	50,477	0	157,740	15.6
Alberta	105,934	90,485	2,207	220,695	6.2
British Columbia	120,791	65,041	2,323	232,290	5.4
Yukon Territory	5,937	694	154	7,710	23.1
Northwest Territories	1,333	2,751	4,232	21,160	51.9
Nunavut	274	0	27,086	27,360	86.3

[a]Includes the Aboriginal groups (First Nations [term used on NHS—North American Indian], Métis, and Inuit), multiple Aboriginal responses, and Aboriginal responses not included elsewhere. The Aboriginal identity population comprises those persons who reported identifying with at least one Aboriginal group, that is, First Nations (term used on census—North American Indian), Métis, or Inuit, and/or who reported being a Treaty Indian or a Registered Indian, as defined by the Indian Act of Canada, and/or who reported being a member of an Indian Band or First Nation.
[b]Includes percentage of total population, including all Aboriginal and non-Aboriginal populations.
Source: Statistics Canada (2013b).

the population counts were the highest in the country, with 301,430 and 232,290 Aboriginal residents, respectively. The Aboriginal population coupled with those of early British and French origin has influenced the composition of the Canadian population from early times.

Founding Nations

In 1871, the first Canadian census identified 3.5 million people living in Canada, with 92% of either British (61%) or French (31%) origin and 6% German (Driedger, 2003). As this census covered the four original Canadian provinces in the east, an estimated one-half million North American Indians, scattered over the northwestern territories, were not included.

According to the 2011 NHS, the ethnic origins of the Canadian population had shifted considerably over the ensuing 145 years (Table 11.2). By this time, 41.2% of the Canadian

TABLE 11.2 Canadian Population by Selected Ethnic Origin[a]

	Total Responses	Single Responses	Multiple Responses[b]
Canada			
Total population	32,852,320	19,036,295	13,816,025
Ethnic Origin			
Canadian	10,563,805	5,834,535	4,729,265
English	6,509,500	1,312,570	5,196,930
French	5,077,215	1,170,620	3,906,595
Scottish	4,714,970	544,440	4,170,530
Irish	4,544,870	506,445	4,038,425
German	3,203,330	608,520	2,594,805
Italian	1,488,425	700,845	787,580
Chinese	1,487,580	1,210,945	276,635
First Nations (North American Indian)	1,369,115	517,550	851,565
Ukrainian	1,251,170	276,055	975,110
East Indian	1,165,145	919,155	245,985
Dutch (The Netherlands)	1,067,245	297,885	769,355
Polish	1,010,705	255,135	755,565
Filipino	662,600	506,545	156,060
British Isles n.i.e.[c]	576,030	128,090	447,945
Russian	550,520	107,300	443,220
Welsh	458,705	28,785	429,915
Norwegian	452,705	44,075	408,630
Métis	447,655	68,205	379,445
Portuguese	429,850	250,320	179,530
American (USA)	375,575	32,923	339,640
Spanish	368,305	66,575	301,730
Swedish	341,845	26,080	315,770
Hungarian	316,765	80,540	326,220
Jewish	309,650	115,640	194,010
Jamaican	256,915	142,870	114,040
Greek	252,960	141,755	111,205

[a]Ethnic origin: refers to the ethnic or cultural group(s) to which the respondent's ancestors belong. An ancestor is someone from whom a person is descended and is usually more distant than a grandparent. Ethnic origin pertains to the ancestral "roots" or background of the population and should not be confused with citizenship or nationality.
[b]Multiple ethnic response: occurs when a respondent provides two or more ethnic origins. As a result of increasing intermarriage between persons of different ethnic backgrounds, an increasing proportion of the population of Canada report two or more ethnic origins.
[c]n.i.e.: not included elsewhere.
Source: Statistics Canada (2013c).

population reported more than one ethnic or cultural group to which their ancestors belonged. Over 10 million residents, or 32.2%, reported a Canadian ethnic origin; 49.4% reported British (English, Irish, Scottish, Welsh) ancestry; and 15.5% reported French ancestry. Ethnic origins from other European countries, Asia, Africa, and Latin America are noted in Table 11.2. By 2011, 13 ethnic origins had passed the one-million mark (Statistics Canada, 2013c).

Immigrants

In 2013, over 258,000 people immigrated to Canada according to Citizenship and Immigration Canada (2014). The total number of new immigrants reached a high of 280,689 in 2010. The primary objectives of Canada's immigration program are reuniting families, contributing to economic development, and protecting refugees. Canadian immigrants are considered either permanent or temporary residents. In 2013, the 258,953 permanent residents included 79,684 in the family class; 148,181 as economic immigrants; 24,049 as refugees; and 7,039 as other immigrants. Table 11.3 illustrates the top 10 source countries that generated the permanent resident immigrant population of Canada in 2013 and the immigration trends for these 10 source countries for the three-year period from 2011 to 2013. In 2013, the majority of immigrants came from the People's Republic of China, which surpassed the Philippines for the first time and India for the second time in as many years. Pakistan and Iran surpassed the United States for the first time, now being ranked fourth and fifth respectively and the United States ranked sixth overall.

Permanent resident immigrant population for 2013 by place of birth, province, and territory is provided in Table 11.4. The majority (40%) of this population resided in Ontario, with 20.1% in Quebec and 14.1% in Alberta. In 2012, 1,091,876 immigrants were temporary residents in Canada, including 491,547 temporary foreign workers; 328,672 foreign students; 122,569 humanitarian population/refugees; and 149,088 others (Citizenship and Immigration Canada, 2014).

Visible Minorities

Some 6,244,800 NHS respondents, or 19.1% of Canadians, identified themselves as members of a visible minority (Statistics Canada, 2013c), an increase of 19.1% since 2006. In Canada,

TABLE 11.3 Permanent Resident Immigrant Population of Canada by Top 10 Source Countries for 2011–2013

Source Countries	2011		2012		2013	
	N	%	N	%	N	%
China, People's Republic	28,503	11.5	33,024	12.8	34,126	13.2
India	27,509	11.1	30,932	12.0	33,085	12.8
Philippines	36,765	14.8	30,932	12.0	29,539	11.4
Pakistan	7,468	3.0	11,227	4.4	12,602	4.9
Iran	7,479	3.0	7,533	2.9	11,291	4.4
United States of America	7,675	3.1	7,891	3.1	8,495	3.3
France	4,080	1.6	6,280	2.4	5,624	2.2
United Kingdom	6,204	2.5	6,195	2.4	5,826	2.2
Iraq	6,196	2.5	4,041	1.6	4,918	1.9
Korea, Republic of	4,589	1.8	5,315	2.1	4,509	1.7
Top 10 Source Countries	131,700	54.9	144,005	55.6	150,015	57.9
Other Countries	117,048	45.1	113,882	44.4	108,938	42.1
Total	248,749	100.0	257,895	100.0	258,953	100.0

Source: Citizenship and Immigration Canada (2014).

TABLE 11.4 Permanent Resident Immigrant Population, Province, and Territories, 2013

	N	%
Canada	258,953	100
Ontario	103,494	40.0
Quebec	51,983	20.1
Alberta	36,636	14.1
British Columbia	36,210	14.0
Manitoba	13,100	5.1
Saskatchewan	10,679	4.1
Nova Scotia	2,529	0.9
New Brunswick	2,019	0.8
Prince Edward Island	998	0.4
Newfoundland/Labrador	825	0.3
Yukon	316	0.1
Northwest Territories	150	0.06
Nunavut	11	0.004
Not stated	3	0.001

Source: Citizenship and Immigration Canada (2014).

the official definition of *visible minority population* is derived from the *Employment Equity Act*. Members of visible minorities are persons, other than Aboriginal persons, who are not Caucasian. Under this definition, regulations specify the following groups as visible minorities: Chinese, South Asians, Blacks, Arabs, West Asians, Filipinos, Southeast Asians, Latin Americans, Japanese, Koreans, and other visible minority groups such as Pacific Islanders.

In 2011, 96% of the visible minority population resided in a census metropolitan area (an urban core with a population of at least 100,000), with 52.3% of them residing in Ontario, 25.9% in British Columbia, and 18.4% in Alberta. This diverse cultural landscape of Canada demonstrates the rationale for multiculturalism, including the development and implementation of practices, programs, and policies to support the quality of life and well-being of people and groups who comprise the Canadian mosaic.

KEY CONCEPTS RELATED TO CULTURAL DIVERSITY

Clarification of key concepts related to culture and ethnicity will enhance understanding of cultural diversity and assist in building knowledge and skills for working with people from different cultures. Differentiation among the terms *culture* and *ethnicity* is followed by a discussion of cultural pluralism, universality, and multiculturalism.

Culture refers to the integrated lifestyle, the learned and shared beliefs, values, worldviews, knowledge, artifacts, rules, and symbols that guide behaviour of a particular group of people. Individuals are the primary building blocks upon which cultural groups are based. Culture is transmitted intergenerationally, explains patterns of thought and action, and contributes to a group's social and physical survival. Culture is continuous, cumulative, and progressive (Fleras, 2014). Although culture is most commonly related to ethnicity, a culture may develop within an organization, a workplace, a profession, across a population or group, or within a community. Although this chapter will concentrate on culture related to ethnicity, much of the content may be applied to other cultural aspects and environments.

Ethnicity involves cultural, organizational, and ideational values, attitudes, and behaviours. In its broadest sense, ethnicity refers to groups whose members share a common social and cultural heritage passed on to successive generations. Members of an ethnic group feel a sense of identity, as people are defined, differentiated, organized, and rewarded on the basis of commonly shared physical or cultural characteristics (Driedger, 2003; Fleras, 2014).

Cultural pluralism or *cultural relativism* is the view that beliefs are influenced by and best understood within the context of culture. This theory developed by anthropologists is used to prevent the natural tendency to judge other cultures in comparison with one's own and to promote the collection and analysis of information about other cultures without this bias (Birx, 2006). Cultural pluralism cautions against unfairly condemning another group for being different and promotes respect for the right of others to have different beliefs, values, behaviours, and ways of life. Cultural relativism fosters awareness and appreciation of cultural differences, rejects assumptions of superiority of one's culture, and averts ethnocentrism. While cultural convergence or assimilation involves merging cultures and creates a cultural melting pot, cultural relativism involves respecting culture and honouring diversity, thus generating a cultural mosaic.

For the purposes of this chapter, *multiculturalism* is considered to be a set of ideas and practices for engaging cultures, as different yet equal, for the purposes of living together with those differences (Fleras, 2014). Canada as a multicultural society is ethnically diverse, espouses a set of ideals that celebrate diversity, and advances a social movement that challenges the privileging of any culture over any other. From a political stance, official multiculturalism represents a doctrine and set of practices that officially acknowledge and promote diversity as legitimate and integral to the composition of the country.

MULTICULTURALISM IN CANADA

The history of multiculturalism in Canada begins with the early periods of the country; however, its official beginning starts with the multicultural policy adopted by the Canadian government in 1971 (Dewing, 2013). Since the adoption of this stance, Canada's approach has evolved through legislation and policy. Multiculturalism offers a theoretical, ethical, and practical framework for community practice and working toward the improvement of human rights and social conditions in Canadian communities.

Multiculturalism Within a Bilingual Framework

In 1971, Canada officially became the first country to adopt a multicultural policy, a policy that has been touted as a model taken up by other countries seeking a pluralist route. In his affirmation of multiculturalism and rejection of the monocultural or assimilation model, Prime Minister Pierre Trudeau (1971) declared:

> ...there cannot be one cultural policy for the Canadians of British and French origin, another for the original peoples and yet a third for all others. For although there are two official languages, there is no official culture, nor does any ethnic group take precedence over any other (p. 1).

The concept of Canada as a multicultural society can be interpreted descriptively as a sociologic fact, prescriptively as ideology, politically as policy, and practically as a set of dynamic intergroup processes and actions (Dewing, 2013).

Canadian Charter of Rights and Freedoms

In 1982, the *Canadian Charter of Rights and Freedoms* located multiculturalism within the wider framework of Canadian society and empowered the courts accordingly. The Charter stated that its contents should be interpreted in a manner consistent with the multicultural heritage of Canadians and declared the equality of every Canadian, including the right to equal protection and equal benefit of the law without discrimination based on race, national or ethnic origin, colour, religion, sex, or mental or physical disability (Dewing, 2013).

Canadian Multiculturalism Act

In 1988, the *Canadian Multiculturalism Act* was adopted by parliament, making Canada the first country in the world to pass a multiculturalism law. The Act acknowledged multiculturalism as a fundamental characteristic of Canadian society and sought to assist in the preservation of culture and language, reduce discrimination, enhance cultural awareness and understanding, and promote culturally sensitive institutional change at the federal level (Dewing, 2013). While many espouse the benefits and achievements of multiculturalism, others extol its shortcomings and disappointments; most, however, will agree that much has been achieved and much remains to be done.

Benefits of Multiculturalism

In his working paper for the Economic Council of Canada, cross-cultural psychologist John Berry (1991) identified the social benefits of multiculturalism. Berry articulated the goal of the multiculturalism policy as the support and encouragement of groups and individuals to adopt an integration strategy, following a midcourse between the alternatives of assimilation and separation, and moving away from the social and psychological pathologies associated with marginalization. The policy emphasizes human rights, social participation, and equity, in addition to group maintenance and intergroup tolerance, thus demonstrating concern for individual as well as group choices and freedoms. Berry identified the balancing act between collective rights and individual rights as well as between two sets of collective rights, those of the dominant society and those of the various constituent groups.

Benefits of multiculturalism identified by Berry (1991) include:

- The existence of the policy demonstrates concern for the quality of human relations in Canada and makes people aware that their ethnocultural and individual needs are not being ignored, psychologically contributing to morale, self-esteem, and positive group relations.
- The policy is a primary prevention program with the intention of giving every individual and ethnocultural group a place and a sense of belonging in Canadian society.
- Diversity is a resource: The greater the variance in a population, the greater the capacity of that population to deal effectively with changing circumstances. The maintenance of ethnocultural diversity at home may be seen as important in Canada's ability to participate abroad.
- Multiculturalism, in principle, permits Canada to better meet its national and international obligations with respect to human rights. While most agree with the need for improvement (Aboriginal rights, culturally sensitive health and education, reduction of bias in policing and delivery of justice), this policy offers an ethical framework for working toward the improvement of human rights and social conditions in Canada.
- Multiculturalism has potential to promote social and psychological well-being of Canadians. Potential benefits of multiculturalism and integration must be judged in relation to potential costs of the alternatives, including the denial of the right to be different (assimilation), the rejection of persons who pursue that right (segregation), or both (marginalization).

BARRIERS TO MULTICULTURALISM

The focus of the traditional transcultural care theory and relationships with the individual client render less visible and less apparent for discussion the broader context and social practices that perpetuate racism, sexism, and other systematic oppressions (Gustafson, 2005).

Discussion of the barriers to multiculturalism opens that dialogue and encourages health professionals to expand their thinking as they extend their work to the broader community.

Prejudice

Prejudice involves negative and preconceived notions about others. Though often unconscious, these attitudes are irrational, unfounded, and run counterproductive to existing evidence. Refusal to modify beliefs in the face of contrary evidence distinguishes prejudice from ignorance (Fleras, 2014). Prejudice is a function of group dynamics, with social and historical roots and dimensions of ethnocentrism and stereotyping.

Ethnocentrism

Ethnocentrism is a tendency to see reality through one's own cultural perspective—a culture, which is deemed necessary, normal, and desirable. With this preferred cultural lens comes a faith in the superiority of one's ethnic or cultural group and a privileging of its values and views, beliefs, and behaviours (Fleras, 2014). The existence of ethnocentrism in people's lives, the books they read, and the television shows they watch perpetuate the influences of ethnocentrism as a social norm and value. Replacing ethnocentrism with tolerance has potential to facilitate multiculturalism and respect for all cultural groups.

Stereotyping

Categorization of things has been considered characteristic of the thinking of all people. Categorizing of people or stereotyping may reflect prejudice, although it need not (Fleras, 2014). Stereotyped thinking can be functional for the person who uses it to organize and simplify a wealth of information, leading to accurate predictions about others to the extent that the stereotypes contain accurate generalizations. Even innocuous and accurate stereotypes can be dysfunctional. Tolerant individuals suspend stereotypes when appropriate, while intolerant ones probably do not.

Racism

Racism is an ideology that ascribes beliefs of inferiority to physical and cultural differences among people, places people in a hierarchy, and perpetuates inequality and privilege. Racism involves ideas and ideals of normalcy or superiority of one social group over another because of perceived differences, together with the institutionalized power to put these beliefs into practice with the intent or effect of denying or excluding (Fleras, 2014). Racism can be expressed in terms of culture and power. Racism related to culture emphasizes cultural superiority and uniformity beneath a mask of citizenship, patriotism, and heritage. Dominant groups are considered culturally appropriate, and minorities are dismissed as culturally inappropriate and incompatible (Fleras, 2014). Racism as an expression of privilege and power is part of the very structure of society and can be defined as any exploitation or process of exclusion that institutionalizes and privileges the dominant group at the expense of others.

Discrimination

Discrimination occurs when individuals or groups of people are denied equality of treatment because of race, ethnicity, gender, or disability and is often viewed as the behavioural counterpart of prejudice that is considered attitudinal. A popular equation summarizes the components of racism: racism = prejudice × discrimination × power (Fleras, 2014). Four levels that demonstrate a continuum of prejudice and discrimination include differential treatment, prejudicial treatment, disadvantageous treatment, and denial of desire. The differential end of the continuum refers to a predisposition to prejudice, and disadvantageous treatment represents blatant discrimination (Racher & Annis, 2007). Differential treatment might include ethnic jokes, while vandalism is disadvantageous treatment. Denial of the desire for equality may be apparent in housing or employment opportunities.

FACILITATORS OF MULTICULTURALISM

Federal, provincial, and local governments as well as organizations, agencies, and individuals take action to promote multiculturalism and integration among people of all cultural groups. Programs and activities that support knowledge exchange and the development of understanding and participation across cultures are valuable resources for health professionals engaged in community practice. Building skills that facilitate knowledge exchange and cultural awareness encourage inclusion and participation and assist in developing projects and initiatives with people from across different cultures.

Government Programs and Policies

In support of the national policy on multiculturalism, programs are offered by federal and provincial governments (Government of Canada, 2015) to provide English and French language education and training, Aboriginal languages maintenance and revitalization, and interpretation and translation services. Young people learn about and share in the cultural diversity of Canada through government-sponsored youth forums and youth exchange programs. Governments offer grants designed to increase access for Canadians to performing, visual, and media arts; museum collections; and heritage displays. Research funding is provided to identify socioeconomic and cultural barriers and to inform the development of policies and practices intended to foster and promote an inclusive society (see Box 11.1).

Critical Thinking Exercise 11.1

Comparing Research Methods and Considering Use of the Findings

Consider the different methods for conducting research on culture and health used in the studies noted in Box 11.1. What are the strengths of each method of data collection? What are some of the limitations? How might the results of each study contribute to the practice of health professionals working with the community and to the health of the community?

Community and Organizational Initiatives

Many communities have multicultural groups and organizations that undertake activities and sponsor events designed to celebrate diversity and promote cultural understanding. For example, *Folklorama,* sponsored for 2 weeks each year by the Folk Art Council of Winnipeg, Manitoba, boasts of being the largest and longest-running multicultural event of its kind in the world, with more than 40 cultural pavilions spread throughout the city (Folk Arts Council of

---

Box 11.1 Studies on Culture and Health Reveal Useful Findings

1. McKeary and Newbold (2010)
   - Capturing the perspectives of recent immigrants and refugees to Canada is critical for ensuring culturally appropriate health and social services. The voices of new Canadians are often not well captured, particularly among refugees. Semistructured, in-depth interviews with health and social service professionals identified systemic barriers encountered by both refugees and service providers. Five recommendations were identified from the interviews to enhance service delivery: increasing interpretation services and ensuring providers have adequate time for appointments requiring translation, enriching the cultural competency of service providers, creating and supporting forums to reduce social isolation of refugees, and increasing knowledge about health insurance coverage available for refugees.
2. Jardine and Furgal (2010)
   - Northern communities pose different contexts for health and social service provisions compared to southern counterparts. The research was designed to be community-based, ensuring research findings are shared with the local communities and integrated into local planning. To enhance the understanding of public perceptions of health risks in northern areas, surveys were conducted in two northern Aboriginal communities. Local community workers delivered questionnaires to residents, allowing participation in local languages. To further the identification of health risks and engage discussions about the risks, residents participated in a Photovoice exercise. This participation allowed residents to take photographs of situations they believed to pose a risk in their community. These methods facilitated trust building between researchers and the community members. The results were utilized to develop additional community-based initiatives to examine risks to health in northern communities.
3. Setia et al. (2011)
   - Arriving in a new country comes with opportunities and challenges that impact quality of life. Given the wide variety of countries from which new immigrants arrive (see Table 11.3), they are bound to adjust to life in Canada in different ways. Data from Statistics Canada's Longitudinal Survey of Immigrants to Canada were examined to identify ways that new immigrants adjust to life in Canada. Adjustments by immigrants to life in Canada differ by sex, marital status, and source country. Women, single immigrants, and immigrants arriving from countries with lower development indices often required more and different health services.

Winnipeg, 2015). First Nations often host cultural events to celebrate and share their cultures through sports competitions, native art festivals, and powwows.

Organizations are striving to be culturally sensitive in reviewing their structures, policies, and practices. For example, the Pan West Community Futures Network (2015) has developed and continues to refine a board training module on cultural awareness. Communities are using such tools as *An Inclusion Lens: Workbook for Looking at Social and Economic Exclusion and Inclusion* (Shookner, 2002) in an effort to foster inclusion and participation of residents through a philosophy of valuing members of all cultures and their contributions.

Professional and Individual Responsibilities

Community practice built on ethical foundations facilitates multiculturalism. The ethical foundations of public health and community practice as discussed in Chapter 3 include inclusion, diversity, participation, empowerment, social justice, advocacy, and interdependence. These ethical foundations facilitate multiculturalism when health professionals incorporate them into the values that underpin their practice and apply them consistently in the work they do. Community health workers must identify and work to redress prejudice, ethnocentrism, stereotyping, racism, and discrimination as barriers to multiculturalism.

Community health workers have a responsibility to encourage and actively support integration and multiculturalism in the organizations that employ them and the agencies and communities with which they work. Community health teams that demonstrate a thirst for knowledge, an open and enduring curiosity, and consummate critical reflection facilitate inclusion and foster respect for the cultures of all Canadians.

Critical Thinking Exercise 11.2

Cultural Sensitivity and Traditional Medicine

In 2014, health practitioners encountered cultural challenges in delivering services to two young First Nations children diagnosed with leukemia. In both instances, the children and their families decided to discontinue the chemotherapy treatment to pursue traditional medicine. In the first case, the McMaster Children's Hospital filed a court motion to have the Children's Aid Society intervene and compel the continuation of the chemotherapy treatment. The Ontario Court of Justice ruled against the motion and stated that Aboriginal people have the right to practice traditional medicine according to the Constitution. This unprecedented ruling created a new dynamic in the culture of care. How do these recent developments influence cultural competence in community practice?

Listen to the CBC Radio's Day 6 program on Cultural Sensitivity related to a situation involving traditional medicine: http://www.cbc.ca/player/AudioMobile/Day+6/ID/2649638393/

COMMUNITY PRACTICE: ATTUNING PRACTICE TO DIVERSITY

Theory that underpins community practice in multicultural environments continues to evolve. There is diversity, and increasing diversity, in health professionals in Canada. Cultural competence, conceptualized as a commendable goal for health professionals, is viewed from an organizational perspective. Cultural attunement, a more recently developed approach, and cultural humility are explored concerning their application in community practice. Both serve to facilitate the ever-changing diversities of Canadian communities.

Cultural Competence in Community Practice

Cultural competence is a common goal sought by health professionals as they work with individuals from cultures that differ from their own. Unlike traditional definitions of cultural competence that function at an individual level, the National Centre for Cultural Competence (NCCC) has developed the *Cultural Competence Continuum* (Goode, 2004) to generate guidelines for achieving cultural competence at a system or organizational level (Pumariega et al., 2005). More recent considerations of cultural competence look at the concept more as a process in addition to an outcome and recognize that achievement is a lifelong struggle. According to the NCCC definition:

Cultural competence requires that organizations:

- Have a defined set of values and principles, and demonstrate behaviours, attitudes, policies, and structures that enable them to work effectively cross-culturally.

TABLE 11.5 Cultural Competence Continuum for Systems and Organizations

Level of Competence	Application
Cultural destructiveness	The organization is characterized by system attitudes, policies, structures, and practices that are destructive to a cultural group.
Cultural incapacity	The organization demonstrates a lack of capacity to respond to needs, interests, and preferences of culturally and linguistically diverse groups.
Cultural blindness	The organization exhibits a philosophy of viewing and treating all people as the same, encourages assimilation, and ignores cultural strengths.
Cultural precompetency	The organization demonstrates awareness within the system of strengths and areas for growth to respond effectively and values the delivery of high-quality services to culturally and linguistically diverse populations. Hiring practices support a diverse workforce.
Cultural competence	The organization demonstrates acceptance and respect for cultural differences; works effectively cross-culturally; values diversity; and advocates for and is culturally sensitive in community engagement that results in reciprocity between all collaborators, partners, and stakeholders.
Cultural proficiency	The organization holds culture in high esteem and uses this foundation to guide all endeavours, including research, organizational practices, knowledge transfer, resource development, employment practices, advocacy, and partnership development.

Adapted from Goode (2004).

- Have the capacity to value diversity, conduct self-assessment, manage the dynamics of difference, acquire and institutionalize cultural knowledge, and adapt to diversity and the cultural contexts of the communities they serve.
- Incorporate the above in all aspects of policy making, administration, practice and service delivery, systematically involve consumers, key stakeholders, and communities (Goode, 2004, p. 1).

Six levels span the *Cultural Competence Continuum* (Table 11.5), from very negative circumstances of cultural destructiveness and cultural incapacity, through cultural blindness and cultural precompetency, to positive circumstances of cultural competence and cultural proficiency. When an organization reaches cultural proficiency, it is seen to hold culture in high esteem and use this perspective as a foundation to guide all of its work: endeavours including practice, research, advocacy, and partnerships. Community health workers have responsibilities and opportunities to influence the agencies and systems within which they work, and the groups and organizations within their community practice, to strive to reach these laudable goals.

Cultural Attunement

Cultural competence can be viewed as content knowledge, as community health workers learn about unique customs, rules, rituals, and norms of specific ethnic groups—the concrete knowledge passed from one generation to the next (Hoskins, 1999; Racher & Annis, 2007). While continuous learning about groups, their beliefs, and customs is important, Hoskins warns about this kind of objectification of groups leading community health workers onto dangerous ground. Not all Chinese people have the same values, beliefs, and experiences, neither do all Pakistani or all First Nations, Métis, or Inuit people. Community health workers, educators, and others must move beyond the superficial knowledge of a culture to seek and consider the personal meanings that individuals ascribe to their own ethnicity. Carefully "attuned" listening is required to understand meaning; "cultural attunement" is a way of "being" in relation to the "other."

Hoskins (1999) encourages movement from content knowledge to relational processes. Out of these relational processes, she offers principles to use "when entering into the spaces between self and other, particularly when they, us, and we, are worlds apart" (p. 77). From her experience as a teacher, she generated five principles to assist people in working toward cultural attunement including:

- Acknowledging the pain of oppression
- Engaging in acts of humility
- Acting with reverence
- Engaging in mutuality
- Maintaining a position of "not knowing"

Acknowledging the Pain of Oppression

Although there are aspects of Canadian history such as Canadian Residential Schools and The Chinese Head Tax and Exclusion Act that many would prefer to deny or forget, acknowledging the pain of oppression is essential. Such misuses of power, often perpetuated through a reluctance to share power, must be acknowledged in order for people to be able to take responsibility for their contributions, seek to grow from them, and change oppressive tendencies. Recognizing that privilege, particularly white privilege, is constantly operating to some degree and creating situations of power imbalance (Chavez et al., 2008) is crucial in honest communication that builds trust and respect.

Engaging in Acts of Humility

Humility is an act of control, restraint, temperance, and modesty. Community health workers strive to resist the inclination to privilege their own cultures, their own perspectives in their work. Hoskins (1999) challenges those who seek to achieve cultural attunement to engage in acts of humility. She challenges them to allow themselves to be vulnerable in reaching into the space between self and other, although that effort may not be well received by those who have been marginalized by the dominant culture. She urges those who work across cultures to recognize that reaching toward others without a guarantee of reciprocity requires courage and willingness to abandon a position of social comfort. Reaching forward effectively requires acquiescence to the other and surrender of cultural perspectives, biases, and expectations of specific behaviour.

Acting With Reverence

Respect for difference is a common quality espoused by health professionals. Hoskins (1999) argues that movement beyond acting with respect for difference (which implies judgment) to acting with reverence, honour, and regard is preferred. "Homage can be paid to courageous lives, and people's initiatives to fight poverty, sexism, and racism can be honoured and discussed. Reverence can be lived, modeled, and taught so that when differences arise a deeply felt sense of awe moves one beyond basic 'respect for difference' to nurture souls and spirits" (p. 80).

Engaging in Mutuality

When similarities are shared in the development of a relationship, feelings of connection emerge. Kirkham (2003) found that seeking common ground and emphasizing shared humanity were common practices used by nurses in intergroup interactions. Engaging in mutuality, identifying similarities, and sharing likenesses from one's own world are effective in building connections and establishing meaningful relationships. These meaningful relationships become the foundations on which partnerships are developed and groups work together to achieve mutually determined outcomes. Connections through difference can thus become the ideal that shapes a revisioning of intergroup relationships.

Maintaining a Position of "Not Knowing"

Cultural competence often conjures up visions of knowing, competency, proficiency, and mastery. Such is not the case with culture (Chavez et al., 2008). Assumptions of knowing can lead to decreased efforts to learn. Rather, effective learning in relationships is facilitated when coming from a place of "not knowing." Abandoning a desire for certainty, closure, and control in relationships and replacing it with efforts to be tentative, experimental, and open-ended is useful in community practice. The desire "to learn" and "to understand" replaces the desire "to know" and "be proficient." Competence may also be problematic if it implies that certain skills can be learned in order to deal with certain situations. Building bridges to connect diverse worlds is not merely a set of strategies but is an all encompassing "way of being" that comes from an ethic of care, an ethic of cultural attunement (Hoskins, 1999). The most critical role of the community health worker is that of learner: learner seeking to gain understanding when working with community members to facilitate change (Gutierrez & Lewis, 2012).

 Critical Thinking Exercise 11.3

Applying the Principles for Working Toward Cultural Attunement

Consider the five principles for working toward cultural attunement as discussed in the previous section. Can you identify examples of situations where these principles were being applied? Can you identify situations where the principles were not applied but may have been useful had they been applied? How might use of these principles contribute to your practice?

Cultural Humility

Minkler (2012) contributes to this dialogue on cultural attunement with a definition and discussion of "cultural humility" and its application at the community level. She defines cultural humility as a lifelong commitment to self-evaluation and self-critique to redress power imbalances and develop and maintain mutually respectful and dynamic partnerships with communities. She challenges those who work with communities to recognize and confront the many courses of white privilege and invisible systems of conferring dominance. Minkler suggests that although community health workers can never become truly competent in another's culture, demonstrating humility in one's outsider status, along with openness to learning and making one's best effort, can be quite effective in cross-ethnic group interactions. Based on their experiences in the healthy neighbourhood program, Ellis and Walton (2012) learned a key capacity of community health workers is the ability "to suspend beliefs long enough to hear and accept the truth of another" (p. 134). Building culturally sensitive relationships of mutual respect and trust is essential before becoming immersed in collaborative planning and decision making related to community initiatives. Refer to Box 11.2 for touchstones of working with diverse communities.

Box 11.2 Touchstones for Working With Diverse Communities

- *Reframing cultural diversity as a benefit* and understanding the multiple and varied cultural contributions to community and society decreases the potency and counters the negative conceptualization of cultural diversity.
- *Creating spaces for voices to be heard and groups to be represented* produces opportunities to break down resistance and facilitate social change. Community health workers have both opportunity and responsibility to take action in creating such spaces.
- *Understanding concepts of health, health practices, and health promotion used by different cultures* expands the knowledge base of community health workers. Sharing knowledge across cultures creates a foundation for new ideas and the evolution of effective strategies to achieve and sustain health.
- *Community health workers have the responsibility to facilitate alliances and partnerships across different cultures* in order to develop needed programs, confront exclusionary practices and marginalization, and advocate for integration and the promotion of full participation by all cultural groups in the larger society.
- *Effective community practice requires the ability to differentiate* between (1) facilitating discussion between people with diverse perspectives to reach a single outcome and (2) facilitating acceptance of multiple different cultural perspectives within an inclusive framework so that outcomes do not require the relinquishing of cultural ideologies by participants nor do they privilege one culture over another.
- *Knowledge of language is necessary but is not sufficient* for effective communication; community health teams have the opportunity to develop programs that involve interpreters who have knowledge of language and culture rather than translators of language only.
- *Community health teams working with Aboriginal communities need to share their experiential learning,* speak about their work, and publish it. The capacity of community health workers to facilitate and support change is growing; education and training to support work with Aboriginal communities is early in its development, and advocacy for its extension is pivotal.
- *Examining the cultural awareness and sensitivity of organizations* within the health care system and beyond offers opportunity for change and growth. Recognizing democratic racism, action from positions of exclusion, or unequal power relations within systems are important step toward change. Self-assessment by organizations builds organizational commitment to be inclusive, open, and progressive in meeting the needs of clients from different cultures. Community health workers are advocates and resources for this work.
- *Effective, committed community health workers examine their cultural attunement and humility;* grow as lifelong learners and reflective practitioners; and critically determine how they chose "to be" in their relationships with individuals, groups, and communities of multiple cultures.

Summary

Embracing the value of diverse cultures, along with the perspectives and insights they generate, builds new ways to achieve social change and community well-being. Capacity building, civic engagement, inclusion, and participation are keys to health promotion and social transformation within communities. The lens through which individuals, organizations, and communities see each other informs their response to health and social problems as well as their action in building community.

Cultural pluralism, as it honours culture and diversity, generates the cultural mosaic that is Canada. Multiculturalism acknowledges and promotes diversity as legitimate and integral to the composition of the country. Discussion of prejudice, racism, and discrimination opens a dialogue that encourages community health workers to expand their thinking as they extend their work to community and the broader society.

In response to this open dialogue, an increasing number of community organizations are striving to establish processes of cultural competence and proficiency, while more community health workers are seeking cultural attunement and humility. Social change is becoming more apparent as health professionals grow in their emphasis of shared humanity and reverence for cultural diversity. Community health workers are pursuing new visions of intergroup relationships and building bridges to connect diverse worlds. For more and more community health workers, cultural attunement and cultural humility are becoming an encompassing "way of being" situated within the ethic of a caring community practice. Interpreting culture is not sufficient in community practice; one's practice must change to fit the diversity.

REFERENCES

Berry, J. W. (1991). *Sociopsychological costs and benefits of multiculturalism* (Working Paper No. 24). Ottawa: Economic Council of Canada.

Birx, H. J. (2006). *Encyclopedia of anthropology.* Thousand Oaks, CA: Sage.

Chavez, V., Duran, B., Baker, Q. E., Avila, M. M., & Wallerstein, N. (2008). The dance of race and privilege in community based participatory research. In M. Minkler & N. Wallerstein (Eds.), *Community-based participatory research for health: From process to outcomes* (2nd ed., pp. 91–106). San Francisco: Jossey-Bass.

Citizenship and Immigration Canada. (2014). *Facts and figures 2013—Immigration overview: Permanent residents.* URL=http://www.cic.gc.ca/english/resources/statistics/facts2013/index. asp

Dewing, M. (2013). *Canadian multiculturalism* (Background paper). Ottawa: Library of Parliament. URL=http://www.parl.gc.ca/Content/LOP/ResearchPublications/2009-20-e.pdf

Driedger, L. (2003). *Race and ethnicity: Finding identities and equalities* (2nd ed.). Don Mills, ON: Oxford University Press.

Ellis, G., & Walton, S. (2012). Building partnerships between local health departments and communities: Case studies in capacity building and cultural humility. In M. Minkler (Ed.): *Community organizing and community building for health* (3rd ed., pp. 130–152). New Brunswick, NJ: Rutgers University Press.

Fleras, A. (2014). *Racisms in a multicultural Canada: Paradoxes, politics, and resistance.* Waterloo: Wilfred Laurier University Press.

Folk Arts Council of Winnipeg. (2015). *Folklorama.* URL=http://www.folklorama.ca

Goode, T. D. (2004). *Cultural competence continuum.* Washington: National Centre for Cultural Competence. URL=http://cssr.berkeley.edu/cwscmsreports/LatinoPracticeAdvisory/Cultural%20Competence%20Continuum.pdf

Government of Canada. (2015). *Culture, history & sport.* URL=http://www.canada.ca/en/services/culture

Gustafson, D. (2005). Transcultural nursing theory from a critical cultural perspective. *Advances in Nursing Science, 28*, 2–16.

Gutierrez, L. M., & Lewis, E. A. (2012). Education, participation, and capacity building in community organizing with women of color. In M. Minkler (Ed.), *Community organizing and community building for health* (3rd ed., pp. 215–228). New Brunswick, NJ: Rutgers University Press.

Hoskins, M. L. (1999). Worlds apart and lives together: Developing cultural attunement. *Child and Youth Care Forum, 28*, 73–85.

Jardine, C., & Furgal, C. (2010). Knowledge translation with northern Aboriginal communities: A case study. *Canadian Journal of Nursing Research, 42*(1), 119–127.

Kirkham, S. (2003). The politics of belonging and intercultural health care. *Western Journal of Nursing Research, 25*, 762–780.

McKeary, M., & Newbold, B. (2010). Barriers to care: The challenge for Canadian refugees and their health care providers. *Journal of Refugee Studies, 23*, 523–545.

Minkler, M. (2012). Introduction to community organizing and community building. In *Community organizing and community building for health* (3rd ed., pp. 5–26). New Brunswick, NJ: Rutgers University Press.

Pan West Community Futures Network. (2015). *Welcome to Community Futures Leadership Institute: Module contents: Module 9: Cultural awareness.* URL=http://cfleadershipinstitute.ca/bd/module-contents.php

Pumariega, A. J., Rogers, K., & Rothe, E. (2005). Culturally competent systems of care for children's mental health: Advances and challenges. *Community Mental Health Journal, 41*, 539–555.

Racher, F., & Annis, R. (2007). Respecting culture and honouring diversity in community practice. *Research and Theory for Nursing Practice, 21*, 255–270.

Setia, M., Lynch, J., Abrahamowicz, M., Tousignant, P., & Quesnel-Valle, A. (2011). Self-rated health in Canadian immigrants: Analysis of the Longitudinal Survey of Immigrants to Canada. *Health & Place, 17*, 658–670.

Shookner, M. (2002). *An inclusion lens: Workbook for looking at social and economic exclusion and inclusion.* Halifax: Health Canada, Population and Public Health Branch.

Statistics Canada. (2013a). *Canada (Code 01) (table). National Household Survey (NHS) Profile. 2011 National Household Survey. Statistics Canada Catalogue no. 99–004–XWE.* Ottawa. URL=http://www12.statcan.gc.ca/nhs-enm/2011/dp-pd/prof/index.cfm?Lang=E

Statistics Canada. (2013b). *Aboriginal peoples in Canada: First Nations people, Métis, and Inuit.* National Household Survey, 2011. Ottawa: Author. URL=http://www12.statcan.gc.ca/nhs-enm/2011/as-sa/99–011-x/99–011-x2011001-eng.pdf

Statistics Canada. (2013c). *Immigration and ethnocultural diversity in Canada.* National Household Survey, 2011. Ottawa: Author. URL=http://www12.statcan.gc.ca/nhs-enm/2011/as-sa/99–010-x/99–010-x2011001-eng.pdf

Trudeau, P. E. (1971). *Federal government's response to Book IV of the Royal Commission on Bilingualism.* Ottawa: House of Commons.

ONLINE RESOURCES

Please visit thePoint at http://thepoint.lww.com/Vollman4e for up-to-date Internet resources and additional learning materials on this topic.

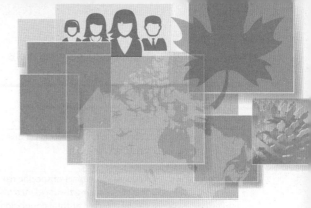

CHAPTER *12*

Population Health Action: Prevention and Harm Reduction

Nancy C. McPherson, Kathy L. Belton, and Gaynor Watson-Creed

LEARNING OBJECTIVES

After studying this chapter, you should be able to:

1. Describe the differences between levels of prevention and levels of care

2. Define primordial prevention

3. Discuss the application of primordial prevention to the determinants of health

4. Apply injury prevention theory to community health practice

5. Define the key principles of harm reduction and apply them to community health practice

Introduction

The leading causes of death and disability in Canada are chronic diseases. Four main risk factors that contribute to chronic disease are unhealthy diets, lack of physical activity, tobacco, and alcohol use. Addressing these risk factors through preventive action can reduce the incidence of disease, delay onset, and offer more disability-free years to people's lives. In addition, preventable injuries (e.g., falls, motor vehicle crashes, poisoning, burns) are leading causes of morbidity and mortality among children and youth. Environmental risks, communicable diseases, and occupational health and safety risks are similarly preventable. This chapter focuses on prevention: levels of prevention for disease and injury, injury prevention theory and practice, and harm reduction. Levels of care are introduced along with policy implications in prevention action.

PREVENTION AND CARE

Public health systems exist to prevent or reduce the occurrence of disease in populations. The conceptualization of prevention activities has been evolving since the 1940s (Leavell & Clark, 1965). Over the ensuing years, modifications to the concepts have been proposed, and more

157

TABLE 12.1 Levels of Prevention

Level of Prevention	Description	Example
Primordial Prevention	Prevention of risk factors for disease from existing	Removal of access to tobacco products and environmental tobacco smoke from public venues
Primary Prevention	Reduces the impact of specific risk factors, thereby reducing the incidence of disease, and can be directed at total populations, selected groups, or even healthy individuals	Protection of health by personal and communal efforts, such as enhancing nutritional status, immunizing against communicable diseases, smoking cessation, and reducing environmental risks
Secondary Prevention	Reduces the prevalence of disease by shortening its duration, and are directed at high-risk individuals not yet accessing health care, or at patients already receiving care	Screening programs for early detection and prompt intervention to control disease and minimize disability
Tertiary Prevention	Reduces the impact of long-term disease and disability by eliminating or reducing impairment, minimizing suffering, and maximizing potential years of useful life	Rehabilitation expertise aimed at people with advanced disease
Quaternary Prevention	Identifies people at risk of medical mishaps (e.g., over-medicalization), protects from new medical treatments that are untested, and suggests interventions that are ethically acceptable	Quality assurance in health care programs that ensure patient safety and best practices

continue to emerge (Frieden, 2010). The core concepts outlining three levels of prevention (primary, secondary and tertiary) are now well described in population health literature (Katz & Ali, 2009; Association of Faculties of Medicine of Canada [AFMC], 2015). A fourth level of prevention—quaternary—has been added more recently and we suggest that a fifth level—primordial prevention—be added as well, as illustrated in Table 12.1.

Effective prevention efforts require detailed understanding of the risk factors that precede the development of health issues. If risk factors are understood, the prevention effort is enhanced, and it becomes easier to reduce the risk of disease occurrence. Consider, for example, childhood obesity. If a risk factor for obesity is poor nutrition, perhaps in the form of a high-fat and high-sugar diet, then dietary advice to lower excessive caloric intake, and even the prescription of a specific diet, become appropriate secondary preventive interventions for the already obese patient (i.e., preventing serious damage from obesity), and also appropriate primary prevention for the patient who is not yet obese and wishes to avoid becoming so. But there are larger population health questions that emerge as one considers this example.

- What are the risk factors for the *existence* of high-fat high-sugar diets?
- Where do such diets come from in the first place?

These questions become answerable by examining primordial prevention. Primordial prevention is best defined as preventing risk factors for disease from even existing (Strasser, 1978). As such, primordial prevention is frequently aimed at whole populations and requires the use of comprehensive health promotion tools, most notably policy development tools. It can therefore be regarded as even more proactive (i.e., upstream) than primary prevention (Fig. 12.1). Many public health practitioners specifically employ primordial prevention, rather than—or in addition to—primary prevention strategies.

There exists some confusion between the concepts of levels of prevention and levels of care. Levels of care refer to the mix of health human resources (i.e., family physicians, specialist and subspecialist physicians, advanced practice nurses, allied health professionals, etc.) operating within a given care setting (Table 12.2).

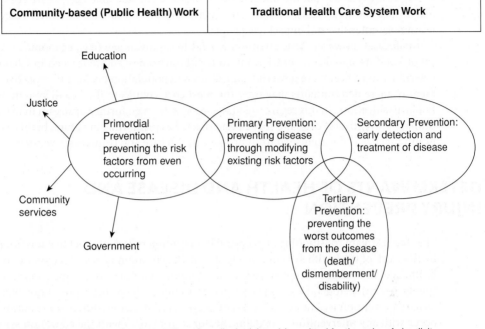

Note: Quaternary Prevention (prevention of medical mishaps) is omitted for the sake of simplicity.

FIGURE 12.1   Primordial prevention and the public health sector in relation to the traditional health care system.

Primary care and primary health care systems (e.g., community health centres and public health clinics that incorporate the primary level of care with the determinants of health) are the main deliverers of primary prevention strategies in the Canadian health system. Strategies for primary prevention of disease employed at this level of the system include health promotion strategies as well as provision of primary prevention interventions (e.g., immunization, tobacco cessation) and advocacy efforts toward supportive environments for health and health equity.

Over the past decade, there has been an appropriate shifting of health care efforts and resources to primary prevention, and thus to primary health care reform, in an attempt to reduce the incidence of disease and corresponding health system costs. Primary prevention has broader potential than secondary or tertiary prevention to promote health and avoid negative impacts on population health as well as to minimize health system use and costs. Secondary prevention

TABLE 12.2 Levels of Care

Level of Care	Description	Example
Primary care	First point of contact with the health system—health promotion, illness prevention, screening, early detection, diagnosis and treatment	Providers include community-based physicians, nurse practitioners, nutritionists, physiotherapists, etc.
Secondary care	Treatment and care provision during an illness episode or injury	Hospital- or specialty clinic-based providers that include specialist physicians/surgeons, advanced practice nurses, pharmacists
Tertiary care	Highly specialized and high tech "state of the art" care provided in centralized teaching hospitals	Focused care settings provided through subspecialists (e.g., cancer centres, pediatric hospitals, trauma centres)

strategies are effective but are understood to produce considerable health care costs (e.g., for diagnostics and treatment). Tertiary and quaternary prevention are extremely resource- and technology-intensive and impact few people.

In all cases, however, little attention is paid to disadvantage (e.g., economic, social, education) and its significant contribution to health outcomes. As we learned in Chapter 1, the determinants of health are powerful contributors to population health and proactive management of these determinants may offer the *most* cost savings to the health system over time. Public health efforts in this regard are understood to be even further upstream than traditional primary prevention efforts, and so are best reflected as primordial in nature. In this way, public health practice is distinguished from primary health care and primary prevention strategies.

DETERMINANTS OF HEALTH AND DISEASE AND INJURY PREVENTION

The "far upstream" positioning of primordial prevention reflects the fact that it is not necessarily the work of the health system (see Fig. 12.1). The community-based sector and traditional health system work is conceptualized as a continuum, with the work of the community-based (public health) sector addressing primordial and some of the primary prevention efforts. Quaternary prevention touches on all levels of prevention in that it addresses the harms that can occur with any intervention. The public health sector works with the education system (e.g., school boards), justice system (e.g., police departments, courts), government (e.g., municipal government planning departments), and other governmental and nongovernmental social services (e.g., social welfare, employment) to address upstream issues that can have a downstream effect on health. Using the example of childhood obesity, the availability of high-fat high-sugar foods is related to policies such as municipal zoning policies and provincial and federal regulations. For instance, municipalities with limited lot sizes may favour fast food restaurants with small footprints over larger grocery stores; provincial and federal regulations do not limit the amounts of sugars and fats in foods; and advertisers are not restricted in promoting nutrient-poor foods to vulnerable populations. It becomes evident that the root causes of the "high-fat high-sugar" diet are rooted in sociopolitical and environmental systems and determinants of health that are well outside the control of the health system (see Chapter 1, Table 1.3). What is most notable about the determinants is that the health system is recognized as only *one* of the determinants contributing to health. In 2009, a Canadian Senate report defined that only 25% of health outcomes can be attributed to the health system, regardless of the size of financial investment into the system (Senate Subcommittee on Population Health, 2009).

Despite understanding the determinants of health as root causes of mortality and morbidity at a population level, the concept of primordial prevention has not been well described or well accessed by public health workers. This deficit may be attributed to the concern that any work that exists outside of the direct influence of the health system (i.e., service delivery) is difficult to access or manage. Primordial prevention efforts require the sharing of work with multisectoral nonhealth actors that the public health sector is well suited to do.

PUBLIC POLICY AND PREVENTION

Public health practice has been described as existing at the intersection between societal attitudes, government policy, and people's lives (Falk-Rafael, 2005). To exist in that realm effectively requires public health to do a few things, including to know the other actors who are present in the policy realm and to have data regarding health outcomes, antecedent determinants, and risk factors where possible. By using these data to expose impacts that large social

---

Box 12.1 Jason's Story

Why is Jason in the hospital?
Because he has a bad infection in his leg.

But why does he have an infection?
Because he has a cut on his leg and it got infected.

But why does he have a cut on his leg?
Because he was playing on a poorly maintained playground next to his apartment building and there was some sharp broken edges there that he fell on.

But why was he playing on a playground with old, broken equipment?
Because his neighbourhood is kind of run down. A lot of kids play there and there is no one to supervise them.

But why does he live in that neighbourhood?
Because his parents can't afford a nicer place to live.

But why can't his parents afford a nicer place to live?
Because his Dad is unemployed and his Mom is sick.

But why is his Dad unemployed?
Because he doesn't have much education and he can't find a job.

But why...?

Source: © All rights reserved. *Toward a Health Future: Second Report on the Health of Canadians, Public Health Agency of Canada, 1999.* Adapted and reproduced with permission from the Minister of Health, 2015.

---

systems (e.g., education, justice) in communities have on health, the public health sector can effectively advocate for the changes in those systems so that positive health outcomes can occur. The systematic and iterative inquiry undertaken by the public health sector to expose outcomes, risk factors, and policy opportunities is often exemplified in the telling of "Jason's Story" (Box 12.1).

Several excellent examples of how the public health sector undertakes asking the "why" questions can be found in practice. One such Canadian example is the national Enhanced Street Youth Surveillance project (ESYS), hosted by the Public Health Agency of Canada (PHAC). This longitudinal survey examines the prevalence of sexually transmitted and blood borne infections (STBBI) in street-involved youth, and then works with those youth through detailed interviews to uncover first the risk factors for infection, and second the risk factors for their initial street involvement (PHAC, 2006). The stories uncovered by the study often highlight the need for changes to systems of education and justice, among others, but not necessarily to the health system, to help prevent street involvement in the first place, as well as to prevent its health-related outcomes. This information can be shared with those other systems, especially at the local public health level, for their review and ultimately for their reform.

The skill sets and strategies deployed by those working in primordial prevention include action on policy development and reform, advocacy, and evaluation. By being available to public (nonhealth) policy discussions, community health workers can ensure that the impacts of public policies on health are not missed (see Chapter 9). Primary prevention of disease and injury, through management of risk factors, also includes public health, health promotion, and primary health care service delivery efforts based on the knowledge of the determinants of health as an important context for prevention of disease in individuals, families, aggregates, and communities.

Critical Thinking Exercise 12.1

Levels of Prevention

- Review "Jason's Story".
- What elements of Jason's Story could be managed by tertiary prevention? Where would that occur? What elements of Jason's Story could be managed by secondary prevention? Where would that occur? What elements of Jason's Story could be managed by primary prevention? Where would that occur? What elements of Jason's Story could be managed by primordial prevention? Where would that occur?

INJURY PREVENTION IN CANADA

Injury prevention in Canada has a strong foundation and a vibrant future. In 2012, four national organizations—Safe Communities Canada, Safe Kids Canada, SMARTRISK, and ThinkFirst Canada—amalgamated to provide a unified national voice for injury prevention in Canada: *Parachute*.

Injury is often called a silent epidemic in Canada. This lack of recognition stems from a universal misconception that injuries are "just accidents," or that they are the result of a simple cause and effect relationship such as risk taking or poor judgement. But injuries are not accidents; 90% of the time injuries can be predicted and therefore prevented (Parachute, 2015).

Canada has made some progress in decreasing the burden of injury over the past twenty years; the overall injury mortality rate from 1990 to 2010 decreased from 47.3 to 40.5 per 100,000 population. Over the same time period, Canada has also seen substantial declines in the motor vehicle death rate from 13.2 to 6.4 per 100,000 population and in the suicide rate from 12.4 to 10.9 per 100,000 population. Despite this progress, the injury rate associated with falls and unintentional poisonings continues to rise, increasing from 4.5 to 8.2 per 100,000 population and from 2.1 to 4.3 per 100,000 population, respectively. As a result, injury remains one of the largest public health issues that Canada faces and is a major burden to the health care system (Parachute, 2015).

Defining Injury

Injury is defined as bodily harm resulting from a sudden transfer of energy that exceeds the human body's capacity for resistance or from the absence of energy essentials such as heat and oxygen. The energy transferred is most often mechanical or kinetic (e.g., fracture from a fall), but it may also be thermal (e.g., burn), electrical (e.g., electrocution), chemical (e.g., intoxication), or radiant (e.g., sunburn). Injuries can also be the result of a sudden loss of energy or vital element (e.g., frostbite, drowning, strangulation) (Lavoie et al., 2014). Injuries are further classified as intentional or unintentional. Intentional injuries are injuries that are deliberate such as violence and self-harm. Unintentional injuries are those that occur without intent to do bodily harm such as motor vehicle crashes and falls.

Injury Prevention Theory

The theory of injury prevention originates mainly from the work of four researchers: Hugh DeHaven, John Gordon, James Gibson, and William Haddon and recognizes that injuries are associated with human behaviour within an environment (Waller, 1989). DeHaven, in 1942, studied cases in which persons fell 15–45 meters without sustaining serious injury, discerning that injuries could be reduced by distributing energy across the body (Waller, 1989). His discovery led to engineering designs that prevented or modified energy exchange, such as seat belts, dashboard padding, automobile crush zones, and bicycle helmets. Seven years later, Gordon suggested that injuries, like classic diseases, could be explained through the epidemiologic triad of host, agent, and environment (Waller, 1989) (see Chapter 4, Fig. 4.1). The host is the person or people to whom an injury happens; the agent is the object that transfers energy and causes the injury; and the environment includes all the physical, social, and economic factors that surround the injury event. There must be interaction between all three components of the triangle for an injury to occur. For example, in the case of an inexperienced driver (host), an icy road (environment), and summer tires on the motor vehicle (agent), you complete the triangle, meaning that all the factors are present, and there is potential for a collision causing injury to the driver, passengers, or others (e.g., pedestrians, drivers/passengers in other vehicles). If we change a factor, for example effectively plowing/salting roadways or having snow tires on the car, the risk to which the driver is exposed is reduced.

Gordon also noted that injuries—as other diseases—can be characterized by epidemic episodes, seasonal variation, long-term trends, and demographic distribution (Waller, 1989). In 1961, Gibson, an experimental psychologist, applied traditional epidemiologic methods to the study of injuries and concluded that injuries to a living organism can be produced only by some form of energy exchange (Waller, 1989). His work helped clarify the energy transfer theory of injury causation, the basis for how injury is defined today. Haddon, an engineer and public health physician—and often considered the father of modern injury epidemiology—extended Gibson's work to the development of preventative approaches and offered a framework for understanding injury events and determining strategies for prevention (Waller, 1989).

The Haddon Matrix

The Haddon Matrix is a two-dimensional phase-factor matrix to help conceptualize an injury event (Runyan, 1998). The first dimension comprises the three factors influencing injury: host, agent, and environment. The second dimension is the injury phase divided into pre-event, event, and post-event. By using the Haddon Matrix we can analyze an injury event by the influencing factors over time, which makes it possible to identify factors related to the host, agent, and environment within the phases before, during, and after the event that might be explanatory and contribute to injury prevention strategies.

The pre-event phase is prior to an injury event and includes all factors that determine whether the event will occur. The event phase captures an event as it happens and includes all factors that determine whether an injury will result from an event. The post-event phase occurs following an injury event and includes all factors that determine the extent of injury.

Runyan (1998) adds a third dimension to the model to assist with prevention decision-making (Fig. 12.2). This dimension includes criteria such as equity, cost, stigmatization, freedom, feasibility, preferences, and effectiveness.

We present an example of a completed two-dimensional Haddon Matrix in Table 12.3. The value of the matrix is the identification of factors—not making sure that they are accounted for in the correct box. And while any factor in the Haddon Matrix can be targeted for intervention, some may be easier and more effectively targeted than others.

Haddon's assertion that injury prevention depends on the control of energy shifted the focus of injury research from behavioural psychology to engineering and epidemiology. In the context of impeding energy transfer during the phases of an injury event, Haddon developed ten injury countermeasures (see Box 12.2).

The ten injury countermeasures are not intended as a formula for injury prevention interventions; they provide a framework to examine possible interventions logically and systematically. A

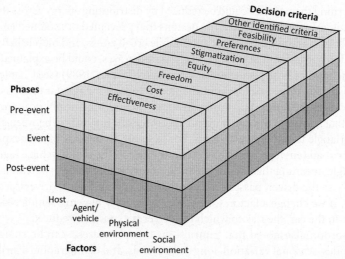

FIGURE 12.2   The three-dimensional Haddon Matrix. (Adapted by permission from BMJ Publishing Group Limited. Runyan, C. W. (1998). Using the Haddon Matrix: Introducing the third dimension. *Injury Prevention, 4,* 302–307.)

guiding principle of injury prevention is that effective injury prevention relies on a combination of intervention strategies. Using a mixture of strategies will broaden prevention efforts across all phases of the injury event and look beyond human behaviour to energy agent and environmental factors. Intervening successfully in injury prevention most often involves a combination of the four E's—*Education* for behaviour change, *Engineering* and technology to make the healthy choice

TABLE 12.3   The Haddon Matrix: An Example

	Person	**Cause**		
	Preschool Child	*Chemical Energy Medication*	**Environment: Physical**	**Environment: Social**
Pre-Event *Will the poisoning occur?*	Age Sex Skill level of child	Type of medication Amount of medication available	Was the medication within reach? Where is medication stored (in a purse or briefcase?) Type of container (blister pack versus bottle)?	What is the caregiver's knowledge regarding the effectiveness of "child resistant" packaging? Manufacturer packaging and standards Pharmacy disposal programs
Event *Will injury occur as a result of the poisoning?*	Age Health of child Physical size (weight)	Type and amount of medication consumed (adult vs. pediatric dose, liquid vs. solid) Tablets coated or not Size of pill Taste of medication	Was ingestion witnessed? Was child supervised? How long was the child unattended?	Does caregiver recognize that poisoning has occurred? Proximity and type of supervision
Post-Event *What will be the outcome?*	Age Health of child Physical size (weight)	Can the medication's effects be reversed or treated? Did level of medication in bloodstream remain at toxic levels after initial assessment and treatment?	Proximity of medical care EMS response time Access to telephone Access to acute care Medical staff knowledge of how to treat poisoning in children	Knowledge caregiver has regarding what to do in an emergency situation Access to 911, Poison Centre, toll free help line Level of public awareness

Source: Pike et al. (2015), Chapter 2.4.

Box 12.2 Haddon's Ten Countermeasures and Examples

Pre-Event (Primordial and Primary Prevention)

1. Prevent the creation of the hazard

   For example, ban the manufacture of wheeled baby walkers; ban three-wheeled all-terrain vehicles

2. Prevent the release of the hazard

   For example, prevent the sale of wheeled baby walkers; introduce graduated drivers licences

3. Separate the person and hazard in time or space

   For example, implement segregated cycle lanes; locate high volume roadways away from residential neighbourhoods

4. Place a barrier between the person and hazard

   For example, implement mandatory four-sided pool fencing; create safety guards on work-related machinery

Event (Secondary Prevention)

5. Reduce the amount of the hazard

   For example, reduce speed limits; decrease water temperatures on hot water tanks

6. Modify the rate or spatial distribution of the hazard

   For example, bicycle helmets; blister packaging for medication; seat belts; air bags

7. Modify the basic qualities of the hazard

   For example, implement energy absorbing surfacing in playgrounds; replace roadway lighting infrastructure with breakaway light poles

8. Strengthen the resistance to the hazard

   For example, implement a warm-up program for sport and recreational participation; implement standards with building and fire codes

Post-Event (Tertiary Prevention)

9. Begin to counter the damage already done by the hazard

   For example, install smoke detectors; provide rapid treatment such as first aid

10. Stabilize, repair, and rehabilitate the object of the damage

    For example, provide/have access to emergency medical facilities; acute care and rehabilitation facilities

Source: Christoffel and Gallagher (2006).

---

the easy choice, *Enactment* of legislation, and *Enforcement* to penalize noncompliance. A good example of these four interventions can be seen in child vehicle restraints. In Canada, legislation was enacted that requires children below the age of four to be restrained in approved child safety seats. The child safety seat is an engineering countermeasure that is proven effective when used properly. Parent education is needed to ensure that the child safety seat is used consistently and properly. Fines penalize those that are not in compliance with the law.

Take Note

The Haddon Matrix is a useful framework to plan prevention intervention strategies for many risks associated with injury. There are several examples of the Haddon Matrix related to childhood injuries including burns, falls, and playground safety on the Parachute website: http://www.parachutecanada.org/child-injury-prevention

Injury prevention countermeasures are often hidden from everyday view, for example, collapsible steering columns in motor vehicles and automatic fire sprinkler systems in public places. These "passive" measures protect us automatically without requiring any action on our part. "Active" measures require some protective action by the person, such as wearing helmets for biking and using seatbelts in vehicles.

There has been tremendous growth in the number of people and organizations focused on injury prevention that has led to an increase in the knowledge base of Canadian research and evidence-informed injury prevention practice. In 2015, *Parachute,* in collaboration with Canada's longstanding network in injury prevention—the Canadian Collaborating Centres for Injury Prevention—and over 60 authors, published the first Canadian resource on injury prevention. This online resource provides a more in-depth examination of injury prevention theory and practice (Pike et al., 2015).

Critical Thinking Exercise 12.2

Levels of Prevention and Haddon's Matrix

- Measles afflicted many people, primarily children, before the measles vaccine became licensed in 1963. Based on related epidemiologic and public health activities, use the levels of prevention and discuss how these apply to measles.
- How could you use Haddon's Matrix to guide the development of a prevention program for measles? What other models might be applicable?

HARM REDUCTION

Harm reduction is a practical approach aimed at reducing or minimizing the adverse consequences associated with high-risk behaviours. According to the International Harm Reduction Association (IHRA, 2010), "Harm reduction refers to policies, programmes and practices that aim primarily to reduce the adverse health, social and economic consequences of the use of legal and illegal psychoactive drugs without necessarily reducing drug consumption" (p. 1).

The harm reduction movement began in the Netherlands and the United Kingdom in the 1970s as a more compassionate approach to support for individuals engaged in illicit drug use rather than traditional punitive tactics through law enforcement. In the mid-1980s, harm reduction was embraced on a large scale in the UK for the first time. The emergence of a heroin epidemic in Liverpool and surrounding area including Merseyside and Cheshire led to the development of the Mersey Model of Harm Reduction. This model focused on the delivery of user-friendly and nonjudgemental services, including needle exchange programs that were attractive to drug users. Three guiding principles formed the basis for the model: initiate contact with the entire population at risk; maintain contact with the drug users in an effort to influence their behaviour; and support changes in their high-risk behaviour (Ashton & Seymour, 2010). The success of the Mersey Model of Harm Reduction was a catalyst for international reform through the development and acceptance of harm reduction in the UK, Europe, North America, and Australia.

The HIV crisis that escalated through the 1990s, particularly among injecting drug users, resulted in harm reduction becoming a global social movement (Lee et al., 2011; McKeganey, 2011). The focus of governments shifted from perceiving drug use as a criminal justice issue based on the illegal nature of the activity to a public health threat for injecting drug users and the wider population that doesn't use drugs. "Preventing the physical disease of AIDS has now been given priority over concerns of drug problems. In this paradigm, prevention takes on a new meaning—the key prevention task is not the prevention of drug use, but the prevention of HIV infections and transmission" (Stimson, 1990 as cited in McKeganey, 2011, p. 180).

Box 12.3 Everyday Harm Reduction

You have a meeting two hours away from your home tomorrow morning. Your risk reduction strategies are:

1. Make sure the car is full of gas
2. Listen to the road report to assess travel conditions
3. Set the alarm clock to allow enough time for travel

The next morning, you ignore your alarm and oversleep. Your compensatory plan of action is to exceed the highway speed limit in order to reach your destination on time, thus engaging in a higher risk activity. Your risk reduction strategies will include:

1. Before leaving home, text a colleague to alert the committee that you may be late
2. Wear a seatbelt
3. Choose a different route to access a highway with a passing lane
4. Reduce your speed in areas with frequent police radar and deer crossings

To exceed the highway speed limit in an effort to arrive at the meeting on time is an informed decision with associated risks. The strategies used to mitigate those risks illustrate a harm reduction approach to an everyday problem.

Harm reduction is a practical response that focuses on the harms associated with high-risk behaviour, rather than on the behaviour itself. Although the concept of harm reduction is most often associated with illicit drug use, many harm reduction initiatives have been incorporated into conventional public health programs such as sexual health clinics and safer drinking campaigns for youth. Harm reduction efforts are also supported by legislation at federal, provincial, and municipal levels such as seatbelt and bicycle helmet laws and smoking bans in public places to reduce exposure to second-hand smoke (Canadian Nurses Association [CNA], 2011). Harm reduction offers an effective approach to disease and injury prevention because the immediate focus is on keeping people safer while engaging in higher risk activities.

It is important to distinguish the direct harms from consuming substances from the indirect harms of policies that seek to manage those same substances. The Canadian Public Health Association (CPHA) (2014) notes: "The policy of prohibition has failed to be an effective deterrent to substance use and is increasingly recognized as having many harmful consequences" (p. 6), among them criminalization, stigma, marginalization, and increased use of health services.

Harm reduction approaches to mitigate heightened risk are often used by the general population in daily life. Box 12.3 provides an example of a harm reduction approach applied to an everyday situation.

Key Principles of Harm Reduction

Several key principles provide the foundation for harm reduction efforts (Winnipeg Regional Health Authority [WRHA], 2011; Marlatt & Witkiewitz, 2010; British Columbia Ministry of Health, 2005). While these principles are rooted in illicit drug use, they may be easily applied to a wide range of public health issues.

Pragmatism

Harm reduction recognizes that risk taking is inherent to the human experience. There will always be a portion of the population that engages in higher risk activities. Therefore, services must be accessible while an individual engages in high-risk activities as opposed to withholding services until the individual abstains from the harmful behaviour.

Human Rights/Autonomy

Harm reduction is based on the inherent belief in the dignity and respect for all people and is not influenced by moral issues associated with high-risk behaviours. Harm reduction recognizes the rights and abilities of individuals to make their own choices. The focus is the provision of meaningful support while minimizing punitive measures related to the behaviour.

Focus on Harms

Interventions must focus on the harms associated with high-risk behaviour, rather than efforts to stop the behaviour. These harms may be related to health, social, or economic factors that affect the individual, family, and broader community. Harm reduction emphasizes a change to safer behaviour that may lead to abstinence in time.

Maximize Intervention Options

Harm reduction recognizes client uniqueness and the need to accommodate personal goals and capacity for change. Effective harm reduction efforts must be tailored (rather than general) and encompass a broad range of strategies.

Priority of Immediate Goals

Harm reduction recognizes that people engaged in high-risk behaviours often lead complex and chaotic lives. Harm reduction focuses on "where people are at," recognizing the influence of the determinants on health.

Client Involvement

Active participation of individuals involved in high-risk behaviour is integral to harm reduction. Individuals who are most impacted by risk reduction strategies have valuable insight from their personal experiences and are well positioned to help design effective interventions.

Examples of Programs and Policies

Six examples of programs and policies that illustrate effective approaches to harm reduction for people involved in high-risk substance use are provided next. Note that the principles of effective harm reduction programming are embedded in these examples.

Needle Exchange Programs

Needle exchange programs distribute sterile needles and syringes and collect used injection equipment. The focus of a needle exchange program is to ensure every injection is performed with sterile equipment. These programs are relatively simple and cost-effective and achieve significant health gains for injection drug users (British Columbia Ministry of Health, 2005).

Methadone Maintenance Therapy

Methadone maintenance therapy (MMT) is used for treating heroin addiction. Methadone is a legal opioid medication prescribed by physicians and usually administered by community pharmacists or addiction treatment centres. MMT reduces the use of other opioids, health risks associated with injection practices, mortality, and drug-related criminal activity (British Columbia Ministry of Health, 2005).

Education and Outreach

Education materials with a harm reduction focus provide valuable support for individuals engaged in risky behaviours. These materials teach how to engage in safer injecting practices and reduce associated risks. Effective outreach programs, often in nontraditional settings, offer information, resources, and services to hard-to-reach populations.

Law Enforcement

Harm reduction efforts depend on strong partnerships between the health and justice systems. While each system is unique in its mandate and models of service delivery, there is considerable overlap and benefit in working together on common issues.

Supervised Consumption Facilities

Supervised consumption sites are legally sanctioned and medically supervised facilities where users are able to inhale or inject illegal substances. These facilities provide an opportunity to engage in high-risk behaviours in a safe and supportive environment with access to health care providers.

Naloxone for Lay People

In order to deal with overdoses by people who inject opioids, Naloxone kits are being distributed by several provincial health ministries to users and lay people (e.g., friends and family members) who might witness an overdose. Training is provided along with the kits so that Naloxone is used correctly. Naloxone slows the progress of opioids, giving more time to get overdose victims to a hospital, thus reducing the mortality that often accompanies overdose.

Challenges for Community Health Workers

Despite the benefits of harm reduction approaches to disease and injury prevention, many community health workers are challenged to provide empathetic, nonjudgemental care for individuals engaged in high-risk behaviours. For some, the notion of harm reduction conflicts with their moral values; for example, they cannot accept that drug users are allowed to continue using substances rather than focusing on abstaining from drug use (Marlatt & Witkiewitz, 2010). For others, harm reduction may be in opposition to their religious or cultural beliefs. Successful harm reduction efforts take time to support people through incremental change. Perhaps the greatest challenge is the absence of harm reduction in many health education curricula resulting in health workers not having the knowledge and skills to integrate the concept of harm reduction into their practice.

Critical Thinking Exercise 12.3

Harm Reduction

Scenario: You are working as a community health worker and the principal of a local high school has called you to discuss his concerns with drug use among the students.

- What information do you need to gather?
- Who will you involve in the planning process?
- What role will students/health care providers/parents/school staff assume?
- What actions will you take to address the various drug-related issues?
- How will you know if you have been successful?

Summary

In this chapter, you have been introduced to the concepts of levels of prevention and injury prevention theory with an emphasis on far upstream approaches, advocacy, and public policy in the context of the determinants of health. The concept of harm reduction is presented as a meaningful approach to disease and injury prevention. Examples of these concepts in community health practice illustrate the complexity of prevention activities, the unique role of the public health sector, and the value of intersectoral and multidisciplinary involvement in addressing prevention at the program and policy levels.

REFERENCES

Ashton, J. R., & Seymour, H. (2010). Public health and the origins of the Mersey Model of Harm Reduction. *International Journal of Drug Policy, 21*, 94–96.

Association of Faculties of Medicine of Canada (AFMC), Public Health Educators' Network. (2015). Chapter 4: Basic concepts in prevention, surveillance, and health promotion. In *AFMC primer on population health*. URL=http://phprimer.afmc.ca/Part1-TheoryThinkingAboutHealth/Chapter4BasicConceptsIn PreventionSurveillanceAndHealthPromotion

British Columbia Ministry of Health. (2005). *Harm reduction: A British Columbia Community Guide*. URL=http://www.health.gov.bc.ca/library/publications/year/2005/hrcommunityguide.pdf

Canadian Nurses Association (CNA). (2011). *Harm reduction and currently illegal drugs: Implications for nursing policy, practice, education and research*. Ottawa: Author.

Canadian Public Health Association (CPHA). (2014). *A new approach to managing illegal psychoactive substances in Canada*. Ottawa: Author. URL=http://www.cpha.ca/uploads/policy/ips_2014-05-15_e.pdf

Christoffel, T., & Gallagher, S. S. (2006). *Injury prevention and public health: Practical knowledge, skills and strategies*. Gaithersburg, MD: Aspen Publishers.

Falk-Rafael, A. (2005). Speaking truth to power: Nursing's legacy and moral imperative. *Advances in Nursing Science, 28*, 212–223.

Frieden, T. (2010). A framework for public health action: The health impact pyramid. *American Journal of Public Health, 100*, 590–595.

International Harm Reduction Association (IHRA). (2010). *What is harm reduction? A position statement*. London: Author.

Katz, D., & Ali, A. (2009). *Preventive medicine, integrative medicine and the health of the public*. Washington: Institute of Medicine of the National Academies.

Lavoie, M., Maurice, P., & Rainville, M. (2014). Prévention des traumatismes : une approche pour améliorer la sécurité des populations [Injury prevention: An approach to improve the safety of people]. In *Injury Prevention Media Kit of the Institut national de santé publique du Québec (INSPQ)*. URL=http://www.inspq.qc.ca/prevention-traumatismes/une-approche-pour-ameliorer-la-securite-des-populations

Leavell, H., & Clark, E. (1965). *Preventive medicine for the doctor in his community: An epidemiologic approach*. New York, NY: McGraw Hill.

Lee, H. S., Engstrom, M., & Peterson, S. R. (2011). Harm reduction and 12 steps: Complementary, oppositional, or something in-between? *Substance Use & Misuse, 46*, 1151–1161.

Marlatt, G. A., & Witkiewitz, K. (2010). Update on harm-reduction policy and intervention research. *Annual Review of Clinical Psychology, 6*, 591–606.

McKeganey, N. (2011). From harm reduction to drug user abstinence: A journey in drug treatment policy. *Journal of Substance Use, 16*, 179–194.

Parachute. (2015). *The cost of injury in Canada*. Toronto: Author. URL=http://www.parachutecanada.org/costofinjury

Pike, I., Richmond, S., Rothman, L., & Macpherson, A. (Eds.). (2015). *Canadian injury prevention resource*. Toronto: Parachute.

Public Health Agency of Canada (PHAC). (2006). *Street youth in Canada: Findings from enhanced surveillance of Canadian street youth, 1999–2003*. Ottawa: Author.

Runyan, C. W. (1998). Using the Haddon Matrix: Introducing the third dimension. *Injury Prevention, 4*, 302–307.

Senate Subcommittee on Population Health. (2009). *A healthy productive Canada: A determinant of health approach*. Ottawa: Author.

Strasser, T. (1978). Reflections on cardiovascular diseases. *Inderdisciplinary Science Reviews, 3*, 225–230.

Waller, J. A. (1989). Injury control in perspective. *American Journal of Public Health, 79*, 272–273.

Winnipeg Regional Health Authority (WRHA). (2011). *Position statement on harm reduction*. URL= http://www.wrha.mb.ca/community/publichealth/files/position-statements/HarmReduction.pdf

ONLINE RESOURCES

Please visit thePoint at http://thepoint.lww.com/Vollman4e for up-to-date Internet resources and additional learning materials on this topic.

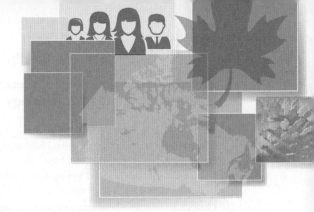

CHAPTER 13

Community Mental Health Promotion

J. Renée Robinson

LEARNING OBJECTIVES

After studying this chapter, you should be able to:

1. Discuss the importance of mental health promotion in public health practice

2. Describe public health issues that represent a threat to mental health

3. Identify initiatives directed toward addressing threats to mental health

4. Discuss ways in which mental health can be integrated into existing public health practice to address threats to mental health

5. Identify personal strategies to build skill and embed skills into practice

Introduction

Mental health problems and illness are very common, and the level of disability associated with mental illness is significant. In any given year, one in five adults lives with a mental illness. Injury rates for people with mental illness are 26 times the rate in the general population (Centers for Disease Control and Prevention [CDC], 2011). The World Health Organization (WHO) identifies unipolar depression as the leading cause of disability in developed countries. The cost to the Canadian economy is at least $50 billion annually (Mental Health Commission of Canada [MHCC], 2013a). The cost to individuals with mental health issues, their families, and communities is immeasurable.

 Take Note

More than 6.7 million people in Canada are living with mental health issues today. By comparison, 2.2 million people in Canada have Type 2 diabetes (MHCC, 2013a, p. 1).

Mental health and mental health issues (see Box 13.1) are experienced by individuals, but arise largely from the broader social, political, economic, and cultural environments

> **Box 13.1   Defining Terminology**
>
> The phrase "mental health problems and illnesses" is the phrase specifically chosen by the MHCC to refer to the full range of mental health and illness concerns (MHCC, 2012, p. 14). When used separately, the term "mental illness" is used to refer to diagnosable disorder, and "mental health problems" is used to refer to negative effects that may or may not be diagnosable. "Mental health issues" is a bridging term that refers to both mental health problems and mental illness.

in which individuals live. The broader environment influences mental health status at all levels. Social conditions determine the extent to which members of a community flourish or languish. Social conditions also influence the prevalence of some mental health issues, such as anxiety disorders and depression in women and substance abuse in men. Promoting health involves creating healthy environments in which citizens can thrive. Preventing mental illness involves a combination of reducing stressors and enhancing coping. Successful treatment, rehabilitation, and recovery are facilitated through attention to the psychosocial environment.

Take Note

Mental health and well-being are fundamental to our collective and individual ability as humans....The promotion, protection, and restoration of mental health can be regarded as a vital concern of individuals, communities, and societies throughout the world (WHO, 2014, p. 1).

The purpose of this chapter is to illustrate the importance of attention to mental health promotion in public health practice, describe public health issues that represent a threat to mental health, and provide examples of how the strategies for health promotion can be applied to addressing some of these mental health threats. Integration into public health and personal practice will also be discussed.

EVOLUTION AND CURRENT STATUS OF MENTAL HEALTH PROMOTION IN CANADA

Achieving health for all: A framework for health promotion (Epp, 1986) is a foundational document for health promotion in Canada and internationally. Minister Epp also released a parallel document titled *Mental health for Canadians: Striking a balance* (Epp, 1988). The intent of the second document was to ensure that "ideas and practices concerning mental health and mental disorder...keep pace with this emerging vision of health, which so clearly accentuates the importance of mental and social well-being" (p. 5). The document proposed a broad and positive definition of mental health, described a two-continuum model for mental health, and applied the framework for health promotion to a series of challenges in mental health. *Mental health for Canadians* has been highly influential, and the concepts outlined in that document continue to shape current thinking about mental health and mental health promotion.

In 2006, a Senate Standing Committee Chaired by Senator Michael Kirby (known as the Kirby Commission) released an extensive report on mental health and addiction in Canada.

Out of the shadows at last: Transforming mental health, mental illness and addiction services in Canada (Senate Standing Committee on Social Affairs, 2006), also referred to as the Kirby Report, made a number of recommendations including improving mental health promotion and preventing mental illness. The document emphasized the importance of action on the determinants of health using strategies identified in the Ottawa Charter (1986) and the Bangkok Charter (2005), both detailed in Chapter 1 (see Table 1.2).

The MHCC was established in 2007 with a 10-year mandate to serve as a catalyst for change. The Commission used extensive consultation processes to develop the first mental health strategy for Canada, and to tackle a number of priority topics. Some of these priorities, such as social inclusion, housing, and workplace health, will be described later in this chapter.

Changing directions, changing lives: The mental health strategy for Canada (MHCC, 2012) identifies six strategic directions for improving mental health in Canada. The document includes core background information, strategic priorities, and recommendations for action on each of these priorities. The first strategic direction is to promote mental health across the lifespan in homes, schools, and workplaces, and prevent mental illness and suicide wherever possible.

The national strategy for mental health provides a roadmap for action, but taking action requires people across multiple systems working together (i.e., intersectoral collaboration) to make change happen. The most recent initiative of the MHCC is to engage stakeholders in creating a mental health action plan.

MENTAL HEALTH CHALLENGES

People who live with mental illness are influenced by the same public health issues as other members of society. However, some public health issues pose particular challenges to mental health and to people who live with mental illness. The following is not meant to be an exhaustive discussion of these issues, but rather presented as illustrative examples.

STIGMA AND SOCIAL EXCLUSION

Social inclusion means providing all individuals and groups in society with access to resources such as employment, housing, health care, and education (Shookner, 2002). The term also implies connectedness to other community members. Social exclusion and discrimination occur when people are prevented from participating fully in the economic, social, and political life of the society in which they live. Stigma is social exclusion.

Stigma, and associated discrimination, may be the single largest issue in the mental health field today: it leads to many of the problems faced by people with mental illness. Stigma serves as a barrier to seek or participate in treatment, leads to social isolation and self-stigma, and results in discrimination in housing and employment. Further, stigma is viewed as being responsible for structural barriers such as lack of attention to mental health in research funding, professional education, and service delivery. Stigma often extends to family members and service providers, influencing their ability to advocate for change.

Stigma and discrimination have a huge negative impact on people living with mental health problems and illnesses, affecting all aspects and stages of their lives—dealing with friends, family, communities, educators, employers, mental health service providers, and the justice and health care systems…stigma and discrimination frequently have as great an effect on people as does their mental health problem or illness itself, seriously impeding their ability to fully participate in society and attain the best possible quality of life (MHCC, 2009, p. 90).

Lack of Safe and Affordable Housing

Shelter is one of the most basic human needs. As part of the built environment, housing design (e.g., accessibility) and neighbourhood characteristics (e.g., physical and social environment, proximity to services, safety) have a direct effect on how people interact, what social opportunities are available, and what resources and supports are available. Housing then has a substantial effect on health and quality of life.

Lack of safe and affordable housing can lead to mental health issues. For individuals who are experiencing mental health issues, lack of safe and affordable housing exacerbates mental health problems and may lead to additional challenges such as homelessness. Inadequate or unsafe housing also impedes recovery.

Affordable housing is in short supply across Canada. Overcrowded housing is common in First Nations communities. In other communities, the stock of social housing, where rent is geared to income, has declined over time and waiting lists can be lengthy. The cost of renting in the public market is often substantially beyond the resources of people who live with disabilities. With limited housing available, landlords can be selective, and vulnerable people, including youth, visible minorities, and people with mental illness, often experience discrimination. Housing that people are able to obtain may be unsuitable, in need of major repairs, or located in areas where safety is of concern.

Unemployment

Employment has a variety of meanings in a person's life. Aside from income and lifestyle, employment offers social position and prestige, provides meaning and purpose in life, and a sense of contribution. Employment is a source of social connection and self-esteem and also provides structure. People with mental illness often experience a number of barriers to meaningful employment, including discrimination in hiring and failure to provide reasonable accommodations (i.e., adaptations to working conditions to allow people with disability to perform the essential duties of their jobs).

Unhealthy Workplaces

Individuals who are employed may also experience challenges to their mental health. Seventy percent of Canadian employees expressed concern about psychological health and safety in their workplace (Great-West Life Centre for Mental Health in the Workplace, 2012). Mental health issues are the leading causes of both short-term and long-term disabilities, and account for about 30% of disability claims. However, to date, attention to mental health issues has not been a core element of occupational health and safety programs.

Family Violence

Interpersonal violence is a pervasive mental health problem, and a serious public health issue. Violence, abuse, and trauma are risk factors associated with mental health issues and substance abuse. In addition to physical injury, experiencing or witnessing abuse can lead to a wide range of health and social problems over the course of a lifetime.

Interpersonal violence is very common. One in four adults reported physical abuse in childhood. More than 25% of all reported crime in 2011 resulted from family violence. Three in four murder-suicides involved family members, and 70% of victims of family violence were women and girls (PHAC, 2015).

Bullying

Bullying can lead to a wide range of emotional, behavioural, and relationship problems (Craig & McCuaig Edge, 2012). Awareness of bullying in schools, neighbourhoods, and workplaces is increasing. One in three Canadian adolescents reported being recently bullied, and the rate for lesbian, gay, bisexual, transgendered, and questioning (two-spirited) (LGBTQ) youth is three times higher. Forty percent of Canadian workers reported being bullied on a weekly basis (Canadian Institutes of Health Research [CIHR], 2012). Intervention by others can make a difference, but intervention rates are low.

Suicide

Depression and mental illness can lead a person to consider ending one's life. Suicide is one of the ten leading causes of death in Canada. Among all ages and including both sexes, suicide rates have been consistent from 2008 to 2012 at just over 11 per 100,000 population. In 2012, the suicide rate for youth aged between 9 and 15 years was 10.2 per 100,000 population; the highest rate, 17.6 per 100,000 population, was in the age range of 55 to 59 years (Statistics Canada, 2015). Suicide rates among Aboriginal populations are alarming: Aboriginal youth commit suicide about five to six times more often than non-Aboriginal youth, and the suicide rate for First Nations males is 126 per 100,000 population compared to 24 per 100,000 for non-Aboriginal males (Health Canada, 2015). Federal legislation (Bill C-300) recognizes suicide as a serious public health problem and a priority for action.

Cultural Discontinuity

Intergenerational effects of colonization continue to be experienced by Aboriginal people. Disruption of families and communities through forced relocation, attendance at residential schools, and apprehension of children in the "Sixties Scoop" have led to substantial problems with identity and self-esteem. These disruptions have contributed to high rates of mental health issues, addiction, and suicide among Aboriginal people.

Justice System Issues

People with mental illness are at increased risk of coming into contact with the justice system, often due to minor poverty-related concerns such as shoplifting, loitering, or panhandling. Once in contact with the justice system, people with mental illness are more likely to be arrested, and more likely to be convicted than other people. People with mental health issues are disproportionately represented in jails and prisons, and the number has been increasing rapidly. The Office of the Correctional Investigator of Canada (2012) identified that 45% of the total prison population and 69% of incarcerated women experience mental illness. While the stated purpose of imprisonment is rehabilitation, resources to support treatment and rehabilitation are minimal. The prison environment often compounds existing mental health issues and, once people are released, few community resources are available.

Limitations of Existing Health and Mental Health Services

People who live with mental health issues die earlier than other Canadians and have almost twice as many medical conditions as people who do not have mental illnesses (Martens et al., 2004). Mental health issues receive inadequate attention in primary care settings. Lack of access to specialized services and fragmentation of service have been consistently identified as problems for people who live with mental health problems.

As with other areas of health, existing services have been oriented toward inpatient care and biomedical approaches. Resource allocation for health promotion and for psychosocial interventions has been very limited and is often vulnerable to budget reductions. Services tend to be provider-oriented rather than being recovery-oriented. Practice realities are far removed from the goal of true partnership with clients, and support for self-determination.

PROMOTING MENTAL HEALTH

The WHO describes mental health as "a state of well-being in which the individual realizes his or her own abilities, can cope with the normal stresses of life, can work productively and fruitfully, and is able to make a contribution to his or her community" (WHO, 2014, p. 1).

> *The Public Health Agency of Canada defines positive mental health as: the capacity of each and all of us to feel, think, act in ways that enhance our ability to enjoy life and deal with the challenges we face. It is a positive sense of emotional and spiritual well-being that respects the importance of culture, equity, social justice, interconnections and personal dignity (PHAC, 2014).*

Mental health and mental illness are often viewed as part of a single continuum, but evidence supports a two-continuum model (Keyes, 2007) with one continuum being presence or absence of mental illness, and the second continuum anchored by flourishing and languishing. Keyes identifies the dimensions of flourishing as emotional well-being (positive affect and reported quality of life), psychological well-being (self-acceptance, personal growth, purpose in life, autonomy, mastery, and positive relations with others), and social well-being (social acceptance, social actualization, social contribution, social coherence, and social integration). The two continuums are correlated, but people with mental illness can flourish, and people without mental illness can languish. Complete mental health means absence of illness and a state of flourishing. Anything less than complete mental health is associated with increased impairment and disability (Keyes, 2008). Promoting mental health then requires both preventing mental illness and promoting flourishing.

Promoting flourishing involves creating supportive environments that enable people to be productive and experience personal growth; a sense of purpose and satisfaction in life; and positive relationships with friends, family, and community members. A healthy environment both promotes mental health and reduces challenges to mental health (see Chapter 7).

PREVENTING MENTAL HEALTH ISSUES

Preventing mental health issues involves both population-level and targeted interventions. The window of opportunity for prevention occurs early in life. About half of all mental illnesses emerge by the age of 14, and 75% are present by the age of 24. Symptoms typically precede diagnosis by 2 to 4 years. Proven approaches to preventing mental illness include strengthening families, strengthening individuals, preventing specific diagnoses, promoting mental health in schools, and promoting coping through health care and community programs (O'Connell et al., 2009).

Preventing mental illness also involves addressing factors known to pose a risk to mental health (see Fig. 13.1). Adverse circumstances often compound over time and lead to a range of negative outcomes that will contribute to additional problems. For example, bullying can cause psychological damage, particularly for students predisposed to emotional difficulties. These difficulties lead to problems in learning and potentially leaving school, which impacts educational outcomes and in turn impacts future life opportunities. In this example, reducing exposure to bullying would help to prevent psychological injury as well as future social and

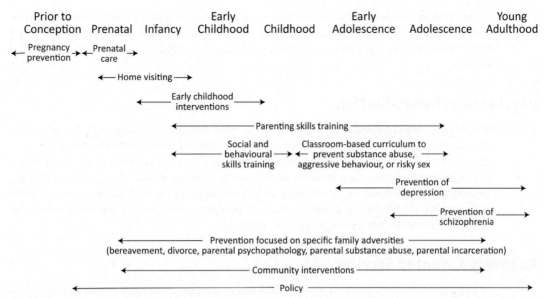

FIGURE 13.1   Mental health issue prevention interventions by developmental phase. (Reprinted with permission from *Preventing mental, emotional, and behavioral disorders among young people: Progress and possibilities, 2009 by the National Academy of Sciences*. Courtesy of the National Academies Press, Washington, DC.)

economic disadvantage. Other risk factors to be addressed through targeted intervention include gambling, interpersonal abuse, stressors related to housing or unemployment, stressors in the workplace, and cultural discontinuity.

PROVIDING EARLY INTERVENTION

Recognizing when people are struggling and assisting them to better manage mental health issues can avert more serious problems or connect people with resources and supports. For instance, early intervention services for psychosis limit disruption caused by illness and may fundamentally alter the trajectory of illness. Providing early intervention can be a challenge since most people who are experiencing difficulty are not connected with mental health services, and their natural supports may not have the knowledge or skill to help. One strategy to enhance the knowledge and skills of natural supports is Mental Health First Aid (MHFA).

Like other forms of first aid, the purpose of MHFA is to provide support to a person who is experiencing difficulty until more specialized services can be engaged. More than 100,000 Canadians have been trained in MHFA. Training assists participants to recognize common mental health issues and to refer people to appropriate supports. People who have been trained in MHFA extend helping networks into schools, workplaces, and communities. In addition to providing direct aid to individuals, building these skills increases community capacity and cohesion.

IMPROVING QUALITY OF LIFE FOR PEOPLE WHO LIVE WITH ENDURING MENTAL HEALTH ISSUES

Interventions intended to create supportive environments are also essential to facilitate recovery. Better housing, employment opportunities, and inclusive environments provide the conditions needed for recovery. Tertiary prevention strategies are also needed to limit disability and restore people to their maximum capabilities. Reorientation of health services and creating supportive environments are needed to support people who are recovering. For people who live with mental health issues, tertiary prevention also involves psychosocial rehabilitation and recovery-oriented services.

Psychosocial Rehabilitation

The mission of psychosocial rehabilitation is to help persons with long-term mental illness and disability increase their functioning so that they are successful and satisfied in the environments of choice, with the least amount of ongoing professional intervention. The process of psychosocial rehabilitation involves working with clients to identify their goals, identifying existing and needed skills and supports to achieve those goals, and building needed skills and supports. Additional information about the practice of psychosocial rehabilitation can be obtained from PSR Canada (http://psrrpscanada.ca).

Recovery-Oriented Services

In the mental health context, recovery does not mean cure. Recovery means living well in the presence or absence of illness. Recovery is, or should be, the goal of the mental health system.

> Recovery is a deeply personal unique process of changing one's attitudes, values, feelings, goals, skills and/or roles. It is a way of living a satisfying, hopeful and contributing life even with limitations caused by illness. Recovery involves the development of new meaning and purpose in one's life as one grows beyond the catastrophic effects of mental illness (Anthony, 1993).

The recovery movement was initiated by people with mental illness. The recovery vision is a major driver for improvement in mental health service delivery across Canada. A recovery-oriented service system is designed to support people in their recovery. This means shifting from largely provider-centred and medically oriented services toward partnerships with patients. Recovery-oriented services are designed to build on people's strengths, empower them to make their own choices, and support them in achieving their goals. In essence, the goal of mental health services is to create environments in which recovery can take place.

APPLYING STRATEGIES FOR MENTAL HEALTH PROMOTION

Strategies for health promotion outlined in the *Ottawa Charter* also apply to promoting mental health, preventing mental health issues, and supporting people in recovery from mental illness. Each health challenge is complex, so multiple strategies and intersectoral collaboration are required for most issues. For instance, family violence can be prevented by creating supportive environments, building mental health and resilience, strengthening community action, developing policy, and reorienting services. Solutions require coordinated efforts from health and social services, justice, education, and other sectors. The example strategies that follow cannot fully describe the range of interventions needed to address each specific issue, but do provide an illustration of actions to improve mental health.

Creating Supportive Environments

Supportive environments are central to promoting flourishing, preventing mental health issues, and facilitating recovery. The ecologic perspective on creating supportive environments for health described in Chapter 7 is useful for considering the complex relationship between

TABLE 13.1 Psychosocial Factors Affecting Mental Health in the Workplace

Psychosocial Factor	Defining Features
Psychological support	Coworkers and supervisors are supportive of employees' psychological and mental health issues, and respond appropriately as needed.
Organizational culture	The organization is characterized by trust, honesty, and fairness.
Clear leadership and expectations	Effective leadership and support helps employees know what they need to do, how their work contributes to the organization, and whether there are impending changes.
Civility and respect	Employees are respectful and considerate in their interactions with one another, as well as with customers, clients, and the public.
Psychological competencies and requirements	There is a good fit between employees' interpersonal and emotional competencies and the requirements of the position they hold.
Growth and development	Employees receive encouragement and support in the development of their interpersonal, emotional, and job skills.
Recognition and reward	There is appropriate acknowledgement and appreciation of employees' efforts in a fair and timely manner.
Involvement and influence	Employees are included in discussions about how their work is done and how important decisions are made.
Workload management	Tasks and responsibilities can be accomplished successfully within the time available.
Engagement	Employees feel connected to their work and are motivated to do their job well.
Balance	There is recognition of the need for balance between the demands of work, family, and personal life.
Psychological protection	Employees' psychological safety is ensured.
Protection of physical safety	Management takes appropriate action to protect the physical safety of employees.

Source: Samra et al. (2012).

individuals and their environments. Political, economic, and sociocultural environments need to be considered as influences on health and as targets for intervention.

Creating better housing conditions involves advocacy with others for social housing and income assistance rates that enable access to housing; working with clients, landlords, and the local building inspectors, to ensure that housing meets safety requirements; and working with landlords to reduce discrimination and increase access to housing.

Creating a supportive work environment involves taking action on the 13 factors known to influence psychological health in the workplace (Table 13.1). GuardingMinds@Work was commissioned by The Great-West Life Centre for Mental Health in the Workplace (Samra, 2012) and provides free tools to assess psychological health in the workplace and resources to support planning and implementing workplace change.

Creating healthy schools involves providing a school environment that fosters both learning and health. Education is an important determinant of health. However, academic success is only one element of the foundational knowledge needed for success in life. A whole school approach involves expanding learning to include development of the social and emotional competencies necessary to flourish in life.

Creating a healthy society involves reducing stigma and building social inclusion. Traditional strategies for addressing stigma, such as public education, have had limited effect. More recent initiatives emphasizing the biologic perspective, the "disease like any other" approach, have not been effective and may actually increase stigma against people with mental health issues (Read et al., 2006). Targeted education, contact-based education, and legislative measures have been more successful in addressing stigma.

The MHCC Opening Minds campaign has identified four groups for targeted education. Health professionals are one of these target groups, since people with mental health issues report health professionals as the source of the most deeply felt stigma. Contact-based education and skills training can improve the attitudes of students in professional programs.

Critical Thinking Exercise 13.1

Members of the public are relatively well informed about mental health issues and treatment for mental illness. They also report relatively positive attitudes. Attitudes are less positive when social distance scales are used. How comfortable would you be in working as a colleague with someone who has a mental health issue? Do you have friends with mental health issues? Would you feel comfortable receiving health services from someone with mental health issues? Would you be comfortable knowing that your child's teacher has a mental health issue?

Mental health issues are very common. Many of the people you know, work with, and receive services from, live with a diagnosed mental illness. Stigma and fear of discrimination keep people from disclosing their diagnosis. If you don't know people with mental illness or mental health issues, consider what keeps people from being open with you. What actions can you take to remove barriers to disclosure? What actions can you take to reduce the fear and secrecy associated with mental health issues and build an environment where people with mental illness feel safe and included?

Action to prevent suicide is another aspect of creating supportive environments. The PHAC is working on a framework for suicide prevention that includes increasing public awareness, defining best practices, and promoting integration of best practices into service delivery. Provinces and territories are undertaking additional initiatives. The Canadian Association for Suicide Prevention and the Centre for Suicide Prevention are working with governments and agencies to reduce the suicide rate.

Action is also required at the local level since conditions that increase or mitigate risk will be unique to each community. For instance, while the suicide rate in the Aboriginal community is high, communities exhibiting greater cultural continuity had lower rates of suicide (Chandler & Lalonde, 2009). Any national framework will need to be tailored to the unique circumstances of each community.

Building Personal Skills

Skill building for primary care providers and training in MHFA are examples of building personal skills. Police training is another example of developing skills to improve system response. Police have very little information in their training on how to respond to people who are experiencing mental health issues. The MHCC commissioned a report and recommendations on improving interactions between police and people with mental health issues (Coleman & Cotton, 2014). Strategies include using contact-based education and partnership with community mental health services to decrease undue use of force, and to facilitate an empathic response, de-escalation, and connection of the person with community agencies and services.

Strengthening Community Action

Information, resources, and community mobilization are core strategies to strengthen community action. The MHCC was established to serve as a catalyst for change in the mental health system and in the attitudes and behaviours of Canadians. The goal is to take mental health "out of the shadows forever."

Many of the MHCC initiatives involve creating new knowledge through knowledge synthesis and through research directed at key questions. The MHCC Knowledge Exchange Centre provides a mechanism for sharing information, identifying better practices, and facilitating application of new knowledge. Projects such as the Multicultural Mental Health Resource Centre provide information and resources for a range of stakeholders, including service providers, policy makers, families, and people with mental health issues. Other projects involve providing training to build capacity in adopting better practices.

Foundational work by the Kirby Commission, development of the framework for the mental health strategy, and the strategy itself each involved extensive consultation and engagement of a wide range of stakeholders to build a shared vision for mental health. The Mental Health Strategy for Canada (MHCC, 2012) serves as a blueprint for action. Work continues on a range of issues to provide people with the information and resources to take action at all levels, including developing a Network of Ambassadors to assist in disseminating information and developing a mental health action plan.

Developing Healthy Public Policy

Healthy public policy, which is discussed in detail in Chapter 9, refers to using policy levers such as legislation and financial strategies to promote and protect health or prevent illness (see Chapter 9). Policy levers are also used to promote mental health and protect people from risks to mental health. Public policies favouring mental health also address poverty reduction, safe and affordable housing, and a whole school approach in education.

Developing a national standard for psychological health and safety in the workplace complements the creation of supportive workplace environments by generating a requirement for action. The MHCC and the Canadian Standards Association developed the National Standard on Psychological Health and Safety in the Workplace (MHCC, 2013b) accompanied by an implementation guide. The purpose of the Standard is to engage employers in identifying and addressing known risks to psychological safety, control risks that cannot be eliminated, and create structures to support the development of a healthy workplace.

Mental health policy documents routinely identify a need for increased engagement of people with mental health issues, and their families, in every aspect of service planning. Involvement in program development, delivery, and evaluation is increasingly required by funders. Providing ongoing financial support to consumer organizations is a mechanism to facilitate engagement of people who live with mental health problems and their families in these important tasks.

Reorienting Mental Health Services

Limitations of the existing mental health service system are numerous, and reorienting services is a substantial undertaking. Some of the strategies include improving skills of front-line service providers, evaluating relevant elements of services, and addressing barriers to recovery.

Tools such as the Recovery-Oriented Services Inventory (Dumont et al., 2012) measure domains relevant to providing quality services. Incorporating these domains into routine evaluation provides a foundation for ongoing program development. Incorporating expectations into accreditation standards would establish a requirement for adopting recovery-oriented practices.

Primary care settings are the entry point for health and mental health services. Efforts to improve mental health knowledge among primary care providers have been helpful. Shared-care, where primary care providers and mental health professionals work together to offer complementary services, has been demonstrated to improve service quality (Fuller et al., 2011).

Mental health services have been focused largely on clinical treatment. Supporting recovery also requires service providers to take action on barriers to recovery, such as discrimination (e.g., in work, housing), stigma, and poverty.

IMPLICATIONS FOR PRACTICE

Promoting mental health and preventing mental illness are increasingly recognized as critical to good health, and to public health services (CDC, 2011). Integration of mental health promotion and prevention of mental health issues must occur at both systems level and individual level.

Integration into Public Health Practice

The CDC (2011) describes a national framework for action on integration of mental health into public health practice in the United States. The framework operates on every level, from increasing awareness of the public to policy integration and systems integration. Education of health professionals and program integration are also key strategies. Education for health professionals includes recognition of mental health symptoms and increasing awareness of implications for physical health. Education also includes protective factors and strategies for mental health promotion. Program integration refers to integrating traditional public health with mental health promotion and mental illness services.

In practice, these recommendations suggest integrating more mental health content into traditional public health programs and full integration of health promotion and prevention programs. Increased awareness and ability to meet a broader range of needs and connections with mental health services that provide easy access to specialized services will provide more holistic care. The CDC recommendations also suggest a need to integrate greater attention to medical concerns in mental health services. Since people with mental illness experience a disproportionate number of medical conditions, greater ability to recognize and address concerns and to engage the medical care system as needed, will also increase capacity for holistic care.

Integration into public health services has received less attention in Canada, but some initiatives have been undertaken. For instance, the PHAC (2011) funded a number of innovation projects to support positive mental health. These projects are intended to address issues such as bullying and suicide while strengthening families and communities. The goal is to use the results of these projects to shape future projects and inform mental health programs. In addition, the MHCC emphasizes the need for improved awareness and action by identifying mental health promotion, illness and suicide prevention, and stigma reduction as the first goal of the national strategy for mental health.

Integration into Personal Practice

Applying knowledge about community mental health issues and strategies for health promotion to everyday practice requires community health workers to build their own personal knowledge and skills and to embed use of these skills in everyday practice. Contributing knowledge and skill to collective efforts to address challenges at the program and system level is also essential.

Personal growth is an ongoing process. The CDC (2011) recommends that health professionals be educated to increase their awareness of the relevance of mental health in overall health, the importance of protective factors, and strategies for health promotion. Some ways to build personal knowledge and skills include:

- educating yourself about work being done by the MHCC and considering how you can contribute to this important work (see Box 13.2)
- taking MHFA training to assist in recognizing and addressing common mental health issues, and ability to refer people to appropriate supports
- becoming familiar with education resources for yourself, your clients, and their families
- learning about and declaring your commitment to recovery (see Box 13.3)

Box 13.2 Selected Mental Health Commission of Canada Initiatives

At Home/Chez Soi conducted a $110 million research project in five Canadian cities to test application of the *Housing First* model with a range of populations to identify what works for people experiencing homelessness and mental health issues.

Opening Minds engaged in a systematic effort to change the behaviours and attitudes of Canadians toward people with mental illness, to address discrimination and promote social inclusion.

Mental Health Strategy used an extensive consultative process to develop the first national strategy for mental health in Canada. Work is also under way to develop an action plan and indicators to evaluate progress toward goals.

Knowledge Exchange Centre was established to synthesize existing knowledge, facilitate knowledge exchange, and build capacity for people to work together in order to facilitate implementation of best and promising practices.

National Standard on Psychological Health & Safety in the Workplace collaborated with the Standards Bureau to develop standards for mental wellness in workplaces, and to develop tools to assist in implementing the standard.

Work on a Wide Range of Topics developed resources related to concerns including caregiving, child and youth, diversity, Aboriginal health, legal issues, seniors, and suicide prevention.

Additional information at www.mentalhealthcommission.ca

Mental health is intrinsic to health and a critical factor in many conditions. Factors such as self-efficacy, coping, and depression influence, and are influenced by, the presence of other conditions such as arthritis. Mental health is a key element of how illness is experienced, the ability to engage in self-care, and the trajectory of illness. Embedding mental health into all aspects of community health practice involves, for example, considering mental health and environmental stressors as well as diet and exercise in addressing obesity.

Embedding mental health into practice means:

- assessing emotional, psychological, and coping skills as well as psychosocial environment and functioning
- investigating potential mental health challenges such as housing, family violence, bullying, and suicide
- using a recovery-oriented framework for practice
- using MHFA skills to identify mental health issues and refer when needed
- building connections between public health and mental health services to support service access

---

Box 13.3 The Mental Health Commission of Canada Declaration of Commitment to Recovery

The MHCC identifies that "the concept of 'recovery' in mental health refers to living a satisfying, hopeful, and contributing life, even when there are on-going limitations caused by mental health problems and illnesses."

The Declaration "outlines key recovery principles," is "designed to help foster ongoing dialogue on recovery and build momentum for change," and is "intended to encourage and support individuals and organizations to engage in the promotion of recovery-oriented practices at all levels of the mental health system."

Read more at http://www.mentalhealthcommission.ca/English/document/25671/recovery-declaration-brochure

Many of the mental health challenges identified in this chapter, such as supporting inclusion and addressing stigma and discrimination, or working to address housing challenges, require action at the program and system levels. Community health workers can contribute by participating in collective efforts to address health challenges.

Summary

Mental health is a significant public health concern based on prevalence, disability, and implications for the health of the community. The importance of action on mental health is increasingly acknowledged, and current initiatives by the MHCC are exerting significant influence on Canadian society. Taking mental health from an individual problem to a collective challenge for all sectors of society is critical. Applying health promotion strategies to promoting mental health, preventing mental health issues, and facilitating recovery provides a vehicle for improving the health of all members of our communities. Mental health promotion is an integral aspect of community health and community health practice. Everyone has a role to play.

Critical Thinking Exercise 13.2

Occupational Health Officers are usually responsible for diagnosing and treating people who are injured in the workplace, providing case management, assisting with disability claims, and facilitating return to work. Activities such as pre-employment testing (e.g., physicals, vision screening), ongoing monitoring (e.g., immunizations, workplace hazardous materials information system [WHMIS]), and implementing health and wellness education programs are also part of the role. Review the 13 factors known to influence psychological health and safety in the workplace and consider how Occupational Health Officers can expand their role in promoting mental health.

REFERENCES

Anthony, W. A. (1993). Recovery from mental illness: The guiding vision of the mental health service system in the 1990s. *Psychosocial Rehabilitation Journal, 16*(4), 11–23.

Canadian Institutes of Health Research (CIHR). (2012). *Canadian bullying statistics.* URL=http://www.cihr-irsc.gc.ca/e/45838.html

Centers for Disease Control and Prevention (CDC). (2011). *Public health action plan to integrate mental health promotion and mental illness prevention with chronic disease prevention, 2011–2015.* Atlanta: U.S. Department of Health and Human Services

Chandler, M. J., & Lalonde, C. (2009). Cultural continuity as a moderator of suicide risk among Canada's First Nations. In L. Kirmayer & G. G. Valaskakis (Eds.), *Healing traditions: The mental health of aboriginal peoples in Canada* (pp. 221–248). Vancouver: UBC Press.

Coleman, T., & Cotton, D. (2014). *TEMPO: Police interactions: A report towards improving interactions between police and people living with mental health problems.* Ottawa: Mental Health Commission of Canada.

Craig, W., & McCuaig Edge, H. (2012). Bullying and fighting. In J. G. Freeman, M. King, & W. Pickett (Eds.), *The health of Canada's young people: A mental health focus* (pp. 167–183). Ottawa: Public Health Agency of Canada. URL=http://www.phac-aspc.gc.ca/hp-ps/dca-dea/publications/hbsc-mental-mentale/bullying-intimidation-eng.php

Dumont, J. M., Ridgeway, P., Onken, S., Dornan, D., & Ralph, R. O. (2012). Recovery oriented systems indicators measure (ROSI). In T. Campbell-Orde, J. Chamberlin, J. Carpenter, & S. Leff (Eds.), *Measuring the promise: A compendium of recovery measures (Vol II).* Cambridge: Human Services Research Institute. URL=https://www.power2u.org/downloads/ROSI-Recovery%20Oriented%20Systems%20Indicators.pdf

Epp, J. (1986). *Achieving health for all: A framework for health promotion.* Ottawa: Health and Welfare Canada.

Epp, J. (1988). *Mental health for Canadians: Striking a balance.* Ottawa: Minister of Supply and Services.

Fuller, J. D., Perkins D., Parker, S., Holdsworth, L., Kelly, B., Roberts, R., et al. (2011). Effectiveness of service linkages in primary mental health care: A narrative review part 1. *BMC Health Services Research, 11,* 72.

Great-West Life Centre for Mental Health in the Workplace. (2012). *GuardingMinds@Work. A workplace guide to psychological health and safety.* URL=http://www.guardingmindsatwork.ca/info

Health Canada. (2015). *First Nations and Inuit health: Mental health and wellness.* URL=http://www.hc-sc.gc.ca/fniah-spnia/promotion/mental/index-eng.php

Keyes, C. (2007). Promoting and protecting mental health as flourishing: A complementary strategy for improving national mental health. *American Psychologist, 62,* 95–108.

Keyes, C. (2008). Towards a mentally flourishing society: Mental health promotion, not cure. *Journal of Public Mental Health, 6*(2), 4–7.

Martens, P., Fransoo, R., McKeen, N., Burland, E., Jebamani, L., Burchill, C., et al. (2004). *Patterns of regional mental illness disorder diagnoses and service use in Manitoba: A population-based study.* Winnipeg: University of Manitoba, Manitoba Centre for Health Policy.

Mental Health Commission of Canada (MHCC). (2009). *Toward recovery and well-being: A framework for a mental health strategy for Canada.* Calgary: Author.

Mental Health Commission of Canada (MHCC). (2012). *Changing directions, changing lives: The mental health strategy for Canada.* Calgary: Author.

Mental Health Commission of Canada (MHCC). (2013a). *Making the case for investing in mental health in Canada.* Calgary: Author.

Mental Health Commission of Canada (MHCC). (2013b). *National standard of Canada for psychological health and safety in the workplace.* URL=http://www.mentalhealthcommission.ca/English/issues/workplace/national-standard

O'Connell, M. E., Boat, T., & Warner, K. E. (Eds.). (2009). *Preventing mental, emotional, and behavioral disorders among young people: Progress and possibilities.* Washington, DC: The National Academies Press.

Office of the Correctional Investigator. (2012). *Annual report of the Office of the Correctional Investigator. 2011–2012.* URL=http://www.oci-bec.gc.ca/cnt/rpt/annrpt/annrpt20112012-eng.aspx

Public Health Agency of Canada (PHAC). (2011). *Harper Government announces funding to support positive mental health in communities across Canada* [News Release]. URL=http://www.phac-aspc.gc.ca/media/nr-rp/2011/2011_0608-eng.php

Public Health Agency of Canada (PHAC). (2014). *Mental health promotion.* URL=http://www.phac-aspc.gc.ca/mh-sm/mhp-psm/index-eng.php

Public Health Agency of Canada (PHAC). (2015). *Family violence: How big is the problem in Canada?* URL=http://www.phac-aspc.gc.ca/sfv-avf/info/fv-problem-eng.php

Read, J., Haslam, N., Sayce, L., & Davies, E. (2006). Prejudice and schizophrenia: A review of the 'mental illness is an illness like any other' approach. *Acta Psychatrica Scandinavica, 114,* 303–318.

Samra, J., Gilbert, M., Shain, M., & Bilsker, D. (2012). *Psychosocial factors.* Vancouver: Centre for Applied Research in Mental Health and Addiction. URL=http://www.guardingmindsatwork.ca/docs/abouts/Psychosocial_Factors.pdf

Senate Standing Committee on Social Affairs. (2006). *Out of the shadows at last: Transforming mental health, mental illness and addiction services in Canada.* Ottawa: Government of Canada.

Shookner, M. (2002). *An inclusion lens: Workbook for looking at social and economic exclusion and inclusion.* Halifax: Health Canada, Population and Public Health Branch.

Statistics Canada. (2015). *Suicides and suicide rate, by sex and by age group (Both sexes rate) [table].* URL=http://www.statcan.gc.ca/tables-tableaux/sum-som/l01/cst01/hlth66d-eng.htm

World Health Organization (WHO). (2014). *Mental health: Strengthening our response* (Fact Sheet No. 222). URL=http://www.who.int/mediacentre/factsheets/fs220/en/

ONLINE RESOURCES

Please visit the Point at http://thepoint.lww.com/Vollman4e for up-to-date Internet resources and additional learning materials on this topic.

CHAPTER 14

Social Media and Health Promotion

Cameron D. Norman

LEARNING OBJECTIVES

After studying this chapter, you should be able to:

1. Identify the thinking strategies required to approach social media use in health promotion

2. Distinguish the unique characteristics for communication and the related opportunities and challenges that social media presents for health promoters

3. Discuss the skills and capacities that are required for health promotion to use social media effectively

Introduction

When future generations of health promoters look back on the early 21st century they will see two eras demarcated: health promotion before and after social media. This was the period when media, that is information delivered by the Internet, and mass public engagement came together through an emergent set of tools, technologies, and practices organized under the term social media. Social media represents more than just a set of tools and technologies that connect people to information and each other; it is a means of connecting to the roots of health promotion through a paradigm shift in health communications (Norman & Muzumdar, 2013). The fundamental tenets of the field as outlined in the Ottawa Charter (World Health Organization [WHO], 1986) place particular emphasis on strengthening community action, developing personal skills, and creating supportive environments, while contributing to a reorientation of health services and a wider discussion on the definition, creation, and implementation of healthy public policies. Social media offers health promotion a vehicle to contribute to all of these goals simultaneously, drawing on the power of networked technology and social interaction.

Social media is defined as "any networked ICT (information and communications technology) tool or platform that derives its content and principal value from user engagement and permits those users to interact with that content as part of a larger movement in communications organized under Web 2.0" (Norman, 2012, p. 3). Web 2.0 is the name given to user-generated content and channels that permit wide-scale distribution, editing, usability, and interoperability. Organized under the term *social media* are tools or platforms such as

TABLE 14.1 Sample of Social Media Platforms

Multimedia Platforms

Platform	Description	Media
Facebook	Multimedia platform for sharing content. World's most widely used social media service	Text, photographs, video, audio, web links
LinkedIn	Network aimed at creating, maintaining, and promoting connections between professionals	Text, photographs, video, audio, web links
Twitter	Short message (140-character) service that enables distribution of linked content that appears in a stream and is open to the public	Text, photographs, video, web links
Tumblr	Content curation site mixes together aspects of blogs, media-sharing, and reposting of other sources	Text, photographs, video, audio
Google+	Multimedia site allows for blogging, distribution of most forms of media with easy links to the Google platform of services	Text, photographs, video, audio, web links

Media-Specific Platforms

Platform	Description	Media
Pinterest	Users create topic-specific "pin-boards" to share images collected from the Internet	Photographs
Instagram	Original photos shared via mobile device are shared and tagged in a constant stream of content	Photographs, video
Vine	Short 6-second video clips are uploaded and repeated on a loop	Video
Flickr	Photograph-sharing network designed for sharing original content from any source	Photographs, digital artwork
YouTube	Video sharing website that combines source content from private, professional, and public sources	Video
Reddit	Content curation board that enables users to share links, images, and text on topic-specific issues from around the world	Text, photographs, web links
Soundcloud	Audio sharing tool designed to facilitate exchange and distribution of podcasts, music, and other recordings	Audio

Facebook, LinkedIn, Instagram, and Twitter. In Table 14.1 some of the popular social media tools in use at the time of this writing are profiled.

FROM TOOLS TO PLATFORMS

Social media is not a single entity, but a constellation of tools and technologies that support peer-to-peer conversation and cocreation. For health promotion it is important to focus on the fundamental qualities of what a particular technology offers rather than the specific tool or platform, particularly because the features of each tool can adapt and change over time. Blog-style tools that provide platforms for sharing original work are useful for developing in-depth information, allowing others to offer commentary and reposting of material to other sources. Microblog services like Twitter enable users to quickly share ideas, links, and observations to the global community and connect quickly on a global scale with short-form content, ideal for spreading information at a rapid pace. Twitter is an open system and can be thought of as a tool to find answers to questions that may not have occurred to someone from a source that was never known in the first place, making it a powerful tool for building and extending professional networks and for outreach to diverse, previously inaccessible or hidden communities. Wikis like Wikipedia and editable documents like Google Docs allow mass collaboration and cocreation of textual content. Programs that emphasize a single media form like YouTube (videos), Instagram (photos), and SoundCloud (audio) provide means for sharing simple content that goes beyond text, whereas multimedia platforms like Facebook and Google+ allow for the distribution of content in a variety of forms.

Social media provides the means for person-to-person conversation that operates on human scale like a conversation yet takes place on a global space across time. Social media brings together elements of a face-to-face conversation with its attendant emergent properties and an asynchronous component akin to email. Health promotion's principal challenge with social media is not technological, but social. The *social* component of social media requires rethinking the way health promotion organizations and activities are organized, thus the emphasis on ways of thinking about communication and messages are as important as the actual techniques and tools involved. With social media, health promoters have an opportunity to engage diverse audiences, connect to ones that have remained elusive, and create networks of influence and practice using tools that may reside in our pockets and reach people wherever an Internet connection resides.

SOCIAL MEDIA: PAST, PRESENT, AND FUTURE

Social media is both an old and new concept (Standage, 2013). Since humans started using media to communicate, they have consistently sought to rework, manipulate, and share content to exchange ideas and spread knowledge. As Standage (2013) notes, social media has been around for more than two millennia, it just takes a different form now, and is simply a step in an evolutionary process of human communication. Yet, there are qualities of modern social media that make it quite distinct from what has come before it and are worth noting. Powered by Internet-driven networks, social media has made the process of creating, editing, extending, and distributing content and making social connections considerably faster, more widespread, and more mobile than anything that has come before it. Unlike the distribution of pamphlets or the posting of messages on boards, social media enables individual messages to reach across the globe in an instant. What also makes it different is that it provides simultaneous mechanisms for communication at different levels to different audiences from one-to-one, one-to-many, and many-to-many to anyone, anywhere someone is connected to the Internet and has the tools and literacy to use them.

The scope, implications, and magnitude of this shift are without historical comparisons. Through social media, individual citizens have the means to connect to anyone. Even the Prime Minister of Canada has a Twitter account (@JustinTrudeau) where he tweets in both English and French. Justin Trudeau and his supporters are not novices to social media as it was Trudeau's effective use of social media as a mobilizing tool for supporters that contributed to his election. Whether it is to raise awareness of health or social causes (e.g., Ice Bucket Challenge in 2014), mobilize resources (e.g., relief efforts in Haiti following the 2012 earthquake), create community (e.g., the Canadian Virtual Hospice program in Canada), provide a voice for the disenfranchised or marginalized (e.g., the Idle No More movement by Aboriginal peoples in Canada), or advocate for policy changes, social media has demonstrated itself to be a powerful tool that health promotion professions need to consider in their practice options. But as US President Barack Obama's first official presidential tweet in 2015 showed, this unparalleled connection to the world has consequences; he received many hate-filled, racist, and offensive tweets in response (Davis, 2015).

As these technologies proliferate and become more widely used across social groups, we are seeing that social media resembles a lot of what health promotion has always done, only in novel forms. This chapter will explore the ways in which social media has shaped health promotion practice and research and how these socially driven *high tech* tools actually reflect core, long-established health promotion values (and challenges) in their use.

HEALTH PROMOTION 2.0: NEW THINKING ABOUT CREATING CONVERSATIONS ABOUT HEALTH ONLINE

Social media is as much about a shift in mindset as it is about technology. Traditional health communication emphasizes planned, structured messaging that is largely unidirectional from health professionals to the public. The foundation of this approach can be found in the historical framing of language on information behaviour as noted in the shift in language from concepts such as dissemination and diffusion to knowledge translation and exchange through knowledge integration (Best et al., 2008).

Traditional health communication approaches have been designed around an expert-driven linear model, and the language surrounding the way professionals speak about how knowledge contributes to action supports this (Best et al., 2008). A review of the factors that support knowledge-to-action research using cancer research as a case illustrates the generational shift in the way knowledge is thought to support effective action (as illustrated in Table 14.2) (Best et al., 2008). This shift is one that started with linear models and has evolved to one of systems models even though the language of each model is still in use.

Systems Thinking

The shift from individuals to systems fits with the manner in which social media is used as a tool for health promotion, and this requires systems thinking (Norman, 2011). *Systems thinking* is an interdisciplinary field that has emerged out of disciplines such as biology, physics, engineering, and sociology to explore the interconnections and patterns of influence between actors operating at a distance. It has been argued that health promotion, at its core, is about

TABLE 14.2   Three Generations of Knowledge-to-Action Models

Time Frame	Language	Key Assumptions
Generation 1 1960–mid-1990s **Linear models**	• Dissemination • Diffusion • Knowledge transfer • Knowledge uptake	• Knowledge is a product • The key process is a handoff from knowledge producers to users • Knowledge is generalizable across contexts • Degree of use is a function of effective packaging
Generation 2 mid-1990s to present **Relationship models**	• Knowledge exchange	• Knowledge comes from multiple sources—research, theory, and practice • The key process is interpersonal, involving social relationships—networks of research producers and research consumers who collaborate throughout the knowledge production-synthesis-integration cycle • Knowledge is context-linked, and must be adapted to local setting • Degree of use is a function of effective relationships and processes
Generation 3 **Systems models**	Knowledge integration	• The knowledge cycle is tightly woven within priorities, culture, and context • Explicit and tacit knowledge need to be integrated to inform decision making and policy • Relationships mediate throughout the cycle and must be understood from a systems perspective, in the context of the organization and its strategic processes • Degree of use is a function of effective integration with the organization(s) and its systems

Reprinted from Best, A., Hiatt, R. A., & Norman, C. D. (2008), with permission from Elsevier applying systems thinking to health because of the nature of the problems it deals with (and their unintended consequences) and the manner in which they are addressed (Mittelmark, 2014; Naaldenberg et al., 2009; Norman, 2009). Concepts such as the social determinants of health can be illustrative of the impact of both proximal and distal forces on health and well-being, connecting disparate concepts like social position, neighbourhood, employment, education, gender, race, and others together when the direct influence of any single variable may be difficult to connect.

Systems thinking as a connected collection of theories, methods, and tools can provide a means to see these relations, determine potential causal pathways, and explore ways in which structural and localized actions influence health and well-being. Some of the most important systems concepts in systems science relevant for health promotion are (Norman, 2011):

- **Networks:** Social media is predicated on the ability to connect people together and form, extend, or transform networks of influence through those connections.
- **System dynamics:** The central tenets of system dynamics are found in social media where influence pathways are often nonlinear and multidirectional, include delays and accumulations, and also produce an environment where the impact of a social media action may be felt far from the source within the system.
- **Complexity:** The variety of actors engaged in social media and their diversity of position, knowledge, and influence combined with the multiple forms of media, adaptation potential, dynamic boundary conditions, and nonlinear paths for influence can be understood partly through the application of complexity theory which delves into such things.

eHealth Literacy

Among the areas that health promotion has been seeking to directly influence is health literacy, and social media may play a role contributing to this effort. While health promotion has been held to account for many health-related outcomes that it is only partly able to influence, health literacy is one of the few areas where it has the ability to directly influence. In the context of using ICT for health, health literacy is compounded by a series of other literacies that are needed to use the tools available online and include basic prose literacy and numeracy, computer literacy, information literacy, media literacy, and science literacy. Together these are a part of a meta-literacy called *eHealth literacy,* which is defined as: "the ability to seek, find, understand, and appraise health information from electronic sources and apply the knowledge gained to addressing or solving a health problem" (Norman & Skinner, 2006b). Figure 14.1 outlines the eHealth literacy model and how various literacy skills are organized.

The eHealth Literacy Scale (eHEALS) was developed to measure this multi-dimensional skills set and has been translated into multiple languages and is used worldwide (Norman & Skinner, 2006a).[1] The eHEALS is currently the main instrument used to assess eHealth literacy, although it may require some further development and adaptation to account for the unique cocreative and mobility aspects of social media (Norman, 2011).

Public and Professional Engagement

Social marketing has been one of the principal approaches used by health promoters for connecting to the public and engaging them through health communications (Lefebvre, 2013). The

---

[1]Note that the eHealth Literacy Scale is provided as an appendix to the cited article, and can be downloaded as a word document (http://www.jmir.org/2006/4/e27/).

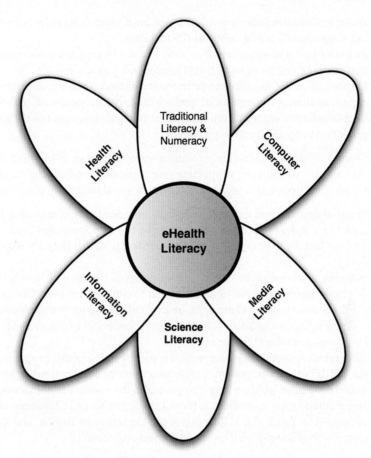

FIGURE 14.1   eHealth Literacy "Lily" Model. Norman, Skinner (2006b).

nationally recognized ParticipACTION program in both its current and previous incarnations was one of the most notable examples of social marketing in action (Tremblay & Craig, 2009). ParticipACTION (http://www.participaction.com) has been a notable leader in the use of social media tools such as interactive blogs, Twitter, and Facebook. Other programs, such as the EatRight Ontario (http://www.eatrightontario.ca), have also provided examples of ways in which social media can be used to gain feedback on client-focused materials to provide rapid-response mechanisms for quality improvement.

Marketers Chris Aarons and Geoff Nelson looked at case studies where social media did not produce desired results for organizations and noted some themes to serve as lessons for organizations (Lefebvre, 2013):

● Good strategy results in messages *going viral,* but viral is not a strategy in itself.
● Social media is less about command and control, and more about engagement with audiences.
● The social aspect of social media is both the content and the vehicle for sharing it. Marketers must recognize that audiences have many different motivators for action, however recognition or compensation will likely to lead to higher levels of engagement.
● Relationships and knowledge are the best social currency, not money.

- Social media creates the ongoing and sustained interest between news and launches and can supplement a public relations (PR) strategy.
- Promoting your message requires work, not just buying advertisements; the more reach that you seek, the more work that is needed, not just money.
- Each social media site needs to be treated as distinct: random, unplanned tactics to engage audiences through social media will likely turn people off or fail to engage them.
- Social media is a strategic amplifier of a campaign's message, not the entire campaign, given that people will act on and offline.

Communication and health promotion campaigns can take different forms and social media can play a leading or supporting role depending on how the campaign is structured. There are three orders of interventions in which social media can play a part:

1. **Stand-alone:** The tool designed to operate independently of any other resource is considered a first-order intervention. (For example, the Stop Smoking Centre developed by V-CC Systems and the Centre for Addiction and Mental Health [http://www.stopsmokingcenter.net].)
2. **Adjunct:** A second-order intervention is designed for use with another type of resource (e.g., a telephone helpline) or as an adjunct to clinical treatment. Unlike first-order interventions, these types of campaigns are explicitly designed to complement other methods. (For example, the Canadian Cancer Society's Smokers' Helpline website in Ontario [http://www.smokershelpline.ca].)
3. **Integrated:** A third-order intervention is part of an integrated program of delivery where the ICT is but one component. Unlike second-order interventions, a third-order intervention is embedded within a larger program and the resource is not viewed as integral to the larger initiative nor apart from it. (For example, the Virtual Classroom on Tobacco Control, developed by Youth Voices Research at the University of Toronto and TakingITGlobal [http://www.takingitglobal.org/tiged/projects/tobacco//].)

See Norman (2007) for further explanation of how the examples fit the orders of interventions.

Equity and Access

Concerns regarding the use of technology for health promotion often focus on the *digital divide*—the gap between those with the means to access technology and those without. While such access issues are important, the level of overall reach and ability to use social media in Canada is high with over 70% of Canadians reporting to be active users of social media (Media Technology Monitor, 2015) following a decade of development that made Canada a leader in putting ICT in schools as part of an effort to create a technology-adept population. Nonetheless, as Skinner et al. (2003) note, it is important to pay attention to the quality of access, not just absolute access. While inequities exist, there remain few alternatives that offer the same level of connectivity and diversity of means of sharing content for low cost as social media.

What social media can offer is a direct means to find and engage diverse populations on different issues in ways that have few parallels for similar costs. Within any particular campaign, social media can be used to identify and engage members of different populations through appropriate search strategies and tailored engagement approaches that draw on health promotion values and methods. What makes it different is that social media can allow for a very open, public, transparent, and immediate means of connecting with these populations in a manner that affords them as much control and influence in the interaction as the health promoter. Rather than addressing an audience, the health promoter is generating a conversation with and cocreating *audiences* (Norman, 2012).

Social media has been used effectively to engage hard-to-reach populations on key health topics across the spectrum of issues, including HIV, food security, tobacco cessation, and mental health. The portability, high reach, and low barrier to access has made social media a key tool for engaging hidden populations or groups who are unlikely to engage with traditional health promotion programming.

SOCIAL MEDIA AND HEALTH COMMUNICATION

The field of health communication encompasses a variety of theoretical positions that deal with issues such as knowledge gaps, message framing and processing, agenda setting, risk communication, and information processing. These models, while useful in understanding the way health messaging is sent, received, and processed, do not offer a complete account of the manner in which knowledge is cocreated, remixed, edited, and distributed via social networks through social media, often in real time and mediated through technology. New theories are required to build upon the foundation of traditional health communication messaging that take into account the properties of social media. Further, these theories need to account for the unique features and challenges that social media introduces.

Transparency

For organizations seeking to shape their communications, social media can be as problematic as useful. Transparency has a downside in that it can lead to public denunciation that may be disproportionate to the issue, making the risks associated with using social media worth serious consideration (Ronson, 2015). Transparency also introduces new challenges for how messages get received and the unintended consequences of carrying out conversations in full view of the entire social media world.

Case Study: Anti-Vaccination Messages

Jenny McCarthy, a celebrity television host, author, and model, was one of highest profile individuals to support Andrew Wakefield's fraudulent research that claimed to link vaccines with autism, research that was falsified and has been thoroughly disproved (Flaherty, 2011).

On Monday, March 13, 2014, McCarthy posted on Twitter the following question:

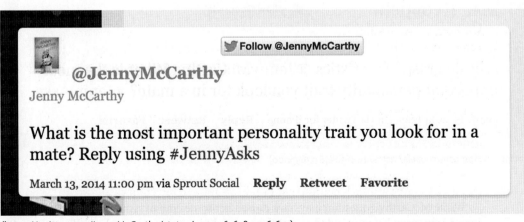

(https://twitter.com/JennyMcCarthy/status/444246562844061697)

The response from Twitter users included answers to her question that included comment on her stance on vaccines and autism that included:

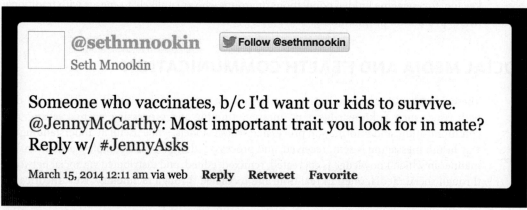

@sethmnookin　　Follow @sethmnookin
Seth Mnookin

Someone who vaccinates, b/c I'd want our kids to survive.
@JennyMcCarthy: Most important trait you look for in mate?
Reply w/ #JennyAsks

March 15, 2014 12:11 am via web　**Reply　Retweet　Favorite**

(https://twitter.com/sethmnookin/status/444626925013983232)

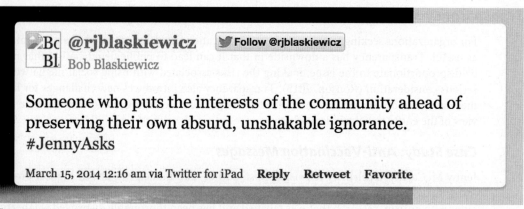

@rjblaskiewicz　　Follow @rjblaskiewicz
Bob Blaskiewicz

Someone who puts the interests of the community ahead of
preserving their own absurd, unshakable ignorance.
#JennyAsks

March 15, 2014 12:16 am via Twitter for iPad　**Reply　Retweet　Favorite**

(https://twitter.com/rjblaskiewicz/status/444628277890514944)

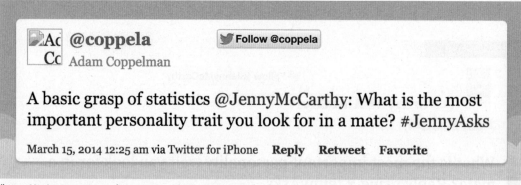

@coppela　　Follow @coppela
Adam Coppelman

A basic grasp of statistics @JennyMcCarthy: What is the most
important personality trait you look for in a mate? #JennyAsks

March 15, 2014 12:25 am via Twitter for iPhone　**Reply　Retweet　Favorite**

(https://twitter.com/coppela/status/444630546333696000)

While McCarthy's question may have caused her some embarrassment due to the unanticipated response, the unintended consequences might have done as much good to her profile as she noted in a post four days after the original question was asked, referring to a rise in a marketing metric score:

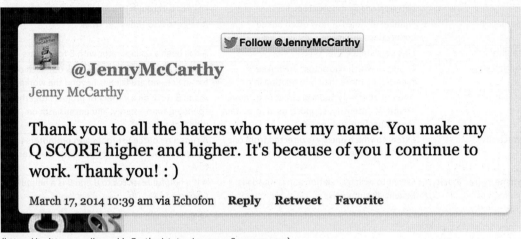

Follow @JennyMcCarthy

@JennyMcCarthy

Jenny McCarthy

Thank you to all the haters who tweet my name. You make my Q SCORE higher and higher. It's because of you I continue to work. Thank you! :)

March 17, 2014 10:39 am via Echofon   **Reply   Retweet   Favorite**

(https://twitter.com/JennyMcCarthy/status/445509784973094912)

This case represents some of challenges that social media poses for organizations where debates are held in public for many to see and traces of the conversation can live on through indexed web pages and screen captures made even if the original post or comment is deleted. For health promoters operating in areas of responsibility, potentially as a perceived authority on health matters, and with organizations who share that status, two notable risks present themselves. The first risk is having messages skewed or misrepresented or unintentionally mistaken causing potential reputational harm. The second risk is related to disengaging from audiences due to a lack of authenticity or relevance or through a presentation of content in a manner that is not attractive to target groups, alienating health promoters from the public. The risk is that the public can disengage from health promotion if they feel that the messages and communications do not reflect their needs, desires, and preferences.

Networks

The potential of social media is realized through networks, as illustrated in the McCarthy example (positively and negatively). The most central feature of networks is ties: connections between individuals or entities, or *actors*. The manner in which these ties are formed and maintained and the role that actors play are all part of a series of concepts represented in network theories (Monge & Contractor, 2003). Network theories focus on various elements of relationships and motivations for engaging in and acting through those relationships. Some of the most relevant concepts in social networks include:

- **Cliques:** Cliques are measured through shared network connections and clustering of links (e.g., three or more individuals connected to each other).
- **Network strength:** This is assessed by the emotional or intellectual intensity, intimacy, or reciprocity or amount of time invested in interactions. For example, posts and reactions to posts are one source of determining network strength. As the quality and quantity of the posts change and evolve, so too will the overall strength of the network.
- **Symmetry:** Symmetrical relations in social networks are assessed through bi-directional ties, whereby interactions are mutually beneficial. A network that has many symmetrical

TABLE 14.3 Typical Social Network Measures of Ties

Measure	Definition	Example
Indirect links	The path between two actors is mediated between one or more actors	A is connected to B and B to C; thus A indirectly links to C through B
Frequency	Number of times or how often linked connections are made	A talks to B 10 times per week
Stability	Link persistence over time	A has been a collaborator with B for 3 years
Multiplexity	Extent to which two actors are linked together by more than one relationship	A and B are colleagues, they seek out each other for advice and are friends beyond the workplace
Strength	Amount of energy and resources (e.g., time, emotional intensity, support) used to sustain the connection, link, or tie	A and B work on a variety of projects together, spending time, energy, and enthusiasm on different projects
Direction	Extent to which energy is directed from one actor to another through a link	A runs a resource list for health promoters that B receives, but B does not provide resources to A
Symmetry (reciprocity)	Extent to which a relationship is mutually beneficial, supportive	A is a helpful resource to B and B is a helpful resource to A

Adapted from Brass, D. J. (1995).

relations within it is more likely to be robust in its ability to sustain engagement and achieve impact.

- **Frequency:** The number of transactions that take place and the frequency of interactions are indicators of overall engagement on a social network.
- **Role:** Exploration of the various roles that users play, including an assessment of the overall diversity of the network characteristics, allows for determination of the type and impact of different roles within the network.

The manner in which network ties are measured is often observation and surveys looking at the number, type, and purpose of the connections through measures are described by Brass (1995) in Table 14.3.

The need to create networks of health promoters was made clear as a priority for health promotion in the 2007 Bangkok Charter for Health Promotion (see Chapter 1, Table 1.2). The Charter identified the need to empower communities and build health promotion capacity globally through collective action. It proposed a framework for a set of strategies across all sectors and settings designed to support advocacy, address the determinants of health, build health promotion capacity, promote policies protecting the vulnerable, and build alliances and partnerships among diverse sectors for sustainable action. Social media has an opportunity to directly influence all of these goals and serve the capacity-enhancing mission outlined in the Bangkok Charter. One of the ways social media is able to do this is through the power of networks; understanding how knowledge is exchanged, generated, and distributed through such networks is central to using social media with health professionals and creating the right messages.

Media and Messaging

Social media embodies Marshall McLuhan's (1964) statement "the medium is the message." The medium for social media can be desktop or laptop computers, tablets, mobile handsets, and soon other objects as the *Internet of Things* leads online access through a diversity of platforms such as household appliances, automobiles, and even living creatures (Oriwoh & Conrad, 2015). These platforms will enable social engagements that reflect an embodiment of the messages they facilitate and produce. It is not surprising that the rise and evolution of social media has directly paralleled and indeed supported mobile Internet development and tools in a symbiotic relationship. Mobile technologies that bring together telephones, text, and video-supported messaging, with audio, photographic, and video recording capability, enable anyone to play the role of a participatory citizen journalist (Bulkey, 2012).

Message development for this mobile, multifaceted social media engagement space requires something more than adopting the explicit planning-focused models of traditional health communications due to the inherent complexity in health promotion related to the diversity of need, context, and social circumstances. Norman and Muzumdar (2013) provide four key recommendations for health promoters who are seeking to engage audiences through social media, particularly on issues of social determinants of health:

1. Have a distinct, clear message; be authentic; and share what you know.
2. Create space for conversation, not just one-sided, unidirectional messages.
3. Whenever possible, make connections among people, concepts, and content: hyperlink, mention, and tag.
4. Sensitize yourself to the needs of both health promotion organizations and audiences.

Social media communication is itself part of the complexity that encompasses health promotion, thus requiring communication strategies that are adapted for complexity in their design (Norman, 2012).

DESIGNING FUTURE HEALTH PROMOTION SYSTEMS THROUGH SOCIAL MEDIA

"Everyone designs who devises courses of action aimed at changing existing situations into preferred ones." —Herbert Simon (1996)

Health promotion is fundamentally about change, whether it is change the status quo, or working with change to preserve and protect what is currently in place; thus, health promoters are fundamentally designers. The multidisciplinary field of design brings together tools and perspectives from art, architecture, biology, business, engineering, psychology, and social science to shape the thinking and practice of creating products (objects, processes, spaces, and systems) that change the way things are done. The design approach is particularly relevant to social media where communication patterns are emergent and nonlinear rather than prescriptive and controlled. Van Alstyne and Logan (2007) believe that design operating in complex systems needs to attend to and facilitate emergence, arguing that having a clear purpose is key, aligning the proper materials and catalyzing them into a process of design that allows for self-organized patterns to develop to achieve the design.

Design Thinking

Design thinking is a concept that emerged as a way of aiding nondesigners to apply the same thought processes to social and human systems more readily (Cross, 2011). Although the tools and technologies that facilitate social media use (computers, handsets, tablets, websites, and software applications (i.e., apps)) are already designed, what concerns health promoters is the design of the experience of using these technologies through social media. Skinner et al. (2006) outlined a design process for eHealth communications—the Spiral Technology Action Research (STAR) model—that has been widely adopted as a guide for health promoters about how to develop tools for online health promotion. The STAR model entwines iterative development cycles with technology design and community involvement to generate products that are responsive to changing needs and the values of the populations being engaged (Skinner et al., 2006) (see Fig. 14.2).

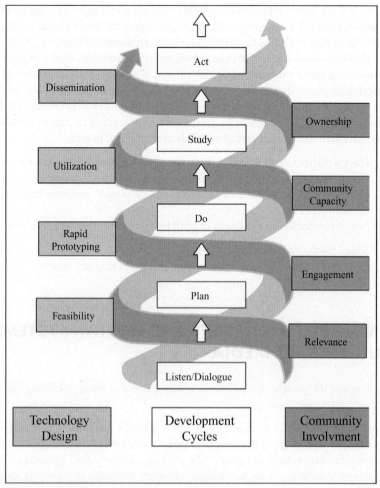

FIGURE 14.2   STAR model showing the interplay among technology and community involvement through successive development cycles (Skinner et al., 2006).

Social Media Futures

Social media will continue onward, although it will likely look quite different even into the near future given the rapid evolution of the technologies that power the media and the messages. While Facebook, Twitter, and the other current popular platforms may drift away or evolve into new things, it is likely is that the trend toward more visual, rich media will continue. Photo and video sharing will remain popular, largely because it conveys a lot of information to users. The trend toward providing quick, portable, "byte-sized" content accessible from nearly any device, anywhere, is also likely to prove robust over time. Other trends we may see that will influence social media include:

- **Blending local and global perspectives.** *Glocal* patterns of interactions (Thörn, 2007) will allow us to engage in global health promotion with ease, although the risk is that we collectively spread our attention too thin. There will be great pressure to develop better information filters, behaviours, and tools that will enable us to sort through the volume of content created as more of the global population goes online and uses social media.
- **Local engagement, focused engagement.** Things like meet-ups, news, and online coalitions will continue to develop at local and global levels simultaneously as community

groups, not-for-profit organizations, public health institutions, and governments learn how to use social media more effectively to reach new audiences and learn from one another around content organized around contexts.

- **Greater engagement and lesser privacy and control.** As technologies allow greater customization including location awareness, the risks to privacy and security increase as well. Munson et al. (2013) examined social media and health, and noted the tension between privacy and sharing, policy information credibility, accessibility, and tailoring in social spaces as the key sociotechnical challenges.
- **Narrowing perspective instead of choice.** Zuckerman (2013) has discussed the paradox of how tools like social media allow us to connect to anyone and see any perspective, yet we often find ourselves more insular and at risk of engaging with content that simply reinforces our currently held beliefs rather than exposing ourselves to alternative perspectives.
- **Keeping pace.** The speed at which change takes place is not congruent with the academic system of funding, peer review, and publication. Evidence needs to be generated faster and published in alternative sources (Norman, 2012).

Summary

Social media tools will change and evolve, but the central concepts and ideas around connecting people together, cocreating, and globally distributing content will remain. People have always enjoyed sharing what they learn and having conversations. They have also wanted more freedom, flexibility, speed, and reach and therefore we are likely to see social media—in whatever forms it takes—continue. Learning to think about it and adapt to it is key to using it for health promotion practice.

REFERENCES

Best, A., Hiatt, R. A., & Norman, C. D. (2008). Knowledge integration: Conceptualizing communications in cancer control systems. *Patient Education and Counseling, 71*, 319–327.

Brass, D. J. (1995). A social network perspective on human resources management. *Research in Personnel and Human Resources Management, 13*, 39–79.

Bulkey, K. (2012). The rise of citizen journalism. *The guardian.* URL=http://www.theguardian.com/media/2012/jun/11/rise-of-citizen-journalism

Cross, N. (2011). *Design thinking: Understanding how designers think and work.* Oxford: Berg.

Davis, J. H. (2015). Obama's Twitter debut, @POTUS, attracts hate-filled posts. *The New York Times.* URL=http://www.nytimes.com/2015/05/22/us/politics/obamas-twitter-debut-potus-attracts-hate-filled-posts.html?_r=0

Flaherty, D. K. (2011). The vaccine-autism connection: A public health crisis caused by unethical medical practices and fraudulent science. *The Annals of Pharmacotherapy, 45*, 1302–1304.

Lefebvre, R. C. (2013). *Social marketing and social change.* San Francisco: Jossey-Bass.

McLuhan, M. (1964). The medium is the message. In *Understanding media: The extensions of man.* URL=http://web.mit.edu/allanmc/www/mcluhan.mediummessage.pdf

Media Technology Monitor. (2015). *Media technology adoption Fall 2014.* Toronto: CBC/Radio-Canada. URL=https://www.mtm-otm.ca/Download.ashx?req = 405

Mittelmark, M. B. (2014). Unintended effects in settings-based health promotion. *Scandinavian Journal of Public Health, 42*(Suppl 15), 17–24.

Monge, P. R., & Contractor, N. S. (2003). *Theories of communication networks.* New York, NY: Oxford University Press.

Munson, S. A., Cavusoglu, H., Frisch, L., & Fels, S. (2013). Sociotechnical challenges and progress in using social media for health. *Journal of Medical Internet Research, 15*(10), e226.

Naaldenberg, J., Vaandrager, L., Koelen, M., Wagemakers, A-M., Saan, H., & de Hoog, K. (2009). Elaborating on systems thinking in health promotion practice. *Global Health Promotion, 16*(1), 39–47.

Norman, C. (2007). Using information technology to support smoking-related behaviour change: Web-assisted tobacco interventions. *Smoking Cessation Rounds, 1*(6).

Norman, C. D. (2009). Health promotion as a systems science and practice. *Journal of Evaluation in Clinical Practice, 15*, 868–872.

Norman, C. (2011). eHealth literacy 2.0: Problems and opportunities with an evolving concept. *Journal of Medical Internet Research, 13*(4), e125.

Norman, C. D. (2012). Social media and health promotion. *Global Health Promotion, 19*(4), 3–6.

Norman, C. D., & Muzumdar, P. (2013). How can social media support knowledge exchange on the social determinants of health? URL=http://nccdh.ca/blog/entry/SDH-social-media-blog3

Norman, C. D., & Skinner, H. A. (2006a). eHEALS: The eHealth literacy scale. *Journal of Medical Internet Research, 8*(4), e27.

Norman, C. D., & Skinner, H. A. (2006b). eHealth Literacy: Essential skills for consumer health in a networked world. *Journal of Medical Internet Research, 8*(2), e9.

Oriwoh, E., & Conrad, M. (2015). "Things" in the internet of things: Towards a definition. *International Journal of Internet of Things, 4*(1), 1–5.

Ronson, J. (2015). *So you've been publicly shamed.* New York, NY: Riverhead Books, Penguin.

Simon, H. A. (1996). *The sciences of the artificial* (3rd ed.). Cambridge: MIT Press.

Skinner, H., Biscope, S., & Poland, B. (2003). Quality of internet access: Barriers behind internet use statistics. *Social Science & Medicine, 57*, 875–880.

Skinner, H. A., Maley, O., & Norman, C. D. (2006). Developing internet-based eHealth promotion programs: The Spiral Technology Action Research (STAR) Model. *Health Promotion Practice, 7*, 406–417.

Standage, T. (2013). *Writing on the wall: social media—the first 2,000 years.* New York, NY: Bloomsbury USA.

Thörn, H. (2007). Social movements, the media and the emergence of a global public sphere from anti-apartheid to global justice. *Current Sociology, 55*, 896–918.

Tremblay, M. S., & Craig, C. L. (2009). ParticipACTION: Overview and introduction of baseline research on the "new" ParticipACTION. *The International Journal of Behavioral Nutrition and Physical Activity, 6*, 84.

Van Alstyne, G., & Logan, R. K. (2007). Designing for emergence and innovation: Redesigning Design. *Artifact, 1*, 120–129.

World Health Organization (WHO). (1986). *The Ottawa charter for health promotion.* Geneva: Author.

Zuckerman, E. (2013). *Rewire: Digital cosmopolitans in the age of connection.* New York, NY: W. W. Norton & Company.

ONLINE RESOURCES

Please visit thePoint at http://thepoint.lww.com/Vollman4e for up-to-date Internet resources and additional learning materials on this topic.

The Process of
Community as Partner

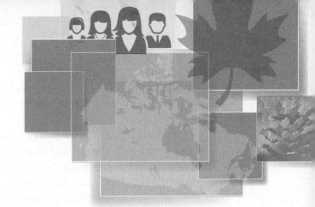

CHAPTER 15

A Model to Guide Practice

Ardene Robinson Vollman

LEARNING OBJECTIVES

Models that serve as guides for practice, education, and research have become important tools for community workers. This chapter, in which we begin our examination of the process as applied to the community as partner, focuses on the use of one model to guide practice.

After studying this chapter, you should be able to:

1. Define *model*
2. Describe the purposes of a model
3. Describe selected models relevant to community practice
4. Define *community* and the aspects of a healthy community
5. Begin to apply a model to community practice
6. Understand the interprofessional and multidisciplinary nature of community work

Introduction

Health disciplines have developed models for practice that provide processes and structures to identify issues and work across disciplines and with communities. Conceptual maps are useful guides for action, particularly when practice focuses on entire communities. The Canadian community-as-partner (CCAP) model provides us with processes, structures, and a conceptual map that will be used throughout this chapter. While a model might look structural, it also encompasses the processes by which the model is enacted. Throughout, we will refer to these processes as well as to the values and assumptions that underpin the practice of working with community as partner.

MODELS

A *conceptual model* is the synthesis of a set of concepts and the statements that integrate those concepts into a whole. A *community process model* can be defined as a frame of reference, a way of looking at a community, or an image of what working in and with a community encompasses. A model is a representation of practice, not a reality. Other types of models that are used to represent realities are model airplanes, blueprints, chemical equations, and anatomic models.

A model with which health workers identified for many years was the medical model, that is, a disease-oriented, illness- and body system–focused approach to patients, with an emphasis on pathology. This model has served us well in our quest to eliminate childhood communicable diseases and common preventable illness. However, reliance on the medical model that focuses on individuals excludes health promotion and the holistic focus that is central to population/public health and community well-being. Additionally, important aspects of care, such as psychological, sociocultural, and spiritual areas, are not explicitly included in the medical model. Thus, a community-as-partner model should encompass all aspects of health and incorporate long-range goals and planning.

As a representation of reality, a model can take numerous forms. Because they describe professional practice, all models are narrative; that is, words are the symbols that are used by workers (e.g., nurses, social workers, nutritionists) to define how they view their practice. And although all models are described in words, many are clarified further through the use of diagrams or illustrations. Diagrams are an efficient and effective way of depicting models; the use of such images allows the model builder to show relationships and linkages among the concepts in the model. The diagram is often thought of as the model itself, with the accompanying text seen as the elaboration or explanation of the model.

The method chosen to depict a model reflects the model builder's own philosophy and preference; no one method is accepted as the best. General agreement exists that four concepts are central to health disciplines: person, environment, health, and the defining characteristics of the specific health discipline (e.g., nursing, social work, medicine, nutrition). *Concepts* are defined as general notions or ideas and are considered the building blocks of models. How each of the four concepts is defined will both dictate the organization of the model and be illustrated in that model. For example, health may be defined on a continuum with wellness at one end and death at the other; as a dichotomy wherein one is seen as well or ill; as the outcome of numerous biopsychosocial and spiritual forces; or as the interaction of these same forces. In the medical model, *health* has been defined traditionally as the absence of disease.

Hancock and Perkins (1985) address the complexity of people's lives and the interactions with the environment in their model of the Mandala of Health (Fig. 15.1). The Mandala resonates with the concepts presented in earlier chapters. It is based in part on an understanding of human ecology as the interaction of culture (including politics) with the natural environment (biosphere) depicted in the outer circle and represents the living planet. Health is understood in a holistic sense, so the health of the population is seen as having body, mind, and spiritual dimensions. The system levels or shells extend outward from the individual and comprise the family, the community, and the built environment, and also include the natural environment as exemplified by the culture/biosphere shell. The social sciences (psychology, sociology, economics, anthropology) are integrated in the upper half of the model (personal behaviour and psychosocial and economic environments), while the physical sciences (physics, chemistry, biology, engineering) are integrated into the lower half of the model with human biology and physical environments as factors that influence health. *Lifestyle* is defined as "personal behaviour as influenced and modified by, and constrained by, a lifelong socialization process and by the psychosocial environment, including cultural and community values and standards" (Hancock & Perkins, 1985, p. 8). The health care system is rightfully given the title "sick care services," a determinant of health that attempts to integrate the physical and social sciences. The Mandala should be viewed as a three-dimensional model in which various components shift in shape and size according to their relative importance over time and in different settings.

Neither the Mandala nor the medical model has an action component, however. For this, we go to a model developed by the Rural Development Institute (Rural Development Institute

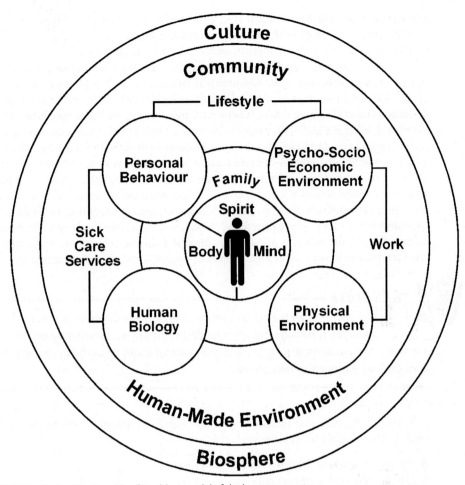

FIGURE 15.1 The Mandala of Health: A model of the human ecosystem.

[RDI], 2005) in Brandon, Manitoba (Fig. 15.2). It illustrates the goal of action (becoming) and the steps along the process—being and belonging.

Being represents those actions that people undertake and involves their interactions with others as they form a collective unit. These interactions lead to a sense of *belonging* or expression by the group of a "sense of community." McMillan (2014) identifies four elements of sense of community: membership, influence, need fulfillment, and shared emotional connections. Belonging leads to *becoming* through the collective action of the community. This community action entails the processes of assessing the community, settings goals and planning for change, implementing change processes, and evaluating both the processes and the outcomes of the actions taken (RDI, 2005). The goal of action is to improve community health. Action

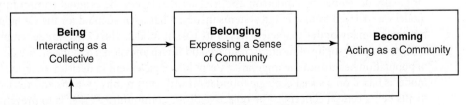

FIGURE 15.2 Being, belonging, and becoming model for a healthy community.

relates to community development (i.e., Ottawa Charter—strengthening community action) with the outcome being healthy people in healthy settings.

Health is one of the four concepts central to health disciplines and is defined for the purposes of this book as "a resource for everyday life, not the objective of living. [It is] a positive concept emphasizing social and personal resources as well as physical capacities" (World Health Organization [WHO], 1986). Üstün and Jakob (2005) call for the WHO to update its definition of health, citing that it fails to take into account the more contemporary notion of well-being. Bircher's (2005) definition—"a dynamic state of well-being characterized by a physical and mental potential, which satisfies the demands of life commensurate with age, culture, and personal responsibility"—is more comprehensive and relevant to today's context. *Person*, in this book, refers to collectives rather than individuals or families, that is, populations, aggregates, systems, structures, and society. The *environment* is conceived as an encompassing concept that includes biologic, psychological, social, emotional, and spiritual dimensions and the contexts or settings where people live, love, learn, work, play, and pray. The mandate of the action of *health disciplines* is preventive, aimed at reducing community and population-level risk factors and stressors, building community capacity, and enhancing resilience.

Take Note

As we proceed through the action components of the community process in this section of the book, you will encounter other models to guide your community practice. Think for a moment of what a model is to you and how a model might be useful in your practice. What does professional practice mean to you?

If you can answer that question, you have begun to describe your model of practice. A model serves the following purposes:

- Provides a map for the problem-solving process
- Gives direction for assessment
- Guides analysis
- Directs community health diagnoses
- Assists in planning
- Facilitates evaluation
- Provides a curriculum outline for education
- Represents a framework for research
- Provides a basis for development of theory

A model is nothing more or less than an explication of practice. A model not only describes what is but also provides a framework for making decisions about what could be.

CANADIAN COMMUNITY-AS-PARTNER MODEL

Originally developed by Anderson and McFarlane (1988), the original community-as-client model was derived from nursing systems theory; it has been adapted for the Canadian context but retains many of the characteristics of its parent model. The CCAP model emphasizes the underlying philosophy of multidisciplinary and interprofessional actions on the determinants of population health and the imperative for public engagement in decision making. The CCAP model is based on a social ecologic foundation with community systems and related environments being central concepts. The objective of the community worker is to prevent fragmentation of services to the population and the community. The community team's goals are to intervene to (1) decrease the potential of the community system to encounter stressors, (2) limit the impact or effects of stressors on the community through prevention interventions, and (3) build the capacity of the community to act on its own behalf.

 Critical Thinking Exercise 15.1

Before you read the next section, write down on a piece of paper what you think community is. Do this again after you have read this section. Are there any differences?

What is community? When we think about community, we think about geographical locations such as towns or neighbourhoods. We also think of settings where people congregate to carry out their daily lives (e.g., workplaces, schools, places of worship) as communities. But groups of people (populations, aggregates) are also referred to as communities (e.g., ethnic communities, farm communities, gay community, professional community, virtual community). When we use the term *community,* we are placing a boundary (real or symbolic) around a group of people that demarcates who is in and who is out of that group. Community refers to people who have a common bond and share beliefs, values, and norms that identify members. People rarely belong to a single community, but may identify with several based on variables such as geography, occupation, and interests. A healthy community, according to the Ontario Healthy Communities Coalition (OHCC, 2015), has the following characteristics:

- Clean and safe physical environment
- Peace, equity, and social justice
- Adequate access to food, water, shelter, income, safety, work, and recreation for all
- Adequate access to health care services
- Opportunities for learning and skill development
- Strong, mutually supportive relationships and networks
- Workplaces that are supportive of individual and family well-being
- Wide participation of residents in decision making
- Strong local cultural and spiritual heritage
- Diverse and vital economy
- Protection of the natural environment
- Responsible use of resources to ensure long-term sustainability

Additional community attributes might include a sense of unity, effective collaboration and communication, judicious balance between utilization and conservation of resources, problem-solving orientation, and the ability to handle crises and conflict (Allender & Spradley, 2005). A healthy community generates and effectively uses its assets and resources to support the quality of life and the well-being of the community as a whole. A healthy community is *resilient*—it responds to adversity and improves its level of functioning as a result of meeting challenges. A healthy community is *participative*—members identify with it, they engage in social interaction and build ties with it and with each other, and they share decision making about the community. The goal of a healthy community is *sustainability*—maintaining the reciprocal relationship among people and the environment (social, economic, physical) over time and through inevitable change (Racher & Annis, 2008). How a community functions determines its health.

Consider the CCAP model (Fig. 15.3). Three central factors underpin this model: a focus on the community as a system, the people in the community as engaged partners in action, and the use of the problem-solving process. The model is described next in some detail to assist in understanding its parts and guiding community practice.

Assessment

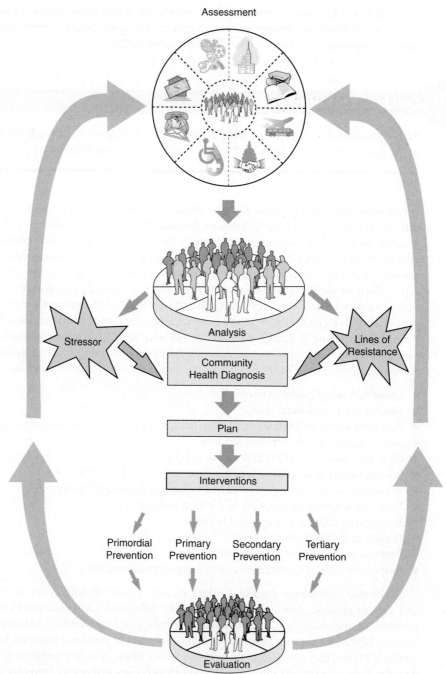

FIGURE 15.3 Canadian community-as-partner model.

The intent of the action phases of the CCAP model is to build community—build the capacity of community members to participate in all aspects of the community so that they can collectively and collaboratively take action to achieve the outcomes they desire for their community and the people living in it. In this regard, the community worker may lead in some parts of the process, but in other parts the community worker will be a bystander, supporting and encouraging community members. This process of developing community assets, capacity, and competence is fundamental to the action component of the CCAP model. Regardless of how a community and a community worker came together, the CCAP process should engage the community, involve its members, and be driven by the issues as viewed by the community itself. The community agenda supersedes the agendas of government, not-for-profit groups, non-governmental organizations, and business interests.

The *core* of the assessment wheel (which is shown in detail in Fig. 15.4) represents the people who make up the community. Included in information to describe the community's

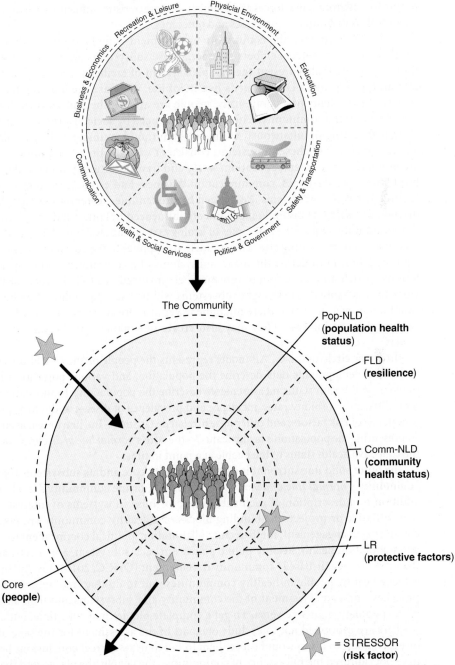

FIGURE 15.4   The community assessment wheel, featuring lines of resistance and defence within the community structure.

core are the population's social demographics (e.g., age, sex and ethnic distribution, culture, education achievement, and socioeconomic status), its values, beliefs, and history, as well as information about the population's health indicators (e.g., mortality and morbidity). Understanding the people is essential in planning community action, and changes in the community demographics must be identified and considered over time. Community development and health-promoting change are dependent upon community workers and teams working *with* a community on actions and issues community members deem critical to the community's health and quality of life. People live in constant and reciprocal interaction with their environments. Environmental forces and population characteristics influence each other and make reciprocal contributions to processes and outcomes.

In the CCAP model, the community environment is divided into several *subsystems* with which community members interact. These subsystems are the structural foundations of society that represent the complex system of facilities, programs, and networks that aim to improve a community's quality of life. They are the building blocks of civil society. As residents of a community, people are affected by and, in turn, influence the subsystems of the community. Citizens are influenced by societal structures at several levels that are acting simultaneously at the neighbourhood, municipal, provincial/territorial, and national levels. These subsystems, consistent with the broad determinants of health, are physical environment, education, safety and transportation, politics and government, health and social services, communication, business and economics, and recreation and leisure. The eight subsystems are divided by broken lines to remind us that they are not discrete and separate but influence (and are influenced by) one another and the people of the community. One of the principles of ecology (see Chapter 7, Fig. 7.2) is that everything is connected to everything else. This premise also applies to the community as a whole. The eight divisions both define the major subsystems of a community and provide the community worker and those community members involved in a CCAP process with a framework for assessment. These eight subsystems will be used throughout this book; readers should, however, note that there might be fewer or more subsystems at work in their own communities of interest. They may also create new names for the various subsystems at play.

The inner circle of the CCAP model represents the people or the *core* of the community. Social and demographic data describe the population, and various population-level epidemiologic and health status measurements describe the population's health status (e.g., birth, mortality, and morbidity rates; incidence and prevalence of disease and injury; presence and prevalence of risk factors; and other health-related statistics). The line drawn around the core (representing the population's health status)—the core's *normal line of defence* (Pop-NLD)—is the collective health status of the people at a point in time.

The outer solid line surrounding the community core and its subsystems represents the community's *normal line of defence* (Comm-NLD), or the community's level of health. In addition to a description of each subsystem, or those subsystems of interest to a particular initiative or project, the building blocks of a healthy community are taken into account: citizen engagement, multi-sector collaboration, political commitment to community and population health, healthy public policies in each subsystem, and asset-based (rather than risk- or deficit-based) community development (OHCC, 2015). Ideally, the goal is to achieve healthy people in healthy communities, but to do that may require stepwise approaches—first an assessment of the community and subsystems and then an assessment of the population, or vice versa. To get a complete picture may take time, but community workers are cautioned not to exclude one part of the assessment for the sake of efficiency or expediency; to do so would cause them to fail to draw correct conclusions because they have not captured the full essence of community—the people, the places, and the structures of the community.

Take Note

Take a moment to examine the selection of subsystems that have been identified. Can you think of any that have been omitted? Think of the community where you live. Would you add faith or spirituality as a subsystem? What about culture, heritage, and the arts?

Within the community subsystems are *lines of resistance* (LR); these are relatively permanent factors and mechanisms within each of the subsystems that act to defend against threats such as risk factors (stressors) penetrating to the community core. Lines of resistance are the protective factors—the strengths and *assets* of the community. The LR exist throughout each of the subsystems, and their strength influences the degree of reaction to a stressor experienced by a community or population aggregate. The stronger the capacities and assets of the community and its people, the more resilient the community and its population are, and the more likely it will fend off any threats (stressors). Strengths include community assets such as community capacity, social capital, and usual patterns of collective coping and problem-solving competencies in each of the subsystems. Networks and harmonious connections among people, associations, government and nongovernmental organizations, faith institutions, and social agencies are examples of community assets that can be mobilized when a stressor threatens the community and its citizens. For instance, if teen pregnancy is an ongoing concern in the community (stressor), having a community-based teen health clinic accessible near public transit routes can offer culturally attuned sexual and reproductive health services and social services to prevent teen pregnancy and to support those teens that are pregnant or parenting. These services and those from other subsystems (e.g., education, social services, housing) along with the community attitudes that support them, represent community assets, strengths, competence, and capacity, that is, the community's LR.

The *flexible line of defence* (FLD), shown as a broken line around the community and its NLD, is a buffer zone representing a dynamic level of health resulting from a temporary response to threats (stressors). It prevents temporary or transient stressors from penetrating through the NLD to either the community subsystems or the core itself. Examples of temporary responses may be that, in the time of an economic crisis, inner-city churches will provide temporary shelter, and the food bank will offer food to a wider clientele when the weather suddenly turns cold. Temporary responses are used until more permanent solutions are found (e.g., the economy recovers and people find jobs and housing or the weather improves). For an example of a FLD in action, see Chapter 24 that relates a flood disaster response. The FLD illustrates the community's *resilience* in the face of challenges. A resilient community bounces back from adversity; the people of the community are mutually supportive through a dense network of social supports. Hard times make people angry, alienated, and disengaged; resilient communities reach out to those who are socially isolated and offer support to those who need a hand.

Stressors are risk factors that have the potential to threaten or cause tension in a community and lead to disruption in relationships, connections, and coping mechanisms. Risk factors and threats may arise from the internal environment, the external environment, or the created environment. Stressors may originate within the geopolitical community, population, or group (e.g., gang activity, graffiti, influx of refugees). They may also be risk factors that are created outside of the community and its people (e.g., poor air quality from distant forest fires, extreme weather conditions, economic recession). Some risk factors can originate from interactions among community subsystems (e.g., low minimum wage, soaring housing costs, school fees) that place burdens on families and strain social services. Risk factors can also be enduring (more permanent, long-lasting) stressors on a community or transient (short term) in nature. For example, the 2013 Calgary flood was transient while the effects of residential schools have had a more enduring impact on Aboriginal population groups.

Take Note

To honour the people, and to develop community capacity, all efforts must be made by community workers to encourage community members to take ownership of the CCAP process to meet the community's goals, and to assume responsibilities of planning and implementing activities. The community is responsible for the outcomes of its actions. The role of the community worker is to assist the people with those things they are not able to do alone—to work *with* the people.

After analyzing the information collected about the community and its population, community workers come to a conclusion about community needs for which action can be taken. Stressors and the degree of reaction they cause on the health status of the population become part of the *community health diagnosis.* To illustrate, the following is an example of the analysis of a Hutterite colony in Alberta. The issue is the community's adaptation to several members of the colony needing special care (a *degree of reaction* by the community core) related to hypertension (*stressor*) caused by a combination of genetic endowment, diet, and physical inactivity. Data that illustrate the health issue were increased physician visits for hypertension, costs of medications and equipment (health and social services subsystem), and need to change the communal cooking practices and menus (physical environment subsystem). There is a regular health promotion service to the colony provided by the public health nurse (*LR,* or protective factor, located in the health and social services subsystem). When this service is temporarily supplemented by a monthly blood pressure clinic and wellness activities (e.g., healthy weight and healthy activity programs) in response to the alteration in the health status of the people in the community (*Pop-NLD*), this service is called the *FLD* and serves to buffer the community's reaction to the stressor and build the community's capacity to respond and become resilient in the face of this health issue. How might the members of the colony become more aware of the precipitating factors related to hypertension and work together to tackle prevention of hypertension by taking action at a community level?

Take Note

The outcome of a stressor impinging on a community is not always negative. Often, it is positive. For example, in the face of a crisis, people may band together and develop a community group to deal with the crisis. This group may continue to function after the crisis is over, strengthening the community and continuing to contribute to its health. Advocacy for gun control laws and the implementation of anti-bullying programs in schools after a shooting at a school are examples of positive outcomes following a stressor.

ASSESSMENT

The goal of assessment is to uncover the community's strengths, capacities, and assets (LR), and learn about the people and how they interact with their environment and its various subsystems. Because community work is founded on the principles of primary health care, public engagement is a critical component of all steps in the CCAP process. A community health team that assesses from a distance will not gain the insider knowledge important to making accurate and appropriate interpretations of what they learn about the people, and about the community as a whole.

The community's core and subsystems comprise assessment parameters. A variety of methods are used to complete a community assessment (described in Chapter 16), and the data are organized in ways to facilitate the understanding of community members and the interdisciplinary community team regarding the people (community core), population health status (Pop-NLD), its history of community resilience (FLD) and its assets and strengths (LR), any stressors, and the community or population response (degree of reaction) to any stressors present or threatening. Assessment might begin with a scenario such as this: Take a large picture view and then focus (depending on the data and its interpretation) on a population group (aggregate) or an issue (need or problem) in the planning stage of the process. However, if a community profile has already been completed, or if a crisis is happening, the community team may begin at the aggregate or problem level and work outward to get a more complete picture of the community as a whole.

ANALYSIS, DIAGNOSIS, AND PLANNING

Once a profile of the community has been developed, the information is examined to find trends and patterns that denote community capacity and any issues the people identify as concerns or stressors. During this phase of the CCAP process, the factors that underpin the strengths of the community are examined so they can be maintained and fostered. The concerns are also examined to determine what the root causes are in order to generate solutions. To be relevant, acceptable, and successful, the process of analysis must include the people, just as the assessment process embraced community participation. The community health diagnosis (see Chapter 17) is the result of analysis by the community health team; it is the collaborative determination of the issues of priority that gives direction to both goal setting and intervention planning. The goals are derived from the impact of stressors (degree of reaction caused) and are aimed to reduce community encounters with the stressor (risk factor) or to limit the effects of a stressor through prevention activities that strengthen the community's normal lines of defence (Pop-NLD and Comm-NLD) and flexible line of defence (temporary buffering services). Planning processes are detailed in Chapter 18 and are built on an understanding of how people make choices (e.g., behaviour change models) so that planning is theory-driven and based on evidence of best practices in health promotion intervention.

Take Note

The term community health diagnosis is preferred over a discipline-oriented diagnosis for three reasons: It is holistic and does not imply that only a member of a particular discipline can address the identified problem; it underscores that work in the community is by nature inter- and multidisciplinary (not only confined to health professions but incorporating many others); and it places the emphasis once again on the community, which is the focus of our practice. For the purposes of planning nursing interventions, however, do use a community nursing diagnosis; for social workers, use a community social work diagnosis, and so on.

INTERVENTION

In this model, all community interventions are considered to be preventive in nature. There are four levels of prevention at which interventions are aimed (see Chapter 12). The process of implementing community interventions is detailed in Chapter 19.

Primordial prevention is the furthest upstream and is in the domain of public health—it seeks the root causes of the stressors, risk factors, and threats to the health of populations and asks why these exist in today's society.

Primary prevention focuses on risk factors and health promotion. Health education and awareness programs that foster social justice, reduce inequities, and encourage healthy lifestyles are examples of primary prevention interventions. These programs assist the community in strengthening its ability to respond to stressors by expanding its FLD. Primary prevention strategies help the community to retain its system stability. Often, the most appropriate and relevant ideas come from collaboration with community members to identify strategies that fit with current lifestyles, culture, and adaptation of existing resources.

Secondary prevention is used after a stressor has penetrated the community subsystems. The focus is on treating responses to stressors and emphasizes early case finding, symptom management, and correction of maladaptive responses. Such interventions strengthen the LR by building on the capacities and assets of the community so that it can attain system stability.

Tertiary prevention activities focus on residual consequences of a stressor's impact by strengthening and re-expanding the FLD to the previous level (or a new level) in an effort to maintain system stability. Tertiary prevention interventions are aimed at re-establishing equilibrium in the community. Again, a reminder—community processes challenge the community team to move from the expert model of doing *to* and *for* the community to a model that facilitates the community to build its capacities and strengths from its already-existing assets, connections, and relationships. No intervention should take place without community involvement in all aspects of its planning and delivery.

The outcome desired by interventions relates to both the health of the people and the development of the community. A model of health and the community ecosystem that integrates in a holistic way the multiple sectors (community, built environment, economy, culture, and the overarching natural ecosystem) that must be involved to achieve a healthy population, in a healthy world is depicted in Figure 15.5.

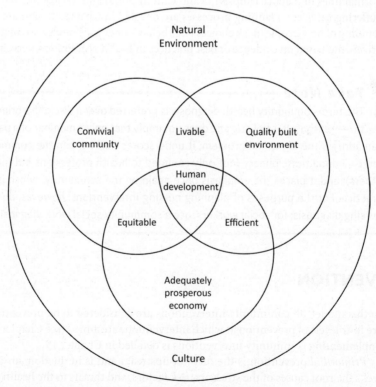

FIGURE 15.5   Healthy community model (Hancock, 1993; revised 2008).

The *community* must be convivial—it needs to have social support networks; its members need to participate fully in community life and live harmoniously together. The *built environment* needs to be both livable—urban design must foster a viable human setting and support conviviality and participation—and it must also be efficient; the use of energy and other resources and the flow of people, goods, and services must be accomplished at minimal cost. To achieve equity, community members must be treated justly and fairly—their basic needs must be met, and they must have equal opportunity to achieve their personal potentials. The *economy* must be adequate to generate enough wealth to enable members of the community to achieve a satisfactory level of health and quality of life while using resources efficiently and protecting the environment in a responsible manner, in order to ensure the sustainability of the economy and environment over time. The model suggests that health is formed at the conjunction of community, environment, and economy and is best achieved when balance exists among the components. It also suggests all this must occur within the context of a *cultural* environment that these days is both local and global and within the constraints of the Earth's *natural ecosystems;* in other words an eco-social approach is needed. The process of governance for health and human development is the process of managing and balancing these sometimes competing interests so as to achieve health for all in a socially just and ecologically sustainable manner (T. Hancock, personal communication, 2015).

Take Note

Many single interventions address more than one level of prevention. The community's capacity to act in concert with health care providers will be enhanced by improved communication networks and mutual trust if future events occur.

EVALUATION

Feedback from the people in the community provides the basis for evaluation of community interventions (see Chapter 20) just as involvement of community people in all steps of assessment, analysis, diagnosis, planning, implementation, and evaluation processes ensures relevance to the community and ownership by the community. The community health diagnosis sets the parameters for evaluation (as described in Chapter 17). The population for the intervention is identified by the reaction of the community to the stressors (risk factors). The goals and objectives of the intervention are related to the stressor that caused the reaction, and indicators for success are established by the manifestations of the reaction as illustrated by a program logic model (see Chapter 18). Such is the process of working with the community as a partner in action. Interconnections, overlap, and interdisciplinary considerations are the rules rather than the exceptions. While the CCAP process appears to be linear, it is in fact iterative. Most community teams analyze the information and data collected on an ongoing basis and that informs further data collection. Also, they evaluate "as they go," asking what is going well, what is not, and what needs to be done differently in each of the stages of the process (see Chapter 20). Left to the end, evaluation suffers because it was not planned for, appropriate data were not collected, and interventions did not match the goals and objectives!

PARTNERSHIP PLANNING AND TEAMWORK

The first step in the CCAP process is to establish a working group that includes community members, stakeholders, program participants, program developers, front-line practitioners, and community leaders. Stakeholders have an interest in the problem or program while also holding divergent views; conflicting interpretations of causality; and different values, goals, and life experiences. Community participants can be unaffiliated residents, community organizations, staff members that work in and with communities, managers, and leaders from community groups. The internal systems that link program planners, implementers, and evaluators are also important to include in either steering committee or working group roles.

Green and Kreuter (2005) list six principles of collaboration:

- Community involvement from the beginning and throughout all stages of the project
- Equally shared influence on the direction and activities of the project
- Respect for diversity in values, perspectives, contributions, and confidentiality
- Time and resources to devote to group function
- Compensation for community participants
- Concern for sustainability, long-term benefit, and development of community capacity

Once a work group is composed, it is important to manage it so that it is productive. The group needs to define its responsibilities and decide how it will make decisions. The group will have two key functions: instrumental (tasks) and expressive (group maintenance and team building). In Chapter 16, the work of the community assessment team is detailed.

Summary

Consider the CCAP model once more (see Fig. 15.3). The goal represented by the model is system equilibrium; that is "healthy people in a healthy and resilient community." The goal implies the preservation and promotion of community health as well as the development of the community and the sustainability of the environment. The CCAP model presents a structure but also comprises a process built on participation—working with the population and community in equal partnership.

Take Note

Health may not be a primary goal of the community (although it may be that of the community health worker). It is, however, an important resource for the community to meet its goals. Realizing that we do not always share the same goals is important for anyone working in the community and must at least be considered (if not reconciled) as we plan, implement, and evaluate programs aimed at improving health.

The CCAP model views the focus of action as the total community, the population, and its aggregate groups and, as such, includes the individuals and families nested therein. The community worker's role is to assist the community to attain, regain, maintain, and promote health, that is, to act as a facilitator, catalyst, and advocate for health so that the community is empowered to regulate and control its responses to stressors that are the sources of difficulty. The intervention focus is the actual or potential disruption experienced by the community or an inability of the community to function. The intervention mode comprises the four levels of prevention: primordial, primary, secondary, and tertiary. The consequences intended in this model include strengthened population health status (Pop-NLD) and community health (Comm-NLD), increased resistance to stressors (FLD and LR), and a diminished degree of reaction to stressors by the community. Said in other words, the outcomes desired of community interventions are convivial and livable communities that are environmentally viable and sustainable and that treat its members with respect and justice. Congruent with the principles of primary health care, it is the community's capacity and competence to deal with its own problems, strengthen its own lines of defence, and resist stressors that dictate the interventions and measure their success. Let us now begin the process.

REFERENCES

Allender, J. A., & Spradley, B. W. (2005). *Community health nursing: Promoting and protecting the public's health* (6th ed.). Philadelphia, PA: Lippincott Williams & Wilkins.

Anderson, E. & McFarlane, J. (1988). *Community as client: Applications of the nursing process.* Philadelphia, PA: Lippincott.

Bircher, J. (2005). Towards a dynamic definition of health and disease. *Medicine, Health Care and Philosophy, 8*(3), 335–341.

Green, L. W., & Kreuter, M. W. (2005). *Health program planning: An educational and ecological approach* (4th ed.). New York, NY: McGraw-Hill.

Hancock, T. (1993). Health, human development, and the community ecosystem: Three ecological models. *Health Promotion International, 8*(1), 41–48.

Hancock, T., & Perkins, F. (1985). The Mandala of Health: A conceptual model and teaching tool. *Health Education, 24*(1), 8–10.

McMillan, D. (2014). *Four elements to creating a "sense of community."* URL=http://thecommunitymanager. com/2014/02/06/4-elements-to-creating-a-sense-of-community-by-dr-david-mcmillan/

Ontario Healthy Communities Coalition (OHCC). (2015). *What makes a healthy community?* URL=http://www. ohcc-ccso.ca/en/what-makes-a-healthy-community

Racher, F. E., & Annis, R. C. (2008). Community health action model: Health promotion by the community. *Research and Theory for Nursing Practice: An International Journal, 22*(3), 182–191.

Rural Development Institute (RDI). (2005). *The community health action model.* Brandon, MB: Author.

Üstün, B., & Jakob, R. (2005). Calling a spade a spade: Meaningful definitions of health conditions. *Bulletin of the WHO, 83*(11), 802.

World Health Organization (WHO). (1986). *The Ottawa charter for health promotion.* Geneva: Author.

ONLINE RESOURCES

Please visit thePoint at http://thepoint.lww.com/Vollman4e for up-to-date Internet resources and additional learning materials on this topic.

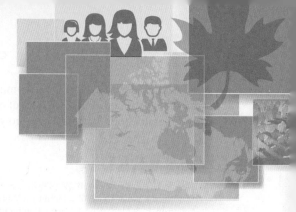

CHAPTER 16

Community Assessment

Ardene Robinson Vollman

LEARNING OBJECTIVES

Preceding chapters have focused on the foundational concepts for community practice. A model was introduced in Chapter 15 to provide a structure and guide the process of working with people and communities. This chapter and the four that follow in this section focus on the application of the Canadian community-as-partner (CCAP) process in the community. Consequently, the objectives are practice oriented.

After studying this chapter, you should be able to:

1. Participate with a community to undertake a community and population assessment using the Canadian community-as-partner (CCAP) model

2. Discuss the challenges of working with communities and population groups

3. Detail the processes that are helpful in overcoming barriers and resistance

4. Describe the various methods of data collection and their strengths and weaknesses

5. Begin organizing data for analysis

Introduction

Community and population health assessment is one of the functions of public health (see Chapter 2). It is a fundamental skill for community workers regardless of their disciplines (Public Health Agency of Canada [PHAC], 2008). Public health departments across the country are, for the most part, mandated to carry out health status reviews on a regular basis. Municipalities, provinces, federal agencies, and special interest groups also conduct studies on certain aspects of population health. Population and community health assessment is a dynamic and ongoing process undertaken to identify strengths (assets) and needs of the population and community and to determine priorities for action.

Community and population health assessment is a systematic process; it is the act of becoming acquainted with a community and its people. The people in the community are our partners and contribute throughout the process; the assessment phase is their point of entry into the processes of inquiry, planning, implementing programs, and evaluating their success. The purpose of a *population health assessment* is to collect, analyze, and present information so that the health of the population can be understood and improved, and to provide evidence to inform health service planning. It provides baseline information about the health status of community residents, tracks health outcomes over time, and helps to identify opportunities for disease prevention, health promotion, and health protection. A *community health assessment* allows an appraisal of the various community subsystems to provide insights into programs, policies, and services that affect the health of people of the community. It helps to identify gaps and duplications in services from other sectors, and determines direction for advocacy and mediation efforts. In both instances, assessment allows the identifications of positive factors (strengths and assets) and risk factors that impinge on people's health. It provides the basis for change and, when the public is engaged in the assessment processes, for empowerment.

Community assessments are used for pre-intervention planning, assessing community readiness and leadership capacity for planned interventions, and stimulating community action.

Take Note

Community health promotion, as a philosophy, entails the fundamental belief that people can identify and solve their problems. As a process, it supports citizens as they find the power to create change. As an outcome, community health promotion involves citizens working together to bring about change in their community. Community health promotion builds capacity and develops communities (Racher & Annis, 2008).

In this chapter, we first discuss the community assessment team[1] and how to enter into the community assessment process, and then we move into sources and types of data and methods that can be used to collect information. We will use the community assessment wheel (Fig. 16.1) as a framework for the assessment itself and the preparation of the data for the next stage in the process—analysis.

THE COMMUNITY ASSESSMENT TEAM

Rarely does a community worker conduct a community assessment alone; rather, it is a team effort that brings together people from different disciplines, perspectives, agendas, and approaches. It is critical to have community members on the team to facilitate the processes of the assessment, analysis, planning, implementation, and evaluation. Remember, we work *with* the community. Teams bring people with diverse knowledge and skills together for a common purpose. The same teams may not work on all aspects of a project together—they may re-form with new members at different stages when different skills are needed. The benefits of teams are that the workload can be shared, more people can be reached, and a project can move ahead more quickly. Members' contacts and networks enhance the capacity of a team, and brainstorming exercises can assist with problem solving as the community process proceeds.

No matter how well intended its members may be, the team will likely experience "growing pains" as it evolves and matures. Teams go through five predictable stages as they develop: forming, storming, norming, performing, and adjourning (Table 16.1). The process of team development is not linear, and gaining or losing a member, making a major decision, or facing

---

[1]Note: In this chapter "the team" refers to the people engaged in community assessment and analysis. This team may differ in its membership (as in its mandate) from the community planning team, which we will also refer to as "the team" in Chapter 18.

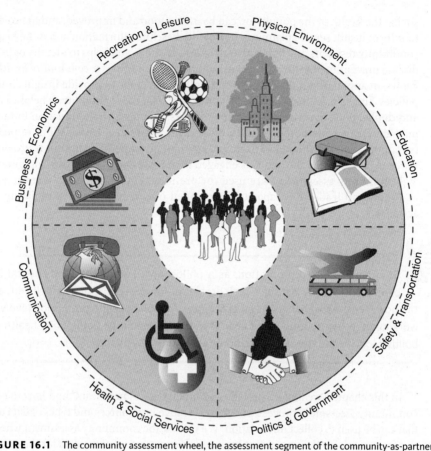

FIGURE 16.1   The community assessment wheel, the assessment segment of the community-as-partner model.

a particular challenge may cause the team to regress in its developmental stage before it can be productive again.

Remember, the full participation of community members is important at all stages of the CCAP process. In fact, assessment is the first stage in building capacity as community members become involved in the various tasks associated with the assessment part of the process.

TABLE 16.1 Five-Stage Team Development Process

Stage	Characteristics
Forming	When the team comes together, people are polite and agreeable and tend not to make clear statements of commitment. The primary tasks are to get to know each other, determine leadership, define the purpose of the team and the goals of its work as well as the skills and contributions of each member.
Storming	As the work begins, differences of opinion can arise, causing subgroups to form. At this point, it is natural to have some tension and perhaps conflict that emerges as challenging, detail and procedural haggling, and personal clashes. Conflicts must be brought into the open in helpful ways to avoid negative impacts later in the project.
Norming	As emotions cool down, practical rules of behaviour can be established, and the team can now focus on group cohesion and effective working relationships and processes.
Performing	This stage is a time of team productivity where members have assumed individual and collective responsibility for finishing the work. They agree on tasks and processes, and most decisions are made by consensus.
Adjourning	As the project comes to an end, reports are finalized; loose ends and unfinished business are cleared up. Celebrations bring closure to the project, and while some people may mourn the "good times," the team adjourns its work.

True partnership and full collaboration will evolve as community members gain confidence and competence throughout the process. The ability of community members to contribute will vary at different points in time, by what formal and informal positions they hold in the community, by what skills they can contribute, and by what is needed by the team.

The report of a community assessment portrays a realistic profile of the community, its people, and its subsystems that allows a meaningful determination of strengths and capacities as well as an identification of risks to population aggregates and the environment. Assessment goes beyond documenting types of needs—it also helps to examine why the needs are occurring, the prevalence and urgency of concerns, and the capacity of the community to address the issues it faces and may point to some possible solutions. By the time the assessment process is complete, one should expect community members to be fully engaged and taking ownership of the project.

BEGINNING TO WORK AS A COMMUNITY ASSESSMENT TEAM

No assessment project can begin without a clear plan from its beginning to its end product. First, the community assessment team must obtain support from the management and leadership in the sponsoring organizations and the communities of interest. In the case of students, this support will be from course professors. Next, the team must determine the roles and responsibilities of each of its members and divide itself into work groups (if needed). The team itself will be responsible for completing the day-to-day work, staying on budget, and adhering to time commitments. At this point, the creation of a work plan, timeline, and budget are critical to ensuring the team's community assessment work goes smoothly. At a minimum, the assessment team's work plan should consider the following steps in some detail:

- Defining the process and scope of the assessment
- Collecting and analyzing the population and community data
- Documenting and communicating assessment results

Community and population assessment projects need funds if they are to be done on a large scale. When putting together a budget, consider if there is already an internal budget for data collection, analysis, and reporting; the size of the community to be assessed; how extensive the data collection process will be (e.g., existing data, surveys, focus groups, interviews); fees for meeting space, catering, and supplies; and support staff costs. Community work is not completed quickly, thus making time commitment, travel costs, child care costs, and other considerations important to volunteers.

An advisory group might be needed to support the community assessment team. If so, try to acquire diverse representation and ensure all participants agree to provide past and current data; identify additional secondary data sources; provide input on primary data collection; motivate support from the community; and assist in organizing meetings, interviews, and focus groups. Regular meetings that are relevant to the partners and the advisory group should be considered to maintain momentum, build rapport and trust, and keep the assessment on track.

Determine whether the team, work groups, and advisory committees need an orientation to the whole assessment process, and if there are training needs to be addressed. Part of community engagement in the assessment is to build capacity—community members may need some development activities to build their skills to carry out their tasks as meeting chairpersons, focus group facilitators, and effective participants in team deliberations. Ongoing support will be needed to get the most benefit from community engagement efforts.

Before actual data collection begins, the team must prepare itself. Early in the process the team should agree on the purposes of the assessment, the goals it wants to achieve, the framework it will use to organize the assessment, and the questions it seeks to answer. Often, because team members do not normally work together, a purposeful team-building process is required to support a successful process and outcome. Setting standards of operation and behaviour allows the team to effectively operate and maintain itself. The team needs to determine how it will function: how often and where it will meet, who will chair or lead, who will take minutes and to whom and how they will be distributed, how people will communicate, and how team members will divide the work. A work plan that sets the timelines, delineates responsibilities, and estimates resources required for each activity will guide the team and keep it on track. Minutes of meetings and decisions will remind people of commitments. Occasionally, taking the "pulse" of the group by self-reflection helps to minimize conflicts and ensure member satisfaction and enthusiasm.

It is essential in community work that members of the population group of interest are included in the process, not only for their opinions, but also for the deliberation process that interprets data and for the action phases of implementation and evaluation of consequent interventions. Efforts to recruit and retain community people on work groups may be challenging; directly involve people and create a working culture that encourages and supports the participation from people across the life span; from diverse cultural backgrounds, income and education levels; and with differing perspectives. Ensure that the process is inclusive and open, and that information is widely shared throughout the assessment process—via newsletters, media interviews, town hall meetings, etc.

GETTING TO KNOW THE COMMUNITY

A key task of the community assessment team at this point is to define the scope of the assessment. Will the focus be on a geographic community? Is there evidence of an issue that needs to be further investigated? Or, will the team focus on a particular aggregate? See Table 16.2

TABLE 16.2   Examples of Community Assessment Questions

Questions	Typical Data Sources
General community profile: What are the characteristics, structure, and history of this community? What geographical features distinguish this community? What are the concerns, agendas, and recent civic actions of this community?	*Secondary sources:* Census, economic development data, social services information, social indicators, historical data, newspapers, minutes of community meetings, or municipal council publications.
Health/wellness assessment: What is the level of health and illness, injury, or disability in the community? What is the wellness level of its residents?	*Secondary sources:* Epidemiologic studies. Health data sources including health status, injury incidence, and health care utilization statistics including pharmaceutical sales.
Health risk profile: What are the behavioural, social, and environmental risks to the population and/or special groups?	*Primary sources:* Targeted surveys, telephone surveys, key informant interviews, and group discussions.
	Secondary sources: National/provincial population health surveys, local health screening surveys, risk factor studies, special registries (e.g., injury, disease specific).
Community health promotion survey: What programs, resources, and provider groups already exist? What is the level of participation in these programs? What are barriers to participation? What possibilities exist for partnership? In what areas are there gaps to be addressed?	*Primary sources:* Key informants from provider organizations and members of the population of interest.
	Secondary sources: National, provincial, and local population health promotion surveys and databases, community resource guides, and local inventories.
Specialized studies: What special target groups exist? Who are the gatekeepers—will they help or hinder the project? Who can facilitate diffusion of program messages? What do these groups want to do?	*Primary sources:* Systematic surveys, key informant interviews, contact (interview, survey) with organizational managers, contact with influential people or groups (champions). Community asset mapping activities.

Adapted from Rissel and Bracht (1999), p. 65.

Box 16.1 Assessing a Population Group

Several years ago six women in a small town not far from a major city formed an interest group on the basis of their small businesses. One owned a café, one a small motel, another took over her late husband's gas station, one owned a salon, another cleaned houses, and the sixth ran a successful home sales business for cosmetics and storage containers. Over the years these women spearheaded a number of social services in their town—school lunches, safe grad, community watch, and a food bank service. "The Six," as they became known, were seen as informal leaders in their town.

Last year a new industry was opened in the nearby city, drawing several hundred temporary workers from several countries around the world. A few families of African origin settled in the town. The children were enrolled in school but were not doing well academically, and there were often incidents of bullying reported. While their husbands worked in the industry, the women were considered unemployable. This did not sit well with "The Six," who could foresee problems if the town did not act to be more accepting of these new community members.

They invited the women to meet with them at the café. They poured tea and served cookies. They asked the six women who joined the group to talk to them about coming to Canada and to this small town. The conversation was stilted; it was more like a question and answer session. In the end, contact information was exchanged and the meeting ended with the group agreeing to meet again in 2 weeks for tea.

Afterward, "The Six" decided they needed to take another approach. Each accepted the role of befriending one of the women. They wanted to learn about their needs and what they thought could be helpful to making their transition to Canada stress-free. When they re-convened 2 weeks later, they brought their friends with them. "The Six" shared what they had learned: the women had trouble dealing with the cold weather; they had trouble making Canadian friends because they did not speak English very well; there was no place for them to worship; they could not find foods with which they were familiar; and they were worried about how their children were doing in school. They reported that the children had been teased and insulted on several occasions.

The women from Africa were proud; they were courageous. After all, they followed their husbands to a foreign land for work, safety, and security. They had survived war, and they wanted their children to grow up in peace and opportunity to aspire to become more than skilled labourers. They did not want hand-outs or welfare; they wanted to become valuable members of the Town.

Around this time "The Six" were approached by a local nongovernmental organization (NGO) that provided services to new immigrants to endorse a program of health promotion with the temporary workers and their families. "The Six" agreed to help, but only if the health promotion action also involved change to the Town and its residents, so it could become more welcoming to families from other countries.

With the agreement of the Mayor and Council, the churches, the school, and the business community, the NGO began a process to assess the community interest, capacity, and ability with respect to immigration. Community members wanted to know more about the immigration experience and life in Africa. The Project Leader asked questions about barriers and challenges to immigration from local and immigrant points of view; what are the indicators of welcome; what resources and knowledge do we need as a community to help new immigrants feel welcome?

Thus began the process of advancing community growth through the first step of community health promotion: assessment.

for examples of assessment questions for each of these foci, and Box 16.1 for an example of a successful approach to assessing a population group. The team will need to understand the rationale for the assessment and the events that lead up to it. The team will also want to understand the goal of the assessment in order to appreciate what others expect from the results—will the report lead to the planning of interventions on an issue, for a population group, or in a community setting? Understanding the purpose for the assessment project will assist the team in clarifying its parameters. Further, understanding the goals and values of the agencies/ groups that support the assessment will often provide some direction for the team with respect to its focus and scope.

Will the community assessment team members be participants in or observers of community life? If present and visible in the community, team members may be asked for their contributions to community decisions, may be requested for advance notice of the assessment findings, or may be made to feel somewhat uncomfortable. If any team members are also members of the community or population, they may be perceived to have a privileged position. Regardless, the presence of the team will have an influence on the community; care must be taken to ensure ethical practice and minimize any potential for bias.

Two of the persistent challenges facing a community assessment team are how to enter the community and gain access to people with information. In many cases, team members will be outsiders—they will not live in the community of interest nor will they necessarily be members of the population of interest. It is essential to get to know the people, how the community is organized formally and informally, and to build rapport and trust. Sometimes, being an agent of an organization is helpful in entering the community; other times, it may be an impediment. For instance, the public health nurse may be a valued outsider with a history of positive engagement in the community who will be accepted more readily than a police officer who may be perceived as a punitive force and a person to be avoided. Building trust and rapport takes time; often, teams do not allow enough time for this important process. For ideas on how this process can be facilitated, the case story in Chapter 33. Key points in the community entry and access process include:

- Select a spokesperson or lead agency that already has a relationship with the community
- Make contact with the formal community leaders who may be gatekeepers to the population
- Be physically present, available, and visible in the community
- Engage with people in nonthreatening ways; be open and honest in your actions
- Communicate—keep the people involved in decisions and processes

Sites and times for informal conversations can be created through informal, unstructured personal contacts (e.g., at coffee breaks). Personal contacts and consultations are critical to a smooth entry into the community and facilitate access to informants and information sources.

A letter of introduction or a proposal for the assessment may be needed to gain access to formal community leaders, reports, and official data. The team needs to have a clear message that states the purpose of the assessment, what it will require of the community, and what benefits it will have to the people involved.

During the assessment process, the team might need to participate in a variety of formal meetings, some of which they will call themselves and others they will attend as guests or participants. For meetings that the team leads, an agenda will help to keep participants on task by keeping track of items that need to be discussed and deciding which team member will speak to them. Handouts help attendees follow presentations and keep track of decisions. Remember to keep lists of contacts from meetings (both formal and informal) with contact information and their relationship to the project for future reference. It is a courtesy to follow meetings with letters of thanks—to the chair of external meetings for giving the team time to meet with them, and to attendees for their participation in meetings called by the team. Remember to file meetings minutes and make an action list of what you agreed to do by what date; attention to these details will help the team with its accountability for outcomes, budgets, timelines as well as the promises made along the way. This data will not only help with evaluation but also with recalling to whom reports were promised at the project's end.

TABLE 16.3 Problems Commonly Encountered in Community Assessment, With Suggested Solutions

Issue	Strategy
Boundaries for data sets do not match	Make inferences regarding the boundaries used for data and determining their accuracy by interview with key informants
Data no longer exist	Move beyond traditional data sources and traditional indicators
Team members are impatient with the data collection process—they want to "do something"	Emphasize the importance of cultivating relationships, building rapport and trust to acquiring community information
Reluctance to report derogatory data	Emphasize the importance of veracity in the context of assessment
Conflicting opinions among vested-interest groups within the community	Ongoing sharing and analysis of information among team members so that all data are noted and discussed
Insider versus outsider views of various community issues	Make certain that a variety of perspectives are obtained during data collection
Community members request conclusions before data collection is complete	Be consistent in messages that premature conclusions may not be correct and may harm the process and the community's trust

Inevitably, something will go awry—weather will impede transportation to interviews, people will not show up for meetings, other work demands will take priority over community participation. When this happens, it is important to recognize it immediately and take action to rebuild relationships and re-establish the momentum of the assessment. Issues related to data generation and strategies to address them are summarized in Table 16.3.

PLANNING THE DATA COLLECTION

To be useful for planning, intervention, and evaluation purposes, a community assessment must be based on the best data available—data that are reliable, accurate, and complete. Data are essential to population and community assessment because without data our knowledge is founded upon opinion and speculation, not facts. At the same time, we have the responsibility to gather opinion and subjective information to draw reasoned conclusions about the community and the people in it. Facts alone are not sufficient for successful health promotion action.

Primary data are composed of information from direct sources specifically for the project—key informant interview data, specific health utilization data, local survey data, and the like. *Secondary data,* on the other hand, are data from sources that collect, store, and report certain information on a routine basis—census, vital statistics, notifiable disease reports, social services reports, crime statistics, education system reports, regional social surveys, local research reports, historical documents, and so on. Often, a review of the literature about the topic or population group of interest, using, for example, the determinants of health as a framework, can help to clarify certain aspects of the project. The review will help the assessment team to see what information already exists in the research literature, policy documents, and elsewhere so that appropriate data collection can be planned to address gaps in knowledge and make the assessment locally relevant. Teams run the risk of attempting to find out "everything" about the focus of the assessment rather than determining what is absolutely necessary to learn and what is "nice to know" but not essential. If the team had unlimited time and unlimited resources, more could perhaps be done and learned—but more often than not, there are time limits and budget restrictions to be considered. Hence, clearly defining the focus of the assessment, its purpose, and expected outcomes will allow the team to refine a work plan and timeline that is realistic and feasible while still allowing time to incorporate community participation.

Data may be numerical or nonnumerical, in other words, quantitative or qualitative. *Numerical* (quantitative) data can be measured on a scale (e.g., weight, blood pressure), analyzed statistically, and displayed graphically. It can be used to calculate rates and other measures that have meaning to population health. Although numerical data have many advantages in terms of reliability, validity, understandability, and comparability over time, they do not provide a full picture of the community. *Nonnumerical* (qualitative) data provide depth and detail to statistics and allow us to interpret the beliefs, values, opinions, and culture of the community or population aggregate (e.g., the meaning of overweight or hypertension to people experiencing it). They provide the context that situates the numerical data in its unique setting. Used together with community stories and history, these two types of data provide a comprehensive community profile that can be used in planning health and social programs.

Many methods can be used effectively to gather information; no single method is perfect, so a team will use a variety of sources to get a complete picture of a community or an aggregate within the population:

- Sociodemographic data: from local, regional, provincial/territorial, and national sources (e.g., census reports, registry reports).
- Vital statistics data: from provincial/territorial vital statistics departments that track births, deaths, marriages, etc.
- Health-related data: from a variety of sources such as Statistics Canada, PHAC Health Status Reports, CIHR information, local/regional public health department reports, specific disease foundations.
- Archival materials: specific reports previously commissioned from such sources as health regions, national and international health status reports, royal commissions (e.g., Mental Health Commission of Canada), and reports prepared by special interest groups (e.g., disease associations, population groups).
- Original data: reports of data collected specifically for the assessment (e.g., windshield surveys, key informant interviews, participant observation, photovoice results, questionnaires, surveys).

Much of what is assessed in community work traditionally focuses on problems, barriers, needs, and weaknesses rather than on the strengths or "assets" of a community or its population aggregates. It is important to be as aware of a community's potential as of its issues to avoid portraying a negative image that can have demoralizing effects on the community. Threats and obstacles are real and pervasive, but they do not tell the whole story of how the community uses its assets to turn these into opportunity and rise above the challenges it faces. It is important to be open to hearing how people deal with challenges to become stronger and more resilient.

METHODS OF PRIMARY DATA COLLECTION

Before beginning to assess a community, the team needs to know what information it needs to meet its objectives, where that information can be found, and how it will be collected and organized. All methods of collecting information have strengths and weaknesses. All involve some ethical issues that need to be considered. No one method will give complete information; therefore, multiple methods are recommended, and triangulation of information from one source to another, one type of data to another, and from different methods is needed to ensure the veracity of any inferences or conclusions drawn. Assessment team members are cautioned about jumping to early conclusions without substantiating data. Additional information and specific instructions for each method presented here can be located in Gilmore (2012) if the team wants to develop expertise in the skills and competencies needed for completing a primary data collection for community assessment.

Observation

Observation methods range from being totally unobtrusive to being a full participant in the community. The observer tries to understand the social setting and lives of the people in the community by observing or participating in events that occur in everyday life. Observation is particularly effective if the assessment team members are outsiders and not familiar with the culture of the community or population group. Obviously, an approach that combines both observation and participation allows trust and rapport to build; observation alone does not allow for interpretation of what is observed. Full participation may not permit an objective distance from which to reflect on the meaning of what is occurring in the community. Regardless, the following preparation is necessary to carry out observational surveys:

- Establish written guidelines about what to observe
- Determine the locations for observations
- Decide on the length of observation periods
- Assess and determine the methods for recording observations (i.e., some are more obtrusive than others but offer better opportunity for team analysis)
- Gather equipment to record observations (e.g., audio recorder or video camera, extra batteries, checklist, writing tools, paper for field notes)
- Ensure that any required permissions have been obtained
- Plan for creating systematic field notes and for their transcription
- Plan debriefing sessions with the team
- Use an analytic journal for decision making and interpretation

A windshield or walking survey is a specific observational technique used in community assessment. Using this type of observation, team members make use of a variety of physical senses to capture the essence of a community, determine areas for further investigation, and sense the tone of the community. It is also useful in observing the physical spaces where population groups of interest meet and interact. In Table 16.4 a guide for undertaking a windshield survey is provided. The team might want to complete the entire guide, focus on a few sections only, or add elements to the guide, depending on the purpose and goal of your assessment project. In column 1, key points of interest are listed, with suggested questions to ask. Column 2 provides space to capture observations, and column 3 provides space to take note of information as it is gathered. This chart then becomes part of the raw data that will be analyzed in the next step of the CCAP process.

Preparation for a walking or windshield survey includes mapping out a route, having a checklist (e.g., Table 16.4) from which to work, finding a means to record findings and reactions (e.g., audiovisual recording), a map to chart locations and make reference to field recordings, and proper equipment for the outdoor conditions (e.g., walking shoes, hats, sunscreen, identification). It is advisable to conduct walking or windshield surveys in teams of two for safety purposes and to have mobile communication devices available. Refrain from taking pictures of people, particularly children. If you plan to take photos that might include adults, take appropriate consent forms with you. It is not ethical to take or use photos of people without their consent.

Observations need to be made at different times of the day and different days of the week to fully capture the life of a community. Team members may make use of some of the community's facilities—a coffee shop, a grocery store—while doing the survey. As well, team members

TABLE 16.4 Windshield/Walking Survey

I. Community Core	Observations	Data
1. **History**—What can you glean by looking (e.g., old, established neighbourhoods; new subdivision)? Ask people willing to talk: How long have you lived here? Has the area changed? As you talk, ask if there is an "old-timer" who knows the history of the area.		
2. **Demographics**—What sorts of people do you see? Young? Old? Homeless? Alone? Families? Is the population homogeneous?		
3. **Ethnicity**—Do you note indicators of different ethnic groups (e.g., restaurants, festivals)? What signs do you see of different cultural groups?		
4. **Values and beliefs**—Are there churches, mosques, temples? Are there signs of diversity? Are the lawns cared for? With flowers? Gardens? Signs of art? Culture? Heritage? Historical markers?		
II. Subsystems		
1. **Physical environment**—How does the community look? What do you note about air quality, flora, housing, zoning, space, green areas, animals, people, human-made structures, natural beauty, water, climate? Can you find or develop a map of the area? What is the size (e.g., square kilometres, blocks)?		
2. **Education**—Are there schools, universities, technical institutes, arts education in the area? How do they look? Are there libraries? Is there a local board of education? How does it function? What is the reputation of the school(s)? What are major educational issues? What are the dropout rates? Are extracurricular activities available? Are they used? Is there a school health service? A school nurse? Are there adult education and second-language programs readily available?		
3. **Safety and transportation**—How do people get around? What type of private and public transportation is available? Do you see buses, bicycles, taxis? Are there sidewalks, bike trails? Is getting around in the community possible for people with disabilities? What types of protective services are there (e.g., fire, police, sanitation)? Is air quality monitored? What types of crimes are committed? Do people feel safe? Are there signs of racism or intolerance?		
4. **Politics and government**—Are there signs of political activity (e.g., posters, meetings)? What party affiliation predominates? What is the governmental jurisdiction of the community (e.g., elected mayor, city council with single member districts)? Are people involved in decision making in their local governmental unit?		
5. **Health and social services**—Evidence of acute or chronic conditions? Shelters? Alternative therapists/healers? Are there clinics, hospitals, practitioners' offices, public health services, home health agencies, emergency centres, nursing homes, social service facilities, mental health services? Are there resources outside the community but readily accessible to residents?		
6. **Communication**—Are there "common areas" where people gather? What newspapers do you see in the stands? Do people have TVs, mobile music devices, cell phones? What do they watch/listen to? What are the formal and informal means of communication?		
7. **Business and economics**—Is it a "thriving" community, or does it feel "seedy"? Are there industries, stores, places for employment? Where do people shop? Are there signs that people can find employment (e.g., Help Wanted signs, classified ads)? Are there signs of thrift stores, pawn shops, and other services for people with money issues? How active is the food bank?		
8. **Recreation and leisure**—Where do children play? What are the major forms of recreation? Who participates? What facilities for recreation do you see? Are they in good order or disrepair? Are there signs that pets are welcome? What about the performing arts, and social and other leisure activities (e.g., festivals, zoo, museums, sports teams, etc.)?		

III. Perceptions	Observations	Data
1. **The residents**—How do people feel about the community? What do they identify as its strengths? Problems? Ask several people from different groups (e.g., old, young, unskilled/skilled workers, service worker, professional, clergy, stay-at-home parent, lone parent), and keep track of who gives what answer.		
2. **Your perceptions**—General statements about the "health" of this community. What are its strengths? What community or population-level problems or potential problems can you identify? Who are the gatekeepers to the community and/or population of interest? Who are the champions that might support your work? Who in the community might become a partner in the process? Where will resistance be found?		

Note: Supplement your impressions with information from the census, police records, school statistics, Chamber of Commerce data, health department reports, and so forth to confirm or refute your conclusions. Tables, graphs, and maps are helpful and will aid in your analysis.
Adapted from Anderson and McFarlane (2015), p. 174.

may hold impromptu conversations with people they meet (e.g., person on the street interviews) so have some short questions ready to begin conversations (e.g., "Is this traffic typical of the middle of the day in your community?"). Be prepared to explain your presence to community residents if requested—have your identification and a statement about your assessment project with contact information available to distribute. And remember, use all five senses (and maybe also your sixth sense—intuition) as you observe (Box 16.2).

Key Informant Interview

There are people in the community who have much to offer an assessment team. They have perhaps lived there for a long time or are members of a population aggregate of interest. Others may be in leadership positions (e.g., community association executive) or may serve the community in some capacity (e.g., police, fire, health, school and social services personnel, faith leaders, business people). Their insights can be helpful in interpreting statistical findings or in offering information that other methods cannot capture. A variety of views and opinions can be obtained through key informant interviews that can be considered to reflect the views of the community at large.

To prepare for key informant interviews, the team should meet to:

- Determine who are the key people/positions that should be included in interviews
- Outline the focus of each informant's potential contribution
- Determine the structure, timing, and recording methods
- Outline the questions and prepare the interview guide
- Create the invitation to participate and design the process

---

Box 16.2 Using Your Senses to Collect Information About the Community

Sight—condition of streets, sidewalks, playgrounds; age, sex, racial distributions, clothing, general health condition of the people; housing and services (e.g., schools, businesses) visible

Hearing—noise levels and sources of noise

Taste—types of food supply stores, variety and prices of foods, water quality

Smell—pollutants, odours, sanitation levels

Touch—climate, psychological sense of safety, feeling of openness or oppression, friendliness

- Set the times and venues for interviews
- Invite the key informants to be interviewed
- Send out confirmation letters with the "rules of engagement" clearly specified
- Prepare letters of thanks to send out after the interviews

It is helpful to send questions to interviewees in advance so that they can prepare themselves; be certain to outline the purpose of your assessment and the outcomes you hope to achieve. Offer them something tangible in return for their participation (e.g., a summary of the final report, an invitation to a presentation). As with all inquiry methods that involve humans, you must be sensitive to ethical issues and ensure that no harm comes to your participants. Make sure they know in advance that the interview will be audio- or video-recorded and that you will be keeping notes.

Be certain to choose interview sites that are comfortable, confidential, and quiet. Make certain your equipment works and also take notes in the event of an equipment failure. Respect when your interviewee wants to go "off the record." Sometimes key informants want to give you information on issues about which you have not asked—be open to hearing them because they may be issues that you have either not considered or of which you have not been aware. Be flexible in the interview process! Telephone interviews or the use of electronic surveys may be preferable in some instances, particularly if the questions are very structured or a key informant is not able to attend an interview in person.

The team needs to prepare the information collected for analysis, which will be discussed in more detail in Chapter 17. Analysis of key informant interviews entails teasing out the main themes and patterns in the responses and capturing the essence of any discussion, debate, or differing opinion. If interviews are transcribed, qualitative analysis software can help to identify themes, but in small samples, this may not be necessary. Since data collection and analysis are iterative processes, and the assessment team will most likely be the one engaged in both, it helps to begin organizing the data in such a way that analysis is facilitated.

Group Interview

A group interview is a rapid, cost-effective data collection method that involves the use of direct probing techniques to gather information from several (no more than 8) individuals in a group situation. Group interviews can serve a wide range of data collection purposes: acquisition of background information; generation of ideas and hypotheses for follow-up; and receipt of feedback from the community about assessment efforts. A structured interview guide that lists precise questions should be prepared. Its language should be simple; leading questions and double-barreled questions should be avoided along with questions on controversial topics that can generate strong emotions among the participants. As far as possible, group interviews should be conducted by a team of two because it is extremely taxing for a single interviewer to preside over a meeting, ask questions, probe participants, and take extensive notes. Suggestions about the environment, equipment, and ethics from the discussion of key informant interviews apply also to group interviews. It is helpful, when inviting participants, to give them a letter with a general idea of what the topic and questions will be, and whether or not the meeting will be recorded. Normally, consent is not required—it is implied if people show up to the interview.

Participants should be reminded that they have been invited to provide their opinions and reflections; the group should be encouraged to hold what is said in the meeting in confidence, not revealing outside of the meeting who said what. It is important that the team captures the information provided, but not the name or position of the person that provided it; data from group discussions should be anonymized in reports by the use of aggregation methods. Any follow-up can be done with individuals on a personal basis outside of the group interview at another time as necessary. To prevent a few people from dominating the interview, the interviewer can give nonverbal cues to participants to bring their comments to a conclusion (e.g., look at other participants). The interviewer can also intervene politely, summarize what the person was saying, and then refocus the discussion. To minimize group pressure that prevents people with diverse or opposing viewpoints from expressing their opinions, the interviewer can ask for other ideas, explanations, or recommendations than those already discussed, suggest new ideas for discussion, and look at nonparticipants and encourage them to speak.

Interviewers should be on the lookout for examples of their personal bias that can undermine the value of the group interview. Four types of bias are:

- Hypothesis-confirmation bias: focusing selectively on information that confirms interviewers' preconceived hypotheses.
- Elite bias: tending to give more weight to the views of people in influential positions than to the opinions of others.
- Concreteness bias: giving the impressions from vivid descriptions and statistical data about a few cases that they represent general situations.
- Consistency bias: attempting to draw meaningful conclusions prematurely from conflicting information.

Mapping

An interesting exercise that can be used with people within group interviews is to ask them to map their communities (Dorfman, 1998). This exercise engages people and uses their creativity, and is an active process, not one that relies on verbalizing opinions or feelings. Give each small grouping of three to four people (preferably with the same characteristics—e.g., age, sex) a large piece of paper and coloured markers and ask them to draw a map of their community. Ask them to note several places in their community:

- Landmarks and features
- Where they go for food
- Where they work, where and what they spend their time doing
- Sacred places
- Schools; other places where they learn
- Places of historic importance
- Where they go for health services
- And other points that come to mind

Compare maps—especially compare those of youth and seniors, of various ethnic and cultural groups—and engage participants in discussion about the maps, noting similarities, differences, gaps, and overlaps. This information will be valuable as the team moves to the analysis phase of the assessment.

Focus Group Interview

Focus group interviews are best used when data themes have emerged from other sources and the assessment team wants to add to the understanding of each theme and determine if the themes include a complete and accurate picture of community perspectives. Focus group participants are limited to 8 to 12 homogeneous people (i.e., they share certain characteristics) with a variety of perspectives to facilitate in-depth discussion in an informal atmosphere where participants are encouraged to explore issues and express opinions freely among themselves. Focus group participants build on the comments of others and come to conclusions not considered individually. Additionally, it is possible to reach consensus about key issues and rank-order issues in terms of priority for action.

Focus group interviews need similar preparation as the key informant interview and group interview processes. Decide who is the best source of information to answer the questions that have arisen, invite the community people that fit that description (e.g., youth, seniors, mothers of school-age children), and plan the interview process keeping in mind the purpose of the focus group interview. Also, two skilled and unobtrusive facilitators are required to elicit the best information, ask open-ended questions, draw out reticent people, and keep the meeting on track with the stated objectives. Focus group interviews are usually recorded for later analysis, but a note-taker is important as well to assess interactions and keep track of points raised. It is important that results not be generalized to the whole population because the participants are not selected to be representative of the population.

Community Forum

A community forum or town hall meeting brings members of a community together to discuss an issue or common concern (American College of Emergency Physicians [ACEP], n.d.). These meetings are usually open to the public and audience participation is encouraged. The primary purpose is to provide information and receive feedback. Knowing precisely what the assessment team hopes to achieve from a large community meeting will have a significant bearing on numerous aspects of the planning process (e.g., date, time of day, venue, agenda, public outreach, promotion, panellists, speakers and invited guests, audiovisual equipment, note-takers, crowd control people, refreshments, media coverage). It is important to allow enough time to prepare for this meeting, advertise it, extend invitations, prepare for media briefings, and secure an appropriate venue. Budget needs to be considered for rental costs (e.g., venue, equipment) and refreshments.

A community forum needs an excellent moderator—a skilled facilitator that can keep the meeting on track, on time, and not allow the agenda to be hijacked by either presenters or audience. The moderator needs to have a basic understanding of the issue to be able to insert questions to keep the meeting moving forward to meet its objectives. Panellists with a variety of viewpoints should be invited to speak—an expert on the issue at hand, a person with a dissenting perspective, a decision maker, and a member of the public that has first-hand experience of the issue. Enough time should be allowed in the agenda for adequate participation from the community. After the meeting, the team should meet to reflect and debrief with panellists and the moderator. Be prepared for the media to request interviews following the meeting. Follow up with notes to share with the team and use for analysis.

Surveys and Questionnaires

Questionnaires are tools (also known as instruments) that are used to collect information from people to supplement data from other sources, update information (e.g., demographic), solicit opinions (e.g., satisfaction, beliefs), assess risks (e.g., behaviours), and document exposure to various hazards (e.g., sexual harassment, pollutants). The process of collecting information from groups of people by the same questionnaire is called surveying. People can be surveyed in person (e.g., door-to-door, telephone) or in writing (e.g., mail-in, electronic). If administration methods are properly carried out and the instruments are valid, a large-scale survey can be relatively inexpensive in terms of the amount and quality of data collected for the expenditure of time and resources. Consent to participate is implied by returning a completed questionnaire. Names are not linked to the data for the purpose of confidentiality. In this way, the results are seen as more objective than interview methods.

Before we continue, a few words are needed about composing questionnaires. Everyone is confronted daily with people who are asking questions. Questionnaires arrive in the mail, and people call on the phone. Frequently, the interviewees learn neither the purpose of the questionnaire nor how the information will be used. When you draft a questionnaire, begin with introductory information that states who you are and what the purpose of the questionnaire is. Emphasize that participation is voluntary and that the information given will be confidential. Sign your name, and if the questionnaire is to be mailed, include a phone number where you can be contacted. Write questions that can be answered quickly (the whole questionnaire should not take longer than 10 minutes to complete). Ideally, place all questions on one side of a standard 8½-inch × 11-inch piece of paper that, if it is to be mailed, can be refolded so that a return address shows. Prior to sharing the questionnaire with agencies or community residents, administer it informally to friends and family; any comments made (such as "What do you mean by...?" or "I don't understand...") signal the need for further rewriting and clarification. Remember to check the reading level and language of the questions and allow for costs of translation as needed.

Take Note

How should the questionnaire be administered? Should the questionnaire be mailed to all households? Should the questionnaire be given to a specific group only? Or should the questionnaire be used as an interview guide and given to a selected number of participants at a specific site? (Recall from research that people who have been randomly selected can be considered representative of the total population.) What would you recommend? Before making a decision, list each option and consider the benefits and drawbacks of each. Here is some information for your decision making: Mailed questionnaires have about a 50% return rate that can be increased somewhat with a reminder postcard or telephone call, whereas questionnaires administered as an interview potentially have a 100% return rate. However, interviews require trained people and about 5 minutes per person per page of the survey, whereas mailed questionnaires require less labour but have the financial cost of postage. Decisions...decisions...

The following issues must be considered when planning to conduct a survey:

- *Purpose.* Knowing the goal of the survey will help to decide which questionnaire format to use, the target population for the survey, and how many people to include in the survey.
- *Resources.* Conducting a survey will use people, time, money, and support services to create the questionnaire, pilot test it, reproduce it, and administer it, and do follow-up data entry, analyze, and report the data.
- *Information needed.* Instruments to collect data need to be sensitive (i.e., not intrusive), reliable, and valid. Developing or choosing a questionnaire that consistently measures what it is supposed to measure takes time and expertise.
- *Format.* Open-ended questions will provide richer data (e.g., unique perspectives) than fixed-response questions (e.g., true–false, multiple choice, 1 to 5 scale), but they are more difficult to analyze.
- *Response rate.* In certain cases, a representative sample whose responses can be generalized to a wider population is desirable. At other times, the survey may need to reach everyone in a target group. Different methods to collect data and improve response rates may be used to ensure that the results are not biased.
- *Training.* People who conduct the survey need to be trained so that there is consistency among them. Data need to be recorded and input appropriately to facilitate analysis.
- *Analysis.* Responses to open-ended questions are analyzed qualitatively, seeking patterns and themes in the data. Results of fixed-response surveys are easily put into electronic form and analyzed statistically.

It is beyond the scope of this text to teach survey research, but excellent references are available to support the community assessment team (e.g., Canadian Public Health Association [CPHA], 2012). Also, you may want to seek out the expertise of a statistician and appropriate software programs to support both qualitative and quantitative analyses.

Other Assessment Strategies

The preceding is not an exhaustive list of methods that can be used to collect information about a community or population aggregate. Other methods can be found described in the literature (e.g., photovoice method—for examples, see case stories in Chapters 22 and 38). Additionally, the literature can be critically examined as issues arise and potential target populations surface. The community assessment team must meet frequently during data collection to share information and determine the scope and depth needed for analysis. Community members can be helpful in suggesting sources for further information (particularly regarding historical or recent events) and in providing evidence of community capacity and assets.

SECONDARY DATA SOURCES

Several forms of secondary data are collected in the course of everyday life: census, vital statistics, morbidity and mortality statistics, population health surveys, records of community services and schools, clinic records, screening records, environmental information (e.g., air and water quality), and the like. Many of these are in the public domain, but issues like confidentiality, data access, and quality of data must be assessed.

Population data can be used to establish baselines for the purposes of making comparisons, determining which indicators have enough support for their use, and setting benchmarks for measuring progress on goals and objectives, and when combined with critical reviews of the literature, they can be used to make program-related decisions.

Local data are often available from the municipality, health and social services departments, chambers of commerce, and similar groups in reports and on websites. Also, government ministries at both the provincial/territorial and national levels release population status reports that are available in local libraries or on the Internet. Health Canada and the PHAC regularly conduct a National Population Health Survey and make a variety of health-related reports available to the public. Statistics Canada also releases reports on population issues that may be of interest to the team for comparison purposes.

Until 2010, the Canadian census was mandatory for all Canadian households. It was discontinued and replaced by a voluntary system in 2011—a short form and a follow-up National Household survey of a sample of Canadian households*. Statistics Canada compiles reports from the voluntary short form census, household survey, census of agriculture, and the community health survey. These reports are located on the Statistics Canada website. In addition, community profiles are available on its website for census metropolitan areas (large cities), census divisions (smaller cities, counties), and census subdivisions (towns). Demographic reports are also available by provincial/territorial health regions. It is worth scrolling around on www.statcan.ca to see what information is available about the community and population of interest.

ELEMENTS OF A COMMUNITY ASSESSMENT

Begin by identifying your community. A system is a whole that functions because of the interdependence of its parts. A community, too, is a whole entity that functions because of the interdependence of its parts, or subsystems. The community assessment wheel (see Fig. 16.1)

---

*In November 2015 the mandatory long-form census was reinstated by Prime Minister Justin Trudeau.

will be your overall framework. The assessment wheel can be used to assess *any* community, regardless of size, location, resources, or population characteristics. It can also be used to assess a "community within a community" such as a school, an industry, or a business. In addition, this guide can be used to assess a population aggregate (i.e., a defined group within the community [e.g., teenagers, lone parents, people of an ethnic group of interest, people living with a particular condition]) by providing the context in which this group is located. The *process* of assessment, regardless of where it is applied, always remains the same.

The use of the assessment wheel of the CCAP model to guide the assessment of a community, neighbourhood, population, or a population aggregate assists with the organization of the assessment process and of the data collected. This section will examine the data that describe the core, the subsystems, and the functions of the community according to the assessment wheel in Figure 16.1. The community assessment team will want to create its own process for data management based on the resources available and the skills of the team (e.g., epidemiologist, biostatistician, geographic information specialist, qualitative and quantitative analysts).

Community Core

The core of a community is its people—their history, characteristics, values, and beliefs. The first stage of assessing a community, then, is to learn about its people to gain insight into their life experience. In fact, collaborating with people in the community is an integral part of working with the community. In Table 16.5 the major components of the community core

TABLE 16.5 Community Core Data

Components	Sources of Information
History	Library, historical society, museum, newspaper archives
	Interview "old-timers," town leaders
Demographics	Census of population and housing
Age and sex characteristics	Planning board (local, county, province)
Racial distribution	Chamber of Commerce
Ethnic distribution	City Hall, archives
	Observation
Household types by	Census (municipal, national)
Family	
Non-family	
Group	
Marital status by	Census (municipal, national)
Single	
Separated	
Widowed	
Divorced	
Vital statistics	Local and provincial territorial departments of health (distributed through health department reports and websites); provincial/territorial vital statistics
Births	
Deaths by	
Age	
Leading causes	
Values and beliefs	Personal contact
	Observation
	Observation
Religion	Telephone book

are listed along with suggested locations and sources of information about each component. Because every community is different, information sources available to one community may not be available to another.

The community core is described through information on sociodemographic, economic, and cultural variables and factors that describe social support. Lifestyle factors, employment patterns, resource production and consumption, and population-level personal health be-haviours help to understand the people of the community and how their values influence the choices made. Indices of social cohesion or isolation, examples of stigma, prejudice or bullying, and predominant values and attitudes toward diversity are also signals of the health of the core/population of interest.

To begin the process, experienced community workers might find it helpful to write thumb-nail sketches that succinctly describe the community (or communities) and populations (or population aggregates) of interest.

Population Description

Sociodemographic characteristics provide a good snapshot of the population. Knowing how many people live in the community, the number in each age group by sex, ethnicity and lan-guages spoken, religious affiliations, housing, education, income, and marital status can assist the community assessment team to uncover assets and also some potential issues or needs. But be cautious; for instance, just because there may be a number of lone parent families in a community does not mean that it is a problem that needs to be addressed. Consider also the strengths of the community—employment rates, income and education levels—that might already be used to support lone parenting families. You need more evidence, usually from different sources, before you can come to any conclusions about any of the characteristics of the community.

Total Population

Knowing the total number of people living in a neighbourhood or in a group of neighbour-hoods allows the team to make certain judgements and comparisons between and among communities. Information that allows us to understand the elements of the community core is found in sociodemographic data that are captured in the census.

Age Distribution

How a population is apportioned by age often provides important clues to potential issues that might be faced. For example, a neighbourhood with a high proportion of seniors will need different services and resources than a neighbourhood where young children predominate. Further, knowing about some characteristics that can have an effect on health and well-being is important. Making a population pyramid for the community and comparing it to the city or province can tell a great deal about how the community is apportioned (see Chapter 17, Tables 17.4 and 17.5).

Social Inclusion

Geopolitical communities provide opportunity for the development of informal and formal social ties. Communities with people who are interested in their neighbourhoods, aware of resources available, and involved in the safety and health of the community are strong com-munities. Those communities that lack connection to people risk social isolation and underuti-lization of available resources to prevent negative physical and economic outcomes. It takes time to develop an attachment to a community; hence, those communities with high mobility and recent in-migration may have lower participation rates in community life. Individuals who lack fluency in the official languages of the country face further risk of social or economic isolation. The census provides information about immigration and mobility, languages used in the home, and facility with official languages.

The census also provides information as to marital status and the number of people living in a dwelling. Adults who live alone (e.g., seniors), board with non-family members, and lone parent families must bear social and financial stress on their own. Furthermore, they are more likely to have incomes below the low-income cut-off (LICO). Seniors and those with disabilities may also face difficulties accessing services due to their frailty.

As the team gets to know the people in the community through observation and interviews, it can put context around the statistics gleaned from the census and develop a deeper understanding of their lives.

Education, Employment, and Income

Certain demographic characteristics are strongly linked. Education is linked to people's ability to gain employment; generally the higher the population's education level the better the job opportunities and the better the rates of pay. The census provides information about education attainment (e.g., less than high school to post-secondary diplomas, certificates, and degrees). The census also provides information about the types of jobs people in the community hold and if those represent full- or part-time employment. As team members engage more fully with population, the more the team will begin to appreciate the effects of education and income on how people are able to cope with the demands of life.

Household Structure

In the 2011 Canadian Census, information was collected that allowed Statistics Canada to publish a portrait of family structures in Canada and tables that illustrate trends and changes over time (Statistics Canada, 2012). Understanding family composition and household structure allows a determination of the complexity of the lives of people in the community. Trends (e.g., increasing numbers of same-sex couples with children) require services that respect diversity in family composition and structures. Linking family structure to the community subsystems, education for example, helps us to understand the family complexities that need to be considered by schools.

Shelter

The ability to afford adequate housing contributes to the health of individuals, families, and communities. Families with low incomes may divert money from other necessities to cover shelter costs or may become homeless. The percentage of income devoted to shelter is a useful measure of housing affordability.

The 2011 Canadian Census collected information about the sorts of dwellings in which Canadians lived (Statistics Canada, 2015). In May every year, many communities in Canada conduct a point-in-time count of homelessness that informs social and health service agencies about the number and characteristics (e.g., age, sex, lone parent, family) of people who are not housed. Assessing the circumstances of the places people call home are important to understanding whether or not shelter is adequate, appropriate, safe, and accessible (Gaetz et al., 2014). Statistical data will form only a part of your assessment; windshield and walking surveys will provide you a more detailed picture of housing quantity and quality in the neighbourhoods and community being assessed.

SUBSYSTEMS

A review of a community's subsystems reveals the context in which people live, love, learn, work, play, and pray. It provides insights into factors that influence how people live, what choices they make, and why. A subsystems analysis focuses on the external environment such as the sociopolitical and economic contexts and the infrastructures of the community and how these have an impact on the population. When we assess the subsystems, we are seeking to find if there are any stressors acting on the population and what flexible lines of defence (temporary responses) and lines of resistance (strengths) are in place to protect the community core.

Physical Environment

It is important to collect information about where and how the community and population are situated within the physical space to understand how the various elements have an impact on community life (e.g., weather, terrain, placement of services, population density, diversity). Such information allows us to assess availability, affordability, appropriateness, acceptability, adequacy, and access to services, housing, green space, and so forth and associated issues of safety, utilization, and community capacity. Note also the roads, transit, location of leisure, recreation and cultural venues, faith institutions, as well as the location of health services (e.g., clinics, physiotherapists, pharmacies) as well as food sources (e.g., markets, fast food outlets, food bank). Maps and photos are valuable methods that visually illustrate the data collected.

Education

Education is closely linked with employment and the economic status of a community and its population. The infrastructure for learning—basic, specialized, literacy—is what comprises the education subsystem. The number of children below school age is an important indicator of whether a school will be fully occupied or if a new school, or portable classrooms, will be needed. If there is in-migration of families who do not speak English to a community, it is an indicator to the school system that English as a Second Language (ESL) classes may be needed in response.

To supplement this broad assessment, information is needed about major educational sources (e.g., schools, colleges, libraries, ESL classes) located both inside and outside the community that people use for formal as well as continuing education and personal interest purposes. In Table 16.6 is a suggested guide for assessing a community's educational sources.

TABLE 16.6   Indicators and Sources of Information for the Education Subsystem

Indicators	Sources of Information
Educational Status	
School enrollment by type of school	Census data
Dropout/completion rates	School board data
Educational Sources	
Intracommunity or extracommunity (collect data for each facility)	Local board of education reports and websites
Services (educational, recreational, communication, and health)	School administrator (such as the principal or director) and school nurse
Resources (personnel, space, budget, and record system)	School administrator
Characteristics of users (geographic distribution and demographic profile)	Teachers and staff
Adequacy, accessibility, and acceptability of education to students and staff	Students and staff

It is sometimes difficult to decide which educational sources to include in an assessment but community usage is probably the most important indicator. Primary and secondary schools attended by the majority of youngsters in a community, regardless of intra- or extracommunity location, are major educational sources and require a thorough assessment, whereas schools composed primarily of students from outside the community do not require such an extensive appraisal. A line of resistance to look for is whether or not children go to school in their own neighbourhood. If children, particularly elementary school children, are required to go outside their community for school, it can be a sign of a community stressor.

Safety and Transportation

Without a safe and secure environment based on public order and respect for property, people will be fearful of participation in community events. Structures in this subsystem exist to reduce fear or anxiety and promote a sense of safety in a community and its population. Hence, the availability of fire, police, sanitation, sewage, recycling, and solid-waste services as well as those that protect air quality, monitor dangerous goods, and protect us from animals are assessed. Public and community services that offer health promotion, injury and disease prevention, and health protection services are important to the health and well-being of a community.

Community perceptions of safety are important indicators for this subsystem—crime statistics give a picture of the community as do people's perceptions of racism, ageism, stigma, prejudice, and feelings of social isolation. Crime statistics broken down by community are located on police services websites.

How do people travel around the community to work and school and to take part in leisure activities? What transit is available and when does it run? What does it cost? What proportion of households in the community has vehicles? In what condition are these vehicles? These are important questions to assess if people are able to attend school, get to and from work in a timely manner, and if they can manage the costs associated with transportation. Transportation safety measures (i.e., roads and road maintenance; private vehicle safety regulations; public transit, air, and rail safety measures; lighting of public places and roads) protect the public from hazards. Take a look at the community's transportation policies to see if there are policies that place stress on community members, particularly those who work night shifts and weekends.

To examine lines of defence (health status and temporary responses to stressors) and resistance (assets), consider what citizen protection mechanisms are in place: identification of children, seniors, and animals in case they wander from home; Amber Alert program; Block Watch program; volunteer school safety patrols and crossing guards; school and mall security personnel; mall walk programs; and emergency call lines for children (e.g., Children's Help Phone), seniors, and people living with mental illness and experiencing domestic violence.

Politics and Government

The various forms and levels of government are responsible for public policy making through legislation. We need to understand which government is responsible for the portfolios that influence healthy public policy, how special interest groups can influence policy, and how communities and populations gain access to these resources. Influential people in positions of power influence the health and well-being of people and communities: provincial/territorial politicians, mayor and council, school board and trustees, local medical officers of health, and heads of social and community agencies. Within the disciplines that are involved in community work, there are opportunities to bring issues and resolutions forward for action locally, provincially/territorially, and on the national scene. For instance, the CPHA has worked successfully with the various provincial public health associations to influence public policy on gun control, home care, clean air, homelessness, and unemployment issues, among others.

Health and Social Services

A review of this subsystem allows an assessment of the "social safety net" infrastructure and provides insight as to how basic needs are met in the community. The focus is on need and utilization—how needs are met (availability, access, affordability) by services within and outside the community. Various sectors that provide health and services are included in the assessment (e.g., formal [government] and informal [volunteer], publicly funded, private). Health units, social services departments, and hospitals provide utilization reports on a regular basis that can be used for assessment purposes (e.g., notifiable disease reports, restaurant inspections, immunization rates, emergency room utilization).

One method of classifying health and social services is to differentiate between facilities located outside the community (extracommunity) versus those within the community (intracommunity). Once the health and social service facilities are identified, group them into categories, perhaps by type of service offered (e.g., hospitals, clinics, extended care), by size, or by public versus private usage.

Maps are an excellent way to display health and utilization data gathered by the team. A map provides a visual picture that cannot be illustrated by lists of addresses. As geographic information systems (GIS) have become more readily available, mapping has become increasingly important to illustrate distributions across territory. It is important to collect information not only about what health and social services are available in the community itself but also about what services exist in the immediate area that people access. If possible, utilization rates can provide helpful data to the assessment. Planners need to know this information if they are going to avoid duplication, facilitate access, and remove barriers or obstacles to utilization.

Communication

This subsystem details how people communicate within the community on an everyday basis and also how emergency messages are conveyed. Access to communication links determines how well people are informed. Because information is key to awareness of goods and services, lack of a satisfactory means of gathering information can adversely affect access and utilization of needed services. Telecommunication companies publish reports about the number of households with television, Internet and cell phones, by neighbourhood, or local surveys can be conducted to collect primary data.

Communication may be formal or informal. Formal communication usually originates outside the community (extracommunity) as opposed to informal communication, which almost always originates and is disseminated within the community and population aggregates. Salient components of formal and informal communication, as well as sources of data, are presented in Table 16.7. Your observations in the community, interviews with key informants, and conversations with community members should provide a picture of how news gets around the community, how many people have cell phones, and how many people have computers in the homes. If you have a "connected" community, you can use social media effectively to communicate. If, however, there are pockets of people you would like to reach but they are not connected electronically, you will have to use more creative (and potentially old-fashioned) means of contacting them (e.g., posters, brochures, cards).

Business and Economics

The business and economics subsystem includes the "wealth" of a community—that is, the goods and services available to the community—as well as the costs and benefits of improving patterns of resource allocation. It should be evident that extracommunity factors, such as the state of the national and world economies, affect in great measure the local economy.

TABLE 16.7 Indicators and Sources of Information for the Communication Subsystem

Indicators	Sources of Information
Formal	
Newspaper (number, circulation, frequency, and scope of news), Radio and television (number of stations, commercial versus educational, and audience)	Chamber of Commerce
	Newspaper office
Postal service	Telephone company
Telephone status (number of residents with service)	Yellow Pages
	Telephone book
	Canada Post courier services
Informal	
Sources: Bulletin boards; posters; hand-delivered flyers; and religious, civic, and school newsletters	Windshield/walking survey
	Talking to residents
Dissemination (How do people receive information?)	Survey
Word of mouth	
Mail	
Radio, television	Reports, surveys

Nevertheless, intracommunity economic factors impinge on all other subsystems, so they must be included in the assessment.

The economy affects household finances through employment, commerce, and productivity, and measures that describe the labour force (e.g., employment rate, occupations) give insight into the "morale" of a population and the vitality of a community.

In Table 16.8, the suggested areas for studying a community's economy are listed, along with sources of data. The census data can be used to summarize most of these economic indicators. Two key indicators of a community's economic "health" are the percentage of households below the poverty level and the unemployment rate. Data from the business and economics subsystem allow the team to see what indicators have had impact on the community and population aggregates.

Statistics Canada publishes Labour Force Survey data monthly around the 15th of each month in "The Daily" along with regular reports on a variety of labour-related economic topics by subject, province/territory, and census areas. These up-to-the moment reports are invaluable when assessing the business and economics subsystem. The team should also link its windshield survey data with questions about the economy—does the community have a number of second-hand stores, pawn shops, a food bank? These might be signs of a community at economic risk.

In making the links between the business and economics subsystem and characteristics of the community core, it is important to keep in mind that work activity (number of hours and weeks worked per year) is related to income adequacy. Those people that work full time for less than a year, or part time, are almost three times as likely to have incomes below the LICO than full-time workers who worked for the full year. Particularly disadvantaged by earning inequality are women and youth workers.

Recreation and Leisure

The recreation and leisure subsystem allows us to focus on assessing the degree of lifestyle support in the community. We will want to link recreation information with the data on physical environment and safety subsystems for a complete picture, but collecting information on parks, sports facilities, jogging and bicycle paths, as well as resources for social interaction (e.g., special interest clubs, seniors' centres, theatres, art galleries, restaurants, bars, festivals, zoos, museums, sports teams) offers insight into access, affordability, and use patterns that can suggest opportunities for

TABLE 16.8   Indicators and Sources of Information for Business and Economics Subsystems

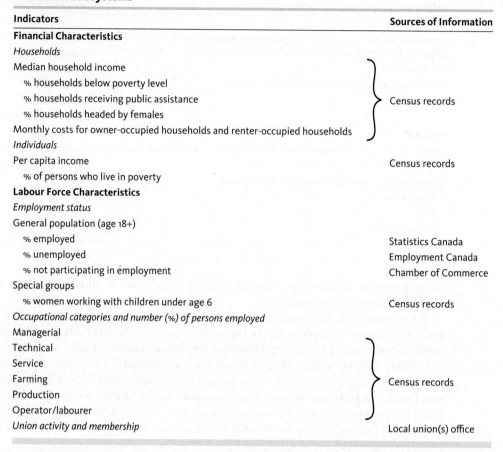

Indicators	Sources of Information
Financial Characteristics	
Households	
Median household income	
% households below poverty level	
% households receiving public assistance	Census records
% households headed by females	
Monthly costs for owner-occupied households and renter-occupied households	
Individuals	
Per capita income	Census records
% of persons who live in poverty	
Labour Force Characteristics	
Employment status	
General population (age 18+)	
% employed	Statistics Canada
% unemployed	Employment Canada
% not participating in employment	Chamber of Commerce
Special groups	
% women working with children under age 6	Census records
Occupational categories and number (%) of persons employed	
Managerial	
Technical	
Service	
Farming	Census records
Production	
Operator/labourer	
Union activity and membership	Local union(s) office

community capacity-building and help to determine activity and social needs of the population. Consider the business and economics subsystem as well—are the leisure and recreation facilities free of charge? If not, are there considerations for people with low incomes? Does business support certain activities through sponsorships? What recreational opportunities are located in community centres, faith institutions? Where people "hang out" are the places the community assessment team should go to interact with the population! (see Table 16.9).

TABLE 16.9   Indicators and Sources of Information for the Recreation and Leisure Subsystem

Indicators	Sources of Information
Sports and fitness	City Parks and Recreation Services will list city-sponsored services; others will be listed under community associations or private business: arenas, playgrounds, bowling alleys, tennis courts, ball diamonds, soccer pitches, bike paths, walking paths, sport associations, fitness clubs, mall walk programs, outdoor skating rinks, water, mountain or forest activities. Professional and semi-professional sports teams (e.g., hockey, baseball, football, basketball, soccer, lacrosse).
Social pursuits	Age-appropriate clubs (e.g., Brownies, Scouts), interest clubs (e.g., stamp collectors), community dances and celebrations, community courses for hobbyists. Library, faith, school-sponsored social events. Places people gather (e.g., coffee houses, restaurants, bars)
Leisure pursuits	Theatres, cinemas, dance, opera, music, artistic appreciation events and sites
Other	Zoo and animal parks, museums, picnic areas

Summary

A community assessment is never complete, because any community and the people who live in it are dynamic and ever evolving; however, we must pause at some point. Because we have addressed all parts of the assessment wheel of the CCAP model, this is where we will stop. Recall that at every step of the assessment, people in the community were included. Not only were "professionals" interviewed (e.g., school nurses, social workers, physicians, principals, police chief, alderman, and so on) but individuals within the subsystems also were included (e.g., parents, shoppers, patients, people on the street). The assessment, like all steps in the CCAP process, is carried out in partnership with the community. The next step is analysis—a process that synthesizes the assessment information and derives from it statements specific to the community.

REFERENCES

American College of Emergency Physicians (ACEP). (n.d.). *Chapter guide to organizing, planning and executing a town hall meeting.* URL=https://www.acep.org/uploadedFiles/ACEP/advocacy/state/Guide%20to%20Hosting%20a%20Town%20Hall%20Meeting.pdf

Anderson, E. T., & McFarlane, J. M. (2015). *Community as partner: Theory and practice in nursing* (7th ed.). Philadelphia, PA: Lippincott Williams & Wilkins.

Canadian Public Health Association (CPHA). (2012). *Guide to questionnaire construction and question writing.* Ottawa: Author.

Dorfman, D. (1998). *Mapping community assets workbook.* Portland: Northwest Regional Education Laboratory, Rural Education Project. URL=http://www.abcdinstitute.org/docs/Diane%20Dorfman-Mapping-Community-Assets-WorkBook(1)-1.pdf

Gaetz, S., Gulliver, T., & Richter, T. (2014). *The state of homelessness in Canada: 2014.* Toronto: The Homeless Hub Press. URL=http://www.homelesshub.ca/SOHC2014

Gilmore, G. D. (2012). *Needs and capacity assessment strategies for health education and health promotion* (4th ed.). Burlington, MA: Jones and Bartlett Learning.

Public Health Agency of Canada (PHAC). (2008). *Core competencies for public health in Canada. Release 1.0.* Ottawa: Author. URL=http://www.phac-aspc.gc.ca/php-psp/ccph-cesp/about_cc-apropos_ce-eng.php

Racher, F. E., & Annis, R. C. (2008). Community health action model: health promotion by the community. *Research and Theory of Nursing Practice: An International Journal, 22*(3), 182–191.

Rissel, C., & Bracht, N. (1999). Assessing community needs, resources, and readiness: Building on strengths. In N. Bracht (Ed.), *Health promotion at the community level: New advances* (2nd ed., pp. 59–81). Thousand Oaks, CA: Sage.

Statistics Canada. (2012). *Portrait of families and living arrangements in Canada: Families, households and marital status, 2011 Census of Population.* Ottawa: Author. URL=http://www12.statcan.ca/census-recensement/2011/as-sa/98-312-x/98-312-x2011001-eng.cfm

Statistics Canada. (2015). *2011 Census of Canada: Topic-based tabulations: Structural type of dwelling and collectives.* URL=https://www12.statcan.gc.ca/census-recensement/2011/dp-pd/tbt-tt/Index-eng.cfm

ONLINE RESOURCES

Please visit the Point at http://thepoint.lww.com/Vollman4e for up-to-date Internet resources and additional learning materials on this topic.

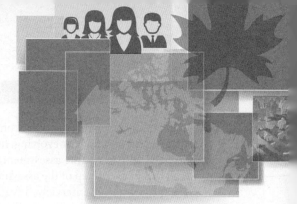

CHAPTER 17

Community Analysis and Diagnosis

Ardene Robinson Vollman

LEARNING OBJECTIVES

This chapter is focused on the second phase of the CCAP process, analysis, and the associated task of forming community health diagnoses. Each of these aspects of the CCAP process needs to include community members if it is to be accurate, appropriate, and acceptable to the community, and if it is to build the capacity of the community to maintain and sustain efforts for health promotion over the long term.

After studying this chapter, you should be able to:

1. Practise within a team environment to critically analyze and synthesize the data collected

2. Classify community assessment data into the categories of the Canadian community-as-partner (CCAP) model

3. Create summary statements and note aspects of incomplete or contradictory information

4. Interpret summary statements in comparison with benchmark data and trends

5. Generate inferences and formulate community health diagnoses

6. Validate information and inferences

Introduction

Analysis is the study and examination of data by the processes of classification, summarization, interpretation, and validation of information in order to write community diagnoses and establish priorities (Helvie, 1998). It is the means by which the community assessment team examines population and social data, plus knowledge of the local context, in order to determine the needs, strengths, barriers, opportunities, readiness, and resources of the community. These data may be quantitative (numerical) as well as qualitative. All aspects of the data collected need to be considered; this is best done with members of the community assisted by the community assessment team. Community members are best informed about the content and context of the life of the community and its residents, its strengths and capacities, but can still benefit from coaching, mentoring, and guidance from team members who will have better access to sociodemographic data and health status information. Analysis is necessary to determine community needs and community strengths as well as to identify patterns of responses and trends in service use. During analysis, any need for further data collection is revealed if there are gaps and incongruities in the community assessment data. The endpoint of analysis is a community health diagnosis.

COMMUNITY ANALYSIS

Analysis, like so many procedures we perform, may be viewed as a process with multiple steps. The phases we will use to help in the analysis are classification, summarization, interpretation, and validation. Each is described and illustrated below.

Classification

To analyze community assessment data, it is helpful to first classify the data. Data can be classified into categories in a variety of ways. Traditional categories of community assessment data include:

- Demographic characteristics (family size, age, sex, and ethnic and racial groupings)
- Geographic characteristics (area boundaries; number and size of neighbourhoods, public spaces, and roads)
- Socioeconomic characteristics (people's occupation and income categories, educational attainment, and rental or home ownership patterns)
- Health and social resources and services (presence and utilization of hospitals, clinics, mental health centres, welfare offices, etc.)

However, models are increasingly being used in the organization and analysis of community health data because they provide a framework for data collection and a map to guide analysis. Because the community assessment wheel (see Fig. 16.1) was used to direct the community assessment, that same model can be used to guide analysis. The community core and each of the community subsystems will be analyzed, and the smaller components within each subsystem will help to describe the categories by which information is sorted.

Take Note

As with community assessment, the process of analysis must be carried out with community members. It is disrespectful to collect information and not use the lens of the community to interpret what it means. To build community means to create trust and rapport—a cardinal rule of community health promotion.

Ultimately, we want to describe the community's normal lines of defence (NLD), that is, the health status of the people (Pop-NLD) and the community (Comm-NLD). We also want to locate sources of risk, threats, hazards, barriers, and challenges (stressors) and identify the flexible lines of defence (FLD) or protective factors that are in place as well as the lines of resistance (LR) that represent the community's strengths, assets, and capacities (see Fig. 17.1). The focus of analysis is the people (community core); the subsystems represent the environment where people live, love, learn, work, play, and pray.

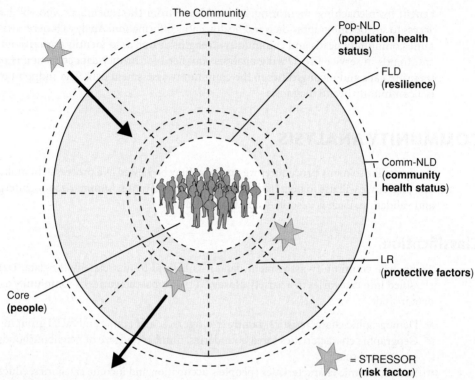

FIGURE 17.1   Analyzing the community assessment wheel—protective and risk factors, stressors, population and community health status.

Summarization

Once a classification method has been selected, the next task is to summarize the data within each category. Both summary statements and summary measures, such as rates, charts, and graphs, are required.

Take Note

Many health care agencies and educational institutions have access to computerized information systems—a system through which formatted data can be retrieved in a variety of forms—including summary health statistics. For example, data entered into a computer system as census figures can be configured into population pyramids, and census and vital statistics information can be programmed to calculate birth, death, and fertility rates. Calculations that previously required hours to complete are now computed in seconds. In your practice, make it a point to inquire as to the availability of computer systems, and if possible, use computer processes to carry out quantitative data analysis. In addition, your local health department may be able to furnish the rates for the team. Note, however, that the denominator used to calculate this rate may not be the community as you have defined it.

Interpretation

To interpret data often requires comparison to established standards or benchmarks, provincial/territorial and national statistics, and the community's own statistics for previous years.

Outcomes of data analysis include the identification of data gaps, inconsistencies, or omissions and the generation of inferences or hypotheses about the findings. Frequently, comparative data are needed to determine if a pattern or trend exists or if data do not seem correct and the need for revalidation of original information is required. Data gaps are inevitable, as are mistakes in recording data; the important task is to analyze data critically and be aware of the potential for gaps and omissions. It is helpful to have professional colleagues as well as community residents review the analysis. Every person has a unique perspective; it is only through the sharing of views that a whole and comprehensive picture of community assessment data can evolve.

Using the data from your community, compare them with other similar data to determine the size of the problem. For instance, you calculate (or discover) an infant mortality rate (IMR) of 12/1,000 live births—how does this compare with other communities? The province? The nation? Is it for the entire infant population of your community, or are there differences among structural or demographic factors? Is the IMR different for different ethnic groups, ages and marital status of mothers, or geographic parts of the community? Have there been any changes for the better or worse in recent years or the past decade? (Note: This is a good time to review Chapter 4 to assist you with epidemiologic reasoning as you try to make sense of your data.)

Other resources for comparison are the documents produced as health report cards by regional health authorities, provinces/territories, Health Canada and Public Health Agency of Canada (PHAC) (and other federal departments such as Environment, Citizenship and Immigration, Employment and Social Development). The PHAC's annual reports on the State of Public Health in Canada (2008–2016) by the Chief Public Health Officer (CPHO) presents national figures, such as incidence and prevalence when available, for our major health concerns. Although Canada does not yet have a specific document regarding population health goals, Healthy People 2020 (U.S. Department of Health and Human Services, 2014), though not Canadian, can be invaluable to you because it contains goals and objectives that help in both data analysis and planning.

Having classified, summarized, and compared the data you have collected, the final phase is to draw logical conclusions from the evidence, that is, to draw inferences that will lead to the statement of a community diagnosis. An *inference* is a conclusion drawn from multiple observations. An inference synthesizes what you have learned about the community and the people—it states what the data *means*. These conclusions or inferences will identify stressors and strengths in succinct phrases; these phrases then form the basis for a community diagnosis. *Synthesis* is the linking of the summary statements from the classification process and formulating hypotheses about the connections among them.

Validation

It is a common complaint of communities that "experts" come in and collect data, make judgments, and then leave. It is important to validate the conclusions you reach and the hypotheses you generate to ensure that they are correct and reflect the community accurately. Often there is only a "sample" of community representation on community assessment teams, so even if the team believes it has carried out a collaborative analysis, it is worth using a validation process with a larger community group to be certain that nothing has been missed or misunderstood. This validation process also creates a broader awareness of the community assessment process underway. Validation requires that the team confirm its information and its interpretation by returning to sources for confirmation or additional data. The team should solicit feedback and check with key sources (e.g., community informants, external experts) to verify that the results of the assessment and analysis processes are appropriate. Town hall or focus group meetings, purposive surveys, or interviews can be used for validation purposes (see Chapter 16).

TABLE 17.1 Team Analysis Issues and Strategies for Solution

Issues	Strategies
Coordinating the sharing of volumes of data	Use electronic tools; sharing information during team meetings
Disagreement in interpretations of data	Ensure that the data are broadly representative of key community perspectives; if gaps exist, seek to fill them with further information
Community-team disagreement on the meaning of data	Include community members in all aspects of analysis
Contradictory data from different sources	Seek further data or clarification; reporting with recommendations for further exploration

Several issues may face the team during its analytic process that will cause argument, conflict and need to be resolved. In Table 17.1 some of these issues are listed, along with suggestions to address them.

The remainder of this chapter will walk the team through the data analysis process so that it can best present and use the data that were collected in the community assessment process.

THE PROCESS OF COMMUNITY ANALYSIS

Normally, data analysis begins with the community core, because it is the core (the people and their health) that is of interest to the community assessment team and the organizations that monitor health status and serve the public with programs to strengthen the Pop-NLD, particularly of groups and aggregates that may be vulnerable to stressors (risk factors). Once the core is analyzed, then the team can move into working groups—one to analyze the data on the community's health status (Comm-NLD) as represented by the subsystems, and another to more deeply analyze the particular health issues that have arisen through the analytic process.

The analytic process is iterative with assessment; it is not unusual to need to return to data collection throughout the analysis process. Here are some practical tips on data analysis:

- Present statistical information as rates or ratios for comparison
- Use trends and projections to display changes over a time period
- Compare local data with other districts or the whole population
- Use graphical presentations for easy understanding

Community Core

Community core data include many population-level sociodemographic measures, data that are especially amenable to graphs and charts. The adage "one picture is worth a thousand words" is particularly meaningful for demographic characteristics. In Table 17.2 examples of selected demographic and health status data are presented as summary statements (Column 1) and in Column 2, relevant inferences are presented.

In Table 17.3 the population by sex and age group for both the community and the province are detailed.

Look how much easier it is to appreciate the differences between the community and the province in the population pyramid illustrated in Figure 17.2. Not everyone can make sense of a table of numbers—visual representations help to bring the data summaries to life.

TABLE 17.2   Summary Statements and Inferences

Data Category	Summary Statements	Inferences
History	• Neighbourhood 1 is the inner city; being revitalized. • Neighbourhood 2 is the industrial centre; very run down. • Neighbourhood 3 has many high-rise buildings; downtown business centre. • Neighbourhood 4 has a large immigrant population; urban. • Neighbourhood 5 is the suburb.	The community is not homogeneous; there is a great deal of variation in terms of neighbourhood history, pride, and attractions
Demographics	• Neighbourhood 5 has the largest population. • More than 43% of the residents over 1 year of age in Neighbourhoods 1 and 2 moved in the past year, above the provincial average of 24%.	The inner city communities have high mobility rates.
Vital statistics	• Data gap: Unable to disaggregate the community vital statistics data by neighbourhood. • From 2010 to 2015, there were 1,901 births. • Crude birth rate: 12.3/1,000 population; Province: 15.6 • Proportion of births to women aged 15–19: 11.3%; in Province: 5.1% • Teen birth rate is twice the Provincial rate. • Community low-birth-weight rate: 8.6%; Province: 6.1% • In the period 2010–14, 688 community residents died. The standardized mortality ratio = 0.9, not significantly different from the province.	Teen women are at higher perinatal risk than other city women as a result of youth, immigration, mobility, and language

Health status	• Causes of death:
	    Cancer (28%)
	    Ischemic heart disease (20%)
	    Respiratory disease (20%)
	    Cerebrovascular disease (8%)
	    Injury (8%)
	• The most frequent reason for emergency room visits is injury (30%). Of these, falls account for the largest proportion.
		Seniors are a risk group
		
		Injuries (e.g., from falls) are a concern, particularly where the senior population is high

The population pyramid is formed of bars; each bar represents an age group. Usually 5- or 10-year age groups are used, although adaptations can be made for smaller or larger age ranges. All age groups in a pyramid should be of the same interval. Bars are stacked horizontally, one on another, with bars for males on the left of a central axis and bars for females on the right. The percentage of males and females in a particular age group is indicated by the length of the bars, as measured from the central axis.

TABLE 17.3   Percent of Population by Sex and Age Group for the Community and Province

Ages (Years)	Males		Females	
	Community	Province	Community	Province
<5	2.5	2.9	2.3	2.9
5–19	6.3	10.3	6.2	9.8
20–24	3.8	4.0	3.9	3.8
25–34	12.3	8.5	10.4	8.3
35–44	10.5	9.7	8.7	9.5
45–54	6.5	7.4	5.8	6.9
55–64	4.1	3.6	3.9	3.6
65–74	3.2	2.5	3.7	2.8
75+	2.2	1.4	3.9	2.3

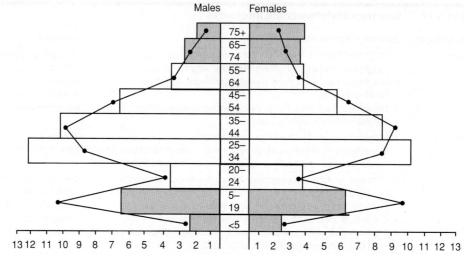

FIGURE 17.2   Population pyramid for the community (bars) with province superimposed (lines).

To construct your population pyramid, use the worksheet in Table 17.4. Determine the community's total population, and then calculate the respective percentages of males and females by age group by dividing the number in each group by the total population. Next use Table 17.5 to draw the pyramid. Note that parts of the population pyramid in Figure 17.2, those depicting people younger than 20 years and older than 65 years, are shaded; this was done to denote the dependent portions of the population. A dependency ratio (Table 17.6) can be calculated when we have information about the size of the dependent population in contrast to those of working age.

TABLE 17.4   Calculations for a Population Pyramid

Community Name, Census Tract, or Geographic Boundaries: _____

Total Population: _____

Ages (Years)	Males		Females	
	Number	Total Population (%)	Number	Total Population (%)
<5				
5–9				
10–14				
15–19				
20–24				
25–29				
30–34				
35–39				
40–44				
45–49				
50–54				
55–59				
60–64				
65–69				
70–74				
75+				

TABLE 17.5 Constructing a Population Pyramid

Population Pyramid for _____: Year _____

Males												Females
					75+							
					70–74							
					65–69							
					60–64							
					55–59							
					50–54							
					45–49							
					40–44							
					35–39							
					30–34							
					25–29							
					20–24							
					15–19							
					10–14							
					5–9							
					<5							
8	6	4	2		0		2		4		6	8

Percentage of Population

The dependency ratio (also known as the Gini coefficient) describes the potentially self-supporting portion of the population and the dependent portions at the extremes of age. It is usually calculated as follows:

$$DR = \frac{\text{population under 20} + \text{population 65 and over}}{\text{population 20 to 64 years of age}} \times 100$$

The dependency ratio is interpreted as the number of persons under age 20 and over age 65 needing support (because of age) for every 100 persons aged 20 to 65 years.

Studying population pyramids for the community as a whole and the province reveals some striking age and sex differences (see Fig. 17.2). If, however, the demographics of each of the five neighbourhoods had been presented separately, we might learn that by aggregating the neighbourhood data as one population pyramid we missed important age and sex differences. They might have been minimized or gone unrecognized, and their associated age- and sex-related needs would be left unmet. Similarly, if the demographics of each of the five neighbourhoods were analyzed separately, significant differences may be detected between them. This hazard in data analysis is referred to as aggregating or pooling the data. It is important to divide data along all possibly meaningful lines so that important information is not overlooked. Be alert to this problem as you proceed with your analysis.

TABLE 17.6 Data for Calculating the Dependency Ratio

Population	n
Total population	51,588
Dependents (age <20 + >64)	12,691
Working (age 20–64)	38,897
Ratio (Gini coefficient)	**33**

As the team studies the data it collected, ask: What inferences can be drawn from our summary statements? Does the built environment have an impact on the lifestyle of the population? Does the large proportion of seniors living alone present any issues relating to health or social isolation? Does a large immigrant population represent a stressor with regard to employment, language, or cultural appropriateness of services? We will need to use other methods of data collection to test these inferences—perhaps by direct observation, key informant interviews, or group interviews with target populations; this is part of the iterative or cyclical nature of data collection, classification, summarization, and interpretation that makes up the analytic process.

Physical Environment

To study the physical components, data were collected by inspection (i.e., windshield surveys) and from written reports prepared by City Hall, Social Services, the Chamber of Commerce, and the regional health authority. Many of these reports are available online.

The team might want to break the analysis into two parts of the environment—natural and built.

Natural environment: In this part of analysis, data such as weather patterns, rainfall trends, extreme weather events, UV index trends, and outdoor air quality trends can be displayed graphically. Summary statements such as the number of smog alerts per month can help to generate inferences about air pollution, for example. Canadian climate data can be presented in many forms (e.g., bar and line graphs) as illustrated on the Government of Canada website that the team might have used for data collection (http://climate.weather.gc.ca).

Take Note

Peel Region in Ontario has conducted surveys regarding people's behaviours around sun safety—observe its website for inspiration on how to display such data that you might have collected in your assessment (https://www.peelregion.ca/health/statusdata/Health Behaviours/sun-safety.asp). What other ways can these data be displayed?

Built environment: The data you collected for this part of the analysis might relate to housing and the different types of accommodation in the community. Rental and ownership rates might inform your analysis, as might the presence of mobile home parks. The availability of green space, parks, and the walkability of neighbourhoods can be helpful in drawing inferences about the built environment and its impact on health. Is there heavy industry near housing? Perhaps there are data that can allow the team to draw inferences about air quality, noise pollution, or safety measures to avoid them.

Summary statements about the physical environment might include:

- There is no heavy industry in the community; commercial enterprises, professional offices, and small businesses are common along main thoroughfares and in strip malls.
- Housing values are higher in Neighbourhood 5 (suburb).
- The proportion of good air quality samples for the community is 95% compared with 87% in the rural industrial area.

From these data, it can be inferred that the five different neighbourhoods will have different health and social needs and concerns, varying capacities to address issues, and different levels of motivation to develop a sense of community. Link this to the previous analysis of the community core to see what impact the physical environment (housing) exerts on the people in the downtown area. Homeless people were found mostly in Neighbourhood 1 (inner city). Who are the homeless? Where are they staying? Can you infer from your assessment data that if there were adequate social housing perhaps many members of this subpopulation would not be homeless?

Continue through each of the subsystems of the community in this manner, writing summary statements, grouping them, drawing inferences, and determining if more data (or different data or data sources) are required to validate your inferences. An example of summary statements for each of the subsystems is located in Box 17.1. In the next section, the focus will be on the health and social services subsystem, because that is the interest in a community health assessment.

Health and Social Services

Health indicators such as morbidity and mortality rates, disability rates, health care utilization rates, and other quality of life indicators can be analyzed according to population characteristics to demonstrate any inequalities or gradients across groups by various demographic indicators.

In health care, a small number of individuals—known as high users—use a large percentage of services and incur a large percentage of costs (Canadian Institute for Health Information [CIHI], 2015). To describe high users of acute care services, three approaches are commonly used: multiples stays (effectiveness of care), length of stay (efficiency of care), and cost (resource use). By all measures, Canadian seniors 75 years and older comprise 25% of the population in acute care. The most frequent causes for multiple hospital stays are chronic obstructive pulmonary disease (COPD), heart failure, and palliative care. For length of stay, mental disorders are the greatest cause and for cost, sepsis and surgical infections are the most frequent causes. High levels of costs are also dedicated to children in the first year of life. Therefore, it behooves the community assessment team to take a close look at the proportions of children and senior populations in the community.

Utilization of social services is primarily by people who require social support for various reasons: low income, lack of shelter, need for support due to disability, and the like. Seniors living on fixed incomes and lone parent families with young children are often the focus for social services. Examine your data to see if you can draw any inferences about these two populations. Are there other groups that require the use of more health and social services than other groups? What about the street-involved population? Can you draw any inferences about their mental health (for example) that might cause them to need services?

Unfortunately, much hospital, social service, and primary health care utilization data are not easily available by community, so the team might have to rely on higher-level (e.g., city, regional, provincial/territorial) comparative information to draw inferences or make decisions. In this instance, the best that can be done is to develop questions for further data collection: do lone-parent mothers regularly receive mammograms? If not, why? What proportion of specific ethnic groups receives annual flu shots? Is there variation among men and women or people in different age groups?

In Table 17.7 several demographic characteristics are presented that indicate there might be stressors or risks to certain populations. See, for example the number of households receiving social assistance. Also see the percentage of seniors who receive guaranteed income supplementation (GIS) on top of their old age security (OAS) payments. This information may be indicators of low income or risks for consequences of poverty in the community.

To understand the capacity of low-income populations, the team will want to examine unemployment rates and level of education because of the links among education, employment, and income. If the team notes low unemployment rates with high incomplete high school education rates, the inference might be that those employed are not making high enough wages to

Box 17.1 Analyzing a Population

Community Core

The new families from Africa were headed by men aged 22 to 26, and women 18 to 22. Most families have two or three children. Children are mostly preschool age or in elementary school. Several of the women are pregnant. All of the men work in the new factory in the nearby urban centre as semi-skilled labour; few have completed high school education but most can communicate in English as their second language. The women, however, are not able to communicate in English and are not literate in their native language either, having been taken out of school before completing Grade 6. They are Muslim and have dietary restrictions as a result of their religion. The women are not able to drive, but the men commute to and from the factory by carpools. They live in rental accommodations that had separate rooms for parents and children.

The townspeople are older on average, with a large proportion of retirees and professionals who commute to the city for work or postsecondary education. They are largely Canadian of European heritage; most have some postsecondary education. Almost all (86%) own their homes and the majority (92%) own at least two vehicles.

Physical Environment

The new families live in close proximity to each other in apartments near the town core, schools, and services. The town has an arena, curling rink, and community centre. There is a ball diamond, tennis court, and outdoor playground shared between the school and the community centre. It is a pleasant and well-kept town. The Team used a map to denote areas of activity in the town.

Education

There is an elementary school and one junior–senior high school. Students have to travel to the city for postsecondary training. The school offers computer classes to the public once a week.

Safety and Transportation

There is no public transit. A provincial police substation serves the town. The fire service is composed of volunteers as first responders. Ambulance services are dispatched from the city. 9-1-1 service is available. Overall, the town is a safe place to live, with crimes against property being mostly mischief and assaults being few (bar fights, domestic abuse).

Politics and Government

The Mayor is well known and most people felt she does a good job for the citizens. The town staff members work with local nongovernmental organizations (NGOs) to provide a range of social services.

Health and Social Services

There is a Health Centre that provides medical services, a laboratory collection depot, community nursing, social services, and some physiotherapy. Prenatal care is available here, as are smoking cessation programs. Alcoholics Anonymous meets at the community centre twice a week, and Weight Watchers once a week.

Communication

The town receives TV and radio from the city; there is a weekly newspaper that is circulated to several small towns. Notices are placed in the grocery store and in church bulletins when people needed to advertise.

Business and Economics

The Chamber of Commerce took the lead to share what they knew about business in the town and what the needs are at present.

Recreation and Leisure

There are recreation facilities for the youth of the town; there is Bingo weekly at one of the churches. All churches are of Christian denominations. The townspeople come out in force for Winter Fest, Fall Fair, Spring Clean-Up, and Summer Festival and for other events. The families from Africa play soccer, but there is no soccer field in town. They are also Muslim and have no place to worship.

TABLE 17.7   Social Characteristics by Percent of Population

Social Characteristic	%
Persons living in low-income households	14.9
Children in social assistance households of total population <20 years old	2.1
Lone-parent families of total families with children	23.7
Seniors on GIS of total on OAS	28.8
Seniors living alone	26.3
Persons >15 without high school	20.1
Tenants spending >30% income on housing	36.4

---

pay housing costs. The team's assessment of the community's health might reveal that different groups of citizens experience very different health status. Therefore, it is extremely important that the team identifies and, if at all possible, quantifies any inequalities in health status according to the determinants of health. To do this, analyze the key health indicators according to population characteristics such as income, education, and employment.

Again, this is the time for the team to write up its summary statements, group them, draw inferences, and determine if more data (or different data or data sources) are required to validate the inferences. Continue to do this for all subsystems, then stand back and see where the inferences are linked, where one may contribute to another, and then you will be able to move to the next step in the CCAP process: coming to some conclusions and preparing a community health diagnosis.

Community Health Diagnosis

In the preceding stages of analysis, the community assessment team will have analyzed the population data as well as information about each subsystem in relation to its effect on the core (the people), the community, and health issues of importance. In each instance, the team will have drawn some inferences and made suggestions for the collection of more data, comparative data, or data from different sources. The final task of analysis is the synthesis of the inference statements into community diagnoses (Neufeld & Harrison, 2000). The purpose of a community health diagnosis is to define existing problems, barriers to health, and gaps in services; determine priorities for action; and set the stage for interventions and evaluation. A community health diagnosis can also be used to describe wellness attributes and community opportunities. Community health diagnoses are action-oriented and are aimed at increasing collective competence and community capacity.

The word "diagnosis" comes from the Greek *dia* (to split apart) and *gnosis* (to learn). It is an act that identifies the nature of something through logic and experience in order to understand. In community health promotion, a diagnosis is a statement that synthesizes assessment data and draws conclusions about the relationships among data. A diagnosis is a label that both describes a situation (or state) and implies an etiology (reason) and gives evidence to support the inference. Some authors, such as Diem and Moyer (2005), prefer to use the term "action statement" and others shy away from using medical terms to describe what are often considered social issues. Regardless, if community members are fully engaged in the assessment and analysis processes, and if the term "diagnosis" is explained, then there ought to be no reason for foregoing its use. On the other hand, if the community prefers to use another term, the community assessment team should find one that is acceptable to all parties. Any statement needs to consider the data, the issues, and the preferred outcomes of collaborative community health promotion action that helps to build capacity and develop community competence.

A nursing diagnosis limits the diagnostic process to those diagnoses that represent human responses to actual or potential health problems nurses are licensed to treat. A medical diagnosis includes those issues a doctor is licensed to treat. A community health diagnosis differs, however, in that it is focused on an aggregate, a population, or a community (rather than on individuals); it requires multidisciplinary action to address; multiple social determinants of health must be considered when planning interventions; and outcomes of action may not be visible in the short term.

Although no standard format exists, most community diagnoses have four parts:

1. A description of the issue, problem, response, or state
2. A statement indicating the aggregate, population, or community of focus
3. Identification of factors related to the issue, problem, response, or state
4. Signs and symptoms (manifestations) that are characteristic of the issue, problem, response, or state

A community diagnosis focuses the diagnosis on a *community*—usually defined as a group, population, or cluster of people with at least one common characteristic (such as geographic location, occupation, ethnicity, or housing condition). To derive a community diagnosis, community assessment data are analyzed and inferences are presented. Inference statements shape community diagnoses. Some inference statements form the descriptive part of the diagnosis; that is, they testify to a potential or actual community problem (risk, hazard, or concern) to a particular segment of the population (i.e., among). An inference statement may also refer to a positive state or issue in the community or among a particular population group. In fact, inferences can be stated both positively (as a capacity or opportunity) and negatively (as a problem, risk, or hazard).

For instance, population health status data (Pop-NLD) may indicate that the low-birthweight rate is higher than a comparison standard (stressor). Literature provides information regarding the causes of low birth weight, and these are compared with the data collected, the conclusions drawn about their applicability to the community of interest, and community resources available to address the issue (LR), and any FLDs (temporary responses to the situation) in place.

Finally, the signs and symptoms of the community diagnosis are the inference statements that document the duration or magnitude of the problem (NLD). Examples of documentation include data from records, census reports, and vital statistics. This final piece of the community diagnosis establishes the relevant data and is linked to the first two parts with an "as manifested by" clause (Box 17.2). In Box 17.3 is an example of a community diagnosis for an aggregate of adolescent pregnant women who reside in the community.

In comparison to taking a "problem" approach (Table 17.8 and Box 17.3) many strengths can be exhibited by a community and the population of interest that offer the opportunity to reframe issues as a wellness or positive diagnosis. For instance, there is opportunity to improve the health status (issue description) of adolescent pregnant women in the downtown (focus) by maintaining attendance at school; receiving social assistance; enrolling in the Best Beginning program; and receiving support (manifestations) for effective parenting, stress reduction, and smoking cessation (etiology).

Box 17.2 Template for a Community Diagnosis

Issue description: risk, concern, issue, state (i.e., potential/actual)

Focus: boundaries of the population segment of interest

Etiology/causal factors: signs and symptoms

Manifestations: data in support of the etiologic inference

Box 17.3 An Example of a Community Diagnosis

Issue Description	Focus	Etiology	Manifestations
Risk of low birth weight	*Among* teen pregnant women living in the downtown area	*Related to* a. Inadequate income b. Use of tobacco	*As manifested by:* a. Insecure housing, use of the food bank, unemployment rates b. Smoking rates among pregnant teens

Although a single problem is stated, the causes and signs and symptoms may be multiple. Also notice that although the problem inferences are drawn from the analysis of one subsystem (such as the health and social services subsystem or the educational subsystem), the causation may be, and usually is, drawn from several subsystems. For example, regarding the issue of low birth weight, etiologic inferences can be derived from four subsystems—educational, health and social services, safety and transportation, and business and economics.

This example sums up the most important lesson of community practice: All community factors (subsystems) join to determine the health status of a community and its residents. No one subsystem is more important or crucial than any other in determining a community's health. Every subsystem has a role in addressing community issues. Refer again to Table 17.8 for examples of community diagnoses.

The process of deriving community diagnoses always remains the same. First, assessment data are classified and studied for inferences that are descriptive of potential or actual problems (stressors that have penetrated the NLD or FLD); next, associated inferences are identified that explain the derivation or continuation of the problem and the community assets or strengths available to address the issue (LR); and last, documentation is (data are) presented to support the inferences. Several community diagnoses may be stipulated; determining the order of priority among them is part of program planning and depends on existing community goals and resources. This important skill is discussed in Chapter 18.

TABLE 17.8 Examples of Community Health Diagnoses

Issue	Population	Cause	Data
Lack of safety	For residents of Neighbourhood 1	Due to crime after dark related to: • The sex trade • Substance abuse • Vandalism	As manifested by Police Service crime statistics about: • Prostitution charges • Incidence of used needles and condoms found in vacant lots near school grounds and parks • Gang tagging graffiti on vacant buildings
Lack of adequate affordable housing	For the residents of Neighbourhood 4	Related to lone-parent families headed by women living in poverty	As manifested by: • The percent of lone-parent families spending more than 30% on housing • The number of children living in homes receiving social assistance • The volume of urban single mothers using food banks, thrift stores, and other community services before month's end
Capacity for instrumental support for community-living senior citizens	By high-school students	Related to the community service requirement at the local high school	As manifested by student-run programs for: • Snow shovelling in winter • Grocery shopping and delivery • Daily telephone contact for at-risk seniors • Friendly visitor support

---

Box 17.4 Creating Community Health Diagnoses for a Population

After engaging not only the new families that immigrated from Africa, but also the long-time community residents in an assessment and analysis process, the project Team came up with the following community diagnoses to support health promotion action.

Improve the ability of the town (focus population is the whole community) to welcome new immigrants (issue) related to (because of) the townspeople's lack of awareness of immigrants' experiences and needs for assistance, as manifested by the stories of the anxiety new families experience (data) and questions posed by townspeople.

Further diagnoses were more specific:

Women who have immigrated to the town from Africa (focus population) have difficulty creating nutritious family meals (issue) caused by their unfamiliarity with Canadian foods and lack of access to familiar foods in local stores as manifested by (data) their stories of failed recipes and refusal of children to eat what they have prepared.

School children (focus population) do not comprehend the history of the new children from Africa (issue) enrolling in their classes. Because they lack understanding of the experiences and skills of the newcomers (symptom), they are often insulting and unkind (manifestation).

Deriving community diagnoses requires critical thinking, decision making, and astute study; it is a challenging and vital task. The completeness and validity of the diagnoses that have been derived will be tested during the next stage of the community process and will form the foundation of that stage—the planning of a health program.

Validating your community diagnoses with the community at large is an important step for establishing and maintaining a genuine partnership. Equally important are the rights of community leaders, organizations, and residents to confidentiality of privileged information and to choose not to participate in planning. Communities have the right to identify their own needs and to negotiate with (and perhaps direct) the community assessment team with regard to interventions and specific programs for implementation (see Box 17.4). In turn, the community assessment team has the responsibility to provide or assist with the development of information needed for this process. This responsibility includes not using jargon when presenting data to community members—what words can you use besides "diagnosis"?

EVALUATION

At every stage in the CCAP process, individuals, teams, and the community should reflect on their collective performance—what went well, what did not, and what should be done differently—as they move to the next phase together. Did you participate honestly, fully, and respectfully? Did you engage others in the process? Did the team experience conflict, and how was it managed? Was the analysis process effective? Were community members fully engaged?

Think back on your analysis. Did you find yourself focusing on community or population deficiencies or strengths? Did you identify ways people could contribute their talents to the community, or did you seek to find services *for* them? Did you impose your ideas on people, or did you foster participation and engagement in ways that empowered people and built their capacity for action on their own behalf? Sometimes, we are so overcome by community needs, challenging issues, or the vulnerability of groups of people that we forget their resilience and competence in the face of adversity. Did you foster a respectful relationship with the community? We need to remind ourselves that we are doing community health promotion *with* people, not *to* or *for* them; that we seek to move people from simply *being* in a community to *belonging* in a community.

At this point, teams that have been constructed to do an assessment and make recommendations for action will adjourn. Remember to file documents for future reference, prepare reports, and send letters of appreciation to your participants and the network of contacts you made. Good will is an important gift that you can give to future teams—the program planners, community developers, and evaluators will thank you for creating a supportive environment! The assessment and analysis processes can be interventions in themselves—they raise awareness and expectations; they build capacity and empower people; they inform providers, politicians, and participants and ignite action that can be an important foundation for the next steps: program planning (Chapter 18), implementation (Chapter 19), and evaluation (Chapter 20). In Chapter 18, the planning process will be detailed.

Summary

Critical analysis of the community and population data collected can be completed using the community assessment wheel as a guide. Community health diagnoses, both relating to community needs as well as strengths, are formulated based on the inferences generated from the analytic process. Although community health diagnoses are relatively new to public health and community practice, community workers have, since the inception of community development and advocacy work, derived inferences from assessment data and have acted on those data. However, the terminology and format that have surrounded these informally produced inferences (diagnoses) have been inconsistent. There is considerable discussion, and some controversy, regarding the structure and terminology that is optimal for community-focused diagnoses. In your practice, you will be exposed to various formats for stating community issues and capacities—evaluate and test the usefulness of each. It is only through collaboration and vigorous testing that a standard format will evolve.

REFERENCES

Canadian Institute for Health Information (CIHI). (2015). *Defining high users in acute care: An examination of different approaches.* Ottawa: Author. URL=https://secure.cihi.ca/free_products/HighUsersAcuteCare_Chartbook_2015_ENweb.pdf

Diem, E., & Moyer, A. (2005). *Community health nursing projects: Making a difference.* Philadelphia, PA: Lippincott Williams & Wilkins.

Helvie, C. O. (1998). *Advanced practice nursing in the community.* Thousand Oaks, CA: Sage.

Neufeld, A., & Harrison, M. J. (2000). Nursing diagnosis for aggregates and groups. In M. J. Stewart (Ed.), *Community nursing: Promoting Canadians' health* (pp. 370–385). Toronto: Saunders.

Public Health Agency of Canada (PHAC). (2008–2016). *The Chief Public Health Officer's report on the state of public health in Canada.* Ottawa: Author. URL=www.phac-aspc.gc.ca/cphorsphc-respcacsp/index-eng.php

U.S. Department of Health and Human Services, Office of Disease Prevention and Health Promotion. (2014). *Healthy people 2020.* Washington, DC: Author. URL=http://www.healthypeople.gov

ONLINE RESOURCES

Please visit thePoint at http://thepoint.lww.com/Vollman4e for up-to-date Internet resources and additional learning materials on this topic.

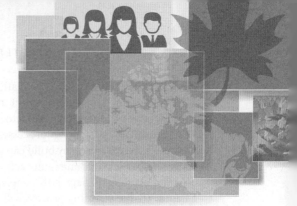

CHAPTER 18

Planning a Community Health Program

Ardene Robinson Vollman

LEARNING OBJECTIVES

After studying this chapter, you should be able to:

1. Use principles of change theory to guide the planning process

2. In partnership with the community, plan a community-focused health program

Introduction

Once a community has been assessed, the data analyzed, and community diagnoses generated, it is time to consider interventions that will promote the community's health and development—to formulate a community-focused plan. Each of the four parts of the diagnosis statement—the population of focus, description of the actual or potential issue, its causes (etiology), and supporting data and/or evidence available—directs planning efforts for the community team. All four parts provide equally important information from which to plan. Figure 18.1 displays the process for deriving a community diagnosis and summarizes how the parts of the diagnosis both describe the community assessment and give direction for program planning, intervention, and evaluation. Community-focused plans are based on the community diagnoses and contain specific goals, objectives, and interventions for achieving the desired population health outcomes. Planning, like assessment and analysis, is a systematic process completed in partnership with the community.

Take Note

Before proceeding, stop and consider the word *partnership* and its implications for community health. Recall that a community is a social group determined by certain boundaries and common values and interests. Community members function and interact within a particular social structure that both creates and exhibits behaviours and values. The normative behaviours and value systems of individuals, families, groups, and the community that you have assessed may be very different from your own behaviours and values as well as the shared values of the community in which you reside. This discrepancy creates a potential conflict.

What may appear to you as a primary health problem of the community or population group may not hold the same importance for the community's residents. They may be far more concerned about another possibility. Hence, there is a real need to prioritize community diagnoses *with* the community and the people involved in the issue.

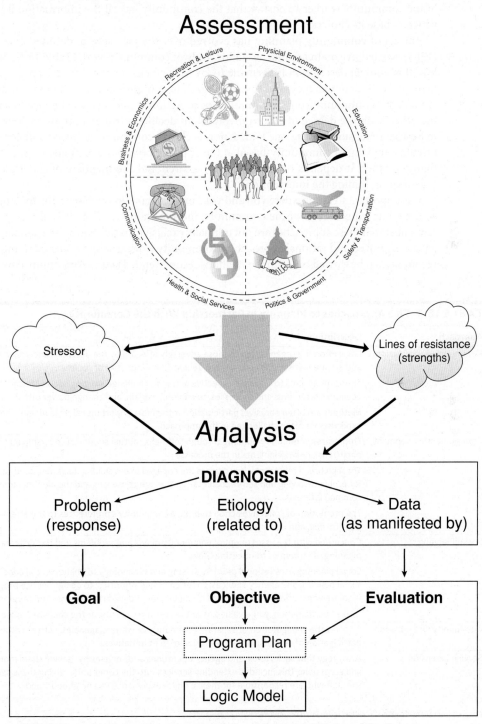

FIGURE 18.1   Relationship of assessment, analysis, and diagnosis with program planning.

PLANNING IN PARTNERSHIP WITH THE COMMUNITY

It is important to validate community diagnoses with the residents and leadership of the community; it is their right to participate in decisions that affect them. The validation process can serve as an important trust-building activity in maintaining the partnership, and it is the role of the community worker to ensure that the community has all the information it needs on which to base its choices.

The art of community planning has evolved over the past several decades since Thomas (1983) isolated five main approaches in his study of community work (Table 18.1). Nevertheless, this seminal description is germane today as we focus on community capacity development, collective competency, and transformation of communities. The Thomas model can be viewed on a continuum from Community Social Action at one pole and Service Extension on the other, with the degree of citizen involvement declining from Community Social Action to Service Extension. At the one end, action is clearly community-centred and community-oriented, moving to community-based at the opposite pole. No one model is more "correct" than the other; it depends on the outcomes desired and the mandate of the leadership or organization leading the intervention.

It is important to know where you and your project stand in relation to the five approaches so that your expectations of the community and the team are clear. It is also important to remember that these approaches are not mutually exclusive. In this book, for example, we present an organized and rational approach to community work (such as social planning), but we recommend it be carried out with the methods recommended by the community development

TABLE 18.1 Five Approaches to Planning in Partnership With the Community

Approach	Description
Community Social Action	Focuses on the organization of those adversely affected by the decisions and policies of public and private institutions and by more general characteristics of society.
	The strategy aims to promote collective action to challenge existing sociopolitical and economic structures and processes, to explore, explain, and change power distributions.
	Methods are often abrasive; participation is the most important value; leadership and expertise are often challenged in this approach.
Community Development	Emphasizes community building through self-help, mutual support. Leadership and education of citizens are key elements in the process.
	Through broad representation, citizens are engaged in developing neighbourhood capacities for problem-solving and self-representation through consensus and the identification of common interests.
	The promotion of collective action to bring a community's preferences to the attention of political decision makers.
Social Planning	Concerned with the assessment of community needs and problems and the systematic planning of strategies for meeting them.
	Social planning uses rational problem solving and technology to analyze social conditions, social policies, and agency services; to set goals and priorities; to design service programs and mobilize appropriate resources; and to implement and evaluate services and programs.
	Citizen participation, while valued, is not necessary. Expertise is the cherished value.
Community Organization	Involves the collaboration of separate community or welfare agencies, with or without the participation of citizens, in the promotion of joint initiatives.
Service Extension	A strategy that seeks to extend agency operations and services by making them more relevant and accessible. This includes extending services into the community, giving these services and the staff who are responsible for them a physical presence in a neighbourhood.

Adapted from Thomas (1983). URL=http://www.infed.org/community/b-comwrk.htm

and social action approaches. As stated previously, to achieve results that are sustainable over time, community workers must be committed to:

- Empowerment—increasing the ability of citizens to influence community circumstances.
- Participation—supporting citizens to take part in making decisions about their community.
- Inclusion—recognizing that some citizens have less influence than others.
- Self-determination—supporting the right of citizens to make their own choices.
- Partnership—recognizing that many agencies can contribute and need to work together to make the most of the available resources and to be as effective as possible.

In addition to forming a partnership with the community, the community worker must consider the influences of social, economic, ecologic, and political issues. Larger policy issues directly and profoundly affect many (if not all) community issues. For instance, the number of injuries due to falls by seniors in the community is related as much to the age and frailty of the people as it is to the condition of the sidewalks, the knowledge of seniors about home safety, the lack of seniors' programs in the community, social isolation, and the nutrition levels of seniors and their access to adequate food. Each of these causes is related to municipal, provincial/territorial, and federal policies and legislation. Consider returning to the discussion of the Web of Causation in Chapter 4 for guidance. No diagnosis can be considered separate from others; all must be considered when doing community-focused planning.

The team involved in community-focused health planning must also consider the needs of populations at risk. Special at-risk groups reside in all communities—people who are homeless, people living with poverty, people with chronic disease and disability, new immigrants, pregnant women, infants, children, and the elderly are groups at increased risk. The health needs of at-risk groups must be considered as part of all community plans.

The community's planning needs must be assessed when determining the membership of the planning team. It may be that the community team formed for assessment purposes and the team pulled together for the planning process will be somewhat different, depending on the nature and priority of the community diagnoses and the scope of the issues of concern. Smith and Maurer (2013) offer the following guidelines for those who should be represented on a planning team, keeping in mind that the team should be neither too large nor cumbersome to manage:

- Broad segments of the community to provide wide base of support to the program
- Leaders with financial and legal authority for the problem
- Champions, people in a position to promote acceptance of the program (e.g., media, community leaders)
- Those who will implement the program
- Those who will be affected by the program (i.e., the target group)
- Those who will most likely offer resistance (i.e., the opposition)
- Specialists in the field who can contribute to understanding and offer alternative solutions

Last, community-focused planning involves an awareness and application of planned change—a process of well-thought-out actions to make something happen. Planned change is discussed in detail later in this chapter.

PRIORITIZING COMMUNITY DIAGNOSES

Not all issues can be addressed at the same time, so priorities must be determined. Many factors can influence the priority of an issue—a life-threatening emergency will take priority over everything else. Other factors are the seriousness of a concern, the desires of the community or population aggregate of interest, time, cost, and availability of resources. Five factors to consider are:

1. Magnitude of concern expressed by members of the community
2. Extent of existing resources to deal with the concern (e.g., knowledge, time, money, equipment, supplies, facilities, personnel)
3. Potential for success in solving the problem with existing resources
4. Need for special education or training
5. Extent of additional resources and policies needed for equitable, cost-effective, and efficient response

Several processes can be used to determine which issue or concern is of the highest priority. For instance, each concern identified can be listed and posted around a meeting room at a community planning workshop. Members of the community and the team could be given a means to "vote" on their top three priorities (e.g., three coloured dots, three sticky notes), and those concerns that receive no "votes" are first removed from the list of priority issues.

In the next step, those issues that receive the most votes are assessed, one by one, according to a predetermined set of criteria, rated on a scale of 1–5, on which the team again "votes" or comes to consensus. The team may decide that community motivation is the most important criterion, and if that is not present to a high degree, action on the issue will fail. Or, the team may decide that quick success is most important, rating the speed criterion the highest. In any event, decisions about how to rate each criterion must be made in advance by the team, before the rating exercise begins.

- How aware is the community of the issue?
- How motivated is the community to resolve the issue?
- How able is the team to influence the resolution of the issue?
- How available is the needed expertise to address the issue?
- How severe are the consequences if the issue remains unresolved?
- How quickly can the team achieve resolution?

As each participant rates each criterion for every issue retained for discussion, scores will indicate the order in which the community ranks its priorities. Discussions can then proceed regarding approaches to addressing the priority issue(s). So, for the first issue, compare the agreed-on issue-weighting criteria with the average of the individual participants' ratings on each criterion by averaging the ratings, then multiplying them by the weighting. The sum of the ranking provides an overall assessment of the priority of the issue. By comparing this score as a portion of the total possible score, priorities among the various issues under discussion can be determined. This ranking process is detailed in Table 18.2.

TABLE 18.2 Ranking Each Issue by Criterion Weight

Criteria	Criterion Weight	Average Rating[a]	Ranking (weight × rating)	Total Possible Score
Awareness	4	5	20	20
Motivation	5	2	10	25
Influence	3	4	12	15
Expertise	4	3	12	20
Severity	5	5	25	25
Speed	1	1	1	5
	Maximum $(6 \times 5) = 30$	Maximum $(6 \times 5) = 30$	Actual score = 80	Maximum score = 110

[a]Rated on a 5-point scale.

> ### Box 18.1 Reinkemeyer's Stages of Planned Change
>
> | | |
> |---|---|
> | Stage 1 | Development of a felt need and desire for the change |
> | Stage 2 | Development of a change relationship between the agent and the client system |
> | Stage 3 | Clarification or diagnosis of the client system's problem, need, or objective |
> | Stage 4 | Examination of alternative routes and tentative goals and intentions of actions |
> | Stage 5 | Transformation of intentions into actual change |
> | Stage 6 | Stabilization |
> | Stage 7 | Termination of the relationship between the change agent and the client system |
>
> Reinkemeyer (1970).

In this way, issues can be examined and compared horizontally (across the row) to determine which criterion has the highest ranking overall and vertically (down the column) to determine which issue is the highest priority for action. As you continue to read this chapter, you learn that the severity of an issue if left unresolved is clearly at a maximum. However, the speed with which the community can address it is at the minimum in the context of relatively low community motivation even though there is relatively high availability of expertise to address the concern. The community can discuss the meaning and interpretation of scores, and effective priorities can be set with efficiency.

APPLYING CHANGE THEORY TO COMMUNITY PLANNING

We all experience change. As you read these words, your knowledge level is changing. Yet planned change differs from change in that actions occur in a definite sequence, with each one serving as preparation for the next. Planned change is a well-thought-out effort designed to make something happen; all efforts are directed and targeted to produce change. (Many theorists have written about planned change; several works are listed on thePoint.) Reinkemeyer's (1970) stages of planned change are presented in Box 18.1. The stages are like a recipe in that to produce the intended outcome, it is helpful to follow them strictly and completely to reach the intended outcomes.

One theorist, Lewin (1958), described three stages of planned change: unfreezing, moving, and refreezing, as shown in Figure 18.2. It is during the unfreezing stage that the client system (in other words, the organization, community, or at-risk population) becomes aware of a problem and the need for change. Then the problem is diagnosed, and solutions to the problem are identified. From these alternative solutions, one is chosen that seems most appropriate for the situation. In the moving stage, the change actually occurs. The problem is clarified, and the program for solving the problem is planned in detail and begun. Finally, the refreezing stage consists of the accomplished changes becoming integrated into the values of the client system.

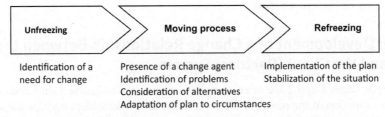

FIGURE 18.2   Lewin stages of planned change and their application to the planning process.

TABLE 18.3   Stages of Change of the Transtheoretical Model (TTM)

Stage of Change	Characteristic
Precontemplation (PC)	Still engages in risky behaviour
	Has no intention of changing within the next 6 months
	May be uninformed, in denial, or demoralized from previous failures
	Defensive and resistant to change, avoids addressing risky behaviour
Contemplation (C)	Engages in the risky behaviour but is aware of problem
	Seriously considering change within 6 months but has not yet made a commitment to take action
	Indecisive, lacks commitment to enact significant change in high-risk behaviour
Preparation (P)	Still engages in high-risk behaviour but intends to take action within the next month
	Has typically taken some significant action in the past year
	Is on the verge of taking action and needs to set goals
Action (A)	Has modified behaviour, experiences, or environment within the last 6 months
	Involves overt behavioural changes and requires considerable commitment of time and energy
Maintenance (M)	Works to prevent relapse and consolidate the gains attained during action
	Is less tempted to relapse and has become increasingly more confident to continue changes
Termination (T)	A continuation, not an absence, of change
	Feels zero temptation and complete confidence
	New, healthier behaviour has become second nature
	Unlikely for most behaviours

In this stage, the idea is established and continues to be influential. Lewin also addressed forces that help or hinder change to occur, labelling them the *driving forces* and the *restraining forces,* respectively.

Theories of planned change are important because they can be used to guide and direct the planning process. Conceptual frameworks that suggest how individuals change their behaviour also inform the planning process. Table 18.3 details the key components of the transtheoretical (stages of change) model (Prochaska et al., 1995). The processes of change addressed by the transtheoretical model (TTM) are located in Table 18.4 (Prochaska et al., 1995). Other models of change are available on thePont.

To validate the priorities and initiate the planning process, Reinkemeyer's stages of planned change (Box 18.1) have been chosen as a guide.

Stage 1: Development of a Felt Need and Desire for the Change

In a social planning approach, to initiate a felt need and desire for change within a community, those people and organizations involved in the assessment phase can be contacted and invited to a meeting to receive a report of the community assessment findings and proposed community diagnoses and to engage in an exercise to validate the findings and discuss priorities. In the community social action or community development approaches, the activity of assessment itself becomes the impetus for change as people become engaged and develop the skills to take action on their own behalf.

Stage 2: Development of a Change Relationship Between the Agent and the Client (Partner) System

Both stages 1 and 2 are often completed during the assessment and analysis phases and the presentation of the report to the community and stakeholders because the team received permission to enter the community and began to establish connections and a trusting relationship

TABLE 18.4 Processes of Change of the Transtheoretical Model

Process of Change	Characteristics
Consciousness-raising	Individuals need to raise their awareness of the negative consequences of their behaviour
Dramatic relief	Individuals need to release and express emotions related to their high-risk behaviour. Life events, such as the death of a close friend or family member, can move people into precontemplation emotionally, especially if the death was related to the high-risk behaviour
Environmental re-evaluation	In precontemplation, individuals need to recognize how the presence or absence of a personal habit affects one's social environment
Self-re-evaluation	This process is most important when the individual is moving from contemplation to preparation, when people assess how they feel and think about the behaviour. People may become aware of their guilt about a particular behaviour
Self-liberation	While preparing for action, individuals need self-liberation, that is, the belief that they can change and the commitment to act on that belief
Reinforcement management	During action, individuals need to provide consequences for taking steps in a particular direction, including the use of punishments for slips or rewards for making positive changes
Helping relationships	Helping relationships can include those with health professionals who are actively involved in assisting the person to change or supportive members of a social network
Counterconditioning	During the action and maintenance stages, individuals need to substitute healthier behaviours for the high-risk behaviours
Stimulus control	People in action or maintenance need to remove stimuli that were associated with the unhealthy behaviour and add stimuli that signal the new behaviour
Social liberation	Social liberation requires an increase in social opportunities or alternatives, especially for people who are relatively deprived or oppressed

with the people in it. At this point, community members (champions) and stakeholders express a desire to become involved in the planning process to address the priority concerns. To preserve momentum and to expedite the planning processes, agencies/groups often delegate a representative to the planning committee. At this point, a member of the community team is usually named to function as a change agent to guide and facilitate, but not to direct, the planning process. Sometimes a co-chair is elected from the community, the committee is given a mandate to plan, reporting measures are determined, and initial meetings are set. At this point, it is important to commit to build community participants' capacity in this process—remember to genuinely involve the community co-chair in all meetings and decisions and to set meeting times that allow this to happen.

Stage 3: Clarification or Diagnosis of the Client System's Problem, Need, or Objective

Now the time has arrived for the planning team to confirm the community diagnoses and compare interpretations of the data with the perceptions of the selected target population. This process can be done by a questionnaire focused on a particular population or neighbourhood; it can be designed as a mail-out or completed as an interview. For instance, lone parents who live in the target neighbourhoods and receive social assistance can be invited by social workers to provide information about the appropriateness of inferences drawn from the data about the need for parenting classes. Lone parents, when they bring their children for immunization, can be approached by public health nurses with suggestions about what services might meet their child-rearing needs. On the other hand, if you are planning to intervene at a community level with a community development project, you may choose to interview community leaders and civic groups (key informants) that are representative of the target population. The word *representative* is very important; the team needs to ensure that they are including the appropriate people in the validation process. For instance, if you are concerned about issues relevant to the well-being of a particular neighbourhood, people from a variety of walks of life, ethnic backgrounds, ages, religions, sex, marital status, family structure, and so forth should be included. Otherwise, a complete picture of life in the community will not be drawn. Validation from professionals and business owners, though informative, will not necessarily provide the most reliable perspective.

Stage 4: Examination of Alternative Routes and Tentative Goals and Intentions of Actions

At this stage, as the results are examined, planning committee members make suggestions about how to address the issues. Inventories of services, resources, and funding already available are compiled. Literature about successful programs in other jurisdictions is examined, program evaluation findings are analyzed, and decisions are made about a preferred approach to the issues.

As details emerge about how to address the issues, the planning committee must make decisions among suggested strategies based on the resources available, likelihood of success, acceptability to the community, and the time it will take to meet the goals.

> ### *Take Note*
>
> Each stakeholder will consider how information and suggested strategies can be assimilated into existing or planned programs. All agencies have budgets and a set number of staff members to deliver services. Agencies must be as cost-efficient as possible and will want to consider how to include new services into an existing program or whether new funding will be needed. Community workers can facilitate this process by becoming familiar with the organizational structure and purpose of each stakeholder to learn as much as possible about their services and decision-making processes to facilitate the planned change interventions.

DEVELOPING A PROGRAM LOGIC MODEL

Now is the time to transform the ideas and proposals of each stakeholder into a community-focused goal and concrete intentions for action. A logic model is a diagrammatic representation of a program (Dwyer & Makin, 1997) that depicts the relationships among program goals, objectives, activities, indicators, outcomes, and resources. It shows how different facets of a program are related and helps to integrate the program planning function with evaluation. The logic model also links back to the data collected in the community assessment phase and the diagnosis formulated in the analysis. There are many ways to present logic models—while each community can use the format that best suits its audience, a standard series of components (sometimes referred to as the "results-chain") should be included in order for the logic model to effectively support an evaluation. These components, which are logically linked, are the program inputs, activities, and outcomes. An important design feature of logic models is that they are, ideally, contained on a single page. As the logic

TABLE 18.5 Parenting Program Logic Model

Overall goal: Parents will be capable of obtaining the support and information they need to maintain and promote the health of their children 0–5 years of age.

Target group: Parents who are young, single, socially or geographically isolated, or who have low income or limited formal education. Participation is voluntary and free of charge. The program is not intended for families in crisis.

Program Components	Support	Education
Short-term objectives	Establish a group for mutual support development. Increased self-help knowledge and skill	Increased knowledge and understanding of children's health, safety, and behaviour. Increased coping skills
Long-term objectives	Increased opportunities to offer aid to other parents in "Parenting Program." Improved self-help, information, and assistance-seeking behaviour. Decreased sense of isolation in parenting	Positive change in parenting knowledge and actions regarding children's health, safety, and behaviour. Improved self-image as a parent. Increased confidence in parenting skill and ability
Short-term indicators	Referred parents will enroll in "Parenting Program." Parents will attend 75% of sessions. Parents will be engaged in session activities. Parents will be satisfied with group process. Parents will be able to articulate sources for self-help and mutual aid	Able to demonstrate learning from each session. Post-test scores greater than pretest scores. Appropriate responses to case study examples. Reported use of coping techniques at home
Long-term indicators	Accepts assistance/advice from group members and facilitators. Provides examples, ideas to group. Actively seeks and accepts support and information from community resources. Feels more connected to the community	Consistently displays positive responses regarding children's health, safety, and behaviour. Views self as a good parent. Is confident in ability to deal with new situations as children grow and develop
Program/Facilitator activities	Recruitment of parents Facilitation of sessions Encouragement of parents Environmental support for learning	Teach, using adult education principles Facilitate session discussions and problem-solving
Resources	Infrastructure for recruitment and registration Physical facility Child care Finances Refreshments "Parenting Program" materials	"Parenting Program" materials Supplies Telephone and other contact resources

model is intended to be a visual depiction of the program, its level of detail should be comprehensive enough to adequately describe the program but concise enough to capture the key details on a single page. In Table 18.5, an example of a logic model for a parent support program is presented.

What is a program? It is an organized set of activities intended to meet specific goals and objectives (outcomes). A program may have a broad series of activities (e.g., a national tobacco reduction program), or it may be smaller and more specifically targeted (e.g., a pre-lunch hand-washing program at a local school).

The program goal is a directional statement that specifies the desired outcome of the intervention. The target group is, as specified in the community diagnosis, the recipient of the program. This recipient group may be defined by age, sex, income level, ethnicity, health characteristics, or geographic location. Groups of activities that go together are called *components* and given a descriptive label. Then, for each component, outcome objectives are written using the SMART formula (i.e., specific, measurable, action-oriented, realistic, and time-specific). Outcome objectives can be short term or long term and represent the desired end results of the intervention. Process objectives specify the activities that are needed to achieve the outcome objectives. Evaluation indicators based on the wording of the objectives need to be specified for each objective. Resources required to successfully carry out the intervention should be listed; they might include personnel, funding, materials, training, and promotional expenses.

Program Goals

A goal is stated as a long-term future condition, situation, or status (Ervin, 2002) of a particular population group that clearly identifies what outcome the intervention is designed to achieve or what change is expected in the target population.

From the setting of the goal, the target of an intervention becomes evident. The focus may be individuals, a group, or the community. When the focus is on individuals, their unique perspectives will govern the level of success attained. For instance, according to the Health Belief Model, the degree of behaviour change achieved may be related to the individual's perceived susceptibility to the condition, severity of the threat to personal health, benefits of acting, barriers to action, and cues to action (Rosenstock et al., 1988). Social support is a factor in how people adapt to situations, and other models (e.g., TTM) define the stages people pass through as they go through the change process.

When the focus of an intervention is a group, people in the group generally fall into five categories: innovators, early adopters, early majority adopters, late majority adopters, and laggards. The focus on a larger community requires different approaches such as those described by Lewin and Reinkemeyer (see Box 18.1 and Figure 18.2). Understanding the processes of change is important for the team when making decisions about what activities to undertake to meet the stated goal.

Program Activities

Program activities map out the actions necessary to deliver the program and thereby reach the goal(s). Choosing an activity requires knowledge of a broad range of intervention strategies. Strategies can be classified as promotion, prevention, or protection and are aimed at education, engineering, or enforcement. Not all strategies are effective on all groups. For instance, an awareness program may be sufficient for action among innovators and early adopters, but personal contact may be needed for laggards. In many instances, a combination of education, policy change, and enforcement may be needed to help populations adopt healthy behaviours (e.g., seat belt campaigns).

Calendar charts are an effective means of planning and documenting program activities. An example is shown in Figure 18.3. Note that the activities are sequenced in a stepwise manner, with start and completion months specified along with the initials of the person responsible to carry out the activity. Such charts are versatile and can show weekly or daily progress, depending on the needs of the program. They may be more or less detailed as required by funding agencies, administration, or working groups.

Program Objectives

Objectives are measurable and describe the behaviour expected in a specific time frame. They describe the step-by-step outcomes that are required to meet the program goal and specify who will perform the behaviour, under what conditions, how well they must perform (standard to be met), and how performance will be measured. The literature relevant to the health issue, population, group, and performance targets will need to be reviewed to ensure that the objectives are realistic in the time allotted.

	J	F	M	A	M	J	J	A	S	O	N	D
1. Invite partners to participate (AA)	0	X										
2. Create steering committee (AA)		0	X									
3. Develop logic model and work plans (All)				0	X							
4. Budget planning (CA)				0	X							
5. Protocols and policy development (DD)					0	X						
6. Develop program materials (CC)					0	→	X					
7. Hiring program staff (AA)						0	X					
8. Training staff (DD)						0	X					
9. Pilot test (CC)							0	X				
10. Evaluate pilot and revise (CC)									0X			
11. Set up demonstration site (DD)										0X		
12. Official launch (AA)											0X	
13. All sites participating (AA)												→

0= Begin task, X= end task (Initials of person responsible)

FIGURE 18.3   A calendar chart for coordinating and tracking planning activities.

Both process and outcome objectives can be written in sequential steps that are required to reach the goal. Alternatively, each objective may have different aspects that, when combined, achieve the goal.

Take Note

The planning team must make every effort to involve community partners in the writing of outcome objectives if the program is to be acceptable to the target group. The team must also weigh the costs of intervention against the outcomes so that the most people can benefit at affordable cost.

Objectives need to be stated in measurable terms. To make statements measurable, use precise words. Examples of precise terms and less precise terms are:

Less Precise Terms (Many Interpretations)

- To know
- To understand
- To realize

- To appreciate
- To be aware
- To lower

More Precise Terms (Fewer Interpretations)

- To identify
- To discuss
- To list
- To compare and contrast
- To state
- To decrease by 20%

In addition, strive for each objective to include:

- A time frame for attaining the change (e.g., "By June 15th…")
- The direction and magnitude of the change (e.g., "Immunization levels at school entry will increase to 95%.")
- The method of measuring the change (e.g., "After the session, each participant will demonstrate…")

Goals and objectives help to clarify a program and establish the expected changes that will result from the program. Although much has been written on the mechanics of writing goals and objectives (several such resources are listed on thePoint), little information exists on the collaborative relationship (Box 18.2) that must exist between the community team and community agencies before meaningful goals and objectives can result. Goals, objectives, and their indicators of success are absolutely crucial to the evaluability of your project. Clear and meaningful statements that articulate what measures will be used to assess achievement are necessary in the next steps of the Canadian community-as-partner (CCAP) process (Box 18.3).

To be effective, each objective needs to be supported by a clear work plan that details the specific steps to be taken in each facet of the planned program. What actions need to be done? How will they be accomplished? For instance, protocols and policies may need to be written to ensure that activities are carried out as designed by front-line workers. What resources are needed? A detailed purchasing or refurbishing plan may need to be developed, in-kind contributions tracked, and training programs developed and undertaken. Who is responsible

---

Box 18.2 Collaboration

What is meant by a collaborative relationship? Could several community concerns be addressed in the same program? If they could, what would be the program goal? The objectives? This process is an example of collaborative planning and is the essence of community health practice. You may be wondering how to establish collaborative planning and inform agencies about the usefulness of goals and objectives. Although you may be convinced of the value of planned change, how do you convince others to agree, especially since planned change is not commonly practised in agencies? Role modelling is probably the best strategy. After reviewing the community diagnoses and validating data with an agency, propose goals and objectives that are congruent with the agency's purpose and organizational structure. Solicit input from the group, and continue to revise the goals and objectives until a group consensus is reached.

The advantages of collaboration include preventing duplication of effort, pooling resources for maximum impact, creating more publicity and credibility than any stakeholder partner could accomplish alone, and increasing opportunities for sharing information.

> ### Box 18.3 Planning: Goals and Objectives for a Population
>
> Below is a community diagnosis from Chapter 17, followed by some suggested goals and objectives to address the issues.
>
> **Community Diagnosis #3:** School children (focus population) do not comprehend the history of the new children from Africa (issue) enrolling in their classes. Because they lack understanding of the experiences and skills of the newcomers (symptom), they are often insulting and unkind (manifestation).
>
> **Goal:** Schoolchildren learn about Africa and appreciate the history of the nation from which the new students have emigrated.
>
> **Objectives:**
>
> 1. By next semester, select classes will study Africa in Social Studies
> 2. The school will have an Africa Day in May to celebrate history and tradition of African children
> 3. By this time next year, reports of insulting and unkind behaviour will be reduced to zero
>
> **Indicators:**
>
> 1. Number of classes that studied Africa
> 2. Evaluation of Africa Day activities
> 3. School reports of respectful behaviour

for each action, when it is to begin, and by when is it to be completed can be detailed using a calendar chart such as in Figure 18.3. The work plan must consider communication methods to ensure that each working group is in concert with every other one. Coordination meetings must be held regularly with full attendance to ensure that the plan runs smoothly and the program is implemented on time. Be sure to keep stakeholder agencies and the community informed of progress along the way.

Resources, Constraints, and Revised Plans

Once goals and objectives are written, the next step is to identify available resources and any constraints to the plan. These are analogous to Lewin's (1958) driving and restraining forces. Last, revised plans are proposed to the planning group. Resources are all the available means for accomplishing a task, including staff and budget as well as physical space and equipment. Recall that part of your community assessment included the identification of strengths. As you consider resources, include those strengths that may facilitate meeting program goals and objectives. For program planning, it is important to identify the resources needed as well as the resources available. Constraints are obstacles that restrict or limit actions and can include a lack of staff, budget, physical space, and equipment. Constraints may be thought of as the difference between needs and resources. Revised plans are actions that are proposed based on the knowledge of resources and constraint.

Take Note

Universal constraints are staff and money—agencies never have enough. An additional constraint is resistance to change. All people are reluctant to change existing routines and patterns of behaviour. Initially, change is uncomfortable, and until new roles are learned, there is anxiety. Making people aware of the natural discomfort associated with change can build rapport and establish a collaborative relationship.

For each constraint identified, a revised plan needs to be proposed, discussed, and adopted. This will become a period of intense collaboration between the community team and community agencies, and only at the completion of this stage will the community be ready for Reinkemeyer's stage 5 of planned change—transformation of intentions into actual change behaviour. This transformation of intentions is the actual program implementation (which is covered in Chapter 19). However, before the plan is implemented, costs must be calculated and the plan recorded.

Budgeting

Several general areas require financing in any program. It is helpful to managers and funding agencies if you use a balance sheet format and specify sources of funds (e.g., new grants, in-kind contributions, funds already dedicated or earmarked for the intervention, donations) as well as the cost centres (e.g., personnel, supplies), staff expenses (e.g., travel, parking), operating costs (e.g., office administration, phone, fax, postage), and meeting expenses (e.g., refreshments, rent). Indicate how anticipated shortfalls or revenues will be managed. Budgets need not be overly detailed at this stage. As the plan progresses, financial expertise may need to be sought to prepare the accounting methods to ensure accountability.

Recording

Community plans must be recorded in standardized, systematic, and concise forms that clearly communicate to others the purpose and actions of the plan as well as the rationale for revisions and deletions of actions. Discuss with each agency its present recording system and decide on a format and system for recording the plan. The format need not be elaborate; a short written memorandum is a key component in the explicit agreement among people and agencies about what they agreed to do. The memo should include a background statement that details the key community assessment findings, the diagnosis, a description of the target population, and the model used for program planning. The components of the logic model should be clearly articulated (goals, objectives, indicators, etc.) along with a description of the program and its related activities. A separate section should present the proposed intervention itself and the details relevant to the delivery of the program. A statement of the available and needed resources, along with the current and anticipated constraints, will set the stage for the budget proposal. It is also a good idea to articulate the anticipated outcomes and impacts of the program without overstating your case and creating expectations that the program cannot be expected to achieve.

Take Note

Remember to keep notes, take pictures, and capture stories from the beginning of the process so that, at the end, you have documented what was, what changed and how, and who was involved.

Summary

The planning process begins with validation of the community diagnoses—a process that establishes the community's perception and value of community health needs. Next, using theories of change, the planning team and the community form a collaborative partnership to establish program goals, objectives, and the program logic model. Then, based on resources and constraints, intervention plans are proposed and revised, work plans and timelines are recorded, and a final plan is adopted. The process of community planning is essentially the same for all programs that are developed. To create programs that are acceptable to the target population, the program planning team must encourage active participation by community representatives.

REFERENCES

Dwyer, J. J., & Makin, S. (1997). Using a program logic model that focuses on performance measurement to develop a program. *Canadian Journal of Public Health, 88*(6), 421–425.

Ervin, N. E. (2002). *Advanced community health nursing practice.* Upper Saddle River, NJ: Prentice Hall.

Lewin, K. (1958). Group decision and social change. In E. Maccoby (Ed.), *Readings in social psychology* (3rd ed.). New York, NY: Holt, Rinehart and Winston.

Prochaska, J., Norcross, J., & DiClemente, C. (1995). *Changing for good.* New York, NY: Avon Books.

Reinkemeyer, A. M. (1970). Nursing's need: commitment to an ideology and change. *Nursing Forum, 9*(4), 340–355.

Rosenstock, I. M., Strecher, V. J., & Becker, M. H. (1988). Social learning theory and the health belief model. *Health Education Quarterly, 15*(2), 175–183.

Smith, C. M., & Maurer, F. A. (2013). Community diagnosis, planning and intervention. In C. M. Smith, & F. A. Maurer (Eds.), *Community/public health nursing: Health for families and populations* (5th ed., pp. 427–449). Philadelphia, PA: Saunders.

Thomas, D. N. (1983). The making of community work. London: George Allen & Unwin.

ONLINE RESOURCES

Please visit the Point. at http://thepoint.lww.com/Vollman4e for up-to-date Internet resources and additional learning materials on this topic.

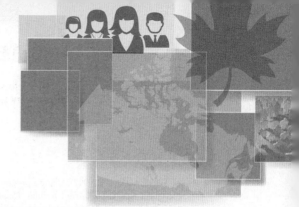

CHAPTER 19

Implementing a Community Health Program

Ardene Robinson Vollman

LEARNING OBJECTIVES

Implementation is the action phase of the community process; it is carrying out the plan. Implementation is necessary to achieve goals and objectives, but more importantly, the implementation of interventions acts to promote, maintain, or restore population health and community well-being.

In this chapter, we discuss the process of implementing a community- or population-focused program. Intervention strategies are presented along with resources that are helpful in program implementation.

After studying this chapter, you should be able to:

1. Suggest strategies to the community for implementation of health promotion programs

2. Working in partnership with the community:
   a. Implement planned programs
   b. Review and revise interventions based on community responses
   c. Use interventions to formulate and influence health and social policies that have an impact on the community

Introduction

Once goals and objectives have been agreed on and recorded during the planning stage, all that remains for implementation is to actually carry out the planned activities to meet those objectives. This probably seems straightforward and simple. Indeed, at this point, the team will have spent considerable time assessing the community (Chapter 16), analyzing the data and coming to some conclusions about issues that need to be addressed (Chapter 17), and planning an intervention to address the priority issue (Chapter 18). The team will be ready and eager to begin. But this very eagerness (and the associated impatience of the intervention stage) is a danger. The team must take time to consider how it can promote community ownership, create a unified program that respects the overall goals of the community, and maintain a clear focus on the target population and the activities planned.

Take Note

This chapter focuses on the process of intervention and provides you with some general resources that may prove helpful in your community work. Many excellent examples of interventions in which community teams work as partners with the community are included in Section 3.

PROMOTING COMMUNITY OWNERSHIP

Essential to achieving the desired outcomes of an intervention is the active participation of the community. The meaning of partnership and collaboration was discussed in prior chapters, but the present concern is ownership of the intervention. The people of the community need to feel a sense of ownership of the intervention (program or event), which can only come with their full participation in the decisions regarding planning as well as their assuming some responsibility for implementation. Herein lies a potential conflict. The human service professions are dedicated to nurturing, sustaining, and caring for others. It is part of those professions to do for others what they would do for themselves if they were able. Indeed, many human service disciplines interact professionally with people during an altered state (crisis) that requires professionals to *do for* others; however, this is not true in community practice. Stepping into the community requires an attitude of doing *with* the people, not doing things *to* them or *for* them. When things are done to people or for them, emotional commitment remains limited and community members become unmotivated.

How might the team ensure community ownership for a proposed program and planned interventions? How can you facilitate involvement?

Take Note

Recall Reinkemeyer's (1970) Stages of Planned Change (Box 18.1). The goal of program implementation is to transform the plan into action so that the aggregate, population, or community of focus can achieve the changes desired (stage 5). Over time, as the program matures by going through several cycles, it will stabilize as part of ongoing community services (stage 6).

Who should be involved in implementation to assist the community to meet its goals? Frank & Smith (1999) propose that effective implementation requires a structure and a process that clearly specify the roles and responsibilities of people involved. Some roles are:

- the prime implementers: responsible for the design and implementation of the community development 2nd population health promotion activities
- the facilitator or coordinator: brings together and coordinates the community organizations and resources that are needed to plan and implement a community development 2nd population health promotion initiative
- a partner: one of several organizations that have formed a community partnership to design and implement community development 2nd population health promotion activities
- the promoter: champions and supports community development 2nd population health promotion activity with knowledge, expertise, energy, and enthusiasm
- the funder: provides the budget funds for community development 2nd population health promotion activities

Having discussed above the importance of community participation and ownership of the program, it remains to consider the delivery of a unified program that respects community goals, focuses on the target population, and emphasizes the activities planned to meet the desired community health goals.

Take Note

Do not panic at this point and feel that you must be knowledgeable about all agencies and their programs in the community that you have assessed. At the implementation stage, refer back to your initial assessment and consider logically which service agencies may have resources helpful to the planned program(s). Then, contact selected agencies, request information on their purpose and current programs, share with the agency your community-focused program plans, and solicit recommendations with regard to materials and resources. Many NGOs have professional staff at the national and provincial levels and an affiliated or community linkage structure. These voluntary organizations have ongoing programs for a wide variety of issues, and most acknowledge health promotion as a vital part of their mission. The Internet is a good way to locate such resources in your community.

IMPLEMENTING A UNIFIED PROGRAM

Because of limited resources, staff constraints, and other situations beyond the control of the planners, many good programs are implemented in a piecemeal fashion that minimizes their impact. A unified program requires collaboration and coordination among the agency personnel who will implement the program, the program's recipients (the target population), and the community. Allowing plenty of time for publicizing the program (and how you perform the mechanics of publicity—the how, where, and to whom) can make a crucial difference in whether people attend and what the subsequent impact will be.

After a time and place have been selected (based on initial input from the survey questionnaires), how might you market a program? Public service announcements, notification in the newspapers and on partner websites, bulletin inserts for civic and religious associations, flyers sent home with school-age children, and posters and notices in community service buildings and local shopping centres are some of the methods to consider.

SETTING COMMUNITY AND POPULATION HEALTH GOALS

The goals of population health promotion are to reduce or eliminate disparities in health experienced by different groups of people, improve quality of life, and add years to life expectancy by strengthening communities and community action on the determinants of health. Provincial/territorial ministries of health and regional health authorities use these goals to establish performance objectives and determine funding priorities.

Many provinces and local health authorities have stated public health goals. Canada's overarching national public health goal, as stated by the Public Health Agency Canada (PHAC) (2006), is: *As a nation, we aspire to a Canada in which every person is as healthy as they can be – physically, mentally, emotionally, and spiritually* (p. 44). See Box 19.1 for other public health goals for Canada.

Take Note

Are the goals and objectives for your community realistic in terms of its past history, current context, and in relation to trends over time? Do the goals and objectives for your community-focused program further regional and provincial/territorial goals and objectives?

Box 19.1   Public Health Goals for Canada

Basic Needs (Social and Physical Environments)
- Our children reach their full potential, growing up happy, healthy, confident, and secure.
- The air we breathe, the water we drink, the food we eat, and the places we live, work and play are safe and healthy—now and for generations to come.

Belonging and Engagement
- Each and every person has dignity and a sense of belonging, and contributes to supportive families, friendships, and diverse communities.
- We keep learning throughout our lives through formal and informal education, relationships with others, and the land.
- We participate in and influence the decisions that affect our personal and collective health and well-being.
- We work to make the world a healthy place for all people, through leadership, collaboration, and knowledge.

Healthy Living
- Every person receives the support and information they need to make healthy choices.

A System for Health
- We work to prevent and are prepared to respond to threats to our health and safety through coordinated efforts across the country and around the world.
- A strong system for health and social well-being responds to disparities in health status and offers timely, appropriate care.

From the PHAC (2006), p. 44.

COMMUNITY HEALTH FOCUS

There is one remaining question to ask before initiating the program plan: Does it focus on community health? This may seem to be a strange question. You might wonder: do not all health programs focus on maintaining, restoring, or promoting health of the community? Frequently, the answer is no. Some community-based programs (i.e., located in the community, not in an acute care institution) focus on individuals and do not take the larger community systems into consideration. Community-oriented and community-focused programs seek to improve the health of groups of people to benefit the quality of life and well-being of the community at large.

Be mindful of the progress being made when implementing a program. It is not hard to become distracted by carrying out activities, going after every competitive funding opportunity announced, and being visibly "involved"; these can easily take precedence over strategic planning, community participation, and collaborative coordination of activities to meet the needs of the community as expressed by the residents of that community and carried out in collaboration with community stakeholders. Remember, we discussed the impatience and eagerness that are often associated with new programs. This situation is normal. Committees tend to overemphasize activities and knowledge and forget the initial reason for the program—to improve community health and quality of life. As activities are successful, more and more people will approach the team with more and more ideas and requests. In an effort to do as much as possible for as many people as possible, team members might find themselves in a state of burnout; community representatives may feel burdened; and programs are begun, carried out once, then fizzle.

It must be remembered that it is the sustained day-to-day use of knowledge and lifestyle practices that improve quality of life. Frequently, a program begins with enthusiastic momentum; media publicity attracts people to the activities—and then the program is over. Objectives are evaluated as having been achieved successfully, and another program is planned and implemented. But was there any real improvement in health? Was there any impact on participants' lifestyle practices? Will the changes be maintained and continued for a week? A month? A year? Most importantly, are the changed lifestyle or health practices supported by the surrounding environment and culture? Without sustained program activity and improvement over time, public policy that supports healthy choices, and social support networks that create a positive environment, population behaviour change and long-term impact on a community's health status will not be achieved.

Take Note

Countless incongruities exist between healthy lifestyles and environmental and cultural practices and policies. Here is an example: A school nurse taught hygiene to the elementary grades, emphasizing the importance of washing hands before meals and after using the toilet. However, the school did not provide soap in the washrooms, and for safety purposes, all taps ran with cold water. Additionally, those students who ate lunch at school were not allowed to go to the washroom to wash their hands before going to the lunch room. The reason? It was too disruptive, and students did not finish lunch soon enough. How would you approach this issue?

The team should take the time now to identify the environmental and cultural practices and policies that resulted from your community assessment and that might be in conflict with the proposed community-focused health program plan. What can be done to increase community awareness of these conflicts, and how can change begin? To focus on health and the maintenance of healthy lifestyles, all of the community must be involved.

The best way to maintain a focus on health and not on the activities of the program is to use the Canadian community-as-partner (CCAP) model as a guide. The CCAP model built and described in Chapter 15 (see Figure 15.4) describes intervention as primordial, primary, secondary, and tertiary levels of prevention. Does the program that you propose address any of these four levels of prevention? (Refer to Chapter 12.)

Recall that *primordial prevention* addresses the far upstream factors that affect population health and prevents stressors from forming. *Primary prevention* improves the health and well-being of the community, making it less vulnerable to stressors. Health promotion programs are primordial and primary prevention, as are programs that focus on protection from specific problems (stressors). *Secondary prevention* begins after a disease or condition is present (although there may be no symptoms). Emphasis is on screening, early diagnosis, and treatment of possible stressors that may adversely affect the community's health and would be considered part of the flexible line of defence against stressors, that is, temporary measures to help people during times of stress. *Tertiary prevention* focuses on restoration and rehabilitation and acts to return the community to an optimum level of functioning.

The distinction between prevention levels is not always clear. Can some programs be primary, secondary, and tertiary depending on the needs of the persons who attend? Certainly. Effective parenting classes for the parent with a child who has a behaviour problem (secondary prevention) will have a different purpose than classes designed for expectant parents of a first child (primary prevention). Few programs are purely at one level of prevention. The important point is to assess your program (the implementation phase of the community process) and ask if the interventions are consistent with the CCAP model.

COMMUNITY INTERVENTIONS

There are four types of interventions: education, engineering, enactment, and enforcement. In this section, we will briefly discuss these, with the focus of interventions being the aggregate, population, or community.

Education

Health education for groups is an effective means of conveying knowledge and supporting behaviour change. Learning can be defined as a measurable change in knowledge, attitude, or behaviour that persists over time. Learning occurs in three different domains: cognitive (memory, recognition, understanding, and application), affective (attitudes and values), and psychomotor (using the muscles and nervous system). For learning to be effective, learners must have the ability to perform and opportunities to practice. The environment needs to be supportive and the teaching format and communication process adapted to the needs of the group.

The health education literature is replete with helpful suggestions for teaching adults. For instance, Onega (2000) has adapted an acronym to describe the process of health education:

T—*Tune in.* Listen before you start teaching. Client needs should direct the content.
E—*Edit information.* Teach necessary information first. Be specific.
A—*Act on each teaching moment.* Teach whenever possible. Develop a good relationship.
C—*Clarify often.* Make sure your assumptions are correct. Seek feedback.
H—*Honour the clients as partners.* Build on clients' experiences. Share responsibility with the client group.

Bryson (2013) suggests several principles to engage adult learners (Table 19.1).

The educational process uses the same steps as the community process, making it straightforward for community educators to assess learner needs, plan and implement teaching interventions, and determine the effectiveness of the process.

- Assessment—Identify the information needs and readiness, barriers to learning, and capacities of the target group.

TABLE 19.1 Principles for Engaging Adult Learners

Adult Learning Principle	Definition
Share responsibility for learning	Education is best seen as a dynamic partnership between teachers and their adult students
Develop a climate of mutual respect	A supportive learning environment in which interaction is low-risk, high-reward, encouraged, and reinforced
Learn through reflection	Being able to think about our thinking and engage in reflection on information to support learning and retention
Apply personal experience	Applying their experience to new learning helps adults make associations that support learning and retention
Learn for action	Recognition of the practicality and relevance of information and how it can be immediately applied
Cultivate a participative environment	When adults participate in learning and work together in groups, they report an enhanced quality and depth of learning
Use self-directed learning	Being offered choice and control over the ways we learn and demonstrate that learning on demand

Adapted from Bryson (2013), p. 26.

- Analysis, Diagnosis, and Planning—State the educational goals and objectives. Select methods, materials, site, time, and market the event.
- Implementation—Carry out the sessions(s) as planned.
- Evaluation—Assess the effectiveness of processes and achievement of outcomes.

Some formats for learning include brainstorming, demonstration, group discussion, lecture, role play, and panel discussion. Strategies to enhance learning may include printed material (bulletin boards, drawings, flash cards), audiovisual material (Powerpoint™ presentations, You-Tube videos, photographs), computer-assisted software and online resources, guest speakers, peer presentations, and field trips. Care must be taken that materials are appropriate to the technology available, the culture, literacy and language levels of the participants, and the size of the group. Pretesting newly developed material is important, and critically assessing print resources for reading level, layout, type font and size, content (verbal and visual), and aesthetic quality is key to ensuring that the resources are appropriate, culturally sensitive, and accurate.

Social marketing is mass media education. In social marketing, mass media are used to "sell" health through particular behaviours or products. With its components of marketing and consumer research, advertising, and promotion, social marketing clearly has a central role to play in health promotion. The social marketing process consists of developing the right product, backed by the right promotion, and put in the right place at the right price. Although a social marketing campaign on its own cannot be expected to change the behaviour of large populations, it can be a potent component in a comprehensive health promotion program.

The *product* is the message and how it is presented. The *price* is not only the cost of producing and publishing the message but also the cost to the consumer of acting on it. *Promotion* is the means of persuasion or the communication function of marketing. *Place* respects adequate and suitable distribution as well as response channels or access to information. In other words, how can people who are motivated take follow-up action?

A systematic approach to mass education, social marketing offers a staged population-focused approach to convert community needs into demand and then provides the means to satisfy that demand (Fig. 19.1). Social marketing is concerned with achieving a social objective. The key components of social marketing are:

- Systematically collecting data and analyzing them to develop appropriate strategies
- Making products, services, or behaviours fit the felt needs of the consumers/users
- Using a strategic approach to promoting the products, services, or behaviours
- Incorporating methods for effective distribution of the message or product so that when demand is created, consumers know where and how to get the products, services, or behaviours
- Improving the adoption of products, services, or behaviours and increasing the willingness of consumers/users to contribute something in exchange
- Pricing so that the product or service is affordable to use or the behaviour is easy to perform
- Social marketing processes include:
  1. *Assessment, data collection, and analysis.* Consulting a sample of people from the target audience to assess their needs, wants, and aspirations (e.g., violence reduction in the community). Community members participate in the development of feasible, attractive solutions to the issues of concern (e.g., focus on schools and bullying) (Box 19.2).
  2. *Market segmentation.* Based on an analysis of the initial data and the community, the target audience is divided into discrete units with common characteristics (e.g., parents, teachers, and children).
  3. *Product and message development.* Products (e.g., posters, pamphlets, t-shirts) and messages (e.g., slogans, public service ads) are developed based on the preferences and characteristics of the relevant segments. These are tested among representative samples

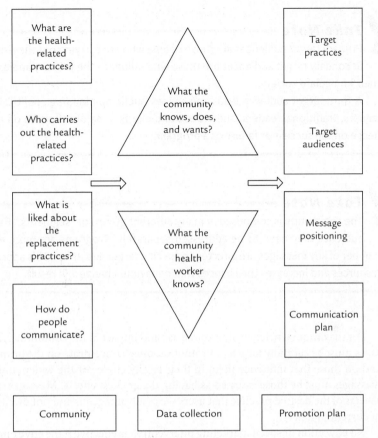

FIGURE 19.1   The process of social marketing. (Adapted from Department of International Development (1998).

of target populations. Products and messages are modified, refined, and re-tested until they are acceptable.

4. *Launch.* The product or service is introduced.
5. *Evaluation.* The performance of the product or service is monitored and evaluated in the market and the strategy, marketing plan, or product itself is revised accordingly.

Box 19.2 Ten Questions for Social Marketing Planning

1. What social or health issue does the community want to address?
2. What actions do community members believe will best address that issue?
3. Who is being asked to take action (target audience)?
4. What will the audience want in exchange for adopting this new practice/behaviour?
5. Why will the audience believe anything we say is true?
6. What is already out there about this issue/message?
7. What is the best time/place to reach the audience?
8. How often and from whom does the intervention need to be received in order to be effective?
9. How can the community integrate a variety of interventions over time in a coordinated fashion to influence the adoption of the desired practice/behaviour by the target group?
10. Do we have the resources to carry out this strategy? Who might be useful partners?

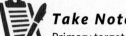

Take Note ————————————————————————————————————

Primary target audiences are those people who are carrying out the risk practices.

Secondary target audiences are those who influence the primary audience and who are in their immediate society.

A third target audience leads and shapes public opinion (e.g., political leaders, religious leaders, traditional leaders, and elders) and exerts a major influence on the credibility and hence on the success or failure of a program.

Take Note ————————————————————————————————————

The community is composed of many different groups or "segments." Each segment of the audience may need to be addressed separately. Programs are more effective if a small number of key messages are directed to specific target audiences. This approach concentrates resources and increases the chances that behaviour change will result.

For maximum efficiency of resource use and impact in the community, audiences and messages must be carefully targeted. Promotion must concentrate on the primary target audience and on those that influence them in their family circles or the wider community. The target messages must be those assessed as having the greatest effects. Messages should bolster those aspects of the desired practice that users see as advantageous and not dwell on negative aspects of current practices.

No education or social marketing intervention is effective if the environment erects barriers to people taking action. In this instance, the community team must act to effect change by creating conditions that support making the healthy choice the easy choice.

Engineering

Engineering is the process of creating an environment that is supportive for change—that is, making the healthy choice the easy choice. For instance, in a context of rising obesity rates, Canadians value fitness and health and believe that healthy eating and activity are important, but they have trouble following through with their intentions to take action. People need support. Hence, the food industry has taken action in many ways: improved product choices on the market; more nutrition information available to consumers on food packages; responsible marketing standards where children are concerned; and governments, media, food producers, and the public working collaboratively to ensure that people have the information, the choices, and the environmental supports to make healthier choices.

Media advocacy, based on the recognition that health is a result of the social and environmental conditions in which people live, uses the mass media to influence the development of healthy public policy through changing the nature of public debate on issues that affect health (Table 19.2). It is a political tool in that it exerts pressure to influence decision makers and legislators.

There are several components of media advocacy. The first step of reframing the debate, or presenting the issue differently than it is usually discussed, results from setting the agenda, shaping the debate, and advancing policy. It involves capturing the attention of the media and demonstrating the newsworthiness of an issue. The second step is to tell the story from the perspective of the population, with emphasis on broad social issues rather than on individuals. The third step involves putting forward the policy solution that you are aiming to achieve

TABLE 19.2 Program Communication Strategies

Strategy	Actions
Interpersonal communication training	1. Strengthen the ability of front-line workers to reach potential targets and to promote the message 2. Provide opportunities for front-line workers to develop communication skills 3. Ensure that quality support materials are available 4. Provide interpersonal support to front-line workers
Mass media	1. Build on existing policies and strengthen government and private-sector capacity for creative presentation of standardized messages
Print media	1. Promote the development and dissemination of a clearly defined program logo to build awareness and aid identification 2. Develop strategies using print media (e.g., billboards, posters, site-signs) and other learning materials, manuals, and program guidelines
Community-based media	1. Use local and social media and employ traditional, community-based entertainment artists (e.g., popular folk singers, actors, and poets)

Adapted from Department of International Development (1998), p. 208.

(Wass, 2000). Community participation plays a key role in media advocacy. To be effective, media advocacy relies on the formation of coalitions that are sustained over a long period of time so that a grassroots movement can gain enough momentum to maintain the issue in the public eye for more than a short time.

Advocacy campaigns consist of providing newsworthy items to the media, writing letters to the editor, preparing media releases, releasing photographs or providing photo opportunities, and doing media interviews (Wass, 2000). Be certain to follow the protocols of your organization before contacting the media, and be prepared for questions that generate controversy!

Enactment and Enforcement

When legislation is in place to require people to act in a certain way (enactment), and there is resistance or lack of compliance, protection services (e.g., police, fire, food inspectors) may enter the community to enforce the law. If community health workers can combine education and engineering with this approach, then enforcement can be most effective. For instance, many health departments collaborate with the police and transportation officials during seat belt checkpoints. If children are unrestrained in a vehicle, or improperly restrained, professionals demonstrate proper restraint methods, provide information on purchasing appropriate restraints, and teach the parents the importance of restraints for child safety.

What kinds of interventions support enforcement efforts? Letters to the editor, policy briefs, petitions, articles in community newsletters, town hall meetings, and knowledge exchange activities assist community health workers to get health messages out to the community, opinion leaders, and policy makers.

EVALUATION

At the conclusion of the planning and implementation phases of the CCAP process, it is important to assess team performance and reflect on individual contributions. Many teams disband at this point if external evaluators enter the process as described by Reinkemeyer (1970) stage 7 (see Box 18.1). A framework for individual reflection is provided in Table 19.3; this can be used to begin a conversation about team function and the participatory process.

TABLE 19.3 Participation Checklist

Personal Behaviour	Never	Occasionally	Often
I suggested a procedure for the group to follow or a method for organizing a task.			
I suggested a new idea, new activity, new problem, or a new course of action.			
I attempted to bring the group back to work when joking, personal stories, or irrelevant talk went on for too long.			
I suggested, when there was some confusion, that the group make an outline or otherwise organize a plan for completing the task.			
I initiated attempts to redefine goals, problems, or outcomes when things became hazy or confusing.			
I elaborated on ideas with concise examples or illustrations.			
I suggested resource people to contact and/or brought materials.			
I presented the reasons behind my opinions.			
I asked others for information and/or opinions.			
I asked for significance and/or implications of facts and opinions.			
I saw and pointed out relationships between facts and opinions.			
I asked a speaker to explain the reasoning that led him/her to a particular conclusion.			
I related my comments to previous contributions.			
I pulled together and summarized various ideas presented.			
I tested to see if everyone understood, and/or agreed with, the issue discussed or the decision made.			
I summarized the progress that the group had made.			
I encouraged other members to participate and tried to unobtrusively involve quiet members.			
I actively supported others when I thought their points of view were important.			
I tried to find areas of agreement in conflicting points of view and tried to address the source of the problem.			
I used appropriate humour to reduce tension in the group.			
I listened attentively to others' ideas and contributions.			

From Annis, Racher, and Beattie (2004), p. 219.

Take Note

Keep track of successes and lessons learned by recording stories, taking photographs, and saving evidence from workshops and gatherings to capture before-and-after intervention circumstances. Such evidence is important for celebrating accomplishments, persuading prospective funders, and making presentations to the media and other communities that want to learn from you.

The program plan and its implementation need to be assessed at this time as well as throughout the process. Throughout, it is important to ensure that the program activities are congruent with its goals and objectives and that the activities target the appropriate audiences and practices. Did you honour the logic model (Chapter 18), or did you make adjustments along the way? Were those adjustments recorded and communicated? Did you collect data on the indicators? Did you collect additional information? Where are these data stored, and who has access to these for monitoring and evaluation purposes? At this time, assess what went well and why in program implementation—celebrate your successes. What did not go well? Try to explain why things went off track or did not turn out as expected. Were there aspects of the process for which you were unprepared? Did you have any surprises—good or bad? There are intended outcomes specified in any project plan; some unanticipated and unintended things happen as well.

Summary

Having considered the importance of community ownership of the program, the need to offer a unified program, and the obligation to maintain focus on the population and activities planned to meet community and program goals, there remains one step in the CCAP process—evaluation. Before an intervention is implemented, the manner in which it is to be evaluated must be established, hence the importance of the logic model. The next chapter explains why this final stage of the community process is best considered before implementation begins.

REFERENCES

Annis, R., Racher, F., & Beattie, M. (2004). *Rural community health and well-being: A guide to action.* Brandon, MB: Rural Development Institute, Brandon University. URL=https://www.brandonu.ca/rdi/files/2011/03/Rural CommunityHealth_and_Wellbeing_a_Guide_to_Action.pdf

Bryson, J. D. (2013). *Engaging adult learners: Philosophy, principles and practice.* Barrie, ON: Author. URL=http://northernc.on.ca/leid/docs/engagingadultlearners.pdf

Department of International Development. (1998). A social marketing approach to hygiene promotion and sanitation promotion. In *Guidance manual on water supply and sanitation programmes* (Section 2.8, pp. 201–219). Leicestershire, UK: Water and Environmental Health at London and Loughborough (WELL), Loughborough University. URL=http://www.lboro.ac.uk/well/resources/Publications/guidance-manual/chapter-2–8.pdf

Frank, F., & Smith, A. (1999). *The community development handbook: A tool to build community capacity.* Ottawa: Labour Market Learning and Development Unit, Human Resources Development Canada (HRDC). URL=https://ccednet-rcdec.ca/en/toolbox/community-development-handbook-tool-build-community-capacity

Onega, L. L. (2000). Educational theories, models and principles applied to community and public health nursing. In M. Stanhope & J. Lancaster (Eds.), *Community and public health nursing* (pp. 266–283). St. Louis, MO: Mosby.

Public Health Agency of Canada (PHAC). (2006). Appendix 4: Public health goals for Canada. In *Sustainable development in public health: A long term journey begins.* Ottawa: Author. URL=http://www.phac-aspc.gc.ca/publicat/sds-sdd/sds-sdd2-app-ann2–3–4-eng.php

Wass, A. (2000). *Promoting health: The primary care approach.* Marrickville, AU: Harcourt.

ONLINE RESOURCES

Please visit thePoint at http://thepoint.lww.com/Vollman4e for up-to-date Internet resources and additional learning materials on this topic.

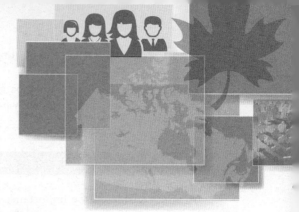

CHAPTER 20

Evaluating a Community Health Program: Collaborative Action Evaluation

Marcia Hills and Simon Carroll

LEARNING OBJECTIVES

After studying this chapter, you should be able to:

1. Identify the purpose of using evaluation to improve community health programs and practices

2. Identify some of the challenges to using evaluation with complex community health initiatives

3. Understand the underlying values and principles of working in an authentically participatory way with community as a partner

4. Use Collaborative Action Evaluation (CAE) as an approach to evaluation

5. Apply methods of data collection and analysis appropriate to CAE

Introduction

> *The cynic is a man who knows the price of everything, but the value of nothing.* —Oscar Wilde

All evaluation should set as its primary task the avoidance of this pernicious cynicism. There is nothing more ruinous and disempowering than forcing good-willed communities into a "gambit of compliance" with a set of reporting requirements that are mutually recognized as absurd, counter-productive, and energy-depleting travesties masquerading as rigorous evaluative technique. If anything, evaluation should be an empowering, supportive inquiry into how best to improve the everyday lives of our fellow human beings. In this mode, cynicism is the enemy that must be harried at every turn.

This may strike the reader of this chapter as a strange beginning, one that is perhaps more appropriate for the conclusion to a much more comprehensive examination of evaluation, not as a comfortable and welcoming start to a benign introductory survey of community health program evaluation. Yet, we leave this here as a provocative application of the maxim that if you need to get one important point across, always be sure to put it at the beginning.

In this chapter, we provide a detailed look at one specific approach to evaluation that we believe addresses the issue raised above: *Collaborative Action Evaluation* (CAE). We also provide some more general background and context in regard to evaluation with communities; however, most of the chapter uses CAE as an exemplary approach that is appropriate for working with the community as a partner.

DEFINING EVALUATION

"Program evaluation is the systematic collection of information about the activities, characteristics, and outcomes of programs to make judgments about the program, improve program effectiveness, and/or inform decisions about future programming" (Patton, 1997, p. 23).

In addition to this generic perspective, community health program evaluation should involve the community as a partner, meaning that all aspects of the evaluation process *should* be participatory, equitable, and empowering. Clearly, this definition places an explicit set of *values* up front as the basis of guiding principles that determine *how* and *why* community health program evaluations are conducted.

The most important preparations to make before engaging with program evaluation are to determine what your working definition of *evaluation* is and to understand the implications of choosing a particular definition.

There are many different approaches to defining the concept and purpose of evaluation in community health programming. One of the broadest is that of Green and Kreuter (1991): "comparison of an object of interest against a standard of acceptability" (p. 248). However, as Rootman et al. (2001) point out, this leaves a great deal to be determined. We do not know the nature of the object, nor the methods used to make the comparison, nor do we know *who* is setting the standard, nor *how* the standard is set. It is once we start to dig deeper into these questions that key ethical and political issues come to the fore.

Without listing all the possible definitions of *evaluation,* we can say that there are two primary dimensions along which most approaches can be plotted. One dimension is about control. Who controls the evaluation process? On this dimension, there is a continuum between external evaluator control on one end and total community control on the other. The second dimension is about knowledge and methods. This dimension has a continuum with established social science methodologies on one end and pragmatic uses of the systematic collection and analysis of routinely produced data on the other.

While it is true that, at its very basis, evaluation is about the judgement of, or the determination of, the worth or value of something (Scriven, 1991), such a definition leaves aside just what is being judged and for what purpose (Patton, 1997). As we shall see, various components of program evaluation and various approaches to these components have different answers to these questions (NCCMT, 2012).

Evaluations that are more community-controlled tend to be focused on pragmatic issues, concerning the ongoing assessment of how well a certain program is being implemented, and see the purpose of evaluation as the collection of evidence to support the immediate improvement of program processes; or at the extreme, the basis for completely changing the focus of the program or replacing it with a more relevant set of activities. Community health workers and community members tend to be less concerned about research and scientific rigour and more concerned that they use the information that they already routinely collect to improve practice.

External evaluations are often initiated by the requirements of large funding agencies and are focused on judging whether the programs or projects they fund are meeting the overall policy objectives that form the basis on which the entire funding stream is constructed and its justification for continued existence. Often with external evaluations of this kind, scientific rigour, based on established methodologic approaches, is seen as a fundamental requirement for credible evaluations.

The community health team often evaluates the responses of the community to a program on an ongoing basis to measure progress that is being made toward the program's goals and objectives. Evaluation data are also crucial for revision of the assessment database and the community diagnoses that were developed from analysis of the community assessment data.

Do we appear to be talking in circles? Evaluation is the final step of the Canadian community-as-partner (CCAP) process, but it is linked to assessment, which is the first step. Professional practice is cyclic as well as dynamic, and for community-focused interventions to be timely and relevant, the community assessment database, community diagnoses, and program plans must be evaluated routinely. The effectiveness of community interventions depends on continuous reassessment of the community and on appropriate revisions of planned interventions. In fact, this has led some writers to argue that evaluation is a process that should take place throughout the life of the program; in other words, as soon as we begin, we should evaluate our progress, so that we can use evidence to implement change immediately, rather than waiting until it is too late for that program, with that community. This principle is driven by the necessity of bringing benefit to each community with which we work, as we work with them. Communities should always be better off having worked with you (Hills & Mullett, 2000).

The purposes of evaluation when working with communities as partners are to determine if threats or challenges to health have been repelled or minimized, if the health status of the population is improved, and if the community's capacity is strengthened as a result of the intervention.

Evaluation is important to community practice, but of equal importance is its crucial role in the functioning of human service agencies. Staffing and funding are frequently based on evaluation findings, and existing programs can be subject to termination unless evaluation evidence can be produced that answers this question: What has been the program's impact on the community? Recent years have witnessed a growing focus on evaluation; training programs on evaluation have become common, and evaluation has become big business. Unfortunately, evaluation is sometimes practised separately from program planning. It may even be tacked onto the end of a program just to satisfy funding sources or agency administration. The problems of such an approach are evident. Effective community practice requires an integrated approach to evaluation; it is a unique aspect of the field.

 Critical Thinking Exercise 20.1

What do you think evaluations should accomplish?

How much control should stakeholders in the community have over the evaluation process?

How strict should an evaluation be in terms of the type of data collection and analysis that is undertaken?

Should evaluators use only well-validated indicators and other forms of measurement?

EVALUATION PRINCIPLES

Congruent with the theoretical foundations of working with the community as partner, we base our program evaluation on principles explicated by the W. K. Kellogg Foundation (1998). These principles are:

1. *Strengthen programs.* Our goal is health promotion and improving a community's self-reliance. Evaluation assists in attaining this goal by providing an ongoing and systematic process for assessing the program, its impact, and its outcomes.

2. *Use multiple approaches.* In addition to multidisciplinary approaches, evaluation methods may be numerous and varied. No single approach is favoured, but the methods chosen must be congruent with the purposes of the program.
3. *Design evaluation to address real issues.* Community-oriented and community-focused programs, rooted in the "real" community and based on an assessment of that community, must design an evaluation to measure those criteria of importance to the community.
4. *Create a participatory process.* Just as the community members were part of assessment, analysis, planning, and implementation, they also must be partners in evaluation. This can be a very difficult process, but not only is it more ethical, it creates enhanced validity for evaluation findings and builds commitment to change for community actors.
5. *Allow for flexibility.* "Evaluation approaches must not be rigid and prescriptive, or it will be difficult to document the incremental, complex, and often subtle changes that occur" (W. K. Kellogg Foundation, 1998, p. 3). The approach should be "able to respond to changing circumstances, opportunities, challenges and priorities" (Rootman et al., 2001).
6. *Build capacity.* The process of evaluation, in addition to measuring outcomes, should enhance the skills, knowledge, and attitudes of those engaged in it, including community health workers and community members alike.

Process or formative evaluation is intended to improve the operation of an existing program or intervention. It answers the question: Are we doing what we said we would do? That is, did we deliver the program or intervention as designed (fidelity), provide a place to meet, include handouts at our meeting, and so forth? Some authors make a distinction between formative and process evaluation by using *process* to denote evaluation conducted during the program and *formative* (as the name implies) at the program formation or pre-program stages.

Outcome (or summative) evaluation is concerned with the impact of a program or intervention on a target group and can be measured at any point in time, but is usually most important at the end point. It answers the questions: Is our program effective? Did we achieve what we intended to achieve? Were our objectives met?

It is in the long-term outcome evaluation, however, that you find out if the changes had a lasting and real effect. Because it is closer to the cause-and-effect question, careful evaluative research is needed to determine the actual contribution of the program to the outcome being measured.

Take Note

An in-depth review of evaluation research is beyond the scope of this text. There are several excellent resources that focus on evaluation research; these are included on thePoint.

SETTING THE CONTEXT FOR EVALUATION

Evaluation is a sense-making process that usually involves making judgements about the worth or merit of health or social programs and/or professional practice. It is a robust arena of activity directed at collecting, analyzing, and interpreting information on the need for, implementation of, and effectiveness of intervention efforts to improve health and quality of life. Evaluation of practice is a professional imperative that allows us to be accountable to the public we serve. Evaluation, as a process of valuing, is essentially a political act that takes place in the public arena.

Early on in modern evaluation research, several key figures developed what was to become the orthodox approach to evaluating health and social programs (Campbell & Stanley, 1966; Cook & Campbell, 1979). At the time, these authors focused on the key question concerning

TABLE 20.1 Differences Between Research and Evaluation

Research	Evaluation
Produces new knowledge	Judges merit or worth
Scientific inquiry based on intellectual curiosity	Policy and program interests of stakeholders paramount
Advances broad knowledge and theory	Provides information for decision-making on a specific program
	Conducted within setting of changing actors, priorities, resources, and timelines

Blome (2009).

whether a program or intervention can be said to have caused the pertinent outcomes of interest. Evaluation design was then built up to address threats to internal validity, meaning that researchers were primarily concerned with avoiding errors of attributing causal force to an intervention, when some alternative factor(s) may have been responsible for the observed changes in outcomes. Although there are many ways to address the problem of alternative causes, the emerging orthodoxy chose to put emphasis on developing quasi-experimental research designs in order to try and (to the extent feasible) rule out these alternatives, and be more certain that it really was the program or intervention that caused the observed changes.

In 1989, Guba and Lincoln published an influential book called *Fourth Generation Evaluation,* arguing strongly for a move beyond the confines of the quasi-experimental orthodoxy they thought had been constraining the field of evaluation. While many did not follow these authors along their particular path, the book is recognized for disrupting the reigning orthodoxy and creating space for new alternative evaluation approaches to emerge and new debates about appropriate evaluation methods to begin.

Evaluation Traditions/Paradigms

In this section, we delve a little deeper into the underlying philosophical or "paradigmatic" foundations for the different evaluation approaches.

There are many ways to conduct an evaluation. Just as there are different approaches to doing research, there are also different approaches to conducting evaluations. Evaluations, from our perspective, are a particular type of research. Most of the principles and rules of good research also apply to good evaluations. The one obvious difference between research and evaluations is that evaluations are more focused on a program or practice while research is generally focused on producing new knowledge. In Table 20.1 several distinctions are outlined.

There are three distinct paradigmatic traditions in evaluation: orthodox, interpretive, and participatory. They are detailed in Table 20.2.

TABLE 20.2 Traditions of Evaluation

	Orthodox	Interpretive	Participatory
Paradigm (world view)	Empiricist/Positivist	Human science/Interpretative	Emancipatory
View of participants	Participant as subject	Participant as informant	Participants as coevaluators
View of evaluator	Evaluator as methodologist	Evaluator as facilitator	Evaluator as social activist
Evaluator's values	Focus on individual	Focus on experience and meaning	Focus on collective
Focus	Behavioural change	Focus on understanding	Systemic change
View of evaluation	Collecting information for decision making	Explicating and understanding participants' experiences	Evaluation as transforming practice and structures

Hills and Mullett (2000).

The interpretive and participatory traditions were developed in reaction to the orthodox approach; both offer strong critiques of the orthodox tradition. One such critique is that the orthodox tradition excludes the people who deliver programs from the evaluation process. Typically, when we talk about evaluation we refer to it as "program evaluation." We talk as if it is the program alone that is to be evaluated, without reference to the people delivering or receiving it. From this perspective, we try to rule out any influence the persons conducting the program might have on the program. So, external consultants are hired to evaluate the program on the assumption that, if an external expert evaluator conducts the evaluation, the results will be more accurate, more reliable, and more trustworthy. We believe, however, that an evaluator needs to consider the question: "What is the relationship between the evaluator and those delivering the program?" We believe it is possible to perform excellent evaluations by collaborating and developing relationships with those who are intimately acquainted with the program or intervention under review.

The remainder of this chapter will elaborate in much more detail how the CAE approach shifts evaluation research to a position where it is much more prepared to live up to the concept of community-as-partner.

Key Concepts

Before moving on, we outline certain key ideas or concepts that emerging alternative evaluation approaches have been able to surface as important. Not all approaches adhere fully to each concept, but there are enough generic affinities to build on and emphasize why these concepts are so essential to consider, especially when thinking of doing evaluations with the community as a partner.

Assets

In parallel with developments within the evaluation literature over the past three decades, there have also been developments within the fields of public health, health promotion, and social interventions that have shifted our thinking. Some key figures within these fields have moved from approaches based on identifying population deficits and needs and aiming to fix their problems, to approaches that identify assets and strengths within communities with the goal of enhancing and reinforcing their effectiveness, thereby building resilience and empowerment. For evaluators this shift gives substance to the ideas of empowering people and communities and developing resources and capacities for self-determination (Hills et al., 2010).

Systems Thinking/Complexity

Another important influence on evaluation has been the recognition that most social and health interventions in communities are themselves complex systems and the settings in which they intervene are also complex systems. The implication is that simplistic models of statistical analysis, measuring the relationship between intervention variables and outcome variables, is likely to miss most of what is going on in an intervention, and worse, is likely to misconstrue what it is that makes an intervention or program work, or not work.

Context

Perhaps more than any other evaluation approach, the interpretive and participatory traditions have integrated how local contexts interact with intervention mechanisms to produce varied patterns in outcomes. It is important to recognize, give attention to, and integrate (in some form) contextual factors into the collection and analysis of evaluation data. Rather than try to hold context in abeyance, as does the orthodox, quasi-experimental tradition, emerging evaluation approaches try to open up the proverbial "black box" to see what is going on inside the program or intervention.

COLLABORATIVE ACTION EVALUATION

Our preferred approach to evaluation, which we call CAE, is situated within the participatory tradition. CAE uses an evaluation process that helps people change the way they think, work, and relate to others. CAE is a form of participatory action evaluation that requires full participation of everyone who has an interest in the program or intervention that is being evaluated. It is an approach to evaluation that does evaluation *with* people; not *on, to,* or *about* them.

The evaluator using CAE plans and simultaneously implements and investigates change through a series of iterations, ensuring that all community health workers and community members are interested in the outcome of the evaluation participate and collaborate in every aspect of the evaluation from its initiation to its conclusion. CAE creates evidence upon which to base practice and catalyzes change to practice. So we ask, "What should be accepted as evidence upon which to base practice?"

CAE is closely aligned with a particular research approach called cooperative inquiry (Reason, 1988; Heron, 1996); cooperative inquiry methods are incorporated in CAE. However, we prefer the word "collaboration" to cooperation:

> Collaboration is the creation of a synergistic alliance that honours and utilizes each person's contribution in order to create collective wisdom and collective action. Collaboration is not synonymous with cooperation, partnership, participation, or compromise. Those words do not convey the fundamental importance of being in relationship nor the depth of caring and commitment that is needed to create the kind of reciprocity that is collaboration. Collaborators are committed to, care about, and trust in each other. They recognize that, despite their differences, each has unique and valuable knowledge, perspectives, and experiences to contribute to the collaboration (Hills & Watson, 2011, p. 71).

Assumptions Underlying CAE

Like any evaluation approach, CAE rests on a number of assumptions.

- Truth comes from the synergy of multiple perspectives (collective wisdom).
- Facts have no meaning except within a value framework.
- Causal relationships can be understood in ways other than probability statistics (theoretical abstractions).
- Phenomena can only be understood within the context in which they occur.
- Evaluators are subjective partners with participants and stakeholders.
- Worthwhile learning is often personal, obscure, and private.
- Only some learning appears as behavioural change.
- Many things that exist are not empirically verifiable.

 Critical Thinking Exercise 20.2

Think about the assumptions that you make about evaluation. Take a piece of paper or a page in a journal and write down your assumptions on the left hand side of the page. Next to each assumption write down how that assumption will impact the way you will do an evaluation.

Characteristics of CAE

CAE is a carefully organized search, inquiry, or examination of an issue or question that is characterized by the systematic collection and analysis of data to create new knowledge or understanding. The emphasis in CAE is on the co-creation of knowledge to bring about change in existing programs, interventions, or systems. Those engaged in the program, intervention, or system form an inquiry team, much like the teams that formed to do the community assessment, planning, and intervention.

Process

CAE uses a systematic process that requires careful planning of each stage. Most CAE inquiry teams begin the evaluation process by asking questions about their program or intervention, the needs of their clients, the effectiveness of their work, whether new ideas are feasible, what options are available as solutions to existing issues or problems, and so on. These are potential evaluation questions and activities. CAE is used to formalize the process of exploring a program, intervention, or systems issue by working with those delivering the program, engaged in the intervention, or who are part of the system to conceptualize the issue or problem as an evaluation question and to systematize the process by which data are collected, analyzed, and presented as results.

Relevance

Because the evaluation questions arise from those delivering and experiencing the program, they are highly relevant to that inquiry team. CAE focuses the evaluation effort in the context of daily work activities in order to solve problems and help make those activities more effective and ultimately more satisfying. The evaluation ought to result in decisions by the key stakeholders (i.e., community agencies, health units, program managers, etc.) or provide information that is in some other way directly useful to the community in which it is initiated.

CAE involves asking questions such as:

- What are the practical problems we are facing in our work? In our intervention? In our system?
- What are some questions and concerns regarding our work and activities within our community setting?
- What issues are the focus of our attention?

Questions such as these guide the selection of meaningful evaluation topics and provide for the development of appropriate evaluation questions for CAE.

Collaboration and Participation

The community health workers and volunteers who deliver the program or are engaged in the intervention or system must be actively involved in and understand the evaluation process. The evaluation is driven by a collaboration among community health workers, community and system decision makers, and evaluators, and tends to be multidisciplinary in nature. It is a collaborative effort involving all relevant parties at all stages of the evaluation process. The level of participant and community involvement may vary at each stage of the evaluation, but CAE involves joint responsibility and decision making during every step. It requires the evaluator(s), decision makers, community health workers, and the community to share power and control throughout the evaluation process.

In CAE, the distinction between the evaluator and the community health worker is minimized or eliminated. This does not necessarily mean that all inquiry team members always do exactly the same thing or that everyone is responsible for exactly the same "tasks." Rather, CAE demands a form of collaboration that is based on mutual respect and trust that maximizes the unique contributions of each team member and that incorporates shared responsibility for the evaluation. It includes responsible reporting of the evaluation results that are sensitive to the community health workers' and community's needs and desires, as well as those of evaluators and academics.

Focus

CAE is designed to illuminate and solve practical problems. CAE uses knowledge gained through the evaluation process to make decisions about how to improve or change practice, programs, and interventions to better meet participants' needs. Often, the evaluation is used to influence decision making at a program or policy level, so CAE can benefit the community not only by the results generated on a specific issue but also in relation to the identification of future actions and policies.

Unlike orthodox evaluation research that focuses on prediction or understanding, CAE seeks to bring about change. It is premised on the belief that engaging in a participatory collaborative evaluation process, and being involved in making decisions about that process, are empowering and transforming. Engagement in the CAE process allows people to develop new ways of thinking and behaving.

Sustainable Contributions

Those taking part in the CAE process should be *better off* as a result of their participation. With many evaluation projects, the interest in an idea wanes when the project ends. In contrast, CAE is designed to continue to make contributions to participants after the project ends. Most significantly, engaging in CAE provides participants with new skills and knowledge that enhances their capacity to engage in future evaluations.

CAE Process

CAE investigates and implements change through iterative cycles of reflecting, planning, and acting. Through reflecting–planning–acting cycles that are designed to reflect the values of participation and collaboration, evaluation is planned and operationalized. The evaluation alliance (inquiry team) reflects on the actions taken to generate more knowledge to be fed back into the process and the cycles continue, all the while building new knowledge and creating change. This process is illustrated in Figure 20.1.

The capacity building and learning that is embedded in this process views learning as the transformation of consciousness and evaluation as relational inquiry (Hills & Watson, 2011).

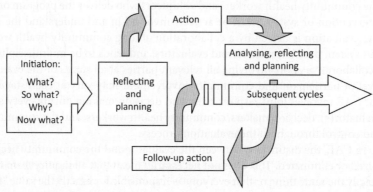

FIGURE 20.1   Collaborative action research cycles.

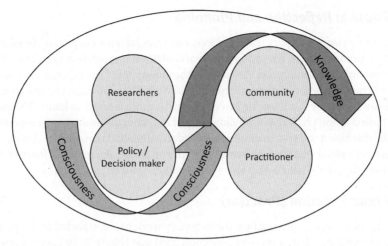

FIGURE 20.2   Knowledge…transformation of consciousness.

Learning occurs at the juncture or intersection when the evaluator and program stakeholders are in a relationship with each other and are engaged in a process of transformational learning in which they co-create knowledge through a complex relational process: relation with subject matter; relation with one's own ideas and personal meaning; relation with peers/social-political dynamics; and through relationships between the evaluator–stakeholder(s). This relational learning leads to new insights, new knowledge, and deeper understandings, resulting in the transformation of consciousness. Transformation of consciousness includes an evolution of consciousness, in that both evaluator and stakeholders experience a higher dimension of integration than before, including a higher consciousness and repatterning of the old into something new (Hills & Watson, 2011).

From our perspective, one aspect of the learning process (evaluator, stakeholder, or knowledge) is not valued over another and the evaluator and stakeholders are engaged in a mutual inquiry process of learning—a relational inquiry process. In contrast to more traditional authoritarian conceptualizations of learning and evaluation in which the evaluator is seen as the expert and transmitter of information, knowledge, and results, the CAE perspective does not permit the evaluator to be viewed as an expert with knowledge to impart, the stakeholders to be passive recipients of the knowledge, or the knowledge itself to be seen as merely information to be transmitted. In Figure 20.2 this transformation of consciousness is represented.

CAE Framework

As shown in Figure 20.1, the CAE framework is cyclical in nature and can be described in six phases.

Phase 1: Initiation

There are two steps involved in the initial phase of a CAE project: identifying the issue and engaging stakeholders. A group or system that is interested in evaluating an intervention, program, or system usually initiates the process. The evaluator's main task in this phase is to clarify with the group what is the specific issue it wants to address; this clarification process may take several meetings and simultaneously builds stakeholder engagement in the evaluation. Together the stakeholders and evaluators, the inquiry team, clarify the program (what?), clarify the stakeholders' values in relation to the program (so what?), discuss their goals and how their goals are related to their activities (why?), and finally identify who the audience is for the program and the evaluation (now what?).

Phase 2: Reflection and Planning

In this phase, the inquiry team develops and articulates the purpose of the evaluation. Then, once the purpose is clear, the inquiry team articulates the evaluation questions. This phase is called reflecting and planning because usually the inquiry team has experience or knowledge about the program so it is not starting strictly with planning. The team begins by reflecting on what it already knows and how this knowing can inform what more it needs to know. The group then plans for the first action phase that will follow. It further refines the evaluation questions for this phase and decides how it will systematically collect information (data) in practice during this action phase. It is in this phase that the inquiry team decides on its specific methods for collecting and analyzing data. The critical issue is that all methods chosen *must be participatory*.

Phase 3: Action (Practice)

This phase occurs in practice; the everyday work of the stakeholders. The inquiry team uses previously decided upon data collection methods (Phase 2) to collect information about the intervention, program, or system that it is evaluating.

Phase 4: Analyzing, Reflecting, and Planning

In this phase, the inquiry team works together to analyze the information that has been collected. Team members reflect on their findings in light of initial (theoretical) understanding and in this way consider propositional and practical knowing. They reflect on their experiences and knowledge and plan for the next action phase. They consider questions such as: *What do we need to know more about? What changes need to occur to change (transform) our current intervention practice? Program? System? What strategies can we use to understand and monitor these changes?*

Phase 5: Follow-up Action (Practice)

The inquiry team implements the recommended changes and then, as in Phase 3, collects information from practice to investigate the intervention, program, or system changes it previously implemented.

Phase 6: Subsequent Cycles

A series of cycles are decided upon. Usually 3 to 5 cycles provide sufficient experience and knowledge development to transform the intervention, program, or system. An advantage of this planning–acting–reflecting approach to evaluation is the building of capacity to continue an ongoing evaluation process as part of everyday work.

 Critical Thinking Exercise 20.3

Consider the six phases outlined above and develop a CAE evaluation plan for a community health program. How will you incorporate the iterative (cycling) nature of the CAE process? Who are the stakeholders in the evaluation and how will they be engaged?

Evaluation Ethics in CAE

Evaluation ethics (just like research ethics) provide the evaluator with a system of moral values or principles to guide decisions in planning the evaluation process. These principles include conforming to accepted professional standards of conduct.

Ethical principles are particularly important in CAE and other emerging evaluation approaches where participants and their personal data and comments may be readily identifiable. In CAE, for example, ethical evaluation includes respecting the participants or community and honouring their involvement and ownership of the project.

The principles of ethical evaluation deal primarily with ensuring confidentiality and preserving anonymity and volunteerism. Related to these are the principles of privacy, right to know, right to withdraw, conflict of interest, informed consent, responsible gathering of personal data, and responsible reporting of evaluation results.

Confidentiality

Evaluators must describe the process they will use to ensure that information collected will be treated confidentially. Confidentiality can be particularly difficult when working in small communities or with small population groups. In some projects it may not be an issue because of the nature of the collaboration and the project; that is, everyone understands that what is shared in inquiry team meetings is to be held in confidence and they feel comfortable with the information they share in the team's reflection meetings.

Anonymity

Participants may want to remain anonymous to others who have access to the information collected. The researchers must describe how they will ensure that all identifying characteristics of individuals will be removed from the data. Again this can be complicated when the participants are engaged in all aspects of the evaluation process.

Volunteerism

Evaluators have the responsibility to inform participants of their rights to withdraw at any time during the evaluation project without any personal negative consequences.

CAE Methods

Determining an appropriate data collection method for CAE is conceptually quite simple yet quite difficult in practice. The only criterion that a method requires to fit with CAE is that it can be made to be *participatory*. In practice, this leaves some methods wanting, as they seem almost impossible to make participatory. However, many of the more accessible and more widely practised methods for data collection and analysis, can, with some reflection and effort, be transformed into vehicles for true participatory evaluation. For more guidance, the National Collaborating Centre for Methods and Tools has resources to support the use of various methods used in evaluation (NCCMT, 2010). Six methods we often use in our own work are: *observation, qualitative interviews, focus group interviews, document review, journals/ self-reports,* and *narrative accounts of practice* (Hills, 1998).

Data Analysis

In reality, you plan how you are going to analyze the data before you actually collect it. However, in learning the evaluation process, it is helpful to separate data analysis methods from data collection methods and deal with them explicitly.

How you analyze the data is directly related to the method you use to collect the data. For example, if you choose to use interviews to collect data, the appropriate analysis method will be already determined—you will either code the data or do a thematic analysis. There are many articles and books written on this process; van Manen (1990), for example, is one author that provides a useful guide.

It is beyond the scope of this chapter to describe numerous data analysis methods; however, you are encouraged to search the literature and choose any data analysis technique that is congruent with your chosen data collection method(s).

Planning for Dissemination of Results

This stage of evaluation is an important and often neglected aspect of planning the evaluation process. Interpreting and communicating evaluation results are explicitly connected to the purpose of the evaluation and to the stakeholder interests and are influenced by principles of evaluation ethics. Personal and social values influence and possibly bias interpretation of evaluation results. It is therefore important to communicate the evaluation results *according to the needs of each stakeholder.* In other words, customize what should be communicated and how to communicate it for each group of stakeholders. For example, community health workers, evaluators, and policy/decision makers require different kinds of reports to share with their respective audiences. A publishable paper will likely be of little use to a decision maker or a community health worker. It is essential to consider all those who should be informed of the results (e.g., funders, those who initiated the evaluation, evaluation participants and intervention or program participants, decision makers, community leaders, media). The goal of CAE is to change things, so the results must be made available to those who can use them most effectively. It may be another community health worker who deals with similar clients in another context; it may be other practitioners dealing with the same issue in other parts of the country. It could also be program directors or policy makers who can make informed decisions based on the results of good evaluation. While planning for the dissemination of results, remember to discuss and suggest the variety of ways through which these groups can be reached with the results (e.g., community meetings, social media, local radio and television programs, newspaper articles, newsletters, professional association meetings).

Summary

We draw attention to the fact that, although this chapter has spent most of its time on a particular approach to evaluation, CAE, we have covered a multitude of important questions concerning philosophical underpinnings, methodologic rationales, ethical dilemmas, and appropriate procedures for collecting and analyzing evaluation data. We hope that the reader will reflect on how implementing an evaluation strategy that truly brings in the community as partner requires thoughtful planning, careful facilitation, and a real commitment to participation in every aspect of the evaluation process.

REFERENCES

Blome, J. M. (2009). Research vs program evaluation (slide 4). In *Measuring value: Using program evaluation to understand what's working – or isn't.* URL=http://publications.nigms.nih.gov/presentations/measuring_value

Campbell, D. T., & Stanley, J. C. (1966). *Experimental and quasi-experimental designs for research.* Chicago: Houghton Mifflin.

Cook, T. D., & Campbell, D. T. (1979). *Quasi-experimentation: Design and analysis issues for field settings.* Chicago: Rand McNally.

Green, L. W., & Kreuter, M. W. (1991). *Health promotion planning: An educational and environmental approach* (2nd ed.). Mountain View, CA: Mayfield Publishing.

Guba, E. G., & Lincoln, Y. S. (1989). *Fourth generation evaluation.* Newbury Park, CA: Sage.

Heron, J. (1996). *Co-operative inquiry: Research into the human condition.* London: Sage.

Hills, M. (1998). Student experiences of nursing health promotion practice in hospital settings. *Nursing Inquiry, 5*(3), 164–173.

Hills, M., Carroll, S., & Desjardins, S. (2010). Assets based interventions: evaluating and synthesizing evidence of the effectiveness of the assets based approach to health promotion. In A. Morgan, M. Davies, & E. Ziglio, *Health assets in a global context—Theory, methods, action* (pp. 77–98). London: Springer.

Hills, M., & Mullett, J. (2000). *Community-based research and evaluation: Collaborative action for health and social change.* Victoria: Community Health Promotion Coalition.

Hills, M., & Watson, J. (2011). *Creating a caring science curriculum: An emancipatory pedagogy for nursing.* New York, NY: Springer.

National Collaborating Centre for Methods and Tools (NCCMT). (2010). *Program evaluation toolkit* (updated April 29, 2011). Hamilton: McMaster University. URL=http://www.nccmt.ca/registry/view/eng/68.html

National Collaborating Centre for Methods and Tools (NCCMT). (2012). *Evaluation module: CIHR resource.* Hamilton: McMaster University. URL=http://www.nccmt.ca/registry/view/eng/149.html

Patton, M. Q. (1997). *Utilization-focused evaluation: The new century text* (3rd ed.). London: Sage.

Reason, P. (Ed.). (1988). *Human inquiry in action: Developments in new paradigm research.* London: Sage.

Rootman, I., Goodstadt, M., Potvin, L., & Springett, J. (2001). A framework for health promotion evaluation. In I. Rootman, M. Goodstadt, B. Hyndman, D. V. McQueen, L. Potvin, J. Springett, & E. Ziglio (Eds.), *Evaluation in health promotion: Principles and perspectives* (pp. 7–40). Copenhagen: World Health Organization.

Scriven, M. S. (1991). The science of valuing. In W. R. Shadish, Jr., T. D. Cook, & L. C. Leviton, *Foundations of program evaluation: Theories of practice* (pp. 73–118). Newbury, CA: Sage.

van Manen, M. (1990). *Researching lived experience: Human science for an action sensitive pedagogy.* New York, NY: SUNY Press.

W. K. Kellogg Foundation. (1998). *Evaluation handbook.* Battle Creek, MI: Author.

ONLINE RESOURCES

Please visit thePoint at http://thepoint.lww.com/Vollman4e for up-to-date Internet resources and additional learning materials on this topic.

Community as Partner in Practice

This section is intended to serve two purposes: (1) to offer an opportunity to share success stories and (2) to provide readers with case stories on which to reflect. Each author has presented a different story—of one community issue, with one target population, in one particular setting. The stories have been written with the Canadian community-as-partner (CCAP) model in mind, but different components of the process have been emphasized along with different actions of the Ottawa Charter (1986). These stories can be used to apply the model components. For instance, you can ask of each:

- What data represent the *community core?* Embedded within the stories are the social, economic, and demographic data relevant to the population or community of interest.
- What is the *normal line of defence?* Health status data are also contained within each story. Recall that the normal line of defence can be drawn around the core to represent population health status (Pop-NLD) or around the assessment wheel to incorporate the subsystems and represent the community's health (Comm-NLD).
- What *stressors* (risk factors) are acting on the population, and what *lines of resistance* (protective factors) are preventing them from invading the community core? What are the community's strengths and assets?
- What *flexible lines of defence* (temporary responses to risk factors) have been erected to preserve the integrity of the core (population) when stressors have affected the community? What information indicates that the community or population is resilient?

In addition, you can observe, vicariously, the processes undertaken in each of the stories. In each instance, assessment and analytic information are presented. Can you derive community health diagnoses from this information? Can you present these diagnoses as problem statements and as positive statements? If you were involved in this project, how would you have presented diagnostic statements to the community or to funding agencies?

As you read about the various interventions, are you able to determine the logic models inherent in the approach and activities? Are the indicators and evaluation processes coherent?

Throughout each of the stories presented in this section, you will see aspects of the community health worker using the strategies of the Ottawa Charter (1986) and the principles of the Declaration of Alma-Ata (1978) as described in Chapter 1. Can you also detect the issues of culture, diversity, ethics, and advocacy that the professionals faced while working in and with those communities?

Critical reflection is an important component of learning. Reflection demands that we use various lenses to critique what we hear, see, and read. Using lenses of population health promotion (Chapters 1 and 2) and epidemiology and demography (Chapter 4), the authors have presented narratives of community practice that represent advocacy and ethical practice (Chapter 3) based on principles of public participation/engagement (Chapter 5), and accountability through evaluation (Chapter 20).

There are many additional settings and population groups of interest to the Canadian community health worker. This section presents a small number of examples for reflection. It is my hope that it will motivate you to do three things: try new strategies in your community practice, share your stories (successes and challenges) with others, and be inspired to contribute to the next edition of this Canadian publication.

I want to express my deep appreciation to the contributors of these case stories, and also to the people and communities with whom they worked to improve quality of life, reduce disparity, and promote social justice and health equity.

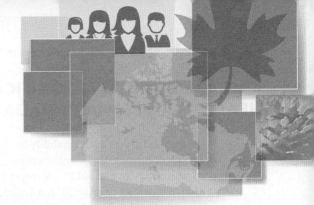

CHAPTER 21

Working With the Community Toward Food Security in Limoilou, Québec City

Sophie Dupéré, André-Anne Parent, Manon Roy, and Gracia Adam

LEARNING OBJECTIVES

After studying this chapter, you should be able to:

1. Understand better how food insecurity is a "wicked" public health problem that is increasing in Canada

2. Appreciate how a certain type of community-based intervention can contribute to addressing food insecurity in the context of an inner-city neighbourhood of Québec City

3. Draw upon the lessons and challenges that emerge from these experiences to improve community development in health promotion

Introduction

Community-based practices are emerging as an alternative to community-placed interventions in the context of complex health and social problems (Minkler & Wallerstein, 2008). They are based on a collaborative process between community members and public health professionals in understanding, identifying, and prioritizing the issues that are important for citizens and their communities. In line with health promotion values, these practices aim to empower citizens in developing solutions that will improve their health, well-being, and living conditions.

The main goal of this chapter is to illustrate this type of practice through two initiatives aimed at improving food security in the inner-city neighbourhood of Limoilou, Québec City, where food insecurity rates are almost three times higher than in wealthier neighbourhoods. After a reminder that food insecurity is a "wicked" public health problem in Canada, we present two projects, highlighting the conceptual components of community development they put in use. Finally, we identify some important challenges emerging from these experiences and reflect upon the lessons we learned from them to improve community development practices.

FOOD INSECURITY: A SIGNIFICANT SOCIAL AND PUBLIC HEALTH PROBLEM IN CANADA

Food insecurity, that is, the inability to obtain or consume quality food in sufficient quantity, in socially acceptable ways, or the uncertainty of being able to do so (Davis & Tarasuk, 1994 as cited in Health Canada, 2012), is a surprisingly serious problem considering the level of wealth in Canada. Indeed, in May 2012, a United Nations Special Rapporteur on the Right to Food examined Canada's situation and was alarmed by the high rates and the severity of household food insecurity. He also denounced the absence of a national food strategy designed to address this human right (UN, 2012).

In 2012, approximately 12% of Canadians experienced moderate or severe food insecurity, which is one in eight households representing 2.8 million individuals including 1.6 million children (Tarasuk et al., 2014). It is a problem that has been increasing in recent years in every province and territory, with the exception of Newfoundland and Labrador (Tarasuk et al., 2013). Québec is not spared; in 2011–2012, 8% of households experienced severe or moderate food insecurity (Maisonneuve et al., 2014). In 2006, in the Limoilou neighbourhood of Québec City, 20.4% of people met or feared to meet food supply difficulties as compared to 7.8% in the wealthier suburb of Sainte-Foy-Sillery-Laurentien (CSSSVC, 2011). Considering that food insecurity has increased in the whole province since then (Maisonneuve et al., 2014), and as observed daily in the continual increase in the use of food banks, it is clear that the situation has worsened in that neighbourhood as elsewhere.

Food insecurity is a growing global problem even in high income countries, with well-recognized consequences on the health and well-being of people and communities. It is considered by many to be a major health determinant (McIntyre & Rondeau, 2009; Mikkonen & Raphael, 2011). Given this context, there have been many attempts by policy makers and public health officials all over the world, including in Canada and Québec, to address this issue (MSSS, 2008). Food insecurity poses significant challenges and is even considered by some authors to be a "wicked" public health problem (McNeill, 2011; Signal et al., 2013) due notably to its complexity and the multi-layered causal factors involved at the individual, group, and social levels (see Boxes 21.1 and 21.2).

Many factors relating to the physical, economic, political, and sociocultural environments contribute to food insecurity (Gorton et al., 2010; Dupéré et al., 2014) making it a highly complex and dynamic issue with no simple solution (Signal et al., 2013). Food security is not just a matter of money to acquire food as can be seen in Box 21.3.

Given what is at stake, interventions that impact people and families as well as diverse environments, from local to global, are usually required to fight food insecurity

---

Box 21.1   What Is a "Wicked" Public Health Problem?

Wicked problems are particularly complex, persistent, and hard-to-resolve. They are commonly encountered in public policy work, and notably within the public health sector. For them the usual linear approaches are not amenable to straightforward solutions. Wicked problems are generally distinguished from tame and complex ones. With *tame* problems, the definition is fairly clear and agreed upon and the point at which they are solved is clear. *Complex* problems are ones where stakeholders agree on the nature of the problem, but not on the solutions. In contrast wicked problems lack agreement on both a definition and a solution, while tames ones find agreement on both.

(Hunter, 2009; Morrison, 2013)

Box 21.2   Definition of Food Insecurity

There are three categories of household food insecurity:

- Households experiencing *marginal* food insecurity reported one food-insecure condition.
- Households experiencing *moderate* food insecurity reported compromise in quality and/or quantity of food consumed among adults and/or children.
- Households experiencing *severe* food insecurity reported reduced food intake and disrupted eating patterns among adults and/or children.
  (PROOF website: http://nutritionalsciences.lamp.utoronto.ca/food-insecurity/)

(Gorton et al., 2010; Dupéré et al., 2014). However, certain authors have questioned the effectiveness of community-based initiatives across Canada to address the problem, advocating primarily for interventions based on structural changes through social policy (PROOF, 2015). Even if policy is tantamount, we believe that to be effective "involving communities affected by food insecurity in research and policy advocacy is critical for linking healthy policy with people's everyday experiences" (FoodARC, 2015, "Community Learning and Development," para. 1), and it is why, through two types of community-based practices, we have developed the initiatives described below.

FIGHTING FOOD INSECURITY THROUGH TWO TYPES OF COMMUNITY-BASED PRACTICES

In the following section, two types of community-based practices are presented—support for the development of communities and the *Sécuribouffe Initiative,* along with an illustration of the activities that emerged from these practices.

In 2003, Québec public health authorities adopted the "Support for the Development of Communities" (SDC) strategy in order to influence actions at the provincial, regional, and local levels (Ministère de la Santé et des Services Sociaux [MSSS], 2008). At the local level, its implementation was given to community organizers who have long practised local and community development in *Centres locaux de services communautaires* (CLSC), the local public health facilities in the province (Parent et al., 2012). The SDC is based on five core concepts: participation of individuals and local communities; empowerment; consensus-building and partnership; reduction of poverty and inequities; and harmonization and promotion of healthy public policies (Leroux & Ninacs, 2002).

Box 21.3   Issues to Address to Ensure Food Security

- Everyone has, at all times, physical and economic access to sufficient food for an active and healthy life.
- The ability to acquire food is guaranteed for everybody.
- Access to simple, reliable, and objective information is ensured so everybody can make informed choices.
- Food is nutritionally adequate and acceptable at the personal and cultural levels.
- Food is obtained in a manner that respects human dignity.
- Consumption and food production are based on social values that are fair, equitable, and moral.
- Food is produced and distributed in a manner respectful of a sustainable food system.
  (MSSS, 2008)

Community participation and empowerment specifically aimed at increasing people's control over their lives and the resources of the community are at the heart of the SDC strategy as per the community-based practices advocated by Minkler et al. (2008). In the area of food security, participation in the planning of activities by citizens, especially those experiencing food insecurity, enhances the success of those activities in reducing food insecurity (Kirkpatrick & Tarasuk, 2009). Hence, the SDC and its core concepts seemed appropriate for action on food insecurity in Limoilou.

Inspired by the core concepts associated with the SDC strategy, the *Sécuribouffe* project was launched in 2008 when a Limoilou food aid organization, *La Bouchée généreuse,* wanted to fight food insecurity beyond the food distribution services they provided. *Sécuribouffe*'s main intention was to explore the needs of the community (particularly for people with few resources) in connection with a healthy diet. The expected outcome was the development of concrete projects to promote healthy eating as well as to foster individual and community empowerment in relation to food security.

From the start there was a strong desire to develop a project rooted in the SDC strategy that, among other things, took the form of a monitoring committee of five local stakeholders, including two citizens accessing the services of *La Bouchée généreuse,* a community organization whose mission is to improve the living environment and the food security of people living in poverty in the region of Québec City. A CLSC community organizer and a community worker from *La Bouchée généreuse* were also involved on a part-time basis for three years. Seed money in the amount of $75,000 over three years was secured from a special budget of the regional public health agency.

The first step was to listen to and engage with the local people through the establishment of new activities (two community kitchens [see Fig. 21.1] and one food purchasing group

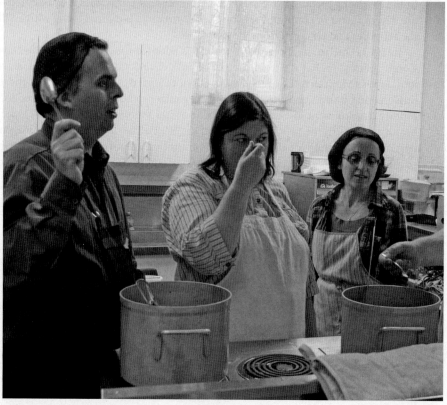

FIGURE 21.1 Collective kitchen.

of 40 members) as well as the use of already existing activities (food tastings and nutritional information sessions). Out of discussions the idea of sharing tips and recipes led to the collective production of a cookbook of easy recipes suitable for small budgets. It generated a lot of pride and empowerment, fostering the interest of participants to get more involved.

This prompted a second wave of action that explicitly pursued specific goals: decrease social isolation and build relationships; develop new skills, including those related to cooking; increase purchasing power for food; eat well with a low budget; and improve health. The activities included: (1) a competition among the recipients of food aid to find a logo for *Sécuribouffe;* (2) a discussion group on the issues raised by food aid; (3) cooking workshops on various topics chosen by participants or specifically adapted for children (5 to 11 years old), with the latter leading to the production of another cookbook designed by and for children; (4) a major collective dinner for Christmas (over 100 people) to celebrate and socialize in an intercultural way (turkey and halal meat); (5) two additional community kitchens: an intercultural one and one for teens; (6) initiation to neighbourhood community gardens; (7) a container gardening project, making use of people's balconies; and (8) a walking club.

The common thread of all these activities was community-identified needs and a commitment to action. *Sécuribouffe* was able to build on, and contribute to, the more general SDC process that was going on in the neighbourhood, addressing other priorities of the community beyond food security (e.g., safety on bike paths, decontamination of polluted grounds). All stages of the activities (needs assessment, planning, and evaluation) were carried out in a participatory manner. The *Sécuribouffe* monitoring committee met regularly to keep track of activities and ensure that they were within the terms of reference of the funding agency. It kept an analytical look at both the outcomes (what was achieved) and the process (how it was done) in order to be able to learn and reflect as the activities unfolded and to react quickly and readjust as needed.

In 2012, the *Sécuribouffe* monitoring committee was transformed into a larger and new team called *À Limoilou, la sécurité alimentaire on en fait notre affaire.* This team realized that a key need pertained to the physical and financial lack of access to fresh fruit and vegetables. This was also a finding of the VAATAVEC research project (discussed later) as well as an explicit concern of other community groups. This need triggered the *P'tit marché solidaire de Limoilou.* Launched in the summer of 2013, this is a mini market offering at low cost fresh fruit and vegetables discarded by farmers because of their appearance through a small fixed stall and two mobile stalls propelled by bicycles (see Fig. 21.2). Limoilou was fertile soil for such a market to take root and grow due to *Securibouffe,* VAATAVEC, and other local initiatives. Some people involved in this market project had also been involved in the beginning of *Sécuribouffe.*

To conclude, Table 21.1 summarizes some of the main challenges and lessons that emerged at *Sécuribouffe* in relation to the key conceptual elements put forward by the SDC.

COMMUNITY-BASED PARTICIPATORY RESEARCH

Community-based participatory action research (CBPAR) has emerged in the last decades, in health promotion as in other fields, as a transformative research paradigm that bridges the gap between science and practice through community engagement and social action in order to increase health equity (Minkler & Wallerstein, 2008).

The CBPAR project about food security and the fight against poverty described below is a "bottom-up" one as it emerged from the request of twenty local stakeholders in the Limoilou and Charlevoix neighbourhoods who contacted two academic researchers. The researchers were successful in getting a grant in the amount of $73,680 for three years through one of the major peer-reviewed granting agencies in Québec.

In this project, three types of actors interacted constantly: academics (including graduate students); community health workers; and people experiencing poverty. A key concept in this

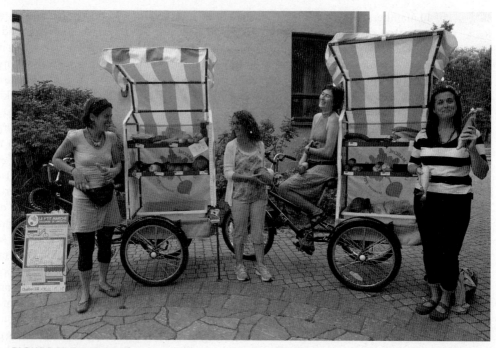

FIGURE 21.2   Mini market.

TABLE 21.1   Challenges and Lessons Learned in the *Sécuribouffe* Project According to Some Principles of the SDC

Principles	Challenges	Lessons Learned
Participation and empowerment	• mobilize the most disenfranchised people • many people have multiple problems • the involved citizens are often the same • tensions existing between citizens and/or organizations outside the project • involved citizens need to go beyond seeing themselves as volunteers working for the professionals and claim more ownership of the project • dealing with failures	• take the time to build the community confidence in the project through sustained individualized contacts • always be willing to integrate new citizens as they show up • at the outset, use the channels and organizations already well known in the community • adopt a little step by little step strategy • try a variety of approaches to mobilize citizens • build on the notoriety of small successes in the community • consciously put in place mechanisms fostering participation • foster mutual aid among the local citizens • acknowledge and celebrate each success
Partnerships/ Intersectoral action	• mobilize actors not used to working together • for individuals, refine their multi-tasking skills • for organizations, push the usual boundaries set by their respective missions despite their respective workloads	• the importance of being able to integrate new interested organizations • the importance of adopting a common vision beyond the various thematic boundaries of each organizations • using an asset-based approach and building on the strengths of the various stakeholders • having a realistic expectations about the involvement of the various partners • step by step strategy
Influencing public policies	• capacity to generate long time funding for these types of projects • feeling of powerlessness by the local citizens toward the more global structural issues • make people realize that reducing social inequities and poverty is an upstream major determinant of food insecurity	• engage dialogue with funders (in this case public health!) so they can understand the context of community development projects and allow budget flexibility • engage local leaders to ensure stability and duration of projects over time • engage with local decision makers

approach was that the respective knowledge of all actors was considered as equal and complementary to understanding the situation and acting upon it. All members of the research team shared the same concerns about the nonutilization of food assistance services by many people who were in need of them and questioned the structural factors influencing food insecurity. Moreover, the researchers were conscious of the fact that people living in poverty have limited access to food and that their voices are rarely heard.

The VAATAVEC (*Vers une autonomie alimentaire pour toutes: Agir et vivre ensemble le changement*) had three objectives: to increase the understanding, *with* socially excluded people, about their food access strategies and about the structural factors linked to these strategies; to explore with a variety of stakeholders (professionals, community decision makers, food industry, people living in poverty) possible lines of action to improve services, programs, and policies to ensure food security for all; and to document the impact of the CBPAR methodology as used in VAATAVEC.

The governance of the project was designed to include the three types of actors mentioned above and comprised a research team (four women living in poverty, two community health workers, and two researchers) that met weekly for two years and a larger research advisory committee (25 partners involved in the project) that met monthly. In order to ensure the input from the people affected, innovative strategies were applied throughout the project [e.g., participatory mapping (Dupéré et al., 2014)].

In our society, scientific research is seen by many as a credible source of knowledge and it can provide legitimacy to information coming from other sources often considered less legitimate, such as people's experiences, in order to assess needs and establish evidence-based interventions. In addition to generating scientific knowledge, VAATAVEC has thus far produced several benefits (i.e., capacity building and social change), illustrating once more how CBPAR can be an important tool for community development.

The project helped stakeholders expand their thinking about food security and the fight against poverty as well as produce an alternative concept to food security—food autonomy (Bélisle et al., 2015). It confirmed the lines of work of several organizations and nurtured intersectoral action, notably at the Quebec City Regional Coordination Table on Food Security, as well as in local activities such as the *Securibouffe* project described previously. It also allowed greater engagement with actors that are generally more difficult to mobilize, such as elected officials and representatives from the food business. Furthermore, the project helped to build bridges among organizations struggling against poverty, those concerned with food insecurity, the ecologic movement, and civic agriculture groups.

Moreover, as an unexpected (and unfunded) benefit, VAATAVEC helped to systematize participatory strategies to work with people in poverty situations. Research team members who lived in poverty situations strongly advocated for the production of a manual describing these strategies (Collectif VAATAVEC, 2014), and it was widely disseminated. Finally, the empowerment experience of the four research team members who were nonacademics and not community health workers has been very significant: one is back in school and the other three are involved in a variety of projects in the community.

Some challenges faced by the project, as well as the key lessons learned are summarized in Table 21.2.

CHALLENGES AND LESSONS LEARNED: GOING BEYOND FOOD SECURITY

As already shown in Tables n.21.1 and 21.2, community health workers and researchers face several challenges when using community-based engagement to fight food insecurity. We offer more general reflections about two of the main challenges associated with such practices.

TABLE 21.2   Challenges and Lessons Learned in the *VAATAVEC* Project According to the Principles of SDC

Principles	Challenges	Lessons Learned
Participation and empowerment	Difficulties in recruiting and sustaining participation of people living in poverty for the project due to: • harsh living conditions (e.g., no phone to follow-up; problems of transportation to attend meetings) • social stigma linked to poverty (e.g., people insulted to have been targeted as "poor" when approached to participate)	• establish and maintain reciprocal and trusting relationships with the participants as key to eliciting meaningful participation and negotiate a precise collaboration agreement • use a variety of strategies to stimulate participation (e.g., perform a stakeholder analysis to understand the dynamics of the communities and identify gatekeepers; "peers recruit peers") • remain sensitive to the participants' needs: no one size fits all approach • provide opportunities for the expression of suffering and offer support • ensure that all members have the tools and knowledge to participate effectively and are provided training or equipment as needed (Collectif VAATAVEC, 2014)
Partnerships/ Intersectoral action	• negotiating the various visions and expectations about the project • dealing with power relationships • engaging with partners not usually included in public health tables (e.g., businesses, food industry)	• understand the local power relationships so as to include marginalized citizens (usefulness of theory and literature) • put forward an iterative process with transparent decision making at each stage • maintain realistic expectations (e.g., do not expect a small business person to come for a full day focus group) • step by step strategy • strong leadership at the table that helped mobilize resources—finding the right person to bring to the table
Influencing public policies	• legitimacy and funding of PAR projects • the difficulty in this place and time of conveying in Canada and Québec that the core issue is fighting poverty and inequities • translating the research findings in a language appropriate for decision makers and concrete policy actions	• building relationships with local policy makers to spark and maintain their interest in the project and garner their support (ideally they should have a role in the research project) • develop a better knowledge of the policy and political contexts (include a policy analyst in the team)

Triggering and Maintaining Community Participation and Empowerment

It can be challenging to engage community participation, especially the ones in which marginalized and socially isolated people live. Food insecurity is frequently accompanied by stigmatization and exclusion of citizenship processes (Pine & de Souza, 2013) and therefore requires innovative outreach strategies. It can also be challenging to sustain the authentic participation of the most marginalized people, beyond the token role to which they are too often confined. The VAATAVEC guide provides several participatory strategies that can help address both of these challenges (Collectif VAATAVEC, 2014).

While participatory processes comprise the basis of empowerment, participation alone is insufficient if building the capacities of community organizations and people (Wallerstein, 2006) is not taken into account. Among many others, Ninacs (2008) has reminded us that the individual empowerment process emerges from the interweaving of four components: participation, abilities, self-esteem, and critical consciousness, with each evolving along a continuum of its own. The community empowerment process also has four interwoven components: participation, knowledge and ability, communication, and community capital (Ninacs, 2008). As argued by authors in health promotion, social theories are grossly underused to understand the social processes underlying participation, and they could be very illuminating in the matter (Potvin, 2007; Marent et al., 2012).

Finally, while participatory research and community development projects do not automatically eliminate social or economic divides, they are at least conscious of them and usually put forward explicit mechanisms to address them (Pine & de Souza, 2013; Knezevic et al., 2014). A major challenge for the future is how public health agencies in Canada, especially at the local level, will be able to develop and maintain meaningful participatory processes (especially with socially marginalized citizens and communities) in a context where they are themselves undergoing significant organizational change in a climate where the fight against inequalities and inequities is not on the agenda of governments.

Facing Complexity

The factors that contribute to food insecurity, as well as to most other "wicked" problems, are numerous and interdependent, creating the need to develop capacity to embrace complexity. The solutions to "wicked" problems do not lie within the boundaries or responsibilities of any single organization. The involvement of a much broader range of stakeholders than those who are usually brought to the table is required. Public health would benefit from the explicit use of theories and frameworks that take complexity into account, such as ecologic models (Richard et al., 2011) or the complexity paradigm (Tremblay & Richard, 2011).

A participative approach that embraces complexity means that one must accept a certain amount of uncertainty. Community health workers implementing CBPAR will be confronted at the outset with the fact that much will remain unclear and undefined and that they might have to do things completely unforeseen. For example, even if the local community organizer never thought she would have to deliver potatoes during her office hours, she had to do so from time to time in order to have the *Sécuribouffe* project run smoothly!

Summary

Both *Sécuribouffe* and VAATAVEC are bottom-up initiatives that emerged from citizens and local actors with input from community organizers and researchers. They show how a community-based participatory action approach can contribute to better understanding of the problem and identification of possible solutions to the problem with the people that experience it, and strengthen community capacity to address the problem. The two initiatives also illustrate the challenges associated with using such an approach when addressing a "wicked" public health problem.

REFERENCES

Bélisle, M., Labarthe, J., Moreau, C., Landry, E., Adam, G., Bourque, M., et al. (2015). Repenser ensemble le concept d'autonomie alimentaire. *Global Health Promotion*, pii: 1757975915585499.

Centre de santé et de services sociaux de la Vieille-Capitale (CSSSVC). (2011). *Portrait de défavorisation du territoire du centre de santé et de services sociaux de la Vieille-Capitale*. Québec: Author.

Collectif VAATAVEC. (2014). *L'AVEC, pour faire ensemble. Un guide de pratiques, de réflexions et d'outils*. Québec: FRQSC. URL=http://www.pauvrete.qc.ca/IMG/pdf/Guide_VAATAVEC.pdf

Dupéré, S., Gélineau, L., Adam, G., Côté, M., Dufour, É., Dumas, A., et al. (2014). Vers une autonomie alimentaire pour toutes: Agir et vivre ensemble le changement (AVEC). *Rapport scientifique*. Québec: FRQSC.

FoodARC. (2015). *FoodARC projects: Activating change together for community food security (ACT for CFS)*. URL=http://foodarc.ca/project-pages/activities-resources/

Gorton, D., Bullen, C. R., & Mhurchu, C. N. (2010). Environmental influences on food security in high-income countries. *Nutrition Reviews, 68*(1), 1–29.

Health Canada. (2012). *Household food insecurity in Canada: Overview*. Ottawa: Author. URL=http://www.hc-sc.gc.ca/fn-an/surveill/nutrition/commun/insecurit/index-eng.php

Hunter, D. J. (2009). Leading for health and wellbeing: The need for a new paradigm. *Journal of Public Health (Oxf)*, *31*(2), 202–204. doi:10.1093/pubmed/fdp036

Kirkpatrick, S., & Tarasuk, V. (2009). Food insecurity and participation in community food programs among low-income Toronto families. *Canadian Journal of Public Health, 100*(2), 135–139.

Knezevic, I., Hunter, H., Watt, C., Williams, P., & Anderson, B. (2014). Food insecurity and participation: A critical discourse analysis. *Critical Discourse Studies, 11*(2), 230–245.

Leroux, R., & Ninacs, W. A. (2002). *La santé des communautés: Perspectives pour la contribution de la santé publique au développement social et au développement des communautés. Revue de littérature.* Québec: INSPQ, Gouvernement du Québec.

Maisonneuve, C., Blanchet, C., & Hamel, D. (2014). *L'insécurité alimentaire dans les ménages québécois: Mise à jour et évolution de 2005 à 2012.* Québec: INSPQ, Gouvernement du Québec.

Marent, B., Foster, R., & Nowak, P. (2012). Theorizing participation in health promotion: A literature review. *Social Theory & Health, 10*, 188–207.

McIntyre, L., & Rondeau, K. (2009). Food insecurity. In D. Raphael (Ed.), *Social determinants of health: Canadian perspectives* (2nd ed., pp. 188–204). Toronto: Canadian Scholars' Press.

McNeill, K. (2011). *Talking with their mouths half full: Food insecurity in the Hamilton community (Doctoral dissertation).* New Zealand: University of Waikato.

Mikkonen, J., & Raphael, D. (2011). *Déterminants sociaux de la santé: Les réalités canadiennes.* Toronto: École de gestion et de politique de la santé de l'Université York.

Ministère de la Santé et des Services Sociaux (MSSS). (2008). *Cadre de référence en matière de sécurité alimentaire.* URL=http://publications.msss.gouv.qc.ca/acrobat/f/documentation/2008/08-208-01.pdf

Minkler, M., & Wallerstein, N. (Eds.). (2008). *Community-based participatory research for health: From process to outcomes.* San Francisco: John Wiley & Sons Publishers.

Minkler, M., Wallerstein, N., & Wilson, N. (2008). Improving health through community organization and community building. In K. Glanz, B. K. Rimer, & K. Vismanath (Eds.), *Health behavior and health education: Theory, research, and practice* (pp. 565–485). San Francisco: Jossey-Bass.

Morrison, V. (2013). *Wicked problems and public policy.* Montréal: National Collaborating Centre for Healthy Public Policy. URL=http://www.ncchpp.ca/130/publications.ccnpps?id_article=927

Ninacs, W. A. (2008). *Empowerment et intervention.* Québec: PUL.

Parent, A.-A., O'Neill, M., Roy, B., & Simard, P. (2012). Entre santé publique et organisation communautaire: Points de convergence et de divergence autour du développement des communautés au Québec. *Revue de l'Université de Moncton, 43*(1–2), 67–90.

Pine, A. M., & de Souza, R. (2013). Including the voices of communities in food insecurity research: An empowerment-based agenda for food scholarship. *Journal of Agriculture, Food Systems, and Community Development, 3*(4), 71–79.

Potvin, L. (2007). Managing uncertainty through participation. In D. V. McQueen, I. Kickbush, L. Potvin, J. M. Pelikan, L. Balbo, & T. Abel (Eds.), *Health and modernity. The role of theory in health promotion* (pp. 103–128). New York, NY: Springer.

PROOF (Research to identify policy options to reduce food insecurity). (2015). *Food insecurity.* URL=http://nutritionalsciences.lamp.utoronto.ca/food-insecurity/

Richard, L., Gauvin, L., & Raine, K. (2011). Ecological models revisited: Their uses and evolution in health promotion over two decades. *Annual Review of Public Health, 32*, 307–326.

Signal, L. N., Walton, M. D., Ni, M., Maddison, R., Bowers, S. G., Carter, K. N., et al. (2013). Tackling "wicked" health promotion problems: A New Zealand case study. *Health Promotion International, 28*(1), 84–94.

Tarasuk, V., Mitchell, A., & Dachner, N. (2013). *Household food insecurity in Canada 2011.* Toronto: Research to identify policy options to reduce food insecurity (PROOF). URL=http://nutritionalsciences.lamp.utoronto.ca/resources/proof-annual-reports/annual-report/

Tarasuk, V., Mitchell, A., & Dachner, N. (2014). *Household food insecurity in Canada 2012.* Toronto: Research to identify policy options to reduce food insecurity (PROOF). URL=http://nutritionalsciences.lamp.utoronto.ca/resources/proof-annual-reports/annual-report-2012/

Tremblay, M.-C., & Richard, L. (2011). Complexity: A potential paradigm for a health promotion discipline. *Health Promotion International, 29*(2), 378–388. doi: 10.1093/heapro/dar054

United Nations (UN). (2012). *Olivier De Schutter, Special Rapporteur on the Right to Food: Visit to Canada from 6 to 16 May 2012.* URL=http://www.srfood.org/images/stories/pdf/officialreports/201205_canadaprelim_en.pdf

Wallerstein, N. (2006). *What is the evidence on effectiveness of empowerment to improve health? (Health Evidence Network report).* Copenhagen: WHO Regional Office for Europe. URL=http://www.euro.who.int/__data/assets/pdf_file/0010/74656/E88086.pdf

ONLINE RESOURCES

Please visit thePoint at http://thepoint.lww.com/Vollman4e for up-to-date Internet resources and additional learning materials on this topic.

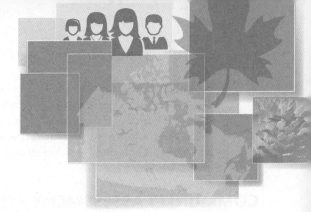

CHAPTER 22

Youth Engagement in Community Planning

Laura Ryan, Sharon Mackinnon, and Alexandria Crowe

LEARNING OBJECTIVES

After studying this chapter, you should be able to:

1. Detail the process of Photovoice as a means for community engagement

2. Discuss how and why community health workers use intersectoral partnerships to create changes in population health through community engagement

Introduction

Community engagement is a recognized process for getting citizens involved in decisions that affect them (Chapter 5). Public participation can be used to inform, communicate, educate, solicit feedback, and work in partnership. Neighbourhood planning can include various forms of community engagement. In this case story, we describe how youth were engaged through photography to give voice to how they feel about their neighbourhoods and what improvements they would like to see implemented.

HAMILTON'S NEIGHBOURHOODS

Hamilton is a post-industrial city with a population of 519,949 (Statistics Canada, 2011). The Niagara Escarpment runs through the middle of the city, separating the lower city and its brown-field industrial belt from the city above the escarpment. To a local, the escarpment is referred to as "the mountain," and for many it unfairly represents both a geographical, economic, and social divide among neighbourhoods. The geography of the mountain is an emotional barrier that unfairly generalizes those living across its peak as socially and economically strong, and those in its shadow as suffering with poverty and crime.

All of the neighbourhoods of Hamilton boast assets, and all struggle to meet their residents' needs. It is because of greater general need in the lower city and core that residents have been cast this way; these same struggles in the mountain neighbourhoods have been rendered nearly invisible.

A number of lower city neighbourhoods house residents that are vulnerable to low income, joblessness, homelessness, and low high school graduation rates. "The primary factors that shape the health of Canadians are not medical treatments or lifestyle choices but rather the living conditions they experience. These conditions have come to be known as the social determinants of health" (Mikkonen & Raphael, 2010, p. 8).

COMMUNITY ASSESSMENT

In 2010, a series entitled "Code Red Hamilton" was published in the *Hamilton Spectator* comparing the life and health outcomes in a number of suburban neighbourhoods to those in the lower city. Life expectancy differences as great as 21 years between some neighbourhoods were reported (Buist, 2010). "Those neighbourhoods with high rates of emergency room visits, no family physician, respiratory-related problems and psychiatric emergencies are the same neighbourhoods, in general, that have the lowest median incomes, lowest dwelling values, highest rates of people living below the poverty line and highest dropout rates from school" (Buist, 2010, para. 27).

The newspaper series started a citywide conversation around the social determinants of health. The City of Hamilton responded by establishing its Neighbourhood Action Strategy (NAS) to work on addressing disparities. The city partnered with and expanded the Hamilton Community Foundation project *Tackling Poverty Together*. This project sought to engage the residents living within low-income neighbourhoods to establish planning teams and then to create neighbourhood master plans aimed at addressing the risks to health and life expectancy. This newly expanded *Tackling Poverty Together* initiative wove the goals developed by existing planning teams into work plans and budget lines across various city departments.

Community developers worked as part of *Tackling Poverty Together* and the NAS in 11 neighbourhoods (see Fig. 22.1) to engage existing resident groups and establish groups

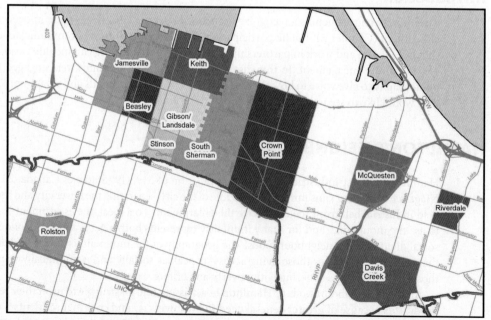

FIGURE 22.1 Hamilton's Neighbourhood Action Strategy Boundaries, showing the Riverdale and Rolston communities. (Reprinted with permission from the Social Planning and Research Council of Hamilton.)

where none existed. The NAS is a resident-led process of community building. Multi-sector planning teams assess their neighbourhoods and write action plans for improving the health of residents. Residents develop asset maps (i.e., strengths) of their neighbourhoods. Quite naturally and intuitively, ideas for change and improvement start to emerge. One of the consistent challenges of these teams was the need for more diverse voices among participants. Many of the plans lacked youth participation, an important perspective that would add to the NAS planning process. A Photovoice project was initiated as a means of inviting youth engagement.

THE PROJECT

"Photovoice is a participatory action research strategy based on health promotion principles" that can be used to give voice to populations and help bring about change in their communities (Wang, 2006, p. 148). Through photographs, participants can be engaged in shaping how they would like to see their community (Wang, 2006). There is a history of using Photovoice as a means of public engagement in Hamilton. Photovoice became an obvious tool to begin expanding the reach of the NAS more deeply into community by validating, enhancing, and identifying emerging issues from developing and existing Neighbourhood Action Plans.

The settings for the Photovoice project were two neighbourhoods in the city of Hamilton: Riverdale and Rolston. According to Neighbourhood Profiles from the Social Planning and Research Council of Hamilton (SPRC), Riverdale has the highest proportion of recent immigrants in Hamilton and 25% of Rolston residents identify with a visible minority (compared to 14% in Hamilton overall). Riverdale and Rolston have high rates of poverty: 35% of the population in both neighbourhoods compared to 18% for Hamilton overall. Additionally in both neighbourhoods 49% of the children under the age of six are living in poverty compared to 26% for Hamilton overall (SPRC, 2012).

The target population for the Photovoice project was youth residing in Riverdale and Rolston who reflected the diverse linguistic, cultural, and religious characteristics of their neighbourhood. The Riverdale youth participants came from two sites: an elementary school ($n = 12$) and a secondary school ($n = 12$). The Rolston youth participants came from three sites: an elementary school ($n = 12$), a middle school ($n = 12$), and a Community House ($n = 18$). The Community House is a single town house unit within a geared-to-income housing complex used for community activities.

The five sites were chosen because there was existing programming in place with leadership committed to supporting the participants during and after the project and because the sites themselves are institutions of importance to the residents of each community. The staff and leaders at these sites assisted the Photovoice project facilitators to select and retain participants, organized logistics for the project, and became change makers for ideas that involved their locations.

Wang (2006) identifies nine steps to implement Photovoice; these steps were used as a framework for our project and are outlined in our Logic Model (Table 22.1).

1. **Select and recruit a target audience of policy makers or community leaders.**
    Photovoice projects are extremely rewarding to participate in, but are not complete until the ideas generated are passed on to community stakeholders who are able to address the concerns raised. Public Health Services (PHS), the SPRC, and NAS are positioned to have extraordinary reach into local government, services, programs, agencies, and organizations. The NAS, because it is positioned within the City of Hamilton and the Hamilton Community Foundation, has a knowledge base to identify resources to fund projects. The many community stakeholder organizations that are members of the planning teams are able to work alongside residents to design and execute projects.

TABLE 22.1 Logic Model for Photovoice in Riverdale and Rolston

Inputs	Outputs			Outcomes-Impact	
	Activities	*Participation*	*Short Term*	*Medium Term*	*Long Term*
What we invest	**What we do**	**Who we reach**	**What the short term results are**	**What the medium term results are**	**What the long term results are**
Students	Partner with school/community leaders	Report results back to the participants and peers	Presentation to the school community at assemblies	Nursing students reported results back to Public Health and Neighbourhood Action Strategy	Impact decision makers within City Council
Parents	Facilitate the process by recruiting participants and obtaining permission	Presentation to the Community Planning Team	Display to school	Created toolkit for communities to use Photovoice for their own populations	Development of a planning work group to move issues forward
School staff (teachers/principal)	Education session with nursing students on process and roles throughout	Nursing students report to Public Health and Neighbourhood Action Strategy	Empower youth leadership attributes	Establishment of a Youth Committee from Photovoice	
Public Health Nurse	Instructional session for participants prior to photo taking	Delegation to City Council and senior staff at General Issues Committee (GIC)	Develop/Foster partnerships with nexus of all involved local leaders	Students validated the existing plans or contribute to a new plan	
Community Developer	Supervised photo taking and journaling	Video of GIC publicly available on YouTube.com	Reinforcing the concerns of present strategy plans or develop new plans	Enhancing physical appearance of environment at Community	
Nursing students	Determining themes from the results and then reporting the themes back to the students to confirm the meaning	Art shows and displays at community events		Housing geared to income housing	
Physical supplies of cameras, banners, and central locations					
Vendors/Exhibitors of results					

2. **Recruit a group of Photovoice participants.**

   Recruitment involves gathering a team of facilitators as well as enlisting participants. The team was co-led by a Community Developer (CD) from the SPRC and a Public Health Nurse (PHN) from the PHS. The team included four nursing students from the McMaster University School of Nursing who were completing a community practicum. The CD and PHN mentored the nursing students throughout the project. The team also included staff members from the five participating sites.

   It was essential that staff members at the project sites assist with the selection of youth participants. The CD met with staff leaders to discuss the goals of the project and requirements of participants, and to get their assistance in generating a list of potential youth to take part in the project. A participant group of 12–15 youth per site was purposively selected from nominees to reflect the diversity in their respective neighbourhoods.

3. **Introduce the Photovoice methodology to participants and facilitate group discussion about cameras, power, and ethics.**

   The CD and PHN met with the nursing students for a full day prior to starting the project to talk about the concepts of Photovoice, community engagement, community development, the social determinants of health, the Ottawa Charter, and logistics for planning and implementing the project. On a subsequent day, the CD and PHN met with the nursing students to do a walkabout in the neighbourhoods of study to familiarize themselves with the areas and identify potential walking routes.

4. **Pose initial theme(s) for taking pictures.**

   The key activities during the first session with participants included introducing the project, asset mapping, and picture taking. During the first session, the CD and PHN introduced the project and then let the nursing students take roles as of primary facilitators. At each site, the session started with an age appropriate icebreaker. The group then moved onto asset mapping in smaller groups of 2–3 participants. Large maps of the neighbourhood were provided by the NAS on which participants were asked to identify assets and needs in addition to mapping key destinations. After each activity, small groups reported their results back to the larger group and common observations and themes were summarized. The mapping exercise helped to inform walking routes for picture taking.

5. **Obtain informed consent.**

   The CD completed the consent process with assistance from administrators and staff at the locations. Youth participants need to have parental/guardian written consent; consent was also obtained to share information, photos, artwork, ideas, and written work for the purpose of promoting project results.

6. **Distribute cameras to participants and review how to use the camera.**

   Cameras were distributed to participants in their groups of two or three to give them the opportunity to familiarize themselves with the functions. Facilitators led a group discussion regarding caution when taking pictures of people and property without permission. Discussions were framed to remind participants to use respectful and inclusive language when describing their community and residents within it.

7. **Provide time for participants to take pictures.**

   Groups dispersed for approximately one hour of picture taking on pre-determined routes. Walkabout routes covered a portion of each neighbourhood, and in some cases were designed to overlap so that several groups had the opportunity to capture photos and discuss areas of particular importance.

   During the walkabout, participants took turns taking pictures and recording observations on a spreadsheet provided. Spreadsheets prompted participants to explain the location, subject, and importance of what they had captured in each photo. These observations became the narrative captions that accompanied images, as well as comprising the list of suggestions brought forward to decision makers.

8. **Meet to discuss photographs and identify themes.**

Between the first and second Photovoice sessions, the nursing students worked with the CD and PHN to extract themes from the pictures and narratives. This activity was done to save some time, recognizing that the process of coding data is sophisticated and would be a difficult task for participants because of their age and developmental stage. The nursing students, with guidance from the PHN and CD, then prepared a presentation to report back to participants to validate the themes.

The key activities during the second session with participants included validation of themes, visioning exercise, prioritizing action items, and presentation back to community. Participants created their ideal vision for the neighbourhood and this vision was used to help prioritize the ideas produced in the asset mapping and photo sessions. Suggestions for action were generated at all stages of the process. Action items were recorded and prioritized in a final exercise. The CD and PHN were able to bring local research knowledge from their respective agencies to share with participants and inform their prioritization exercise. A group vote ranked suggestions in priority order to take to decision makers.

9. **Plan with participants a format to share photographs and stories with policy makers and community leaders.**

Participants selected key photographs and corresponding narratives to represent themes and created a photo gallery exhibit in their neighbourhood. A presentation was also prepared to facilitate reporting back to their communities.

RESULTS OF THE PROJECT

Photovoice projects were managed and celebrated with each participant group, but results were also aggregated by neighbourhood to be used for future planning. The results from each of the five sites in the Riverdale and Rolston neighbourhoods had overlapping themes and in most cases participants identified similar priorities for action. Themes across all five sites included: community health and environment; green space, parks, and open space; interpersonal relationships; and transportation and mobility.

The youth were very conscious of their physical environment. They spoke about the conditions in homes and yards, the activities and behaviour in parks and play spaces, and the sensitivity of the air, greenery, wildlife, and water. Participants at each site produced photos of litter, graffiti, and dumping, and the youth had many ideas about the impact of these features on the people living in and visiting their community.

"[Graffiti] makes us feel unsafe. People might not want to buy houses in this community."

One child expressed concerns regarding graffiti that "spray paint is a pollutant." Another youth suggested that we "need to take care of nature" after finding spray painted graffiti on a tree.

Priority action suggestions included: cleaning up graffiti; creating an art mural; placing more garbage cans in the community; and improving garbage pick-up to address illegal dumping and littering.

Parks, green spaces, landscaped storm catchments, urban forests, and well-manicured private gardens all impressed and inspired the youth; they valued the natural spaces.

"Basketball Court—an asset because it's a place where you can go and be active and have fun with your friends which results in a good health."

A youth described a picture of a butterfly perched on blades of grass in a park: "Nature is beautiful. Parks attract wildlife." Another child described why trees are important: "Then [people] can breathe."

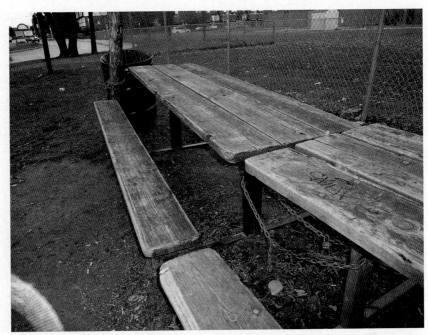

FIGURE 22.2   "During the day moms come to relax. During the night smokers and drunk people come." (Project participant, Neighbourhood Action Strategy, Rolston Neighbourhood 2013.)

There were mixed opinions about the value of an urban forest. Most of the youth did not like to go there alone because of rumoured criminal activity and some unfavourable conditions. "Paths have broken glass. Fires."

Youth participants spoke about the need for stewardship in their community: "We need to take care of nature."

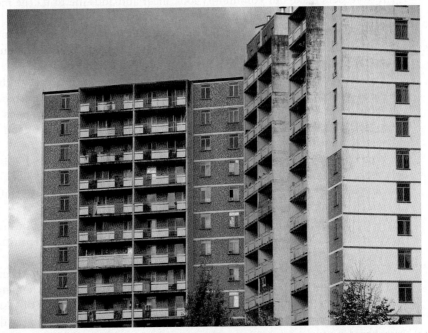

FIGURE 22.3   "The building with new people to Canada [who] are suffering the most." (Project participant, Neighbourhood Action Strategy, Riverdale Neighbourhood 2013.)

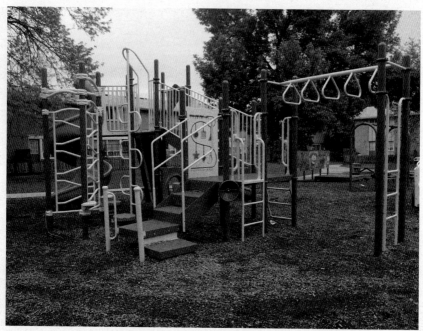

FIGURE 22.4   "[The] park was built with the help of the neighbourhoods…people care about their neighbourhood." (Project participant, Neighbourhood Action Strategy, Rolston Neighbourhood 2013.)

Priority action items developed by participants included: building a tree house; making a soccer field; and adding an outdoor volleyball court.

The most sophisticated observations that the youth made involved interpersonal relationships; there were many stories shared that acknowledged and appreciated a sense of community.

"Bird feeders make our community look nicer and adds life to it. The members of the community should feel safe enough to be able to talk to one another."

"[The recreation centre is] [w]here people come together from the community to enjoy!".

Priority action items suggested by participants included: improving relationships between youth and older adults in the community centre; and addressing bullying.

Transportation and mobility were also common features across each of the sites. While there was concern about safety amid traffic congestion, speed, and road disrepair, there were strengths in the existing transportation features. The two neighbourhoods had excellent parks, sidewalks on most streets, pathways that linked crescents to roads and public spaces, and pedestrian pathways through an urban forest.

"When people drive on the roads [with potholes] it's unsafe because, if it is a big enough hole, a tire could get stuck in it (especially bikes)."

Youth were also concerned about the convenience and safety of pedestrian traffic particularly in winter and inclement weather.

Priority action items developed by participants included: improving bus routes through the communities; improving traffic management around schools; and repairing dirt paths in the playground.

As described earlier, participants identified action items and prioritized them to share with their communities and decision makers. Sharing is a critical piece to wrapping up a Photovoice process. Photography was an effective tool to cultivate sophisticated discussion of change among the youth participants, and between the participants and decision makers. Findings were shared in a variety of venues: art shows, school assemblies, neighbourhood planning meetings, local BBQ, and a delegation to Hamilton City Council's General Issues Committee (GIC).

Regardless of where the results were presented, people were inspired and rallied to address the concerns identified by the youth in their photographs and narratives.

In the Riverdale neighbourhood, the project results were presented by the youth at an assembly dedicated to the topic of citizenship. In the Rolston neighbourhood, the middle school youth, with assistance from the project facilitators, created a report for their school. The school staff were so impressed that a teacher requested that the participants present their results to Hamilton City Council. With the support of school staff and CD, a delegation of 11 participants made a presentation to Hamilton City Council at the General Issues Committee. Their results were received and passed on to relevant departments. The CD was an important conduit as the Photovoice project results made their way through to policy decisions.

Outcomes of this Photovoice process included a rich array of photos and narratives, reports/presentations to the communities, three art displays, a videotape of the delegation's presentation to City Council, a Photovoice toolkit, a Photovoice banner, and a Photovoice poster display to be used at conferences or presentations. Additional outcomes included providing leadership and civic engagement opportunities for youth, and the ability to use the voices of youth to invite adult residents into the planning process. A key strength was the success of the Photovoice process as a method of engaging youth in identifying solutions to develop a healthier community. Findholt et al. (2010) found Photovoice with youth to be an effective method to reach community members and policy makers to advocate for environmental change, and in addition, to provide an opportunity to facilitate youth leadership development. The Ottawa Charter identifies strengthening community action as one of five health promotion actions. In Riverdale, youth participants complemented and reinforced work that adults had already done or were planning to do. In Rolston, youth participants were the first community members to be engaged in the neighbourhood planning process. Their collected data and generated ideas were used to engage decision makers in addressing the needs identified.

Partnering among the NAS, PHS, SPRC, and McMaster University was an additional strength of the Photovoice project. With the Photovoice project completed, the PHN and CD have developed ongoing partnerships with leaders in the participants' neighbourhoods, collected a great deal of data, and leveraged the resources of decision makers to address priorities identified by youth participants. Collaboration across sectors strengthens community capacity to address identified issues. Photovoice is a tool for improving the community health by identifying issues, proposing solutions, prioritizing actions, and sharing results with decision makers for implementation. "At the heart of this process is the empowerment of communities—their ownership and control of their own endeavours and destinies" (WHO, 1986, p. 2).

Summary

We have described a Photovoice project as a method to engage youth in the community planning process; voices that had been missing in many neighbourhood planning efforts. Strengthening community engagement and collaboration across sectors has allowed recommendations to be moved forward as part of the NAS process. Youth participants spoke with loud and clear voices that were heard by many, thereby making their neighbourhoods better for everyone.

Acknowledgements

The Photovoice project described here could not have occurred without all of the participants from both the Riverdale and Rolston neighbourhoods and the level three nursing students from McMaster University. We thank each and every one of you.

REFERENCES

Buist, S. (2010). *Worlds apart. The Hamilton Spectator.* URL=http://www.thespec.com/news-story/2168237-worlds-apart/

Findholt, N. E., Michael, Y. L., & Davis. M. M. (2010). Photovoice engages rural youth in childhood obesity prevention. *Public Health Nursing, 28*(2), 186–192.

Mikkonen, J., & Raphael, D. (2010). *Social determinants of health: The Canadian facts.* Toronto: York University School of Health Policy and Management. URL=http://www.thecanadianfacts.org/

Social Planning and Research Council of Hamilton (SPRC). (2012). *Neighbourhood profiles: Beasley, Crown Point, Jamesville, Keith, Landsdale, McQuesten, Quigley Road, Riverdale, Rolston, South Sherman and Stinson.* URL=http://www.sprc.hamilton.on.ca/wp-content/uploads/2012/03/2012-Report- Neighbourhood_Profiles_March.pdf

Statistics Canada. (2011). *Focus on geography series, 2011 Census.* Census metropolitan area of Hamilton, Ontario. URL=http://www12.statcan.gc.ca/census-recensement/2011/as-sa/fogs-spg/Facts-cma-eng.cfm?LANG =Eng&GK= CMA&GC=537

Wang, C. C. (2006). Youth participation in photovoice as a strategy for community change. *Journal of Community Practice, 14*(1), 147–161.

World Health Organization (WHO). (1986). *The Ottawa charter for health promotion.* Geneva: Author.

ONLINE RESOURCES

Please visit the Point. at http://thepoint.lww.com/Vollman4e for up-to-date Internet resources and additional learning materials on this topic.

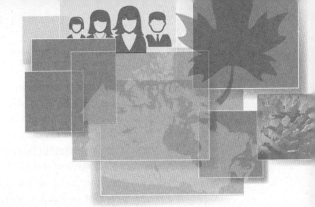

CHAPTER 23

"Together Yet Living Apart": Women Left Behind due to Labour Migration

Christina Murray

LEARNING OBJECTIVES

After studying this chapter, you will be able to:

1. Gain an awareness of outmigration and the factors that contribute to it in Atlantic Canada

2. Identify how being left behind due to labour migration affects women's perceptions of roles and responsibilities within the family unit

3. Recognize how lack of social support can have negative influence on health promotion

4. Understand that creating a supportive environment can promote health

Introduction

Outmigration from Atlantic Canada has become commonplace over the past century as residents from Prince Edward Island (PEI), Nova Scotia, New Brunswick, and Newfoundland and Labrador have left for employment opportunities in other regions of Canada and the United States. In recent decades, there has been a marked rise in the rate of people who have moved away from Atlantic Canada. Of particularly concern has been the increase of youth outmigration. Between 1996 and 2011, 66,000 youth aged 15 to 24 moved from Atlantic Canada for employment in other provinces. From July 2012 to June 2013 alone, 38,812 people moved from Atlantic Canada to other regions of Canada. Ontario and Alberta remain the consistent choices of destination; 77% of Atlantic Canadians who moved from the region from 2000 to 2013 went to one of these provinces (LMSAD, 2014).

For PEI, the negative migration trend has been particularly concerning. Over the past decade, net population losses for PEI have been reported nine out of 10 years. From July 1, 2011 to June 30, 2012, the province experienced a net population loss of 1,252 people. This was the highest rate of outmigration from the province since 1981 (PEI Statistics Bureau, 2013). In

2013–2014, there was a net population loss of 957 people (PEI Statistics Bureau, 2014). The majority of people leaving PEI were migrating to Ontario, Alberta, and Nova Scotia for employment opportunities (PEI Statistics Bureau, 2013; 2014). As of July 1, 2014, the population of PEI was 146,283 (PEI Statistics Bureau, 2014).

In 2012, the federal government instituted changes to the Employment Insurance program that resulted in reduced rates of weekly benefits paid for repeat claimants, a reduction of five weeks of benefits per claimant in a year, a reduction of 50% of allowable earned income while claimants were in receipt of Employment Insurance benefits, and a requirement to accept employment opportunities that were up to a 1-hour commute from the claimant's place of residency (Service Canada, 2013). This was highly problematic for seasonally employed rural residents of PEI who expressed concern that they would be required to travel up to 100 km each way for an employment opportunity that may pay only minimum wage. This federal decision had a devastating impact on many seasonally employed residents in rural PEI, many of whom have worked for generations in industries such as fishing, farming, and tourism. These workers depend on Employment Insurance for income supplementation during periods of time when employment is not available in these industries because of the seasonal nature of such work. Decreased benefit rates coupled with a reduction in the number of weeks being paid per year resulted in economic depression in rural communities. Islanders, politicians, and news reporters believed that these changes to the Employment Insurance program were the catalyst behind the large population loss in 2011–2012.

Take Note

In February 2014, the Employment Insurance program was revised to address the seasonal nature and differing employment opportunities available to residents of PEI who may be living in rural versus urban communities. This was in direct response to the concerns voiced by residents and politicians that the changes implemented to the Employment Insurance program in 2012 were not fair to seasonally employed Islanders living in rural communities. The federal government created two employment classification zones; urban, comprising Charlottetown and surrounding communities; and rural, comprising all other PEI communities. This change was made in acknowledgement that better employment opportunities exist for those who live in the province's capital city and its peripheral communities (Government of Canada, 2014).

All levels of government have voiced concern regarding youth outmigration, low population growth, and increasing age of those remaining in Atlantic Canada. Of particular concern is the potential lack of skilled workers that may be available to replace those retiring from the workforce. Also a concern is the potential increase in support services that will be required as the population ages. Lower population growth results in a drop in government tax revenue that creates challenges in the government's ability to sustain current and future publicly funded services such as hospitals and schools (Beale, 2008; Tam, 2009).

While Atlantic Canada in general, and PEI in particular, have experienced an increase in outmigration for employment, another labour migration trend currently exists that is not statistically recorded. This unrecorded data pertains to individuals who do not permanently move away from one province to another for employment, but rather engage in temporary interprovincial labour migration that involves commuting for employment in one province while retaining residency in another where family members remain. Estimating how many Canadians are engaging in this form of labour mobility is problematic, with most reports being anecdotal or reported by local news media that may under- or overestimate the actual number involved.

With no data and limited research, it is difficult to approximate how prevalent out-of-province work is in communities across PEI. The best estimation available comes from a study commissioned by a local economic development agency that reports 54% of men aged 18 to 55 left the Western Region of PEI at least once for employment out of province between 2005 and 2009 (Atlantic Evaluation Group, 2009). This region comprises one third of the geographic area of PEI and consists of rural communities only. Underemployment and dependence on Employment Insurance may contribute to people's frustration and increased stress as a result of difficulty in meeting monthly household expenses. Such financial challenges are the catalyst for men deciding to migrate for employment in another province, leaving their families behind in PEI. From the literature on labour migration and the narratives of those women left behind, the rationale for leaving is always to take advantage of better economic opportunities available elsewhere (Abrego, 2009; Sternberg, 2010; Hoang & Yeoh, 2012; Maharjan et al., 2012; Wray, 2012). This temporary labour migration results in families who are "together yet living apart."

EXPLORING WOMEN'S EXPERIENCES THROUGH NARRATIVE INQUIRY RESEARCH

To explore the issue of temporary labour migration and the experiences of women left behind, a narrative inquiry research project (Clandinin & Connelly, 2000) was undertaken with the purpose of increasing both awareness and understanding of the experiences of women living in rural PEI communities who were left behind while their partners left home to find work in another Canadian province. I met individually with women participating in this study on five or six occasions. During conversational interviews, the women and I engaged in discussions about who they were, who they were becoming, and how they thought others viewed them. Participants were invited also to share personal photographs; these photographs provided a visual representation of the women's narratives and a deeper understanding of how they experienced their husbands' comings and goings.

The four women who participated in this study ranged in age from 38 to 56 years old and were mothers with two to six children (12 to 20 years old) living at home. The purpose and objectives of this study were discussed in detail with participants; oral and written consent were obtained from each woman prior to beginning the interviews.

All women participating in this study initially believed that their family's experience with labour migration would be short term and temporary. As a result, the women did not accompany their husbands and move their families out of province; they felt that a move would be too disruptive to their family as their husbands' out-of-province employment would be short lived. This, however, proved not to be the case. Within a few years of their initial participation in temporary labour migration, all of the women's husbands had accepted full-time out-of-province employment. At the time when this research was conducted, the women in the project had been experiencing their husbands' repeated comings and goings for a range of 6 to 16 years.

Because of their full time out-of-province employment, the women's husbands were commuting to PEI and being physically present with their families an average of 60 days per year in 2-week visits at 6- to 8-week intervals. This situation has led to family restructuring, creating a paradox by which nuclear families are left behind and evolve in the absence of husbands and fathers.

WOMEN'S PERCEPTIONS OF BEING TOGETHER, YET LIVING APART

In their stories of being left behind due to their husbands' labour migration, women used the term "married-single mother." They acknowledged that although they were married they often felt as though they lived the life of a single mother because of their husbands' frequent and lengthy absences from their families. Women identified a paradox whereby they needed to do everything in their husbands' absences, yet each time their husbands returned home, they had to renegotiate their roles and responsibilities within their families. Women confided that they never felt that they were able to fulfill their roles and responsibilities to the best of their abilities and this situation contributed to feelings of anxiety and worry. For example, the women described that they often felt additional pressure to be overly present in their children's lives to compensate for their husbands' absences.

Women shared in depth about how draining it was to be the person left behind and reported feeling stressed as they attended to multiple responsibilities during their husbands' absences. They acknowledged that other working mothers may also experience such feelings, yet believed that women left behind face additional challenges because although they were married they rarely had the physical and emotional support of their husbands in the day-to-day management of family and household responsibilities. During our interviews, women frequently discussed cycles of "presence and absence" (Wray, 2012) and recognized that they functioned differently in their families during the periods of time that their husbands were away and when they were home. Women explained that their husbands might be at home and with their families for a week or two at a time, and as such, they wanted to have happy homes when their husbands were physically present. Women encouraged and embraced their husbands' participation in household and parental activities while at home, but managed these alone during their absences. Women acknowledged that they loved their husbands and looked forward to their return following a work term; however, some felt that as a result of their husbands' repeated coming and going over many years they were now like visitors who came into their homes every four to six weeks, rather than being an integral part of their family unit.

All women spoke about their sense of connection to rural PEI and how it was this connection that resulted in them not wanting to move away from their communities. They believed that living in a rural community was a great place to raise children; however, they did not believe that rural PEI was a great place for adults due to limited employment opportunities.

The women often felt stigmatized and ostracized by others living in their rural communities because their husbands were working out of province. These experiences had permeated women's lives and had affected their sense of belonging and connection to others in their communities. Women shared multiple examples of how they had been negatively perceived by people because of their higher family incomes. There was gossip about how they had gone out for lunch with friends, to a salon for a haircut, or purchased new furniture or other household goods. They had overheard people in the community embellishing their "extravagant lifestyles" and falsely proclaiming that their husbands were earning double or triple the actual amount of their income. In communities where seasonal economies and part-time employment were the norm, the women felt they were being negatively judged because of their family's better financial situation.

The women's sense of belonging within their communities was affected also by gossip regarding marital fidelity and relationship status. They worried about others in the community who questioned their marriages and the strength of their relationships. Rather than risk gossip, women often chose to stay at home. While this perpetuated feelings of loneliness and isolation, women viewed it to be self-protective. By staying at home with their children and not engaging in adult-only social situations, women were trying to avoid being the targets of gossip.

While women were reluctant to participate in adult social activities offered within their communities, going to watch their children's extracurricular activities presented opportunities to socialize with other adults. They realized how valuable it was to get out of the house and interact with others. Their children's activities became a social outing that the women anticipated and enjoyed. With the children being the primary focus in these events, the women did not have to worry so much about gossip. By attending children's activities, they met other women whose husbands were also working out of province. This common bond contributed to a sense of belonging and presented a springboard for conversations about their mutual experiences.

CHALLENGES TO ADDRESSING HEALTH PROMOTION FOR WOMEN LEFT BEHIND

Women discussed how being "together yet living apart" impacted their health. They reported experiencing multiple emotions associated with being left behind: loneliness, sadness, anxiety, embarrassment, feeling overwhelmed, and fears about how they were being judged by others. All spoke about the overwhelming stress they felt at times and how they tried to manage it. Women described how beneficial exercise was in helping them to take some time away from addressing the needs of others and "clear their heads." However, carving time out for themselves on a regular basis was a challenge because of the demands of their multiple roles, their busy days, and the lack of available child care.

Living in a rural setting also presented a challenge for women looking to exercise indoors at structured group fitness classes or gyms—such facilities are rare in their rural communities. During the winter months, rural PEI can be cold and desolate; frequent storms and frigid temperatures make it difficult for people to exercise outdoors. While women desired to get out of the house for a daily walk, it is not safe to push a stroller or walk with small children on rural roads in the winter. As a result, women often stayed at home and did not engage in health promoting physical activity during the winter months, perpetuating their feelings of isolation and loneliness that, in turn, negatively affected their mental and emotional health.

While acknowledging that scheduling time for exercise could be challenging for all mothers, women felt that being left behind presented additional challenges. If their husbands were working in PEI and home at a certain time each day, the women would have an opportunity to schedule time each week and commit to a fitness regime without having to worry about child care. Some women, however, worried about how they would be perceived by other community members should they use child care to go to the gym on a regular basis. They recalled examples where other women were the subjects of gossip by community members who speculated about why women went to the gym. Participants worried that rumours could start regarding their marital status if they spoke with men at the gym or if they lost weight and made improvements in their physical appearance while their husbands were away from home. Rather than engaging in organized physical activity as a health promoting behaviour, women chose to self-isolate and engage in exercises that they could do alone such as walking or doing an exercise video at home.

ADDRESSING HEALTH PROMOTION THROUGH CREATING SUPPORTIVE ENVIRONMENTS

The Ottawa Charter offers five broad strategies for health promotion (WHO, 1986). The primary intervention to address women's health promotion in this project related to creating supportive environments for health. As I listened to women share their experiences, their common desire for social support was profound. Women spoke about how exhausting and lonely it was for them to be the lone family caregiver for long periods of time. While women appreciated living in a rural community and having an opportunity to raise their children there, worries about how others in their community perceived them had contributed to their decision to isolate themselves. Acknowledging that self-isolation was also a self-protective mechanism, women nevertheless acknowledged that this had a negative impact on their health and perpetuated feelings of loneliness, anxiety, and depression.

Through this project, the women recognized the importance of support for women and children left behind due to labour migration. The women in the project began to conceptualize what support groups would look like and how they could become a reality in rural communities across PEI. Women felt that having an opportunity to come together with others who were also experiencing social isolation would be beneficial and could help develop new support systems. Through support groups women imagined that they could establish a network whereby they could share child care or carpooling services with one another. This intervention could present new opportunities for women to have time away from their children and engage in self-care practices.

In September of 2013, I began meeting with the executive directors of all Family Resource Centres on PEI. I advocated on behalf of the project participants and shared their vision for support groups that address the needs of women left behind. Each executive director acknowledged that the issue of labour migration and families being left behind was common in their communities and an issue about which they had concerns. Many of the families attending their current programs had been directly affected by labour migration. The executive directors expressed a desire to develop and implement programming that could address the specific needs of women and children in their communities whose husbands were working out of province. Through our discussions, the groundwork for *Families of Migrant Workers* support groups became established.

In November 2013, a Family Resource Centre in the Western Region of PEI implemented the first *Families of Migrant Workers* support group. In developing this support group, it was paramount that it be reflective of the needs that had been expressed by women left behind. Women wanted a space that was welcoming and a place where they could share their thoughts and feelings with others without fear of judgement or gossip. Therefore, meetings were held in a room with a door that could be closed during meetings. Confidentiality and respect for each other were principles addressed at the beginning of every meeting.

Prior to implementing the *Families of Migrant Workers* support group, issues relating to accessibility were considered. It was determined that the location for the support group meetings should be at the Family Resource Centre, known to offer a variety of programs for parents and children up to 6 years of age. Its location is central and there is adequate free parking. The Family Resource Centre also committed to paying the wages of two staff members who would be involved in the *Families of Migrant Workers* support group; one being a group facilitator and the other an early child educator. The early child educator provided child care free of charge in the centre while their mothers took part in support group meetings. Children had an opportunity to play and develop new friendships with other children who shared their experiences.

Since its inception, the *Families of Migrant Workers* support group has been well received. It continues to meet bi-weekly and has 20 to 25 women attending each session. Additionally, there is a Facebook group that also provides support for women left behind who are unable to physically attend meetings. The success of this support group has been shared throughout PEI and Atlantic Canada through radio broadcasts and local newspaper reports. Women attending the group meetings or utilizing the Facebook site find the group support helpful and express their appreciation that networks have been established. In particular, women describe how beneficial it is to have a place where they can meet other mothers who understand, firsthand, what it is like to be left behind. Women report that through the support group they have developed new friendships, are feeling supported, and appreciate they are not alone.

Summary

This case story offers an overview of outmigration and current factors that are contributing to temporary labour migration from Atlantic Canada, and in particular, rural PEI. Currently, statistics regarding the number of men engaging in temporary labour migration in other provinces are not available, rendering it impossible to gauge accurately the extent of the issue. A narrative inquiry project was conducted to explore the experiences of women left behind—"together yet living apart." Through this project, women shared their experiences of roles, responsibilities, and family cohesion. They also revealed numerous ways by which they feel unsupported in their communities. Women believed that being left behind was negatively affecting their health status and contributing to their inability to participate in health promoting behaviours. Embracing the Ottawa Charter strategy of creating supportive networks by planning, implementing, and taking part in the *Families of Migrant Workers* program has had a positive impact on women's well-being and has fostered the creation of other supports (e.g., Facebook) for other women left behind.

Acknowledgements

This study received ethical approval from the University of Alberta and the University of Prince Edward Island Research Ethics Boards.

REFERENCES

Abrego, L. (2009). Economic well-being in Salvadoran transnational families: How gender affects remittance practices. *Journal of Marriage & Family, 71*(4), 1070–1085.

Atlantic Evaluation Group. (2009). *Western PEI labour market study summary and recommendations report.* Alberton, PE: Resources West.

Beale, E. (2008). *As labour markets tighten, will outmigration trends reverse in Atlantic Canada?* Halifax: Atlantic Provinces Economic Council.

Clandinin, D. J., & Connelly, F. M. (2000). *Narrative inquiry: Experience and story in qualitative research.* San Francisco: Jossey-Bass.

Government of Canada. (2014). *Government of Canada brings fairness to EI program in Prince Edward Island [archived].* Ottawa: Employment and Social Development Canada. URL=http://news.gc.ca/web/article-en.do?nid=817309

Hoang, L., & Yeoh, B. A. (2012). Sustaining families across transnational spaces: Vietnamese migrant parents and their left behind children. *Asian Studies Review, 36*(3), 307–325.

Labour Market and Strategic Analysis Division (LMSAD), Service Canada, Atlantic Region. (2014). *Environmental scan: Atlantic Region Fall 2013.* Ottawa: Employment and Social Development Canada. URL=http://www.esdc.gc.ca/eng/jobs/lmi/publications/e-scan/atl/atl-escan-fall2013.pdf

Maharjan, A., Bauer, S., & Knerr, B. (2012). Do rural women who stay behind benefit from male out-migration? A case study in the hills of Nepal. *Gender, Technology and Development, 16*(1), 95–123.

Prince Edward Island Statistics Bureau. (2013). *Province of Prince Edward Island thirty-ninth annual statistical review 2012.* URL=http://www.gov.pe.ca/photos/original/fema_asr2012.pdf

Prince Edward Island Statistics Bureau. (2014). *Prince Edward Island population report 2014.* URL=http://www.gov.pe.ca/photos/original/pt_pop_rep.pdf

Service Canada. (2013). *Employment insurance regular benefits.* Ottawa: Government of Canada. URL=http://www.servicecanada.gc.ca/eng/ei/types/regular.shtml#eligible

Sternberg, R. M. (2010). The plight of transnational Latina mothers: Mothering from a distance. *Field Actions Science Reports* [online], Special Issue 2. URL=http://factsreports.revues.org/486

Tam, P. (2009). The battle to keep young workers. *The Ottawa Citizen.* CanWest MediaWorks Publications.

World Health Organization (WHO). (1986). *The Ottawa charter for health promotion.* Geneva: Author.

Wray, D., (2012). "Daddy lives at the airport": The consequences of economically driven separation on family life in the post-industrial mining communities of Cape Breton. *Employee Responsibilities and Rights Journal, 24,* 147–158.

ONLINE RESOURCES

Please visit the Point at http://thepoint.lww.com/Vollman4e for up-to-date Internet resources and additional learning materials on this topic.

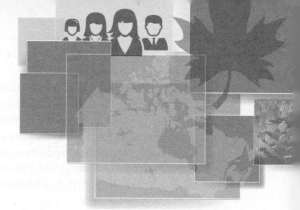

CHAPTER 24

Flood Disaster Response: Calgary, Canada

Gayle Rutherford, Jennifer Langille, J. David Patterson, and Zahra Shajani

LEARNING OBJECTIVES

After studying this chapter, you should be able to:

1. Describe interprofessional public health emergency response in a flood situation

2. Discuss how the Canadian Community-as-Partner model guided the processes used by the health care professional team and linked with disaster response theory

Introduction

No one who has been involved in a disaster is untouched by it. Some populations, such as those who are more vulnerable on a daily basis, are more affected by disasters than others (Baker & Cormier, 2015), but everyone responds to active, genuine interest, and concern that includes practical assistance as well as psychological support (CDC, 2014). Communities, local agencies, and organizations can take a lead in disaster response, "in fact, it often does take a 'village' full of responders to address the multitude of concrete and psychosocial needs following a disaster" (Baker & Cormier, 2015, p. 15). In this chapter, we will explore the experiences of faculty members and students as they provided immediate response to a vulnerable population during a natural disaster.

On June 21, 2013, the City of Calgary and surrounding communities experienced a flood that created disaster conditions for several communities along the Bow and Elbow rivers. Over 100,000 people were forced to leave their homes across Southern Alberta. From an overall population of 1.2 million, it was estimated that 75,000 Calgarians were evacuated due to the flood, 2,000 of whom were housed in emergency centres or dormitories that were used to provide accommodations for some of the displaced (Ogrodnik, 2013). Five days after the flood, 11,000 homes and businesses were still without power in Calgary. Community response to the flood was outstanding as thousands of volunteers helped their neighbours clean up around their homes, and on June 24 2,500 people responded to a call for volunteers to help others whose homes were affected by the flood (Ogrodnik, 2013).

The University of Calgary was officially closed in the late afternoon on Friday, June 21, reopening again on Wednesday, June 26. Up to 450 evacuees from the downtown core, including those from homeless shelters, a women's emergency shelter, and a seniors' apartment building, were evacuated to student residences on the University of Calgary campus. By Monday morning, June 24, those providing support for the evacuees were calling for help. This is the story of the immediate response by the faculty members and students from the Faculty of Nursing and how Nursing students and faculty members came together to provide support within a few hours of the call.

STUDENTS AND FACULTY EXPERIENCE THE FLOOD

The story begins with experiences during the initial stages of the flood, where Nursing faculty members and students were in communities on practicum placements as the waters were rising, making decisions about assisting the communities to meet their immediate need for support and ensuring safety for the students. What started as a typical day in practice took an unexpected turn for students and faculty members, and shaped the learning for the rest of the semester. For JL, her day as a Clinical Instructor started in Cochrane, 37 km west of Calgary, at 6:45 AM in a long-term care centre. By 9 AM, news reports were on the televisions in the residents' rooms about the rising level of Cougar Creek in Canmore, 78 km west of Cochrane, which eventually led to the washout of the TransCanada Highway at Canmore. Many of the students commuted to Cochrane from Canmore and were anxious to check on loved ones.

JDP's day as a Clinical Instructor started in High River, 64 km south of Calgary, at 7:30 AM with a staff meeting at a community health clinic. Students in practice at the clinic were uncertain if they should drive to High River given the notifications they were hearing on the television and radio news. They were advised to attend as usual, not anticipating the risks and validity of these early warnings.

JL, JDP, along with ZS, the course coordinator, spoke often during the morning. JL urged JDP to leave; JDP refused to leave and insisted on ensuring the safety of the students and the practice partners. Both JL and JDP persisted with the clinical day although JL sent her students home at noon in response to their desire to be with their families. As the waters rose, JDP and his students departed from High River in the early afternoon after helping to evacuate residents from the supportive living facility in High River to the local high school.

BACKGROUND AND CONTEXT OF THE NURSING STUDENTS' LEARNING PRIOR TO THE FLOOD

Fortunately, the Faculty of Nursing had a cohort of 100+ students taking classes during the spring/summer semester. These students had begun in January 2013 with initial courses during their first semester focused on nursing at a community/population level, including the use of the Canadian Community-as-Partner model in a community setting. In their current term, they were in community practicum placements with a focus on transition across the lifespan, family-centered care, and interprofessional practice. Thus, the students and faculty members were able to draw from this recent and very valuable education as they moved into action.

RESPONDING TO THE CALL FOR ACTION

In the early morning of Monday, June 24, the Vice-Provost of the University of Calgary reached out to the Faculties of Nursing, Social Work, and Medicine asking for assistance to support the evacuees on campus. The staff at the University residences had been providing support to the evacuees over the weekend, and they needed reinforcement and the professional expertise from these three faculties. In particular, the Vice-Provost requested wellness checks for displaced persons in the student residences to determine overall need for further resources. By 9 AM, an email had gone out to the second year Faculty of Nursing Clinical Instructors asking if any of them and their students would be able to provide assistance, and within an hour a group from the Faculty of Nursing was on its way to begin determining the type of support required. Throughout the first day, there were 17 student volunteers along with five Nursing faculty members. On the second day, we were able to schedule rotating 4-hour shifts of Nursing faculty and students with 24 student volunteers and 8 Nursing faculty members providing support to the students. The focus for the first 2 days of response was primarily on assessing needs, developing resource lists, and determining what basic items could be obtained for the evacuees.

In addition to the Nursing faculty and students, Social Work faculty members joined us at the residence on Monday with additional Social Work faculty and students arriving on Tuesday. A group of second year Faculty of Medicine students, who were involved in a student-run medical clinic at a downtown shelter for the homeless, also joined us on Tuesday. Physicians, registered nurses, occupational therapists, and physical therapists from Alberta Health Services as well as mental health and addictions counsellors were then deployed by the Zone Emergency Operations Centre to the University of Calgary student residences and began providing more direct support by Tuesday at noon. When this additional support arrived, they looked to the Nursing faculty members and students for direction, based on the initial assessments completed on Monday.

ENACTING THE COMMUNITY-AS-PARTNER MODEL

As the many interprofessional faculty members and students came together on Monday, June 24, it was apparent that a systematic assessment and coordinated plan was necessary. Following are the results of the Canadian Community-as-Partner model implementation during the first few days of the Nursing faculty and student intervention.

Assessment

The second year Nursing students initially conducted a needs assessment survey and gathered data by going floor by floor and door to door at the University residences. This was done in partnership with Nursing and Social Work faculty members, Social Work students, and with Medicine students as they became available. The survey focused on gathering a compressed health history as well as providing an overall census of evacuees located on campus. The needs assessment survey included the names of displaced residents, their ages, addresses, additional family members, physical illnesses or injuries, mobility issues, safety concerns, and health concerns. They also assessed the evacuees' overall physical and mental health status to determine the urgency of medical assistance and support required. The initial process of conducting the needs assessment allowed the students and faculty to build trusting relationships with the evacuated residents, many of whom were experiencing distress and emotional uncertainty. Using relational communication skills, the Nursing students listened to the traumatic stories of the evacuees' flood experiences. Many of these stories told of devastation and the uncertainty about the status of homes and previous accommodations.

We met people of all ages, including older adults, pregnant women, children, and even their pets. While going room to room, unmet basic needs were evident in that many people had only the clothes on their backs, no toiletries, no food, no diapers, and no medication. The student teams identified those who were at high risk and a Registered Nurse (RN) from the Faculty of

Nursing would accompany students to further assess the health needs of these individuals. One of the families identified as high risk was a mother who had been assessed in hospital at the beginning of the flood for preterm labor. She was diagnosed with insulin-dependent gestational diabetes and lacked supplies to manage her condition. She was on bed rest, unable to care for her young daughter, and faced barriers in accessing food from the university cafeteria. She was anxious about the health of her unborn baby. A Nursing faculty member, an RN with background in maternity, pediatrics, family, and community health, along with three students, went to the family's room to meet with them. The Nursing faculty member confirmed the health history previously collected by the students and followed up with a more focused assessment based on the mother's needs—a medication review, a review of her recent hospital visit, vital signs and fetal heart rate, nutritional status, and mental well-being. With this information, the Nursing faculty member and students, in collaboration with the family, were able to determine the appropriate interventions to meet the family's immediate needs. They were able to act quickly to provide the immediate assistance required to manage the mother's health issues and family concerns. Students met with cafeteria staff to arrange family access to meals in their room; they contacted a pharmacy to acquire the supplies needed for blood glucose testing and insulin administration.

The Nursing students, with the support from their faculty members, needed to respond immediately to the emotionally and psychologically distressed residents. By actively listening to the experiences and flood stories of the evacuees, the students were able to provide immediate empathic emotional support. The needs expressed were as varied as the populations that were brought together: families; elderly persons; people with addictions; those living with mental illness; and people who were homeless. One of the unexpected things we learned was that some of the evacuees who had been housed in a shelter were actually enjoying their new environment on campus where they were in a private room!

Analysis

During the analysis phase, the Nursing students, guided by Nursing faculty members, were able to identify the issues as listed in Table 24.1 using a strengths, weaknesses, opportunities and threats (SWOT) analysis (Vollman et al., 2013) of the immediate situation.

Diagnosis

During the analysis, a number of protective factors (strengths) were identified along with health risks. In order to capture these, two categories of diagnoses were articulated.

Wellness Diagnoses

1. The Nursing students and faculty members had an opportunity to reduce the impact of the flood disaster for the evacuees as manifested by the number of students and faculty members who volunteered for disaster response and the willingness of the evacuees to participate in the assessment processes.
2. There was a potential for Nursing students to decrease the psychological impact of the flood as manifested by their ability to use relational communication skills and active listening as well as the evacuees' interest in talking with the students.
3. There was an opportunity for the students to increase the availability of resources to meet the initial basic needs, including clothing and personal hygiene products, as manifested by their ability to seek out additional community resources through on-line and social media sites.
4. There were opportunities for Nursing students and faculty members to build collaborative relationships within an interdisciplinary team as manifested by the deployment of physicians, registered nurses, psychiatrists, psychologists, social workers, and community support workers to provide additional support at the university residences.

TABLE 24.1 SWOT Analysis

Strengths	Weaknesses	Opportunities	Threats
Nursing students and faculty members were available to deliver support immediately to the people who were affected by the flood crisis, to optimize wellness and mitigate short-term psychological consequences from the flood trauma. Some evacuees had good coping mechanisms to lessen their feelings of being overwhelmed and helpless. Community programs were available to provide additional support for evacuees who felt isolated, depressed, and anxious.	Increased anxiety and panic related to uncertainty of the situation and the unknown as to where they would be going if their home or shelter were completely destroyed. Crisis situation was causing some individuals to become aggressive and destructive, and show disregard to personal well-being. Evacuees who did not have their medication were becoming confused and medically ill, relapsing in their medical or mental health conditions.	Strengthen collaboration with other health disciplines to expand support for meeting immediate physiologic, psychological, and medical needs. Identify accessible community resources to meet the immediate basic needs of the evacuees. Build trusting relationships and use relational communication skills as early intervention strategies for working with the traumatized evacuated adults and families with young children. Provide emotional support to the Nursing students through debriefing their experiences during and after the disaster response.	Risk associated with the psychological response to the traumatic event for evacuees, students, and faculty members. Risk of students feeling isolated and emotionally numb or overwhelmed due to the extent of the disaster, both personally and professionally. Risk of detachment, reduced sense of hope, and lack of emotional response for the evacuees if adequate support was not provided. Risk for decreased mental health status or medical crisis with lack of access to prescribed medications.

Deficit Diagnoses

1. The evacuees were at risk of psychological crisis related to the traumatic events of the floods in downtown Calgary and their inability to meet their basic needs as manifested by the number of people who had to evacuate their living spaces with only what they were wearing at the time.
2. The Nursing students were at risk of emotional reaction to their disaster response intervention as a result of exposure to the traumatic stories of the evacuees as manifested by the concern of the faculty for the students' well-being and student and faculty members' inability to debrief their responses due to the immediacy of the needs of the evacuees.

Planning

By the second day of disaster response enough volunteers were present so that a schedule with 4-hour shifts could be created. This provided the Nursing students and faculty members with an opportunity to regenerate and to debrief about their joint experiences. At the same time, they were able to develop a plan for next steps and discuss who would take responsibility for the various aspects of the intervention. With the arrival of the additional external support, the Nursing students and faculty members were able to share their findings as a basis for the development of the larger plan. It was amazing to see how quickly the external professionals found the best ways for them to provide intervention, based on the work the students and faculty members had done the day before.

Intervention

By means of the initial assessment, intervention began through active listening to people's stories and continued through ongoing interactions with the evacuees. Our goal was to provide initial and immediate support to the individuals and families who were experiencing trauma from the flood and help them to cope during this intense situation. Through active listening, the students helped the evacuees deal with their immediate thoughts and feelings, assisted them to talk about their trauma and feelings of crisis, and guided them toward gaining some perspective on the reality of what was happening. Many of the residents were in shock and disbelief and were initially disoriented regarding their situation and how to deal with the consequences of the flood. By providing an opportunity for the evacuees to discuss their stories, worries, and crises, the students were able to provide the emotional support needed immediately after a crisis in order to mitigate the increased level of anxiety and intense fear of uncertainty about their future.

The Nursing students worked together to build interdisciplinary teams to meet the complex health needs of individuals and families. The students helped to set up a triage centre where the evacuees were able to seek attention from health care providers deployed from Alberta Health Services as well as medical students, Nursing students, Social Work students, and community crisis support volunteers and workers. The Nursing students partnered with a local community dentist to access oral health essentials such as toothpaste, floss, denture glue, and denture cups.

After seeing the magnitude of need on day 1, on day 2 the students turned to social media. They posted on Facebook and Twitter asking for donations of clothing, toiletries, and games. The response was amazing; colleagues, friends, and families were quickly able to provide clothing, toiletries, and other necessities. The students worked to organize and distribute donations to the evacuees based on their previously assessed needs. While donations poured in, other groups of students investigated a range of community resources that were needed. They contacted the Calgary Humane Society, local dentists, and pharmacists, pooling resources as they were identified. The students also created a list of resources that families might need—nearby banks, grocery stores, shopping malls, transit, and health care—and provided this information to the evacuees.

Evaluation

Although no formal evaluation of the role of the Nursing students and faculty members was done during this immediate disaster response, informal feedback from the evacuees, other professionals, and volunteers was very positive. As with any nursing action, the success of the interventions and adequacy of the ongoing assessment were being evaluated continually. Communication among the team members was continuous and essential to ensure that everyone was working together to reach the goal of immediate support and intervention.

We observed that the Nursing students had developed theoretical knowledge and skills that gave them a strong foundation for their role in this disaster response. During this experience, the Nursing students were able to build trusting relationships with the evacuated individuals and families. They were committed to being physically and emotionally present by actively listening to the difficult situations and providing the emotional support needed. The student teams were very respectful and appreciated the diversity among families. They showed leadership in conducting the initial needs assessment and connecting with people to cultivate a sense of trust, belongingness, and hope. They were courageous in using their abilities and skills; they were able to provide a compassionate, honest, and open approach to support this vulnerable group of people during the crisis.

LINKAGE TO DISASTER RESPONSE THEORY

The 2013 Calgary flood created the need for disaster response through provision of crisis intervention services and immediate support to evacuees across the city. At the University of Calgary, faculty members and students from Nursing, Social Work, and Medicine were able to provide invaluable support to a vulnerable population evacuated from the downtown core. The Nursing students, in particular, were able to enact their previously learned theory related to population health and the Canadian Community-as-Partner model.

Disaster has been defined in a variety of ways but essentially, "it is a destructive event that overwhelms available resources. A disaster may originate as natural or manmade and may be intentional or accidental" (Beach, 2010, p. 1). The disaster cycle has also been delineated in several ways. Baker and Cormier (2015) outlined the stages as prevention, preparedness, response, recovery, and mitigation, while Beach (2010) suggested the cycle involved mitigation (and preparation), response, recovery (and evaluation), and a return to mitigation. All cycles essentially identify response and recovery as two stages that take place after the disaster has happened. Response efforts are immediate and focus on rescuing victims, saving property (Beach, 2010), providing crisis intervention services, and stabilizing the community (Baker & Cormier, 2015). The response phase is "both an organized response by trained personnel and a grassroots effort by victims who may be able to help themselves and those around them" (Beach, 2010, p. 7). The response phase precedes the recovery phase, which is "a slow return to normal life after the disaster" (Beach, 2010, p. 12). In our efforts, we were very focused on the response phase of the disaster cycle in assessing needs and providing short-term intervention services.

The Canadian Community-as-Partner model provided us with a process that guided our response to the request for support after the disaster. Intuitively, as faculty members with experience in public health nursing, we guided the students to begin with the assessment phase, gathering vital information from the evacuees about their needs. Concurrently, we were able to provide an intervention while doing the assessment. We knew that reaching out and listening to the evacuees' stories while assessing their needs made a difference to them. It also made a difference to the faculty members and the students as everyone was either directly or indirectly affected by the flood and felt a need to "do something." As noted by Baker and Cormier (2015), "responding to someone at a point of vulnerability is a privilege. Being with someone when he or she is hurt, afraid, or alone requires a defined skill set, a capacity to be near human suffering, and a desire to make things better" (p. xi). Our students and faculty members surpassed expectations in their ability to provide support and response in this instance: "Your students were unbelievable—professional, confident, compassionate, kind and endlessly helpful" (A. Mackay, personal communication, June 28, 2013).

Our students also experienced interprofessional practice within the intensity of the disaster response. Their work together with faculty members and students from Social Work and Medicine was beyond any other experience that could have been structured within the curriculum. They also viewed highly functioning interprofessional practice among the professionals who were deployed to support the evacuees at the University of Calgary. They enacted and observed the role of nurses within an interprofessional team, recognizing that nurses have an opportunity during a disaster situation to assist those affected through providing psychological support and making appropriate referrals as they worked within an interprofessional team (Sadovitch & White, 2013, p. 84). While providing essential disaster response initiatives, the Nursing students were able to benefit from tying together their theory with practice in a way that could not have been planned.

Four of the Nursing students who had been in High River on June 21 and directly involved in the flood response were interviewed for a University of Calgary daily on-line publication ("In their own words," 2013). They had been unable to return to their practicum placement in High River and had continued to work in flood relief over the following weeks. They reflected on how they had learned about nursing roles in a crisis situation while gaining insight into the full experiences of the evacuees who may have lost everything. They learned how important the question "How are you doing?" was to the evacuees but also as a way to learn more about their needs. The students expressed how this experience had reinforced their selection of nursing as a career and deepened their understanding of the difference nurses can make. One student said, "It is interesting to see what a difference you can make by listening to people and hearing their stories." Another student said, "It felt good knowing that I had made a difference in people's lives when they were experiencing such a difficult transition." Ultimately, they learned that nursing is much more than just hands-on nursing skills, that flexibility and adaptability are fundamentally important along with a lot of listening and caring.

LESSONS LEARNED

- Students and faculty members working side by side in disaster response provides the students with an opportunity to observe their Instructors in action as Registered Nurses. After the assessment with the pregnant mother, the students said that it was amazing to see their instructor practising as an RN. At the same time, the Instructor was able to link theory with practice in a way that was beyond the scope of what could be experienced in their practicum settings.
- The Canadian Community-as-Partner model provides a framework that can be used to guide immediate disaster response.
- Nurses, as members of an interprofessional team, play a unique role in disaster response through their ability to combine relational communication skills with broad assessment skills that encompass physical, emotional, cultural, social, and spiritual health.
- As much as the evacuees benefitted from their interactions with the Nursing students, the students benefitted equally through their learning and exposure to a real-life scenario where they could truly make a difference.

Summary

The 2013 Calgary flood created a disaster situation for many residents of Calgary and surrounding area. Although this was a traumatic situation from many perspectives, the flood also provided opportunities to learn about how a community can come together to support those most affected. From the short-term disaster response described in this chapter to longer term involvement in recovery efforts, our students were able to participate in a learning opportunity that could not be foreseen or planned. They were able to apply their theoretical learning directly to a real-life situation that will become a part of who they are as nurses. They learned first-hand about the importance and relevance of nursing in a community setting, where all of their skills and knowledge are used to their full extent.

REFERENCES

Baker, L., & Cormier, L. (2015). *Disasters and vulnerable populations: Evidence-based practice for the helping professions.* New York, NY: Springer.

Beach, M. (2010). *Disaster preparedness and management.* Philadelphia, PA: F.A. Davis.

Centers for Disease Control and Prevention (CDC). (2014). *Emergency preparedness and response—Natural disasters and severe weather.* URL=http://emergency.cdc.gov/disasters/

Ogrodnik, I. (2013). *By the numbers: 2013 Alberta floods. Global News.* URL=http://globalnews.ca/news/673236/by-the-numbers-2013-alberta-floods/

Sadovitch, J., & White, J. (2013). Human services in disasters and public health emergencies: Social disruption, individual empowerment, and community resilience. In T. G. Veenema (Ed.), *Disaster nursing and emergency preparedness: For chemical, biological, and radiological terrorism and other hazards* (3rd ed., pp. 79–91). New York, NY: Springer.

In their own words: Four nursing students share experiences from the front lines. (2013). *UToday.* URL=http://www.ucalgary.ca/news/utoday/july29-2013/in-their-own-words

Vollman, A. R., Anderson, E. T., & McFarlane, J. M. (2013). *Canadian community as partner: Theory & multidisciplinary practice* (3rd ed.). Philadelphia, PA: Lippincott Williams & Wilkins.

ONLINE RESOURCES

Please visit thePoint at http://thepoint.lww.com/Vollman4e for up-to-date Internet resources and additional learning materials on this topic.

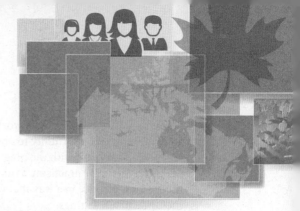

CHAPTER 25

Promoting the Health of Newcomer Mothers to Manitoba

Cheryl Cusack, Gayleen Dimond, and Justine Zidona

LEARNING OBJECTIVES

After studying this chapter, you should be able to:

1. Understand key issues affecting the health of newcomer populations

2. Discuss the role of public health workers in promoting the health of newcomers using strategies from the Ottawa Charter

3. Describe the importance of interprofessional and interagency collaborations in addressing newcomer prenatal and parenting care needs

Introduction

Promoting the health of populations is a foundational tenet of public health practice (CPHA, 2010). One population that the Winnipeg Regional Health Authority (WRHA) works with are newcomers who are pregnant and/or parenting children under 1 year of age. Large groups of women from this population gather weekly in Winnipeg's downtown core for a Healthy Start for Mom & Me (HSMM) group. The intention of the HSMM program is to promote the health and well-being of newcomers and their babies by building personal skills and supportive environments as they transition to their new Canadian home. The HSSM group is the result of collaboration among federal, provincial, regional, and local partners.

POPULATION ASSESSMENT

The province of Manitoba is estimated to have a population of more than 1.2 million and has been growing steadily (Manitoba Government, 2013). A large component of the population growth is due to immigration, with nearly 130,000 people coming to the province over the last 10 years (Manitoba Government, 2015). Nearly two thirds of the province's population live in the capital city of Winnipeg, which ranks between fourth and sixth as the most popular Canadian city for newcomers (Manitoba Government, 2013). The province is known for its low cost of living and housing prices, and cultural diversity (Manitoba Government, 2013).

Box 25.1 Instructions for Newcomers to Canada

All Canadian citizens and permanent residents may apply for public health insurance. When you have it, you do not pay for most health care services as health care is paid for through taxes. When you use public health care services, you must show your health insurance card to the hospital or medical clinic.

Each province and territory has [its] own health insurance plan. Make sure you know what your plan covers.

All provinces and territories will provide free emergency medical services, even if you do not have a government health card. Restrictions may apply depending on your immigration status. If you have an emergency, go to the nearest hospital. If you go to a walk-in clinic in a province or territory where you are not a resident, you might be charged a fee.

Source: Government of Canada: http://www.cic.gc.ca/english/newcomers/after-health.asp

---

Immigration is a key component of economic and community growth in Manitoba. The province is proud to have a 75% success rate for placing newcomers in jobs, the second lowest newcomer unemployment rate in Canada, and an 85% rate of retention within the province (Manitoba Government, 2013).

The process of resettlement is extremely complex; the Government of Canada's Environment, Immigration and Citizenship website provides detailed information and links on a host of topics pertinent to newcomers (Government of Canada, 2015). Understanding fundamental terminology and classifications by which newcomers enter Canada assists community health workers to appreciate some of the basic contexts and experiences that may affect newcomer's health and well-being. In addition, based on their immigration status, newcomers may or may not qualify for different Canadian services and resources (Box 25.1). In most instances (e.g., Manitoba), health care coverage begins on the first day of the third month of arrival in the province.

The Immigration and Refugee Protection Act (IRPA) (2001) defines three criteria by which newcomers may apply to permanently reside in Canada: economic, family, and refugee classes (Government of Canada, 2015). In regard to immigration (i.e., permanent residents), the IRPA stipulates a number of objectives that focus largely on social, cultural, and economic benefits for Canada. *Economic* class immigrants, the largest proportion of Manitoba newcomers, are accepted under the provincial nominee program based on their ability to contribute to the economic growth of the province (Manitoba Government, 2013). The premise of the newcomer *family* class category is family reunification. Adult permanent residents or Canadian citizens not convicted of any crimes and not receiving social assistance may apply to sponsor their spouses, dependent children, parents, and grandparents (Government of Canada, 2015). There are strict criteria on the number of individuals who can immigrate to Canada within this class, and the sponsor is required to gather appropriate documentation, pay fees, and assume accountability for those sponsored (Government of Canada, 2015).

Refugees are the third distinct class of immigrants. Objectives in the IRPA state "that the refugee program is in the first instance about saving lives and offering protection to the displaced and persecuted" (IRPA, 2001, 3.2.a). Refugees are particularly vulnerable to physical and emotional effects of trauma that may have included malnutrition, torture, sexual violence, infectious diseases, and dental health issues (WRHA, 2010). There are both government-assisted refugees (GAR) and private-sponsored refugees (PSR). Individuals or groups can privately sponsor refugees who qualify by signing an agreement and assuming full responsibility for their financial and emotional needs including housing, clothes, and food. If sponsored by the government, resettlement including housing, assistance with employment, food, and clothing, may be supported until the refugee is self-sufficient or to a maximum of 1 year (Government of Canada, 2015).

The proportion of PSRs coming to Manitoba has increased dramatically over time. In 2013, 1,002 or 67.5% of immigrants were PSRs. This was the highest of PSRs per capita in Canada, and represents a substantial increase from 80 PSRs coming to Manitoba in 1998 (Immigrant & Refugee Partners, 2014, p. 33). The majority of the PSRs (81%) arrived from Somalia, Eritrea, and Ethiopia; in comparison, more than half of Manitoba's GARs came from Somalia, Bhutan, Iraq, and the Democratic Republic of Congo (Manitoba Government, 2013). Often associated with trauma experienced in their country of origin, refugees can have up to 10 times the rate of posttraumatic stress disorder (PTSD) than the general population, as well as disproportionate rates of depression and chronic pain (Immigrant & Refugee Partners, 2014).

According to Census data, Canada's female immigrant population grew at more than twice the rate of the total female population (Statistics Canada, 2011). In Manitoba, the newcomer population is also younger, with the largest numbers of immigrants being between ages 25 and 39 with a median age of 28 years (Manitoba Government, 2013), which represents prime childbearing years. Women admitted under the family classification have reported feeling vulnerable not having a secured immigration status and being emotionally and financially reliant on their spouse as sponsor for a minimum of 10 years (O'Mahony & Donnelly, 2013).

THE PROJECT

In early 2000, HSMM experienced a large influx of newcomer women attending programs located at eight sites across the city. Interpreter services were offered at each location; however, the number of interpreters required was increasing at a high rate. To better meet the newcomer women's needs, a specially designed and centrally located program with interpretation services was launched as a pilot in 2004. The group started small with about five women, but attendance has since skyrocketed, with between 40 and 80 women attending weekly. No one is ever turned away. The cultural makeup of this HSMM group is consistent with the profile of immigrants coming to Manitoba, except that the majority of participants tend to be refugee or family class immigrants rather than economic class. The length women in the group have been in Manitoba varies from mere days to as long as 10 years. The diversity of the women's countries of origin accounts for a variety of languages, cultures, and religions, but the common thread of being pregnant or having a young infant in a new country brings them together.

According to the Ottawa Charter "health promotion is the process of enabling people to increase control over, and to improve, their health." Health is promoted by actions that consist of creating supportive environments, developing personal skills, strengthening community action, reorienting health services, and building healthy public policy. Documents guiding public health practice emphasize the role of health promotion in reducing inequities through action at multiple levels that include the individual, community, and government (CPHA, 2010).

Creating Supportive Environments

Health is promoted by linking individuals with their environments using strategies and settings that are safe, enjoyable, and motivating (WHO, 1986) (see also Chapter 7). For newcomers, an important component of the resettlement process is the establishment of social support networks (WRHA, 2010). Lack of support is common because immigrant women are separated from their homes of origin, their husbands are often working long hours, and they do not have connections in their new communities (Higginbottom et al., 2014). A distinguishing feature of the public health role is the prominence of primary prevention activities to reduce inequities and prevent development of future problems (CPHA, 2010). The prenatal and early childhood periods are two of the most critical times to promote health for all women, and especially for newcomer women. A systematic review of 29 studies found that newcomer women are more likely to have inadequate prenatal care compared to their receiving country counterparts (Heaman et al., 2013). In addition to not knowing what health services for which they are eligible, newcomers are unlikely to understand roles of various service providers, functions of programs, and how to access needed health and social services (WRHA, 2010). Language barriers, lack of the ability to communicate effectively, inadequate knowledge, lack of translated information, shortage of interpretation services, and feelings of discrimination have been identified as issues impacting newcomer women's experiences with maternity care (Small et al., 2014). Following the birth of their children, newcomers have been reported to be at increased risk for postpartum depression because of the lack of social support systems as well as issues of poverty, discrimination, and differences in culture (O'Mahony & Donnelly, 2013).

Health programs and policies have to recognize and respond to the complexity of interconnected issues faced by newcomer populations (O'Mahony & Donnelly, 2013). The HSMM team view health as a holistic and culturally based concept, and plan group activities accordingly. Bus tickets are available to those who live at eligible distances from the site location. The newcomer women value the connections and friendships they make with each other. To foster a supportive environment, participants are encouraged to bring support people with them if they choose, and child care is provided. After her first time at the HSMM group, one newcomer exclaimed: "This is great! I can't wait for next week, I loved everything!" Inner city women in Winnipeg have reported that assistance with issues such as transportation, finances, and emotional concerns are positive factors that promote prenatal care (Heaman et al., 2014).

Developing Personal Skills

Developing personal skills enables individuals to make choices that improve their health through access to life skills, education, and information (WHO, 1986) (see also Chapter 6). Often newcomer women have not had past opportunities to make personal choices; therefore, matters associated with pregnancy, birth, and having a newborn can be very overwhelming and confusing. Immigrant women have reported that the biomedical approaches to maternity care in Canada are not consistent with their traditions, beliefs, and cultures (Higginbottom et al., 2014). The HSMM participants may have experienced previous trauma, have low incomes, have little education, and be unfamiliar with the Canadian health system. For some, attending group is the only time they are allowed to leave their house. Women are assisted to increase control and improve their health through specific public health interventions that include pregnancy-testing, referral to culturally appropriate health care providers, and facilitating access to resources such as the provincial prenatal benefit. Community health workers also support the women to access culturally sensitive health care providers, and ensure that interpreter services are coordinated for their appointments.

Each HSMM session consists of presentations, a healthy snack, and a meal. Team members that include public health nurses, public health nutritionist, volunteers, and outreach workers make presentations. Community agencies (e.g., Winnipeg Fire and Police Departments) are also invited to make presentations to help newcomers better understand local services and programs. Various community agencies are invited to the HSMM groups to support participants in feeling safe to access their services. Agencies include primary care and counselling services such as the Sexuality Education Resource Centre of Manitoba, Aurora Family Therapy Centre, and the Women's Health Clinic. The agencies offer a variety of programs and primary care services that are increasingly accessed by group participants on their own or in collaboration with HSMM outreach staff. This approach is consistent with literature citing the importance of familiarizing newcomer women with health care services so that these services can be more engaged and involved in women's care (Small et al., 2014).

Box 25.2 List of HSMM Group Topics

Abortion	Fire safety
Birth control (emergency birth control, tubal ligation, vasectomy, birth control pills, condoms, DepoProvera™)	Food safety
	Hepatitis B
	HIV in Canada
Birthing in hospital (triage process, what to take with you)	Immunization
	Insect repellent
Body changes in pregnancy	Introduction to solids
Breastfeeding	Postpartum depression
Car seat safety	Sleep routine and sleep safety for infants
Caring for your newborn—listening to baby	
Caring for yourself	Summer activities
Comfort measures in labour (medical and nonmedical)	Sun safety
	Tummy time
Dehydration	When to call a doctor (colds, etc.)
Dental care	Winter safety/activities
Diabetes	Yeast infections

HSMM staff has learned that using PowerPoint™ presentations is effective and efficient for these large and diverse groups, and the newcomer women enjoy them. Using slides with pictures and simple English phrases, presenters speak to the topic in English while female community interpreters, who are paid by HSMM, simultaneously interpret it in multiple languages. The HSMM team meets quarterly to organize upcoming sessions and plans topics based on the assessed needs of the group and topics requested by participants. See Box 25.2 for a list of topics that have been discussed in the HSMM group.

A wide variety of important health topics specific to newcomer populations are regularly discussed. Depending on the country of origin, newcomers may have infectious diseases such as TB, HIV/AIDS, and hepatitis; iron deficiencies; parasites and tropical diseases; as well as vaccine preventable diseases not commonly seen in Canada (WRHA, 2010). Public health nurses increase awareness of a variety of health promotion topics, access to vaccination, as well as treatment for and prevention of infectious diseases. The nurses also work with clients on an individual basis to build their capacity to promote their personal and family health. One example is counselling HIV-positive mothers regarding formula feeding. For many newcomers, there is stigma associated with not breastfeeding, as it may be seen as acknowledgement of a positive HIV status. HSMM staff members assist with problem solving by providing anticipatory guidance about infant feeding questions. Given the large group size, HSMM staff is always cognizant of concerns regarding confidentiality pertaining to personal health issues.

The newcomer women are eager to learn about Canadian culture and traditions. The weather is one topic that requires ongoing education, considering the majority of participants come from warm climates and have never experienced snow. Some newcomer mothers and children have come to the HSMM group when it has been −40°C wearing only sandals or with bare feet and without adequately warm winter clothing. Participants may not be aware of how to dress appropriately for the weather or where to access warm clothes for their families. HSMM orders free winter wear specific to family need from *Koats for Kids*. Knowledge of ice and winter safety equips newcomer families to enjoy the many free and low cost winter activities available in Winnipeg, such as river skating and tobogganing.

Food is another key topic for ongoing discussion and skill development. A healthy snack is provided at the beginning of each session, and a meal is provided following the group presentation. The newcomer women are often not familiar with foods found in Canadian grocery stores; they do not know what foods to buy or how to prepare them. Newcomers may have large families with older children in school who want to eat the same foods as their Canadian classmates. HSMM's ready-to-cook "meal bags" are available for $1.50, and contain a simple recipe and the ingredients necessary to prepare it at home. At each session, a public health nutritionist demonstrates how to use the "meal bag" ingredients to prepare the healthy meal, and participants sample it as the group meal provided that day. The nutritionist also offers other food and nutrition suggestions, answers questions, and is available for one-on-one consultation following the group meeting. Some women report that learning how to manage their diet and cook in Canada is the primary reason for attending HSMM. One participant reported that she and her children had anemia, and she wanted to "learn how to eat properly."

Public health nurses have found that newcomer women who never understood about female anatomy, birth control, or choice are now utilizing abortion, DepoProvera™, intrauterine devices, and tubal ligation to manage their fertility and childbearing. The women are taking several hundred of the freely offered condoms each month and openly discussing previously taboo topics such as sexuality, pregnancy, birth control, abortion, genital cutting/circumcision, postpartum depression, and domestic violence. Some women are empowered to make their own choices regarding birth control options rather than relying on their partners for family planning decisions.

Through their group participation, the women are learning and becoming familiar with a variety of different health topics, Canadian customs and foods, and many other important life issues.

Reorienting Health Services

According to the Ottawa Charter, health services are a shared responsibility among "individuals, community groups, health professionals, health service institutions and governments," and must be reoriented beyond a biomedical focus to meet the needs of people holistically (WHO, 1986) (see also Chapter 8). Newcomer families at the HSMM group often have complicated health, legal, and social issues that require highly individualized and interprofessional intervention. Public health nurses collaborate with the HSMM team and professionals from other sectors such as Child & Family Services and Employment & Income Assistance to promote equity by facilitating newcomer access to community resources and services such as housing, income, and child care. These activities highlight the importance of the public health role that focuses interventions on the spectrum of determinants that affect health, not only on health risks or disease.

Moving beyond traditional models of health service delivery is critical to promoting the health of newcomer women and children. Newcomers lack knowledge of Canadian health and social systems, and when compounded by diverse cultures and beliefs from their home countries, it can be difficult for them to access the services and resources that meet their needs (Higginbottom et al., 2014). Other ways that HSMM is reorienting health services for women includes the integration of evidence-based strategies to promote prenatal and postpartum health. With HSMM funding from the Canada Prenatal Nutrition Program, participants are provided with milk coupons during pregnancy and to 6 months postpartum, prenatal vitamins, and Vitamin D for breastfed babies. Each woman who receives vitamins meets individually with a public health nutritionist who provides counselling and supports the woman in understanding vitamin use and administration.

Strengthening Community Action

A community development approach is essential in strengthening community action (see also Chapter 5). The growth of the newcomer population in Winnipeg necessitated an innovative model with access to a variety of languages in one place. It took time, word of mouth, and good

---

Box 25.3 Languages Interpreted at HSMM

Amharic	Dinka	Kirundi	Persian	Tigrinya
Arabic	Farsi	Kurdish	Russian	Urdu
Bulgarian	French	Mandarin	Somali	Vietnamese
Cantonese	Karen	Nepali	Spanish	
Chinese	Kinyarwanda	Oromo	Swahili	

---

spirits but the HSMM group has strengthened newcomer women, the community, and the collaborations among professionals. The success of the group has also highlighted the potential to address inequities and large demographic challenges by working together with women to strengthen community action.

A key to health promotion and strengthening community action is interpretation services. The weekly presentation is interpreted into fifteen languages simultaneously. HSMM staff finds the choreography required to do this both a constant challenge and inspiration. In the past, HSMM groups have had participants speaking as many as 22 languages, necessitating the same number of interpreters. Box 25.3 contains a list of the languages that have been provided at the group. Interpretation is paid fee-for-service work, often done by participants who attended HSMM in the past. Interpretation services, interdisciplinary approaches, and services that are evidence-based have been found to be essential to promoting the health of newcomer populations (Pottie et al., 2014). Language is essential to the development of effective support groups for newcomers, for them to feel comfortable sharing their experiences, asking questions, and developing social support networks (Makwarimba et al., 2013). A research study with Sudanese and Somali refugees in Canada reported that peers and professionals who spoke their language, but were also proficient in the English language and Canadian customs, were especially important and valued by the newcomers (Makwarimba et al., 2013).

Building Healthy Public Policy

Building healthy public policy consists of "coordinated action that leads to health, income and social policies that foster great equity" (WHO, 1986) (see also Chapter 9). Reutter and Kushner (2010) cite policy analysis and advocacy as fundamental in tackling health inequities. Policy analysis is understanding the effect of policy and governance structures in contributing to inequities (Reutter & Kushner, 2010). They argue that public policies that fail to address the social determinants of health are the root cause of inequities.

Public health nurses are ideally situated for this role based on their daily involvement with clients in their homes and community, but they must recognize that policy advocacy and tackling inequities is most effective when working collaboratively (Reutter & Kushner, 2010). One example of building healthy public policy to foster health equity is access to free infant formula for HIV-positive mothers. For most newcomers at HSMM, breastfeeding is the norm but for low-income HIV-positive mothers, access to free infant formula is essential. One of the public health nursing staff at the HSMM group worked in collaboration with the community health nurses at Nine Circles, the main HIV community health centre in Winnipeg, to advocate for the provincial government to make formula available to all HIV-positive newcomer women. Through actions such as collaboration, advocacy, and political lobbying, public health workers contribute to social justice and promote equity by creating change at the organizational, local, national, and global levels (CNA, 2010).

The federal and Manitoba governments have recognized the importance of earliest-possible health and nutrition interventions with high-needs populations by their policy and funding commitments to groups such as HSMM, via the Canada Prenatal Nutrition Program and Healthy Baby of Healthy Child Manitoba. These investments have been proven to make a difference. In collaboration with public health services, new models of collaboration have been developed that contribute to strong social fabric in many Manitoba communities.

Summary

The Canadian Nurses Association states that nurses foster social justice through the promotion of equity and access to health care and other human rights by building capacity, working to reduce poverty, promoting enabling environments, advocating for human rights, and developing partnerships to create change (CNA, 2010). In this case story we described the role of the public health team in promoting social justice and equity for newcomer families at the HSMM site in Winnipeg. The HSMM group is an excellent example of the effectiveness and coordination of multiple services, which can improve health and health outcomes for newcomer women and children.

Acknowledgement

The authors would like to acknowledge the contributions of the HSMM staff in the development and review of this manuscript: Gail Wylie, HSMM Executive Director; Davorka Monti, RD and HSMM Prenatal Program Coordinator; and Lavonne Harms, RD, MEd, Winnipeg Regional Health Authority.

REFERENCES

Canadian Nurses Association (CNA). (2010). *Social Justice…a means to an end, an end in itself* (2nd ed.). Ottawa: Author.

Canadian Public Health Association (CPHA). (2010). *Public health Community health nursing practice in Canada. Roles and activities* (4th ed.). Ottawa: Author.

Government of Canada. (2015). *Immigration & citizenship.* URL=http://www.cic.gc.ca/english/index.asp

Heaman, M., Bayrampour, H., Kingston, D., Blondel, B., Gissler, M., Roth, C., et al. (2013). Migrant women's utilization of prenatal care: A systematic review. *Maternal and Child Health Journal, 17*(5), 816–836.

Heaman, M. I., Moffatt, M., Elliott, L., Sword, W., Helewa, M. E., Morris, H., et al. (2014). Barriers, motivators and facilitators related to prenatal care utilization among inner-city women in Winnipeg, Canada: A case-control study. *BMC Pregnancy and Childbirth, 14*, 227.

Higginbottom, G. M., Hadziabdic, E., Yohani, S., & Paton, P. (2014). Immigrant women's experience of maternity services in Canada: A meta-ethnography. *Midwifery, 30*(5), 544–559.

Immigrant & Refugee Partners. (2014). *Optimizing the mental health & emotional wellbeing of immigrants and refugees in Winnipeg: A conceptual framework.* Winnipeg: Winnipeg Regional Health Authority.

Immigration and Refugee Protection Act (S.C. 2001, c.27). URL= the Government of Canada Justice Laws website: http://lois.justice.gc.ca/eng/acts/I-2.5/page-1.html

Makwarimba, E., Stewart, M., Simich, L., Makumbe, K., Shizha, E., & Anderson, S. (2013). Sudanese and Somali Refugees in Canada: Social support needs and preferences. *International Migration, 51*(5), 106–119.

Manitoba Government. (2013). *Manitoba immigration facts—2012 statistical report.* Winnipeg: Manitoba Immigration and Multiculturalism. URL=https://www.gov.mb.ca/labour/immigration/pdf/manitoba_immigration_facts_report_2012.pdf

Manitoba Government. (2015). *Manitoba is growing through immigration.* URL=http://www.immigratemanitoba.com

O'Mahony, J. M., & Donnelly, T. T. (2013). How does gender influence immigrant and refugee women's postpartum depression help-seeking experiences?. *Journal of Psychiatric and Mental Health Nursing, 20*(8), 714–725.

Pottie, K., Batista, R., Mayhew, M., Mota, L., & Grant, K. (2014). Improving delivery of primary care for vulnerable migrants: delphi consensus to prioritize innovative practice strategies. *Canadian Family Physician, 60*(1), e32–e40.

Reutter, L., & Kushner, K. E. (2010). "Health equity through action on the social determinants of health": taking up the challenge in nursing. *Nursing Inquiry, 17*(3), 269–280.

Small, R., Roth, C., Raval, M., Shafiei, T., Korfker, D., Heaman, M, et al. (2014). Immigrant and non-immigrant women's experiences of maternity care: A systematic and comparative review of studies in five countries. *BMC Pregnancy and Childbirth, 14*, 152.

Statistics Canada. (2011). *Women in Canada: A gender-based statistical report.* URL=http://www.statcan.gc.ca/pub/89–503-x/89–503-x2010001-eng.pdf

Winnipeg Regional Health Authority (WRHA) Research & Evaluation Unit. (2010). *Part two: Developing an evidence-informed response: Understanding the health and health issues of immigrant and refugee populations in Winnipeg, Manitoba and Canada.* Winnipeg: Author. URL=http://www.wrha.mb.ca/research/cha/files/ImmRefug_PART02.pdf

World Health Organization (WHO). (1986). *The Ottawa charter for health promotion.* Geneva: Author.

ONLINE RESOURCES

Please visit the Point at http://thepoint.lww.com/Vollman4e for up-to-date Internet resources and additional learning materials on this topic.

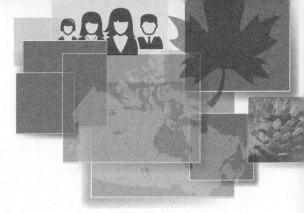

CHAPTER *26*

Nunavut's *Inunnguiniq* Parenting Program

Gwen K. Healey

LEARNING OBJECTIVES

After studying this chapter, you should be able to:

1. Describe the child-rearing philosophy of Inuit people

2. List the five stages of learning described by Inuit Elders

3. Explain the development and implementation of a community-led public health intervention in Nunavut

Introduction

In recent years, communities in Nunavut have drawn attention to the need for parenting support for families (Healey, 2006a; 2006c; 2007). Most of the programs that have been offered in Nunavut have originated from other populations (Healey, 2015b). Parents desire access to programs that reflected Inuit values and knowledge, and that revitalized the parenting perspectives promoted by Inuit Elders. In 2010, the *Qaujigiartiit* Health Research Centre[1] set out to meet this need by developing an evidence-based parenting program based on Inuit childrearing perspectives.

POPULATION ASSESSMENT

Inuit are the indigenous inhabitants of the North American Arctic, whose homeland stretches from the Bering Strait to east Greenland, a distance of over 6,000 km. Nunavut is one of the four Canadian *Inuit Nunangat*[2]: Nunavut, Nunavik (Northern Quebec), Inuvialuit (northern

---

[1]Qaujigiartiit is an independent, non-profit community research centre governed by a volunteer board of directors. Qaujigiartiit Health Research Centre enables health research to be conducted locally, by *Nunavummiut,* and with communities in a supportive, safe, and culturally sensitive and ethical environment, as well as promote the inclusion of both Inuit *Qaujimajatuqangit* (worldview) and western sciences in improving the health of *Nunavummiut* (the Inuktitut term for "people of Nunavut.")

[2]Inuit Nunangat is an Inuktitut term commonly used to refer to the lands occupied by Inuit.

Northwest Territories), and Nunatsiavut (northern Québec). Today, there are 25 communities in Nunavut that range in size from a population of 110 to a population of 7,000. The total population of Nunavut in 2011 was 31,906, of whom approximately 85% are Inuit (Statistics Canada, 2012). Nunavut has a very young population; in 2011, 51% of the Nunavut population was 24 years of age and younger (Statistics Canada, 2012).

Historically, small groups of Inuit families traveled together to different camps and hunting grounds, in *ilagiit nunagivaktangat*.[3] In the Qikiqtaaluk (Baffin) region, for example, Inuit lived in small, kin-based groups in over 100 locations throughout the region (QIA, 2010). Today there are 12 permanent communities in the region. Before formal schooling was introduced, Inuit children learned the skills they needed to carry out their traditional roles by observation and practice (Bennet & Rowley, 2004; QIA, 2010). They acquired knowledge and skills by accompanying parents on harvesting activities (Bennet & Rowley, 2004); preparing skins and sewing clothing; and observing and assisting with childrearing, food preparation, and camp life (Briggs et al., 2000). While specific practices differed among camps/regions in the pre-settlement period (e.g., practices related to childbirth), generally teachings related to family and reproductive health were supported equally by both men and women and embedded in everyday life activities and conversations among the family (Briggs et al., 2000; NCI & QIA, 2011).

A process of relocation to more central sites began as a response by Inuit to the presence of traders, explorers, and missionaries. It took new form with systematic efforts of the government in the 1940s and 1950s to "resettle" Canada's North (INAC, 1996). At the beginning of this period, Inuit in the Central and Eastern Arctic were still involved in the fur trade and were living off the land. Military presence, resource development, and missionary activity were increasing, and tuberculosis and polio epidemics took a toll among Inuit (Tester & Kulchyski, 1994). By 1956, one in seven Inuit was living in a tuberculosis sanatorium in southern Canada for treatment (Sandiford Grygier, 1994). The first government-regulated school for Inuit was opened in Chesterfield Inlet in 1951 (Pauktuutit Inuit Women's Association of Canada, 2007). Inuit parents were asked to place their children in school hostels for all or a portion of the school year while parents and non-school-age siblings returned to their camps. Inuit parents who agreed to schooling did not wish to leave their children alone and often came to the settlement with their families, living in tents until housing was available. However, the majority of children were separated from their parents and sent away. This caused great anguish for both the parents and the children (QIA, 2010). Residential schools for Inuit continued to open into the 1960s, and by 1963, 3,997 Inuit children were attending these schools (King, 2006). In June 1964, 75% of 6- to 15-year-old Inuit children and youth were enrolled in the residential schools. These students are the parents and grandparents, uncles, and aunts of today.

Inuit of northern Canada, as with other indigenous groups in Canada, have experienced a shift in a way-of-living over the last several decades; changes continue to be felt today as well with advances in technology and society. Those people who were medically evacuated for tuberculosis or other medical treatment often returned to their communities up to a year or more later, or not at all (Sandiford Grygier, 1994), and residential school students were away from their families for up to 10 months of the year (King, 2006). These individuals were disconnected from their families, culture, language, and community upon their return (Healey, 2006b; Kirmayer et al., 2009). The reports of physical, emotional, mental, and sexual abuse of children during the residential school era are well documented (Wesley-Esquimaux & Smolewski, 2004). The experiences of resettled Inuit continue to have an impact on many Nunavut residents to this day.

---

[3]*Ilagiit nunagivaktangat* is Inuktitut terminology meaning "a place used regularly or seasonally by Inuit for hunting, harvesting, and/ or gathering."

However, not all Inuit were separated from their families or attended residential school during the relocation events, and each community in Nunavut has a unique settlement history related to, for example, their location, exposure to infectious illness, access to harvesting areas, and presence of authorities or trade (Tester & Kulchyski, 1994). As part of a movement to reclaim and share Inuit knowledge and ways of knowing, *Nunavummiut* have been working most recently to revitalize Inuit perspectives on family and attachments by sharing *inunnguiniq* perspectives through books, DVDs, parenting programs, and resources to make knowledge more accessible to those who do not have access to it through the traditional oral story-telling pathway. Such initiatives include camps and land-based activities that celebrate the role of the land in the holistic Inuit wellness perspective and in the sharing of Inuit skills and knowledge with both youth and adults. Increasingly works are being published that incorporate multimedia, film, information technology, and written text to share Inuit stories, philosophies, knowledge, art, practices, and humour with community members and with the next generation.

Inuit society is founded on a system of kinship relations (Kral et al., 2011; NCCAH, 2011). The kinship group was once the setting for dialogue on family relations and sexual and reproductive health (Ootoova et al., 2001), which has largely been replaced by teachings from the medical community and the school system (Steenbeek et al., 2006).

THE PROJECT

The *Inunnguiniq* Parenting Program is the result of 5 years of research and consultation with many individuals, Elders, organizations, and communities. The first goal of the *Inunnguiniq* Parenting Program is to revitalize the wisdom and practices of *inunnguiniq* (see Box 26.1 and Table 26.1) in our lives today. The second goal is to support healing for program participants and their families. The third goal is to increase the practice of *inunnguiniq* in our communities, strengthening the roles of extended family and community in child rearing.

Program Description

In the *inunnguiniq* learning model, Inuit see everyone in a community as interconnected. In fact, Inuit Elders say we are all both learners and teachers. They say we learn from everyone and everything with which we interact. Traditionally, even young children are both learners and teachers. This is because Inuit believe children carry the souls and personalities of their namesakes (Bennet & Rowley, 2004), so Inuit believe children also carry on their namesakes' knowledge. The idea of continuous learning is also stressed in *inunnguiniq*. Inuit Elders have outlined five stages of learning (Fig. 26.1). People can be at different stages of learning and

---

Box 26.1 Inunnguiniq

Part of Inuit child-rearing philosophy is known as *inunnguiniq*, which literally translates to "the making of a human being" and refers to traditional childrearing wisdom and practices. *Inunnguiniq* is process of socialization and education. The cultural expectation is that every child will become able/enabled/capable so that they can be assured of living a good life. A good life is considered one where you have sufficient proper attitude and ability to be able to contribute to working for the common good—helping others and making improvements for those to come. As such, it describes culturally situated ethical and social/behavioural expectations, specific competencies and skill sets, and an adherence to a well-defined set of values, beliefs, and principles that are foundational to the Inuit life view.

TABLE 26.1 Six Foundational *Inunnguiniq* Principles

Principles	Actions
1. Develop habits for living a good life	• Finish what you start and persevere in life • Continually plan ahead and be well-organized • Take care of your belongings and develop strong skills • Listen to the teachings and apply them in life
2. Rise above hardship by always looking for solutions	• Be adaptable and focus on the future • Be capable so that others will have confidence in you • Identify your needs and do not seek what you do not need • Apply knowledge to experiences • Seek understanding of the things around you
3. Be heart-centred (build a strong moral character)	• Show humanity • Behave ethically • Be self-reliant • Show respect, be responsible, and be accountable
4. Show compassion, serve others, and build relationships	• Anticipate the needs of others • Serve willingly • Show love that is enabling • Discuss openly, communicate well
5. Recognize the uniqueness of each individual	• Set high expectations • Identify skills and nurture them • Never confuse the child • Focus on strengths • Be present in your community
6. Always take steps to make improvements	• Start with sewing the seeds of how to do something • Start with where a person/child is at • Expect progress • Show how to do something and expect the person/child to do what is shown • Never give up on the child/person learn

QHRC, 2014.

Inuit believe this is a positive situation. It means there are those who can benefit from our experiences; at the same time, it means there are others with experiences that can help us. The role of observation is also an important part of the learning model, and Inuit believe practice is essential for the development of proficiency.

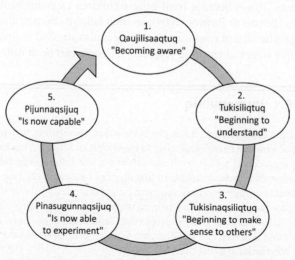

FIGURE 26.1 The five stages of learning described by Inuit Elders (QHRC, 2014).

These traditional beliefs are reflected in the *Inunnguiniq* Parenting Program. The program has an open structure. It can have a drop-in approach. This allows parents to join at any time and engage at any level. They then can take time away from the program and practice what they learned. Parents can return at a later date to join a different module. Other participants may continue directly from one session to the next. In this way, participants are able to move through the program at their own pace.

The basic structure of the *Inunnguiniq* Parenting Program is:

- Pairs of local facilitators, supported by central support coordinators, offer the program together in English, Inuktitut, and Inuinnaqtun as participants require.
- The format is a strengths-based group discussion. Each session begins with a central theme that is explored through a range of activities and dialogue over the course of 2 to 3 hours.
- The target audience is parents/caregivers/foster parents/extended family, anyone who cares for children full- or part-time. This is NOT a program for "high-risk" parents; rather it is designed for ALL individuals who care for children. Group size is approximately 8 to 10 participants, with 2 facilitators and a minimum of 1 Elder.
- The program is not a formal counselling program; referrals are made to mental health counsellors when needed.
- The program consists of 6 modules taught over 19 sessions (offered one to three times per week depending on facilitator comfort and availability).
- Each session is to include an Elder if possible. In some cases, DVDs of Elders speaking or telling stories were incorporated into sessions when Elders were not available or were not comfortable speaking on a particular topic.
- Each program is to incorporate excursions on the land, for example for harvesting animals, fish, berries or eggs, in a minimum of one session, but can expand to more.
- The program provides childcare at each session to support participants.
- Each session incorporates a food component (a snack break). The snack is nutritious and is country food when it is available. Recipe ideas are included in the program.

The resources provided for the *Inunnguiniq* Parenting Program include:

- Each program receives the following documents (two copies in English and two copies in Inuktitut):
  - *Inunnguiniq* Parenting Program Curriculum (Modules 1 to 5 and a separate volume for Module 6)
  - *Inunnguiniq* Parenting Program Handbook (additional material for parents and facilitators that includes additional stories from Elders, supplemental activities, and an appendix of recipes from Nunavut community cooking programs)
  - *Inunnguiniq* Child Development Pamphlets from 0 to 18 years
  - *Inunnguiniq* Evaluation Booklet
- Each program receives a bin of resources (e.g., food guides, DVDs, CDs, posters, pamphlets) to complement the activities in the program.

The *Qaujigiartiit* Research Centre piloted, evaluated, and revised this evidence-based, culturally responsive parenting program prior to releasing it for use in Nunavut. The evaluation was accomplished in two phases. In phase 1 of program development, *Qaujigiartiit* collaborated with the Elder's Advisory Committee to the Nunavut Department of Education. This committee is composed of Elders from across Nunavut who share knowledge and perspectives on various topics and themes at in-person meetings three to four times a year. They permitted access to the knowledge they had about child rearing and Inuit family relationships, which informed the content of the program. In addition, the Nunavut Department of Health and Social Services (NDHSS) contributed to the development of a module about healthy family nutrition. *Qaujigiartiit* secured funding and support for pilot tests in two communities, Iqaluit and Arviat; NDHSS provided funding and program support for six additional pilot sites (Cambridge Bay, Cape Dorset, Clyde River, Coral Harbor, Gjoa Haven, and Rankin Inlet). *Qaujigiartiit* conducted the data collection and evaluation for all eight communities. Based on the findings from Phase 1, the program was revised with the Nunavut Literacy Council to adjust the language and flow of the material to mirror concepts in adult learning theory. The revised curriculum was piloted a second time as part of Phase Two in four of the original communities.

Program Evaluation Process

The evaluation was conducted within an indigenous knowledge framework with a focus on Inuit ways of knowing, specifically the *Piliriqatigiinniq* Partnership Community Health Research Model (Healey & Tagak Sr., 2014). The model highlights five Inuit concepts: *Piliriqatigiinniq,* the concept of working together for the common good; *Pittiarniq,* the concept of being good or kind; *Inuuqatigiittiarniq,* the concept of being respectful of others; *Unikkaaqatigiinniq,* the philosophy of storytelling and/or the power and meaning of story; and *Iqqaumaqatigiinniq,* the concept that ideas or thoughts may come into "one." This framework guided the collaborative, responsive, ethical approach to the implementation of the program and the evaluation. Capturing stories and perspectives of participants was of critical importance.

Information for evaluation was gathered from each of the communities that participated in the pilots of the program. Data collection included: weekly telephone calls between support coordinators and facilitators; evaluation questions completed by facilitators after each session; pre- and postnutrition module questionnaires and an exit questionnaire completed by participants; and teleconferences between the program coordinator and each of the facilitator pairs to discuss program successes and ideas for overcoming challenges.

Criteria that were used to evaluate success of the program were:

- Number of participants/repeat participants
- Involvement of Elders
- Level of facilitator engagement and enthusiasm with program
- Ease of use of the program materials
- Participant comprehension of and responses to the content and its presentation
- Level of participant interaction with other participants in the program
- Participant and facilitator self-reported satisfaction with the program
- Stories articulating positive parenting experiences with family during and after the program

Reflections on the *Inunnguiniq* Parenting Program

Overall, participants reported that they enjoyed the program; they particularly appreciated learning about traditional Inuit perspectives on child rearing and healthy parenting. They reported feeling greater connections with children, stronger bonds, and happier overall.

Not all communities had Elders available to assist with program delivery; those that regularly invited Elders to share Inuit parenting practices had the greatest success. It was reported that their presence had a relaxing effect on participants and facilitators, making sessions more enjoyable. Participants were more engaged when Elders were teaching and sharing stories; they had many questions for the Elders and were keen to learn from them. Elders who understood the purpose of the program and who were comfortable sharing traditional stories were essential to its success.

Participants and facilitators found the session on healing had very strong and emotional responses, and often continued into one to two more sessions. Both facilitators and participants highlighted the need for additional healing support for participants. Facilitators wanted to be responsive to the needs of participants; however, there were insufficient resources (e.g., counsellors, trusted professionals) available in some communities to whom participants could be referred. One facilitator recalled a session that turned into a healing session in which the participants felt compelled to support another participant in need. In this case, the facilitator attempted to re-direct the participants and repeated that healing and counselling was not the intent of the program as no one in the room was trained with the skills to support a seriously distraught person in the event that this was needed (it was not). The participants felt otherwise and stated that their purpose was to support each other. The facilitators consented, and the session was then devoted to supporting the participant in need. All participants hugged at the end of the session and reported feeling lighter and happier. The facilitators also made connections to the community health centre where participants could be referred if they needed additional emotional support.

The strength-based group discussion format was very successful. Facilitators reported that listening and sharing stories with others helped participants feel better about their personal struggles, and that participants provided support to each other. Participants reported transferring this dialogue format into their family life.

Facilitators noted that participants were most comfortable with and responsive to material when they were active and working on something with their hands (e.g., preparing materials for a trip on the land or cooking). When men participated, they participated with more enthusiasm when activities were on the land.

Facilitators and participants both appreciated the food and nutritional components of the program. Some facilitators reported it was the food component of the program that kept parents coming. Snacks, leftovers, and (in some communities) take-home items in the form of a door prize or gift item provided additional, much needed, food in participants' homes. Country food was sometimes difficult to obtain but always appreciated. Activity around food preparation was reported to provide respite for the more strenuous, emotional parts of the program. Participants talked more openly during periods where they were preparing food as a group. They learned how to prepare household budgets as well as plan and budget for family meals that included traditional Inuit country foods and store-bought foods. Parents enjoyed the different types of recipes that were provided by community nutrition projects and the NDHSS.

The implementation of each specific pilot program became adapted to each community; facilitators were responsive to the needs and resources available. Successful delivery was dependent on facilitator literacy level and teaching style, comfort level in leading groups, community resources, and participant needs. There was a wide spectrum of delivery methods: one community read the curriculum directly from the book and, on the other side of the spectrum, one community chose a module topic such as "Living a Good Life" and then asked an Elder to come and share on this topic.

Some groups opened with prayer and took time to do a "round table" check-in about how each participant was feeling and if anything was bothering them or their children. This soft start allowed participants to "get things off their chest" after which they were more clear-minded, not as preoccupied, and more ready for new learning. One group started each session with food and slowly eased into the discussion of program content.

Facilitators noted that participants were more comfortable staying together in a large group. Many chose not to break into smaller groups but rather discussed things together as a whole. This was reported to benefit group unity.

Activities naturally fostered communication and group dialogue. Participants felt more at ease while cooking, interacting with their children, or doing other kinds of activities. Facilitators felt this mirrored traditional and familiar modes of learning in Inuit communities, where a knowledgeable individual would share knowledge, such as the role one plays in a family, to younger members of the community while simultaneously teaching an activity, such as sewing clothing or repairing equipment.

One group felt awkward in the meeting space they were allotted, so they partnered with the Canadian Prenatal Nutrition Program to use their facility with which facilitators and participants were familiar. This change in venue also helped with attendance. The benefits of collaborating with other community programs was noted as helpful in providing a safe space for participants and increasing comfort level as participants felt at ease in a familiar space.

Facilitators reported that when they were responsive to parent needs and flexible with the program material, the order of the sessions, and the mood of the group on any given day, the group was more unified, which resulted in a greater sense of belonging and increased engagement.

A facilitator for the most successful pilot, while leading a group on her own, shared her own feelings about her difficult week, telling participants that "[she] almost did not come, but did so because of the people in the class and that [she] knew [she] would feel better after the group." Parents were very responsive to her honesty and the facilitator reported that they "felt like a little family" as a result.

The most successful group finished the program with a formal sit down dinner open to all participants' family members. Their Elder said a prayer and read out a thank you note in their language. This note was laminated and presented to each participant as a keepsake along with certificates of completion. Some participants made a speech and spoke from the heart. Each participant received a bag with health promotion items to take home.

Summary

Inuit society is relational, founded on a system of kinship relations, and these relations form the basis of a unique attachment philosophy. Many Canadian Inuit families were dispersed and separated during the period of time in which communities were formally created in the Canadian Arctic. Arctic settlement and separation fragmented the very foundation of Inuit society, ways of knowing, language, and knowledge communication. The settlement and residential school era fractured Canadian Inuit family bonds and disrupted parent-child-extended family attachments by separating young children from their parents for extended periods of time (Healey, 2015a).

In reflection upon the relocation and settlement time period in Inuit history, Inuit have since celebrated a collective resilience in the face of such societal devastation. The resilience, strength, and capability of Inuit have become the focus of community-led initiatives to reclaim family relationship perspectives, kinships, creativity, Inuit skills, harvesting, and education. Parents in other studies have described a connection between kinship relations, family attachments, and community wellness (Healey, 2006a; Kral et al., 2011; Healey, 2015a). Public health interventions that mirror community-led initiatives to revitalize *inunnguiniq* are effective and make a positive contribution to Nunavut families by revitalizing and strengthening the family bonds that have been cherished by Inuit for millennia (Healey, 2015a).

REFERENCES

Bennet, J., & Rowley, S. (2004). *Uqalurait: An oral history of Nunavut.* Montreal: McGill Queen's University Press.

Briggs, J., Ekho, N., & Ottokie, U. (2000). *Childrearing practices* (Vol. 3). Iqaluit: Nunavut Arctic College.

Healey, G. (2006a). *Community-identified health priorities for Nunavut.* Iqaluit: Qaujigiartiit/Arctic Health Research Network – Nunavut.

Healey, G. (2006b). *An exploration of determinants of health for Inuit women in Nunavut.* (Masters of Science thesis). Calgary, Alberta: University of Calgary.

Healey, G. (2006c). *Report on Health Research Ethics Workshop and Community Consultation in Iqaluit, Nunavut.* Iqaluit: Qaujigiartiit/Arctic Health Research Network – Nunavut.

Healey, G. (2007). *Report on Health Research Ethics Workshop and Community Consultation in Rankin Inlet, Nunavut.* Iqaluit: Qaujigiartiit/Arctic Health Research Network – Nunavut.

Healey, G. (2015a). *Childhood trauma and the disruption of attachments in Inuit relational society: A study from Nunavut Territory, Canada.* Manuscript submitted for publication.

Healey, G. (2015b). *Inunnguiniq Parenting Program for Nunavummiut: 2010–2015 Final evaluation.* Iqaluit: Qau-jigiartiit Health Research Centre. URL=http://qhrc.ca/sites/default/files/inunnguiniq_parenting_program_evaluation_2010–2015_-_feb_2015.pdf

Healey, G., & Tagak Sr., A. (2014). Piliriqatigiinniq "Working in a collaborative way for the common good": A per-spective on the space where health research methodology and Inuit epistemology come together. *International Journal of Critical Indigenous Studies, 7*(1), 1–14.

Indian and Northern Affairs Canada (INAC). (1996). Relocation of Aboriginal communities. In *Report of the Royal Commission on Aboriginal Peoples (Canada)* (Vol. 1). Ottawa: Government of Canada.

King, D. (2006). *A brief report of the federal government of Canada's residential school system for Inuit.* Ottawa: Aboriginal Healing Foundation.

Kirmayer, L. J., Tait, C. L., & Simpson, C. (2009). Mental health of Aboriginal peoples in Canada:Transformations of identity and community. In L. J. Kirmayer, & G. G. Valaskis (Eds.), *Healing Traditions: The mental health of aboriginal peoples in Canada* (pp. 3–35). Vancouver: UBC Press.

Kral, M. J., Idlout, L., Minore, J. B., Dyck, R. J., & Kirmayer, L. J. (2011). Unikkaartuit: Meanings of well-being, un-happiness, health, and community change among Inuit in Nunavut, Canada. *American Journal of Community Psychology, 48*, 426–438.

National Collaborating Centre for Aboriginal Health (NCCAH). (2011). *The role of Inuit knowledge in the care of children.* URL=http://www.nccah-ccnsa.ca/274/Inuit_Knowledge_in_the_care_of_children__a_fact_sheet_series.nccah

Niutaq Cultural Institute (NCI), & Qikiqtani Inuit Association (QIA). (2011). *Ilaginniq: Interviews on Inuit family values from the Qikiqtani Region* (Vol. 1). Iqaluit: Inhabit Media.

Ootoova, I., Atagutsiak, T. Q., Ijjangiaq, T., Pitseolak, J., Joamie, A., Joamie, A., et al. (2001). *Perspectives on tradi-tional health: Interviewing Inuit Elders* (Vol. 5). Iqaluit: Nunavut Arctic College.

Pauktuutit Inuit Women's Association of Canada. (2007). *Sivumuapallianiq: Journey forward: National Inuit resi-dential schools healing strategy.* Ottawa: Author.

Qaujigiartiit Health Research Centre (QHRC). (2014). *Inunnguiniq Parenting Program curriculum manual.* Iqaluit: Author.

Qikiqtani Inuit Association (QIA). (2010). *Qikiqtani Truth Commission final report: Achieving Saimaqatigiingniq.* Iqaluit: Author.

Sandiford Grygier, P. (1994). *A long way from home: The tuberculosis epidemic among the Inuit.* Montreal: McGill Queen's University Press.

Statistics Canada. (2012). *Nunavut (Code 62) and Canada (Code 01) (table). Census Profile. 2011 Census (Cat. no. 98–316-XWE).* Ottawa: Author. URL=http://www12.statcan.gc.ca/census-recensement/2011/dp-pd/prof/index.cfm?Lang=E

Steenbeek, A., Tyndall, M., Rothenberg, R., & Sheps, S. (2006). Determinants of sexually transmitted infections among Canadian Inuit adolescent populations. *Public Health Nursing, 23*(6), 531–534.

Tester, F., & Kulchyski, P. (1994). *Tammarniit (Mistakes): Inuit relocation in the Eastern Arctic 1939–63.* Vancouver: UBC Press.

Wesley-Esquimaux, C. C., & Smolewski, M. (2004). *Historic trauma and Aboriginal healing.* Ottawa: Aboriginal Healing Foundation.

ONLINE RESOURCES

Please visit the Point at http://thepoint.lww.com/Vollman4e for up-to-date Internet resources and additional learning materials on this topic.

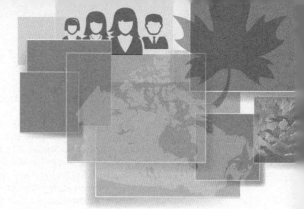

CHAPTER 27

Enhancing the Personal Skills of Service Providers to Promote the Sexual Health of Street-Involved Youth

Wendi Lokanc-Diluzio and Sandra M. Reilly

LEARNING OBJECTIVES

After studying this chapter, you should be able to:

1. Identify the sexual health challenges faced by street-involved youth

2. Compare the sexual health outcomes of street-involved youth to those of mainstream youth

3. Describe an intervention that targets service providers working with street-involved youth

Introduction

On any given day in Canada, thousands of youth live on the streets and face challenges associated with the lack of proper housing and family support. Their financial uncertainty and feelings of powerlessness put street-involved youth (SIY) at risk for negative sexual and reproductive health outcomes, including unintended pregnancy and sexually transmitted and blood borne infections (STBBI) (Alberta Health Services, 2011).

It is important to acknowledge that although SIY face challenges, they also have access to community resources that provide some hope for an improved life. In fact, they go to certain adults at the agencies they access for support. Service providers working with SIY can provide sexual health education and health promotion. However, the special needs of SIY can overtax the capabilities of these providers. As the Canadian Guidelines for Sexual Health Education (PHAC, 2008) points out, SIY have very special characteristics and associated needs. For this reason, we conducted in-depth interviews with SIY and service providers working with them to determine the knowledge that service providers need in order to promote the sexual and reproductive health (SRH) of this high-risk population.

The information collected from the interviews and other assessment data informed the development of two related interventions to develop the personal skills of service providers working with SIY. These are a website resource, Talking About Sexuality in Calgary Communities (tascc.ca), and a 6-hour training program delivered either online or face-to-face.

This case story takes place in Calgary. The interdisciplinary team from the University of Calgary Faculty of Nursing and Alberta Health Services (AHS)—Sexual and Reproductive Health Education and Health Promotion (Calgary Zone) includes nurses, teachers/educators, and health promotion specialists. The AHS team, in its work, provides sexuality education in different settings to a number of populations, and also develops and evaluates resources, and provides in-service education for professionals and parents. In so doing, the team promotes capacity building, working relationships, community engagement, collaboration, and innovation.

To follow, we discuss the assessment and analysis informing the interventions and how we planned, implemented, and evaluated each intervention. It is important to note that although we discuss the process of developing the interventions as linear, it was cyclical, iterative, and evolutionary.

ASSESSMENT

Different types of assessment data informed our interventions. The data included pre-existing literature, anecdotal data, and in-depth interviews with SIY and service providers.

We defined SIY as "young people under the age of 25 who spend considerable amounts of time on the street, hang out with others on the street, and who may live or have lived independently of parents or guardians in marginal or precarious situations" (Worthington & MacLaurin, 2013, p. 163). A 2010 study of 200 SIY, aged 15 to 24 years, in Edmonton described some characteristics of the Alberta-based SIY population (Alberta Health Services, 2011). See Box 27.1.

Box 27.1   Characteristics of Alberta SIY (2010)

- 69% were male; 30.5% were female; 0.5% were transgendered
- 97% were born in Canada; 50.0% were Aboriginal
- Main sources of income: employment (30.1%), government support (24.9%), illicit/unconventional methods (25.9%), and family or friends (18.7%)
- 70% were school drop-outs; 25% planned to return to school
- The majority had experienced some form of abuse in their lives—emotional abuse (81.9%), physical abuse (60.0%), neglect (54.5%), sexual abuse (36.7%)—and witnessed violence (93.5%)
- 40% had used a social worker in the past year; 26% had been in foster care or a group home
- In the three months prior to the study, 40.0% most often slept in a house (e.g., foster care, group home, a relative's home, their own home); 38.5% most often slept in shelters, transitional housing, or hotels; and 21.5% most often slept on the streets or a different place each night
- Over two thirds had been incarcerated at some point
- In terms of sexual orientation, 77.3% were heterosexual, 18.3% were bisexual, 2.5% were "other," and 2.0% were gay
- 25% rated their mental or physical health as fair or poor
- During the year previous to the study approximately 60% had accessed health services through either a walk-in clinic or emergency department
- One third reported they had barriers to accessing health services

---

Source: Alberta Health Services (2011).

A number of SIY partake in lifestyle activities that place them at risk for STBBI and unintended pregnancy. Survey data also indicate that SIY use drugs and alcohol. In the Edmonton study (Alberta Health Services, 2011), 86.4% of SIY reported using alcohol in the three months prior to data collection, with 14.5% of those using alcohol on a daily basis. Additionally, 96.5% used a non-injection drug at least once, 14.0% injected a drug at least once, and over half reported being high on drugs while having sex. Notwithstanding these at-risk behaviours for STBBI, 64.3% of the SIY perceived they were either at no or low risk for acquiring an STBBI, such as HIV or Hepatitis C.

The SRH educators from AHS visit high school Outreach Programs[1] and various agencies to provide SRH education. The topics most commonly discussed include STBBI, relationships, contraception, and safer sex practices. The service providers in these programs and agencies do not have the knowledge, comfort, or skill to deal with the subject matter themselves and the demand for AHS assistance is escalating beyond ability to support it.

To assess the problem, we conducted in-depth interviews with nine SIY and six service providers working at agencies that provide services to SIY. Service providers and SIY alike stated the youth face numerous SRH challenges (e.g., pregnancy and repeated pregnancy, STBBI, unhealthy relationships). Along with their inability to practice safer sex, they suffer from sexual exploitation, substance use, and lack of knowledge about SRH. Further adding to their problems, SIY often experience societal stigmatization and personal embarrassment with regard to their sexuality, and these social problems can certainly inhibit their ability to access services (Lokanc-Diluzio, 2014). Although SIY faced several challenges, it was evident from the interviews that they possessed considerable assets, including a kind of street-sense whereby they learn from their experiences to survive in the face of adversity, and the willingness to make use of community resources (Lokanc-Diluzio, 2014).

Both service providers and SIY reported that relationships play an important role in promoting the SRH of SIY. Because SRH is a sensitive topic and sometimes associated with embarrassment, it is important to build rapport with youth so that they feel comfortable discussing their concerns (Lokanc-Diluzio, 2014).

It was also revealed during the interviews that service providers know they require additional SRH education, specific to SIY. They identified the need for knowledge about community resources and referral mechanisms; pregnancy and contraception; STBBI; safer sex and harm reduction; healthy relationships and communication; substance use and decision making; sexual diversity; sexual exploitation; and facts about anatomy and physiology. They also identified their need for accessible and convenient resources, teaching aids, and tools that contained accurate and user-friendly information, and stressed the importance of connecting with other providers to discuss topics relevant to their work (Lokanc-Diluzio, 2014).

ANALYSIS

The process of analysis entailed comparing the sexual health behaviours and outcomes of SIY to that of mainstream Alberta and Canadian youth (Table 27.1). Comparing the available data illustrated the importance of developing health promotion interventions that could impact the SRH of SIY.

The team decided to focus its efforts on the service providers rather than the SIY for three reasons. First, through the in-depth interviews, the service providers indicated a need and enthusiasm for resources and learning opportunities pertaining to helping SIY about SRH. Second, because street life is transient, the team thought that interventions that targeted SIY and the ability to follow up with them would not be feasible. Finally, the team considered that interventions targeted to service providers would be more sustainable over time and would,

---

[1]Outreach Programs provide many services and a flexible learning environment to high school students whose needs are not met in traditional school settings.

TABLE 27.1 Sexual Behaviours, Substance Use, and Sexual Health Outcomes: Comparison of Street-Involved and Mainstream Youth

	In-Depth Interviews (Lokanc-Diluzio, 2014)	SIY–2010 Edmonton Study (Alberta Health Services, 2011)	Mainstream Youth Aged 15–24 (Canadian Research)
Sexual behaviour	• Many SIY are sexually active	• 98.5% had sexual intercourse at least once • Vaginal (99.0%); oral (91.3%); anal (44.2%)	• 66.0% had sexual intercourse at least once • Age 15–19 (30%); 18–19 (68%); 20–24 (86%) (Rotermann, 2012)
Sexual debut	• Not discussed	• Median age of first vaginal intercourse was 14 years	• 9% of Canadian youth had sexual intercourse prior to age 15 (9.7% males; 8.2% females) (Rotermann, 2012)
Condom use	• Although youth know how to use and access them, condoms are not always used	• During last vaginal sex (47.2%); last oral sex (22.3%); last anal sex (50.6%)	• 72.5% of Alberta youth used a condom during last sexual intercourse (Rotermann, 2012)
Sex trade	• Some SIY have a history of sex trade involvement	• Females (27.0%) and males (2.5%) had sex trade involvement	• Not available
Alcohol use	• Many SIY use alcohol. Alcohol impacts the use of condoms	• 86.4% used alcohol in the last three months	• 79.0% of Canadian youth had used alcohol at least once (Health Canada, 2014) • 71.5% of Canadian youth had used alcohol in the past year (Health Canada, 2014)
Drug use	• Some SIY have a history of drug use and abuse	• 96.5% had tried non-injection drugs at least one time • 56.0% were high on drugs during intercourse during the last three months	• 41.7% Canadian youth had tried cannabis at least once (Health Canada, 2014)
STIs	• Some SIY have either had an STI or been worried they may have an STI	• 12.7% tested positive for chlamydia • 2.0% tested positive for gonorrhea	• 1.5% Alberta youth tested positive for chlamydia • 0.12% Alberta youth tested positive for gonorrhea (Government of Alberta, 2015)
Pregnancy	• Some males have impregnated a partner • Many females have experienced one or more pregnancies • Some females try to get pregnant while on the streets	• 42.6% female SIY had been pregnant at least once	• Not available

in turn, impact more SIY. The team began to plan for two related interventions for service providers: a website and a training program.

Due to time constraints, input from SIY and service providers was limited to the information they provided during the in-depth interviews. With more time, the team could have engaged participants in the planning, implementation, and evaluation phases of both interventions.

THE WEBSITE

The Talking About Sexuality in Calgary Communities website provides a venue for Calgary-based service providers working with SIY to access up-to-date information and resources that reflect evidence-informed practice in SRH education and promotion. The goal is to build service providers' capacity through education and networking. All in all, the website is a platform for on-line education, a vehicle for knowledge transfer and exchange, and a SRH resource for service providers and the youth with whom they work. (Refer to tascc.ca for additional information.)

The design and development of the website took place over approximately 12 weeks and was done on a limited budget. Planning involved meeting with the SRH Education and Promotion Team to create a vision for the website. The team discussed the priorities for website content (as identified in the interviews) and initial ideas for design. Since service providers spoke of needing a "toolbox of resources," the team envisioned a toolbox theme incorporated into the website design. After the team had created a shared vision, they selected a web designer to bring the vision to life. Developing the website content proved time intensive, so the team created a work plan (see example in Table 27.2) to keep things on track. The work plan outlined who had responsibility for writing specific content, who had responsibility for editing or reviewing the content, and the estimated dates for completion.

The website design organized content into the following sections:

- *Who we are:* This section includes the reason and purpose for the website, facts about youth sexuality, key terms, and the models selected to establish credibility of the site.
- *Sexuality topics:* This section includes evidence-informed and current information on 11 topics, as well as case examples and reflective questions to help service providers use the material. The case examples are based upon the stories shared by SIY in their interviews and draw attention to common misunderstandings and myths about sexual health. For a case example related to STBBI, see http://www.tascc.ca/sexuality-topics/sti-hiv.

TABLE 27.2   tascc.ca Website Development Work Plan

Website Section	What	Topic Writer	Topic Editors	Completion Date	Status
Who We Are	Why we developed the site, facts about youth sexuality, key terminology, and theoretical perspectives	AA	BB/CC	Sept 01	Complete
Sexuality Topics	Values	BB	AA/CC	Sept 01	Complete
	Body 101 (Puberty)	BB	AA/CC	Sept 08	Complete
	Pregnancy	CC	BB/DD	Sept 08	Complete
	Birth control	CC	AA/BB	Sept 15	Complete
	Sexually transmitted infections and blood-borne pathogens	AA	BB/CC	Sept 15	Complete
	Relationships	BB	AA/CC	Sept 22	Complete
	Sexual orientation and identity	CC	AA/BB	Sept 22	Complete
	Ages and stages of sexual development	DD	AA/CC	Sept 29	Complete
	Sexual exploitation	BB	CC/DD	Sept 29	Complete
	Sexual decision making	CC	AA/BB	Oct 06	Complete
Training Opportunities	Training opportunities	DD	BB/CC	Oct 06	Under Review
Q & A	Ask a question	DD	AA/BB	Oct 13	Under Review
	Frequently asked questions	CC/BB	AA/DD	Oct 13	Under Review
Resources	Kits and tools	AA	BB/DD	Oct 20	Not Started
	Community referral	DD	AA/CC	Oct 20	Not Started
	Webliography	BB	AA/CC	Oct 27	Not Started
The Latest	Summary of a recent Canadian SRH study	AA	BB/CC	Oct 27	Not Started

---

Box 27.2   Comments About the Website

I think the website is very comprehensive, with a multitude of applicable tools for [service providers] as well as parents. I appreciate the use of non-jargon language as well as some examples of dialogues that will help guide staff and parents in having conversations…I am happy to see relevant as well as current stats being used throughout as often this is difficult to find. The information is factual rather than judgemental and offers a wide variety of options and information without steering the reader towards a specific value or belief system. (Trainer of youth workers)

I love that you can print PDF sheets of information.… There is a lot of information, but it is well organized so I can scan and pick what I need. And there's a lot of real life examples I can think about in relation to clients/youth. (Community educator)

- *Training opportunities:* This section includes workshop and education opportunities for service providers to stay informed about SRH.
- *Q & A:* If service providers or youth have SRH questions, they can submit them to the question box or peruse an extensive assortment of frequently asked questions (FAQs).
- *Resources:* The information and web links in this section can assist service providers to find SRH clinical and education resources.
- *Latest news:* Service providers can read about recent SRH research or news.

Implementation of the website occurred once the development and content were completed. Fifteen individuals representing several professions and disciplines working with various high risk or street-involved youth were asked to formally evaluate the website prior to its launch. Eleven provided oral and written feedback to rate the content, visual appeal, navigation, user-friendliness, and relevance to service providers working with SIY. The overall website rating was 4.9 out of 5. The most common suggestions for improvement related to the website navigation and the need for some sections to have more explanation, and the majority of these were addressed prior to launching the website. Comments from the evaluation are located in Box 27.2.

THE TRAINING PROGRAM

The training program aimed at improving service providers' level of comfort when discussing SRH issues with youth; increasing their knowledge of various SRH topics; and providing educational tools. The logic model for the training programs is illustrated in Table 27.3. The 6-hour program, developed by three SRH education specialists, was devised to be delivered in a 1-day face-to-face training session or over the course of 2 weeks in a series of on-line training sessions.

The design and development of the educational programs occurred over 4 weeks. Once again, a detailed work plan outlined team responsibilities and timelines. Information from the website was used to create the content; the principles of adult education (Knowles et al., 2012) guided the teaching approach. Ultimately, the team used a variety of teaching strategies appropriate to different types of learners. Some of the strategies included:

- *Finding out what participants wanted to gain from the program* allowed the facilitators to respond to participants' expressed needs.
- *Providing teaching aids* such as PowerPoint™ and Adobe Presenter™ provided information both visually (reading the slides) and aurally (viewing slides with voice-over).

TABLE 27.3 Program Logic Model for Training Programs

Overall goal: To enhance the capacity of service providers to promote the sexual and reproductive health of SIY.

Target group: Nurses, teachers, community educators, social workers, and youth workers working at SIY serving agencies/organizations.

Program Components	Face-to-Face Training	Online Training
Short-term objectives	• Increased knowledge related to sexual and reproductive health • Increased comfort addressing sexuality with SIY	
Longer-term objectives	• Sustained knowledge increase related to sexual and reproductive health • Sustained comfort increase in addressing sexuality with SIY • Use of knowledge gained from training program	
Short-term indicators	• Knowledge post-test scores greater than pre-test scores • Comfort post-test scores greater than pre-test scores	
Longer-term indicators	• Knowledge 6-week post-test scores greater than pre-test scores • Comfort 6-week post-test scores greater than pre-test scores • Participants reporting use of knowledge gained from their respective training programs	
Program activities	• Recruitment of participants • Data collection and analysis pre-training, post-training, and 6 weeks post-training • Program facilitation	• Recruitment of participants • Online program facilitation • Data collection and analysis pre-training, post-training, and 6 weeks post-training
Resources	• Facilitators • Training program content • Printed materials • Refreshments • Facility • Computer and LCD projector • Office supplies	• Facilitators • Training program content • Adobe Presenter • Blackboard learning platform • Computer • Surveymonkey.com

- *Doing a Values Quiz* to assist participants in identifying their values and biases about sexuality so they could reflect upon how these could influence interactions with clients. The Values Quiz can be found at http://www.tascc.ca/sexuality-topics/values-and-sexuality.
- *Including examples from SIY and service providers* through quotations and stories to provide context, rationale, and meaning to the content and illustrate that youth need to make decisions that work with their personal life circumstances.
- *Providing a virtual tour* of the Calgary SRH Clinic to inform service providers so that they can explain what youth can expect when visiting the clinic.
- *Using humour and pop culture examples from cartoons, music, and television* to bring content to life and to facilitate discussion.
- *Performing demonstrations* (either hands-on or via YouTube) to allow participants to learn about the use of male and female condoms.
- *Showing relevant short videos* to address sensitive topics; for example, the Canadian video "It Gets Better" that addresses homophobia (ItGetsBetterCanada, 2010).
- *Encouraging questions* throughout the training sessions, either in real time (for in-person sessions) or via an asynchronous discussion board (for online sessions) to promote self-directed learning.
- *Making additional information available* through Internet links, additional readings, and resources to encourage self-directed learning.
- *Facilitating large group discussions* that encourage problem solving and critical thinking and allow participants to share experiences and reflections and learn from each other.
- *Making use of case examples,* experiences that SIY shared during interviews, in order to promote problem solving and reflection.

The face-to-face training program was delivered twice and the online program three times to a total of 92 participants. To measure their level of comfort, participants completed an 11-item questionnaire three times: prior to the training, immediately following the sessions, and 6 weeks later. Using a five-point Likert scale, participants rated their level of comfort in addressing various SRH topics. Fifty-seven participants (62%) completed the questionnaire all three times; scores revealed that comfort levels increased following the training program and were sustained over 6 weeks. To measure knowledge, participants completed a 70-item questionnaire three times, prior to training, immediately following, and 6 weeks later. Fifty-nine participants (64%) completed all three questionnaires; results demonstrated that knowledge improved immediately after the training and while it dipped slightly at 6 weeks, scores remained higher than pre-test levels. Thirteen face-to-face program participants (46.4%) and 21 online program participants (72.4%) reported using the knowledge and skill learned in the training program.

Summary

In this case story, we discussed the SRH challenges that SIY face and compared the sexual health characteristics and outcomes of SIY to those of mainstream youth. Additionally, we discussed how the team planned, implemented, and evaluated two related interventions that built the personal capacity (knowledge, skill, comfort) of service providers that work with SIY. Although the evaluations of both interventions indicate positive results, the interventions remain works in progress. We continuously reassess their relevancy and strive to keep them current, accurate, and meaningful. In so doing, we hope to have a positive impact on the SRH of SIY.

Acknowledgements

This project was funded through a doctoral fellowship awarded by the Alberta Center for Child, Family and Community Research. The University of Calgary ethics identification numbers associated with this study are 22606 and 23554.

The authors thank Heather Cobb, Christine Sturgeon, Tammy Troute-Wood, and Cara Aielo for their hard work under short timelines in developing the website, tascc.ca. We thank Tammy Troute-Wood and Heather Cobb for their outstanding assistance in developing and facilitating the training program. Thank you to the service providers and youth who shared their stories and gave us inspiration.

REFERENCES

Alberta Health Services. (2011). *E-SYS. Enhanced street youth surveillance Edmonton site results (1999–2010).* Edmonton: Communicable Disease Control, Alberta Health Services.

Government of Alberta. (2015). *Health and wellness interactive health data application.* URL=http://www.ahw.gov.ab.ca/IHDA_Retrieval/

Health Canada. (2014). *Canadian alcohol and drug use monitoring survey.* URL=http://www.hc-sc.gc.ca/hc-ps/drugs-drogues/stat/_2012/tables-tableaux-eng.php#t10

ItGetsBetterCanada. (2010). *It Gets Better Canada.* [Video file]. URL=https://www.youtube.com/watch?v=5p-AT-18d9lU

Knowles, M. S., Holton, E. F., & Swanson, R. A. (2012). *Adult learner: The definitive classic in adult education and human resource development* (7th ed.). St. Louis, MO: Routledge.

Lokanc-Diluzio, W. (2014). *A mixed methods study of service provider capacity development to protect and promote the sexual and reproductive health of street-involved youth: An evaluation of two training approaches* (Doctoral dissertation). University of Calgary. URL=http://hdl.handle.net/11023/1507

Public Health Agency of Canada (PHAC). (2008). *Canadian guidelines for sexual health education.* URL=http://www.phac-aspc.gc.ca/publicat/cgshe-ldnemss/index-eng.php

Rotermann, M. (2012). Sexual behaviour and condom use of 15- to 24-year-olds in 2003 and 2009/2010. *Health Reports, 23*(1), 1–5. URL=http://www.statcan.gc.ca/pub/82–003-x/2012001/article/11632-eng.pdf

Worthington, C., & MacLaurin, B. (2013). Promoting health for homeless and street-involved youth: Use and views of services of street-involved youth in Calgary. In S. Gaetz, B. O'Grady, K. Buccieri, J. Karabanow, & A. Marsolais (Eds.), *Youth homelessness in Canada: Implications for policy and practice* (pp. 161–184). Toronto: Canadian Homelessness Research Network Press.

ONLINE RESOURCES

Please visit the Point. at http://thepoint.lww.com/Vollman4e for up-to-date Internet resources and additional learning materials on this topic.

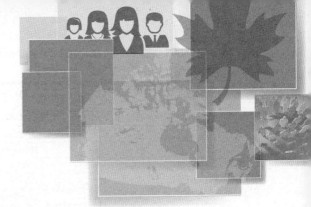

CHAPTER 28

e-Health: Developing Personal Skills for Weight Management

K. Ashlee McGuire and Sasha Wiens

LEARNING OBJECTIVES

After studying this chapter, you should be able to:

1. Describe the challenges and opportunities for the use of technology in client-centred care

2. Describe a process for client engagement and support by using e-health strategies

Introduction

The prevalence of obesity in Canada has increased substantially; individuals with a body mass index (BMI) ≥ 30 kg/m^2 increased 200% between 1985 and 2011 (Twells et al., 2014). The most marked increase is seen in those individuals that are in the higher classes of obesity. Specifically, the number of adults presenting with class III obesity (severely obese) increased by almost 450% between 1985 and 2011 whereas the number of adults presenting with class I obesity (moderately obese) increased by approximately 150% (Twells et al., 2014). Adults with obesity, especially those in higher classes of obesity, are at an increased risk of numerous chronic conditions (e.g., type 2 diabetes / hypertension), poor quality of life, functional limitations, and mental health concerns (Luo et al., 2007) (see Table 28.1). Obesity is also associated with a substantial economic burden that is estimated to be between $4.6 and $7.1 billion annually (Anis et al., 2010; Hodgson, 2011). Annual health care costs associated with obesity are now estimated to be higher than those associated with smoking ($1,330 versus $1,022, respectively per person in 2011) (An, 2015).

Although intentional weight loss of 5%–10% of body weight is associated with a 15% reduction in all-cause mortality (Kritchevsky et al., 2015), adherence to weight-loss interventions is generally poor (Coons et al., 2012). Thus, encouraging and sustaining reductions in obesity and obesity-related health conditions remain challenging for both the health care providers who are expected to counsel and assist clients in this journey and for the clients themselves. Challenges may be due to the complexity of obesity as a condition; in addition, social, environmental, genetic, lifestyle, emotional, and cultural factors all contribute to obesity prevalence (Hodgson, 2011).

TABLE 28.1   Canadian Guidelines for Body Weight Classification in Adults

Body Mass Index (kg/m²)	Classification	Health Risk
<18.5	Underweight	Increased risk
18.5–24.9	Normal weight	Least risk
25.0–29.9	Overweight	Increased risk
30 and over	Obese	
30.0–34.9	Obese Class I	High risk
35.0–39.9	Obese Class II	Very high risk
≥40.0	Obese Class III	Extremely high risk

Source: Health Canada (2003).

TECHNOLOGY AND HEALTH PROMOTION

In recent years, technological advances and increased reliance on automated, energy-saving devices have emerged as key contributors to the increased rates of obesity (Dunstan et al., 2010; Tremblay et al., 2010; Gilmore et al., 2014). Canadians in particular have demonstrated an affinity for the Internet and mobile device usage, which is often captured as "screen time" or "sedentary behaviour" in the literature and associated with negative health outcomes such as obesity (Tremblay et al., 2010). In Canada, 83% of households own a cell phone (Statistics Canada, 2014) of which 57% constitutes smartphone ownership (Canadians Connected, 2014). Canadians are world leaders in Internet usage; on average, Canadians visit 3,731 web pages, spend 41.3 hours surfing the web, and watch videos for 24.8 hours per month. On average, 87% of households connect to the Internet daily (Canadians Connected, 2014).

Despite the negativity surrounding the use of technology and its impact on health, technology in conjunction with the Internet may also present a promising opportunity to assist health care providers to deliver innovative, engaging, and effective care to Canadian adults seeking assistance with obesity management. Indeed, delivering interventions and care via the Internet holds considerable promise as it improves access for people with transportation and/or mobility limitations and for those who live in rural or remote locations, it is readily available at all times, and it can reach a large number of people at low cost. As well, statements such as, "the Internet is part of the day-to-day lives of Canadians" (Canadians Connected, 2014) and "we live in a world wirelessly with almost as many cellular phone subscriptions as there are people on the planet" (PwC, 2014, p. 3) speak to the social acceptability and ubiquity of technology in our current environment.

Internet-based and technology-enhanced interventions and strategies to support weight loss may include a variety of tools such as (but not limited to) text messaging, smartphone applications, internet-based education, peer or provider support, and self-monitoring options. Based on systematic reviews and meta-analyses, there is evidence to suggest that internet-based and technology-enhanced interventions may be effective in or offer promise in promoting significant weight loss (Coons et al., 2012; Kirk et al., 2012; Gilmore et al., 2014; Hutchesson et al., 2015), especially those incorporating a component to address behaviour change, a self-monitoring component using individual data, and a component focused on personalized feedback (Gilmore et al., 2014). However, the mean difference in weight loss demonstrated in a recent meta-analysis of internet-based or technology-enhanced interventions compared to no or minimal interventions, was less than traditional (e.g., face-to-face) behavioural weight-loss interventions (Hutchesson et al., 2015). Additionally, there is significant heterogeneity in program components, length, and specific mode of delivery. This variability makes it difficult to draw concrete conclusions regarding the use of specific tools (i.e., smartphone applications, text messaging), but it does suggest that the tools are simply the vehicle by which to deliver the intervention and their success is determined more by the components included in the intervention and strategies used to encourage both compliance and retention.

Patients in a global study of the use of mobile devices and health care ($n = 1,027$ from 10 countries; representing a variety of economic backgrounds, ages, levels of education, and states of health) report that they expect technology, most specifically mobile technology, to make health care more convenient, improve its quality, and reduce costs (PwC, 2014). Further, patients in the study anticipated using mobile technology to seek information pertaining to specific health conditions, self-manage their health, communicate with their health care providers, and allow their health care providers to monitor their condition and compliance with treatment (PwC, 2014). Interestingly, it is those patients with poorly managed conditions who were most likely to be engaged in and using technology to assist in their management (82% with a poorly managed condition versus 64% of those from the general population) (PwC, 2014). The clear expectations for the use of technology by patients and the promising evidence suggest that incorporating technology-enhanced and/or internet-based tools may prove beneficial for health management. This evidence prompted the Adult Bariatric Specialty Clinic (ABSC) in Calgary to explore the use of internet-based tools to meet increasing demands for their weight management service.

RESPONDING TO CLIENT NEED: CREATING A SUPPORTIVE ENVIRONMENT

Twells et al. (2014) reported that the prevalence of adults living in Alberta with class II obesity is 4.3% and with class III obesity is 1.4% (i.e., they would meet the criteria for entry into the ABSC). Assuming this prevalence in Calgary, approximately 45,000 adults aged 20–64 years (of a total population of 790,061 in this age range (City of Calgary, 2014)) would be eligible to receive weight management support from the ABSC. Presently, the ABSC receives approximately 100 referrals per month. To maintain access to their services and minimize wait lists, the ABSC team began an ongoing process of quality improvement. They chose to integrate key components from the Ottawa Charter (WHO, 1986) and the Knowledge-to-Action Cycle model (Straus et al., 2013) into their clinic process as they recognized the importance of empowering clients to self-manage, developing or adapting their services based on the examination of health needs, current knowledge, barriers and facilitators to treatment, engaging relevant partners, and tailoring of evidence-based practices for local implementation. The use of the Ottawa Charter and model has allowed the team to adapt their program and services as the environment demands and provide clients with individualized care.

Community Assessment

The first step in population health promotion is to understand the issue and the people it affects by conducting an assessment. To begin, the ABSC used postal codes to geo-map (i.e., create a visual representation on a map) where its clients were located. As seen in Figure 28.1, although ABSC clients lived throughout the city, there were distinct areas where there was a higher concentration of clients. Consistent with the literature describing the socioeconomic and social contributors to obesity (Hodgson, 2011), these neighbourhoods also had a high percentage (relative to the Alberta average) of families living below the low-income cut-off point, a high proportion of immigrants, and a high percentage of people without a high school diploma. Additionally, as seen in Figure 28.2, people living in this area of the city presented with a higher incidence of chronic conditions such as type 2 diabetes (Alberta Health, 2013);

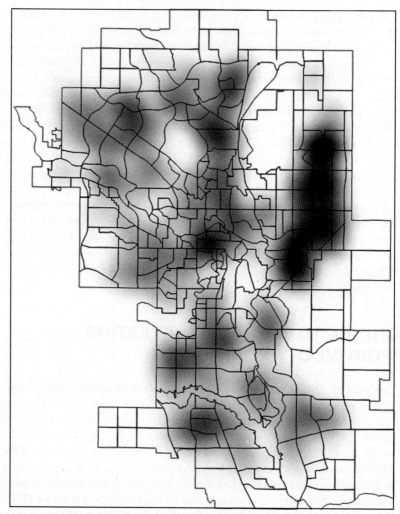

FIGURE 28.1   Distribution of clients (*n* = 3,565) attending the Adult Bariatric Specialty Clinic in Calgary, Alberta. Darker shades indicate a higher distribution of clients in a given area.

this finding also aligns with previous literature (Luo et al., 2007; Hodgson, 2011). The assessment was important for planning purposes and allowed the ABSC to address potential access barriers to its services such as the cost and time of travel and parking, scheduled time away from work, and overall complexity of client situations.

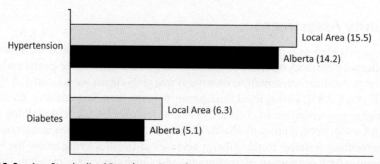

FIGURE 28.2   Age-Standardized Prevalence Rates (per 100 population) of hypertension and diabetes in the local area of Calgary, where a high proportion of Adult Bariatric Specialty Clinic clients reside, compared to Alberta, 2010. (Alberta Health, 2013.)

Client Feedback

Following geo-mapping, clients were surveyed to determine their personal preferences about the location of service and timing of group classes and appointments. Not surprisingly, 75% of clients requested service delivery at a location in the area with the highest density of clients. Consequently, a variety of group classes were offered at the preferred location. Additionally, 50% of clients requested weekend services to accommodate personal schedules; in response, the timing of group meetings was changed from weekday-only to include meetings on evenings and weekends as well.

In alignment with the Canadian Community as Partner Model (see Chapter 15), regular client surveys and focus groups were incorporated into the ABSC evaluation process to allow for the ongoing evolution of services in offering ease of access and a supportive environment. This information helped to shape clinic processes and services. From client feedback, the ABSC also learned that it was difficult for clients to attend all the face-to-face workshops required for program completion. Clients indicated that it would be helpful for them to receive ongoing, regular contact via email or online support from the ABSC team. Based on these suggestions, and the potential to reach a larger proportion of the population at a low cost, the ABSC turned to the Internet as a platform for service delivery, piloting an online education program, and employing a drip marketing strategy.

Take Note

Drip marketing is a concept used commonly in the business world. It is the process of sending prewritten communications (e.g., emails) automatically at designated intervals with the intent of keeping your message at the forefront of the receiver's mind.

Planning and Delivery

Information provided in face-to-face sessions was adapted to suit an online format; for example, the length of each face-to-face session and amount of content provided was dramatically reduced. Vignettes between a client and provider were included to demonstrate key concepts and interactive activities and encourage active learning and self-management skills. Using an automated online service, education sessions and reminders were sent weekly to clients that had subscribed to the service.

The initial pilot of this online education aimed to compare outcomes (weight loss, change in knowledge, and confidence of targeted skills) and demographics (age, rural versus urban) between a group using the online option ($n = 10$) and a group participating in the standard face-to-face education ($n = 42$) and also to assess satisfaction with the online platform. Clients taking the online education were older (49.8 years versus 46.9 years), more likely to live outside of Calgary (60% versus 20%), and lost more weight (7.13 kg versus 5.29 kg) than those in the standard program. After completing the online education they also indicated an increase in knowledge and confidence. Clients liked the convenience of the online option and the ability to start and stop presentations and repeat sessions as needed. These results demonstrated the important role of online education in services provided by the ABSC. Consequently, this education was made freely available on the Internet and to all clients involved with the ABSC in an attempt to increase access to weight management services and ensure consistent messaging across the health care continuum in Alberta.

To satisfy the clients' interest for increased contact from the ABSC via email, the ABSC staff communicated with clients between clinic appointments through twice-weekly purposeful email messages labeled as *News, Nuggets and Nudges*. Development of these messages was a collaborative effort involving multiple teams and portfolios within Alberta Health Services. Once again this service was made widely available, and as of January 2015, over 800 individuals had signed up for this service. In a survey of those clients who received the *News, Nuggets and Nudges,* 96% indicated they were satisfied overall with this service and 87% found it useful. Specific comments included: "I find these emails help me to maintain focus on the days I receive the email" and "It is quick and easy to read, and has a single subject to focus on. One small step at a time, it doesn't overwhelm me with new info." These comments suggest that this low-cost initiative that uses limited resources (compared to face-to-face appointments) is a successful and useful way by which to maintain regular contact with clients involved in weight management programs.

Peer Support

Since clients of the ABSC felt they needed more frequent social contact than what was feasible for the clinic to provide, one of the participating clients fully embraced the concept of self-management and capitalized on the available online opportunities with the creation of *FeelGood Calgary,* a Facebook site. Participation in an online social media site helps people feel more connected to others, especially those experiencing a similar condition or situation (Magnezi et al., 2014) and may support behaviour change efforts (Greene et al., 2013) (see Chapter 14). This project draws upon the principles that health is created by caring for oneself and others, by being able to have control over one's life circumstances, and by ensuring that the society in which one lives creates conditions that allow the attainment of health.

Take Note

In addition to being one of the world leaders in Internet usage and video viewing, Canadians also top the charts for use of Facebook (a free online social platform that allows people to connect with others)—14 million Canadians per day log on to Facebook (Canadians Connected, 2014).

Initially, *FeelGood Calgary,* which aimed to help individuals achieve their goals of becoming healthier and happier while supporting their local community, provided the opportunity for clients of the ABSC to support each other in an ongoing, high frequency, and non-judgemental environment. The Facebook site was a hit with the group because it not only offered increased social support, it also provided the opportunity to garner immediate assistance if needed and allowed those with time constraints, transportation, and mobility limitations the opportunity to experience the camaraderie that was otherwise not available to them. As the needs of this group expanded, the *FeelGood Calgary* website was launched as a multi-faceted site with a blog feature, a community newsletter, community events, and community professionals. This platform allowed for the delivery of more information and sharing of expertise in a well-organized format to a larger audience.

Reflection

Although this initiative is owned and operated by *FeelGood Calgary*'s founder, the importance of sharing responsibility for population health with people and communities has been recognized. In fact, evidence suggests that patients or families working in collaboration with their health care teams have better outcomes and express greater satisfaction with their health care experiences (Hibbard & Greene, 2013). Thus, clients of the ABSC are encouraged to interact with the *FeelGood Calgary* Facebook page and website.[1]

Although the ABSC team is committed to tailoring services to address specific needs of their clients, it is important to consider that this team is part of a large (>100,000 employees) publicly funded health care organization. While the nature of this type of organization ensures that everyone has access to required health care services, it also operates within a restricted budget and lacks the ability to shift resources. Thus, ABSC is unable to fulfill their clients' every request and must seek creative solutions to meet an ever-increasing demand. As well, consideration must be given to the unique needs of the population requesting service. These clients require specialized equipment that is not available throughout the city. Thus, service delivery is limited to specific locations.

Despite the promising potential of technology-enhanced and internet-based solutions to assist the population in weight management efforts (and health care in general), its widespread use will require significant disruption to how health care is currently delivered:

- In general, health care operates within a conservative culture that is highly regulated and fragmented.
- Technology would enable clients to experience greater opportunities for self-management and control of their health whereas health care providers would experience a decrease in control over a client's health, a situation that causes concern among health care providers. Many clients admitted that access to information online had already replaced at least one visit to a health care provider (PwC, 2014).
- The use of technology and internet tools may compromise confidentiality and privacy of health information; many of the information technology systems used by health care organizations are not set up to accommodate the new technology or provide adequate security to comply with privacy laws and regulations.
- These tools may influence the therapeutic relationship between clients and health care providers. Consequently, the adoption of many available technologies and internet-based options will take considerable time or remain unavailable for health care services (PwC, 2014).

Summary

While it has been suggested that the advances in technology and constant availability of the Internet may be responsible in part for the increased prevalence of obesity, evidence indicates that technology-enhanced and internet-based solutions may also play important roles in obesity management. Further, when these tools are used in response to needs identified by clients, their potential impact increases as clients become engaged and empowered. Indeed, pilot projects conducted by the ABSC demonstrate that small changes to clinic processes increase access to services, improve patient outcomes, and lead to patient satisfaction. Importantly, these changes are not resource-intensive and thus may be quite favourable to large health care organizations that need to reach a large population at a low cost.

Although the use of technology-enhanced and internet-based solutions for weight management are currently not widely used in health care, they hold considerable promise; for example, applications for mobile devices may be used to track and transmit data wirelessly, allowing

[1]Copyright © (2015) Ashton Michael. Please note that the *FeelGood Calgary* website and video links referenced by the authors in this chapter with permission from the website owners are maintained by third parties over whom Alberta Health Services ("AHS") has no control. These links have been provided solely for informational purposes as a convenience for the reader and do not constitute an endorsement or approval by AHS of the content of such third party sites and materials. AHS does not make any representation or warranty, express, implied, or statutory, as to the accuracy, reliability, completeness, applicability, or fitness for a particular purpose of these sites or their content.

health care providers to monitor conditions remotely. Clients will not have to wait for face-to-face appointments but will have secure access to health care information on demand, and clients will have the tools and information available to self-manage their health.

REFERENCES

Alberta Health. (2013). *Primary health care community profiles.Government of Alberta.* URL=http://www.health.alberta.ca/services/PHC-community-profiles.html

An, R. (2015). Health care expenses in relation to obesity and smoking among U.S. adults by gender, race/ethnicity, and age group: 1998–2011. *Public Health, 129*(1), 29–36.

Anis, A. H., Zhang, W., Bansback, N., Guh, D. P., Amarsi, Z., & Birmingham, C. L. (2010). Obesity and overweight in Canada: An updated cost-of-illness study. *Obesity Reviews, 11*(1), 31–40.

Canadians Connected. (2014). *The Canadian Internet CIRA factbook 2014.* URL=http://cira.ca/factbook/2014/the-canadian-internet.html

City of Calgary. (2014). *2014 civic census results.* Calgary: City Clerk's Election & Information Services. URL=http://www.calgary.ca/CA/city-clerks/Pages/Election-and-information-services/Civic-Census/2014-Results.aspx

Coons, M. J., Demott, A., Buscemi, J., Duncan, J. M., Pellegrini, C. A., Steglitz, J., et al. (2012). Technology interventions to curb obesity: A systematic review of the current literature. *Current Cardiovascular Risk Reports, 6*(2), 120–134.

Dunstan, D. W., Healy, G. N., Sugiyama, T., & Owen, N. (2010). "Too much sitting" and metabolic risk – Has modern technology caught up with us?. *European Endocrinology, 6*(1), 19–23.

Gilmore, L. A., Duhe, A. F., Frost, E. A., & Redman, L. M. (2014). The technology boom: A new era in obesity management. *Journal of Diabetes Science and Technology, 8*(3), 596–608.

Greene, J., Sacks, R., Piniewski, B., Kil, D., & Hahn, J. S. (2013). The impact of an online social network with wireless monitoring devices on physical activity and weight loss. *Journal of Primary Care & Community Health, 4*(3), 189–194.

Health Canada. (2003). *Canadian guidelines for body weight classification in adults – Quick Reference Tool for Professionals.* Ottawa: Author. URL=http://www.hc-sc.gc.ca/fn-an/nutrition/weights-poids/guide-ld-adult/index-eng.php

Hibbard, J. H., & Greene, J. (2013). What the evidence shows about patient activation: Better health outcomes and care experiences; fewer data on costs. *Health Affairs, 32*(2), 207–214.

Hodgson, C. (2011). *Obesity in Canada: A joint report from the Public Health Agency of Canada and the Canadian Institute for Health Information.* URL=http://www.phac-aspc.gc.ca/hp-ps/hl-mvs/oic-oac/index-eng.php

Hutchesson, M. J., Rollo, M. E., Krukowski, R., Ells, L., Harvey, J., Morgan, P. J., et al. (2015). eHealth interventions for the prevention and treatment of overweight and obesity in adults: A systematic review with meta-analysis. *Obesity Reviews, 16*, 376–392.

Kirk, S. F., Penney, T. L., McHugh, T. L., & Sharma, A. M. (2012). Effective weight management practice: A review of the lifestyle intervention evidence. *International Journal of Obesity, 36*(2), 178–185.

Kritchevsky, S. B., Beavers, K. M., Miller, M. E., Shea, M. K., Houston, D. K., Kitzman, D. W., et al. (2015). Intentional weight loss and all-cause mortality: A meta-analysis of randomized clinical trials. *PLoS One, 10*(3), e0121993.

Luo, W., Morrison, H., de Groh, M., Waters, C., DesMeules, M., Jones-McLean, E., et al. (2007). The burden of adult obesity in Canada. *Chronic Diseases in Canada, 27*(4), 135–144.

Magnezi, R., Bergman, Y. S., & Grosberg, D. (2014). Online activity and participation in treatment affects the perceived efficacy of social health networks among patients with chronic illness. *Journal of Medical Internet Research, 16*(1), e12.

PwC. (2014). *Emerging mHealth: Paths for growth.* URL=http://www.pwc.com/en_GX/gx/healthcare/mhealth/assets/pwc-emerging-mhealth-full.pdf

Statistics Canada. (2014). Residential Telephone Service Survey, 2013. *The Daily,* June 23. URL=http://www.statcan.gc.ca/daily-quotidien/140623/dq140623a-eng.htm

Straus, S., Tetroe, J., & Graham, I. D. (Eds.). (2013). *Knowledge translation in health care: Moving from evidence to practice* (2nd ed.). Hoboken, NJ: Wiley Blackwell and BMJ Books. Also available from KT Clearinghouse, URL=httpy://ktclearinghouse.ca/knowledgebase/knowledgetoaction

Tremblay, M. S., Colley, R. C., Saunders, T. J., Healy, G. N., & Owen, N. (2010). Physiological and health implications of a sedentary lifestyle. *Applied Physiology, Nutrition, and Metabolism, 35*(6), 725–740.

Twells, L. K., Gregory, D. M., Reddigan, J., & Midodzi, W. K. (2014). Current and predicted prevalence of obesity in Canada: A trend analysis. *CMAJ Open, 2*(1), e18–26.

World Health Organization (WHO). (1986). *The Ottawa Charter for Health Promotion.* Geneva: Author.

ONLINE RESOURCES

Please visit the Point at http://thepoint.lww.com/Vollman4e for up-to-date Internet resources and additional learning materials on this topic.

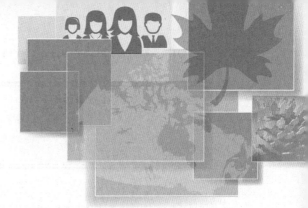

CHAPTER 29

Hearing the Voices of Immigrant and Refugee Women for Planning Postpartum Depression Care

Joyce M. O'Mahony

LEARNING OBJECTIVES

After studying this chapter, you should be able to:

1. Identify how immigrant and refugee women (IRW) make decisions about postpartum care

2. Define barriers and facilitators that influence help-seeking behaviours of IRW

3. Describe the social supports IRW use to address their health needs

4. Discuss strategies for effective and culturally appropriate health services that address postpartum depression (PPD) and care among IRW

Introduction

New immigrant and refugee women (IRW) are at risk to achieve less than optimal health outcomes following childbirth given the social, cultural, and language difficulties and socioeconomic factors that influence their postpartum experiences. This chapter is part of a qualitative research project that explores how IRW seek care to manage postpartum depression (PPD) in the community setting. The objectives of the study are to increase understanding of how IRW make decisions about postpartum care, what factors influence their health seeking behaviour, and what strategies they find helpful. Using the study's findings, we suggest strategies to plan and implement more culturally appropriate and equitable health services for IRW living in Canada.

POPULATION ASSESSMENT

Canada is home to an estimated 6,775,800 immigrants (Statistics Canada, 2013). Immigrants represent one fifth (20.6%) of the Canadian population, the highest proportion in all of the G8 countries (Box 29.1) (Statistics Canada, 2013). The number of immigrants coming to Canada

---

Box 29.1 G8 Countries

| Canada | Germany | Japan | United Kingdom |
| France | Italy | Russia | United States |

---

from non-European countries has increased significantly over the past several decades; Asia (including the Middle East) was Canada's largest source of immigrants in the past 5 years (Statistics Canada, 2013).

Postpartum Depression

PPD affects 3% to 25% of all new mothers globally (O'Hara, 2009; Lanes et al., 2011), and therefore, it is of significant public health importance. Immigrant women in Canada have a higher prevalence of PPD than Canadian-born women (Ballantyne et al., 2013). While there has been research on immigrant women's mental health care experiences, there is limited understanding of how immigrant women access multiple levels of care to deal with mental health issues such as PPD and how contextual factors intersect with race, class, and gender to influence prevention and treatment options.

PPD is a serious mental illness that has far-reaching implications for mothers, infants, and families. There are significant associations between maternal depression and adverse child behavioural and emotional outcomes. A recent meta-analysis including 193 studies reported that maternal depression was correlated with higher levels of internalizing (e.g., depressed mood, anxiety, social withdrawal) and externalizing (e.g., aggression, conduct problems, attention deficit hyperactivity disorder) behaviours, general psychopathology, negative behaviour, and low levels of positive affect in the child (Goodman et al., 2011).

Although the exact cause of PPD is uncertain, psychological and psychosocial factors can predispose some women to this mental illness. O'Hara and Swain (1996) conducted over 70 studies to summarize potential risk factors for PPD. The strongest predictors of PPD included depression or anxiety during pregnancy, recent life stress, personal and family history of depression, poor quality of relationships, and lack of social support. Consistently, results from epidemiologic studies and meta-analyses suggest that lack of social support significantly increases the risk of PPD. They report that the following factors may predispose immigrant women to PPD: lack of friends or a close confident/partner, social isolation, and lack of perceived support from a primary social network.

Treating Postpartum Depression

Treating depression during the perinatal period is challenging; signs and symptoms of pregnancy may mimic the neurologic signs and symptoms of a depressive mental illness. Early recognition of a mood disorder is important because the longer treatment is delayed, the longer the duration of the illness. PPD is a treatable mental illness; prompt intervention improves long-term outcomes. The optimal treatment plan for a woman with PPD involves a coordinated interdisciplinary team and a holistic, family-centred approach. Treatment options include interpersonal psychotherapies and psychopharmacologic therapy. An array of psychosocial and psychological interventions has been found to benefit the prevention and treatment of PPD (Dennis & Dowswell, 2013). Interventions included postpartum home visits, peer-based postpartum telephone support, along with psychotherapy and medications.

In Canada, the Edinburgh Postnatal Depression Scale (EPDS) (Cox et al., 1987) is widely used to screen for PPD in the community. This 10-item self-report scale indicates how the mother has felt during the previous week, and in doubtful cases, it may be usefully repeated after 2 weeks. While the EPDS is a valid and reliable screening tool for identifying women at risk for PPD, a high score on the EPDS does not constitute a psychiatric diagnosis (Zelkowitz et al., 2008). Although there is concern regarding the appropriateness of using the EPDS for non-Western women, this tool has been validated for use in many languages (Tobin et al., 2015).

Immigrant and Refugee Women and Postpartum Depression

Studies reveal that many IRW who suffer serious mental illness such as depression, post-traumatic stress disorder (PTSD), and psychosis often do not receive the care they need (Thomson et al., 2015). New immigrants are 10 times more likely than Canadian-born individuals to identify barriers that prevent or interfere with access to services. Studies show that although IRW are at risk for poor health in the postpartum period, they have difficulty meeting their mental health needs even when health care is universally available. Timely access to needed mental health services can be an issue for IRW because of language difficulties, lack of familiarity or unawareness of the existence of health services, poverty, lack of integration between mental health and other health services, regional disparities, and cross-cultural diversity. An existing shortage of mental health professionals means the demand for service often exceeds supply.

Barriers to Care

Scheppers et al. (2006) reviewed 54 articles from diverse countries to determine potential barriers to health care service usage at individual, health care provider, and health care system levels. At the individual level, barriers were demographic, lack of social support, health beliefs and values, personal and cultural appropriate community enabling resources, personal health practices, and gender. Gender refers to the socially and culturally determined roles, relations, and gendered structures (e.g., government policies). At the provider level, negative attitudes and inadequate skills of the health care provider were reported to be barriers. At the system level, barriers were associated with the delivery of health services (e.g., obtaining appointments, waiting times, lack of appropriately translated material).

Culture

Cultural perceptions at the individual level acting as barriers to health services include fear of stigma and lack of validation of mental health issues within the family and the ethnic community. Mental illness is heavily stigmatized in many cultures. In some cultures it is perceived to be inappropriate to seek external help for mental health issues. Lack of cultural acknowledgment or lack of recognition of PPD may encourage IRW to deny their emotional suffering. PPD may not be viewed as a health problem and therefore professional assistance is not considered appropriate (O'Mahony et al., 2013). Jain and Levy (2013) found, for example, that Indo-Asian mothers suffering from PPD perceived their symptoms to be normal and natural effects of childbirth and therefore were unlikely to access health services. Maternal depression often goes unrecognized in Indo-Asian communities; as a result, the mother remains alone and isolated within her family.

Gender

Gender-based disparities in access to resources, in power and decision making, and in roles and responsibilities can also influence immigrant women's health care practices and access to PPD services. The shifting of gender roles and the underlying power relations within ethnic families greatly influence IRW's access to mental health services. Immigrant women experience complex gender-related problems in accessing health care services alongside the interplay of pre-migration history, socioeconomic opportunities, discrimination, and poor spousal relationships. O'Mahony and Donnelly (2013) compared how immigrant mothers view the influence of their gender role on their PPD care and on their ability to cope with PPD during the vulnerable period after childbirth. Some research participants reported that their traditional gender role was a barrier to personal health care because they were expected to be responsible for all the family caregiving without support. However, some participants viewed traditional beliefs and practices to be important sources of strength and support for IRW and necessary for the maintenance of emotional health and well-being within the family.

Structure

Immigration laws and policies may act as structural barriers to the use of health services for this population. Women who are without secure immigration status or who are emotionally or financially dependent on individual sponsors may face insurmountable barriers in using health services and thus in protecting their health.

At provider level, community health workers can either promote help-seeking behaviour or hinder access to treatment. If a provider minimizes or normalizes an IRW's mental health issues, she may become reluctant to access further care and treatment. Communication skills and provision of translation services are important factors to reduce communication breakdowns. Trust and faith in the therapeutic relationship were found to be essential components to IRW's continued use of a health service. Providers are sometimes frustrated about the passiveness of IRW's participation in available prevention services (Dennis, 2010; O'Mahony et al., 2012).

At the health system level, current evidence shows that many newcomers must struggle to navigate health systems, including maternity services. It is suggested that if IRW's social position, cultural knowledge, beliefs, values, and traditional customs were considered in the provision of culturally sensitive care, their access to health services would be enhanced. Further validation from a narrative systematic review reported that immigrant women experience the broader influences of contextual variables in maternity care, such as race, gender, socioeconomic status, and geographical location (Higginbottom et al., 2015).

Strengths and Resilience

Even with multiple barriers in accessing postpartum care and support, IRW possess strong abilities to act as facilitators in managing and coping with PPD symptoms and related problems. IRW participants in this study spoke of what kept them strong and enabled them to cope with the transitions in and complexities of their environment. Acculturation, being responsible for their own health maintenance, change in mindset, spirituality, collective sharing, and a keen sense of hope for the future were expressed as methods to promote positive emotional well-being. Many women described their resilience in adapting to their often difficult circumstances. They reframed the stressful events in positive terms and as a result experienced growth and a stronger sense of control over their situation. Past hardships such as refugee camps, domestic abuse, and violence had in fact strengthened their coping abilities. Some women found meaningful resources and ways to cope by navigating and negotiating with informal and formal support networks for PPD.

Spirituality

Spiritual well-being can be described as feeling connected to something larger than oneself and having purpose and meaning in life. Spirituality may include religious beliefs and practices as well as the broader values and principles that give meaning to life. Values and belief systems enable the IRW to understand their experiences and to take control of them creatively. Individuals may experience benefits that allow them to adopt healthy lifestyles or cope with adversity and loss depending on the IRW cultural practices and beliefs and inherent in their value system (CIHI, 2009). For some IRW in our project, spirituality was a positive influence that gave them a source of strength, a sense of connectedness to oneself and to other relationships, and a means for coping with problems. Some women found that a new sense of agency was created and that they had more meaning and purpose in their life after having struggled with the negative emotions of PPD. A sense of agency means feeling in control of your life, believing in your capacity to influence your thoughts and behaviour, and having faith in your ability to manage future situations.

Values

Health care providers confirmed the presence of positive coping strategies in IRW. Reliance on strong family and community-centred values, resiliency, strong work ethic, intention to improve their situation, spirituality, and religious practices provided strength and guidance to manage mental health issues in this population (O'Mahony & Donnelly, 2013).

In the next section, we acknowledge the insights and knowledge of IRW based on their struggles and experience of PPD. It is important to recognize this knowledge and the implications it has for health care providers and practice, and how PPD care and treatment is offered to IRW during the perinatal period.

IMMIGRANT AND REFUGEE WOMEN'S PERSPECTIVES ON HEALTH PROMOTION

Qualitative methodologies such as critical ethnography were used in this project to learn about the appropriateness and useful content of community resources and health care services for immigrant women. We explored how IRW make decisions about health care practice, how they manage living daily with illness, how inequity and unequal social relations influence immigrant women's accessibility to health care services, and how the wider social and cultural environments shape immigrant women's health and health care practices. We examined social, political, historical, and economic factors that shape immigrant women's PPD experiences.

Rather than portraying IRW as helpless, we wanted to give voice to their experiences and knowledge, which illustrate both their struggles and their strengths. With IRW, we co-created stories through dialogue that was based on our commitment to listen and respect the participants' voices. We wanted to reveal IRW's values, beliefs, and positive qualities by listening and sharing through dialogue. Further, we recognized the importance of representing IRW not as "other mothers" who are different from the mainstream. IRW have been positioned through patriarchy to be looked upon as subordinate and their experiences dismissed or viewed as insignificant. Stereotyping discourses have labelled IRW as being passive and without agency. Engaging IRW in community-based research and exploring social inequities is critical to inform policies and programs that address social determinants of health (Ganann, 2013).

IRW in the project offered suggestions about the kind of supports they preferred when coping with PPD. They identified appropriate health promotion and prevention strategies to assist IRW during the perinatal period. Their suggestions also included offering information in multiple languages, community outreach, streamlining broad ranges of postpartum services, inclusion of partner and family members, and education for health service providers.

Support for IRW with PPD

IRW identified informal support (i.e., from family, friends, and community) as the preferred way of receiving support to manage and cope with mental health issues. IRW also perceived formal community-based support as being very important. For some, the opportunity to get out of the house, connect with other people, and share their feelings provided a lifeline to improved health. Participants described postpartum home visits, support group meetings, and telephone support as helpful to obtain formal emotional, informational, and instrumental support.

A collaborative interdisciplinary home visiting program for families experiencing PPD was suggested for providing emotional support for mothers, arranging referrals to community-based PPD support programs, and offering educational materials and resources. Additionally, in-home respite support would allow IRW to converse with another person about their issues.

The majority of IRW preferred individual therapy over support group meetings partly because of low English language skill and uneasiness in opening up to others. Most agreed that receiving pamphlets or written material was less effective than personal contact in providing support for mental health issues.

Telephone-based services and language support were essential components of successful care of IRW with mental health issues. The privacy of a telephone intervention provided a higher comfort level. Peer-based (lay) telephone support provided the opportunity to talk about feelings with someone who genuinely understood their situation. The importance of feeling connected to others, normalizing their issues, and hearing that other women experienced similar feelings was reassurance that there was hope that they would be well again.

Health Promotion and PPD Prevention

PPD awareness and education is desirable during the perinatal period. IRW suggested that awareness and information about PPD be offered numerous times throughout pregnancy and postpartum so that all women have opportunity to develop personal skills so that they are able to recognize symptoms of depression and know about available PPD support interventions and services. Exercising more control over decisions to manage PPD and the health care practices they employ will enhance future services and treatment strategies for this population. Knowledge may also decrease the powerful stigma attached to PPD.

Communication

The fact health information is not offered in multiple languages emphasizes the inequality that many IRW face. Past research conducted with health care providers questioned whether lack of interpreter services, or providers choosing not to use these services, was a form of discrimination against immigrant women. A participant with extensive experience with counselling and human rights for women felt that it was a form of systemic discrimination: "Non-provision of translation services [is discriminating]...people are receiving a different kind of service because things aren't explained clearly...in order to be expedient." IRW described how not speaking English could lead to overwhelming isolation and the inability to explain feelings or ask for help. They had difficulty accessing language classes because they had no transportation or child care. IRW indicated that language and communication difficulties and unfamiliarity with community care and support influenced whether they chose to seek help for mental health issues. Interpreters were not often available and women could not easily express their concerns or understand instructions and information provided. To reach out to IRW and offer appropriate mental health services providers must address the importance of language translations and the use of interpreters. Higginbottom et al. (2015) found that communication difficulties for IRW extended past language competency to issues of nonverbal communication, and its relation to shared meaning, migration history, and cultural practices.

Community Outreach

IRW suggested that if information about community services were distributed in community places of worship it would be accessible and would encourage them to seek support; such information dissemination would also generally promote awareness of health promotion and service availability. Spiritual and religious practices sustain many IRW whose resettlement has caused a loss of pre-existing support networks. Closer links with community spiritual organizations, and support from community leaders, could increase immigrant women's awareness of and access to mental health services.

Postpartum Services

Providing a broad range of postpartum services within the same community agency could streamline access to mental health services for IRW. IRW explained that convenient access to a variety of types of health and support services would encourage and attract new mothers and would lower the stigma associated with visiting a mental health professional if services included on-site therapeutic counselling. Most IRW want more information about postpartum diet and infant feeding from a nutritionist. IRW who are mothers could be engaged by incentives such as free diapers, formula, or discount coupons. Information about other health and social services could be offered on site, enabling the IRW to obtain treatment of mental health issues.

Role of Partner and Family Members

IRW strongly emphasized the importance of receiving support and assistance from their partners. They suggested that more attention be directed to educating their partners about PPD, enabling them to provide better support and care.

It is imperative to offer information to all family members because they often do not understand the seriousness of PPD or how to support someone who is depressed. Family members can be advocates for instrumental and emotional support and can make a difference in whether or not IRW will access support for PPD. IRW who are depressed are not likely to go against the wishes of their family or cultural beliefs to seek help independently. Rather, encouragement to use mental health services needs to come from the family.

Education for Health Service Providers

Culturally appropriate health service for IRW necessitates an awareness of the issues they face that cause IRW to feel powerless, dependent, isolated, and oppressed. These feelings must be mitigated if health care is to be successful. Unique cultural identities must be respected and nurtured. A shift away from understanding culture as a social characteristic of IRW toward recognizing culture as a fluid and dynamic process that is important to the everyday situation of IRW is required. Promoting safety requires turning providers' attention to understanding the ways culture can shape IRW's responses to health and illness and adapting their practices accordingly.

Summary

Social determinants such as social support, socioeconomic status, and discrimination affect IRW's health and their health care practices. Strategies that are evidence based, such as actively engaging IRW with PPD and utilizing their experiences to guide change and innovation, are necessary. Through listening to IRW's stories we can increase our understanding about the ways in which social determinants impact their mental health and well-being. Understanding IRW and PPD from the context of their lives rather than labelling them as mentally ill is a step toward decreasing stigma. The complex factors that affect the preferences of IRW regarding postpartum health services need to be understood before measures can be taken to better reach this group of women. Information about IRW's health service preferences can be used to develop culturally appropriate strategies to meet their needs. Health care providers who work with IRW in the child-bearing years need such information to make appropriate referrals.

Acknowledgements

The author acknowledges the immigrant and refugee women who participated in this research study and Dr. Tam Donnelly. The Alberta Heritage Foundation for Medical Research and the Canadian Institutes of Health Research supported this work.

REFERENCES

Ballantyne, M., Benzies, K. M., & Trute, B. (2013). Depressive symptoms among immigrant and Canadian born mothers of preterm infants at neonatal intensive care discharge: A cross sectional study. *BMC Pregnancy and Childbirth, 13*(Suppl 1), S11.

Canadian Institute for Health Information (CIHI). (2009). *Improving the health of Canadians: Exploring positive mental health.* Ottawa: Author.

Cox, J. L., Holden, J. M., & Sagovsky, R. (1987). Detection of postnatal depression: Development of the 10-item Edinburgh postnatal depression scale. *British Journal of Psychiatry, 150*(6), 782–786.

Dennis, C. L. (2010). Postpartum depression peer support: Maternal perceptions from a randomized controlled trial. *International Journal of Nursing Studies, 47*, 560–568.

Dennis, C. L., & Dowswell, T. (2013). Psychosocial and psychological interventions for preventing postpartum depression. *Cochrane Database of Systematic Review,* Issue 2, Art No: CD001134.

Ganann, R. (2013). Opportunities and challenges associated with engaging immigrant women in participatory action research. *Journal of Immigrant and Minority Health, 15*(2), 341–349.

Goodman, S. H., Rouse, M. H., Connell, A. M., Robbins Broth, M., Hall, C. M., & Heyward, D. (2011). Maternal depression and child psychopathology: A meta-analytic review. *Clinical Child Family Psychology Review, 14*, 1–27.

Higginbottom, G. M., Morgan, M., O'Mahony, J. M., Chiu, Y., Kocay, D., Alexandre, M., et al. (2015). Immigrant women's experiences of maternity-care services in Canada: A systematic review using a narrative synthesis. *Systematic Reviews, 4*, 13.

Higginbottom, G. M., Safipour, J., Yohani, S., O'Brien, B., Mumtaz, Z., & Paton, P. (2015). An ethnographic study of communication challenges in maternity care for immigrant women in rural Alberta. *Midwifery, 31*(2), 297–304.

Jain, A., & Levy, D. (2013). Conflicting cultural perspectives: Meanings and experiences of postnatal depression among women in Indian communities. *Health Care for Women International, 34*(11), 966–979.

Lanes, A., Kuk, J. L., & Tamim, H. (2011). Prevalence and characteristics of postpartum depression symptomology among Canadian women: A cross-sectional study. *BMC Public Health, 11*, 302.

O'Hara, M. W. (2009). Postpartum depression: What we know. *Journal of Clinical Psychology, 65*(12), 1258–1269.

O'Hara, M., & Swain, A. (1996). Rates and risk of postpartum depression - a meta-analysis. *International Review in Psychiatry, 8*, 37–54.

O'Mahony, J. M., & Donnelly, T. T. (2013). How does gender influence immigrant and refugee women's postpartum depression help-seeking experiences? *Journal of Psychiatric and Mental Health Nursing, 20*(8), 714–725.

O'Mahony, J. M., Donnelly, T. T., Raffin-Bouchal, S., & Este, D. (2012). Barriers and facilitators of social supports for immigrant and refugee women coping with postpartum depression. *Advances in Nursing Science, 35*(3), E42–E56.

O'Mahony, J. M., Donnelly, T. T., Raffin-Bouchal, S., & Este, D. (2013). Cultural background and socioeconomic influence among immigrant and refugee women coping with postpartum depression. *Journal of Immigrant and Minority Health, 15*(2), 300–314.

Scheppers, E., van Dongen, E., Dekker, J., Geertzen, J., & Dekker, J. (2006). Potential barriers to the use of health services among ethnic minorities: A review. *Family Practice, 23*(3), 325–348.

Statistics Canada. (2013). *Immigration and ethnocultural diversity in Canada.* National Household Survey, 2011. Ottawa: Author. URL=http://www12.statcan.gc.ca/nhs-enm/2011/as-sa/99-010-x/99-010-x2011001-eng.pdf

Thomson, M. S., Chaze, F., George, U., & Guruge, S. (2015). Improving immigrant populations' access to mental health services in Canada: A review of barriers and recommendations. *Journal of Immigrant Minority Health, 17*(6), 1895–1905.

Tobin, C., Di Napoli, P., & Wood-Gauthier, M. (2015). Recognition of risk factors for postpartum depression in refugee and immigrant women: Are current screening practices adequate? *Journal of Immigrant and Minority Health, 17*(4), 1019–1024.

Zelkowitz, P., Saucier, J., Wang, T., Katofsky, L., Valenzuela, M., & Westreich, R. (2008). Stability and change in depressive symptoms from pregnancy to two months postpartum in childbearing immigrant women. *Archives of Women's Mental Health, 11*(1), 1–11.

ONLINE RESOURCES

Please visit the Point. at http://thepoint.lww.com/Vollman4e for up-to-date Internet resources and additional learning materials on this topic.

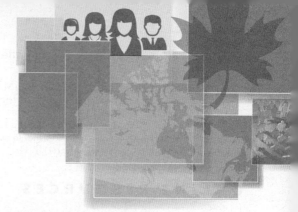

CHAPTER 30

Participatory Action Research: Mosque-Based Exercise for South Asian Muslim Women in Canada

Ananya Tina Banerjee and Jennifer A.D. Price

LEARNING OBJECTIVES

After studying this chapter, you should be able to:

1. Discuss the barriers South Asian Muslim women face with respect to physical activity
2. Detail the benefits of implementing a physical activity program in a mosque
3. Highlight how a physical activity program can empower South Asian Muslim women through participatory action research (PAR)
4. Discuss how PAR promotes culturally sensitive practice
5. Understand how PAR facilitates successful outcomes of an intervention

Introduction

In this chapter, we demonstrate how a mosque-based physical activity program is an ideal avenue for reaching minority populations, particularly South Asian Muslim women, who have disproportionately high rates of diabetes and face unique barriers in being physically active. Taking a participatory action research (PAR) approach in the design and implementation of such a health promotion program is an educative function, which raises the consciousness of its participants and plans for action to improve the quality of lives of women (Reason & Bradbury, 2001). In addition, PAR seeks to transform fundamental societal structures and relationships in order to "redress inequality and redistribute power" (Sarri & Sarri, 1992, p. 100).

Specific reference is made to a PAR project with a group of South Asian Muslim women participating in a physical activity program within a mosque located in Toronto. This case example illustrates a physical activity intervention model with tools and outcomes to be shared with health promotion practitioners working with Canadian Muslim communities. The successful outcomes, empowerment of Muslim women and the commitment of researchers to be culturally sensitive, are examined.

Please be mindful the content of this chapter does not reflect any one South Asian Muslim woman nor does every South Asian Muslim woman necessarily hold the same cultural beliefs and perceptions in relation to physical activity. Instead, the content describes the data and perceptions derived from a group of South Asian Muslim women participating in a physical activity intervention within a mosque and represent the salient findings that have emerged from this project.

SOUTH ASIAN MUSLIM WOMEN IN CANADA

The immigrant population in Canada is diverse and growing. South Asians (i.e., people with ancestral origins from Pakistan, India, Bangladesh, or Sri Lanka) make up one of the largest non-European ethnic origin groups in Canada (Statistics Canada, 2006). South Asians include a number of different ethnic, cultural, and religious backgrounds. In Canada, women of the Islamic faith (the religion of the Muslims, a monotheistic faith regarded as revealed through Muhammad as the Prophet of Allah) represent a significant proportion (approximately 22%) of the South Asian population, making them the second largest religious group after Christianity and the fastest growing religion in Canada (Statistics Canada, 2013). As with immigrants in general, South Asian Muslim women have come to Canada for a variety of reasons, such as higher education, security, employment, and family re-unification. Others have come for religious and political freedom, safety, and security, leaving behind civil wars, persecution, and other forms of civil and ethnic strife (Khan & Watson, 2005). Immigration for South Asian Muslim women is a life change made to improve one's overall quality of life and well-being. However, it entails profound challenges that may culminate in compromised physical health (Banning & Hafeez, 2009).

Risk for Type 2 Diabetes

South Asian Muslim women living in Canada have considerably higher mortality and morbidity from type 2 diabetes compared to the general population (Chiu et al., 2012). The causes of this disease are not fully understood. However, risk factors most common in South Asian Muslim women, which are postulated as important, include obesity, low high-density cholesterol, and insulin resistance coupled with immigration and settlement challenges in Canada that cause stress (Chiu et al., 2012). Women of this ethnic group, particularly those of low income, often describe rigid gender roles and hence experience constraints when taking care of their health. The evidence suggests South Asian Muslim women have been insufficiently engaged in defining their health goals and prevention practices that include regular physical activity to help attenuate their risk for diabetes and related conditions (e.g., cardiovascular disease).

Burden of Physical Inactivity and Associated Barriers

The case to promote physical activity in South Asian communities for the management and prevention of diabetes has been made for over a decade (Sriskantharajah & Kai, 2007). For those with or at risk for type 2 diabetes, physical activity reduces both mortality and symptoms and improves disease control and quality of life (Chudyk & Petrella, 2011). However, low levels of physical activity have been reported in people of South Asian origin (Bryan et al., 2006), particularly in South Asian Muslim women (Williams et al., 2011). Studies suggest that they participate in less physical activity or recreational exercise compared to other South Asian women (Carroll et al., 2002). On the premise of these findings, there have been several qualitative studies exploring barriers to engaging in physical activity among this population group (Lawton et al., 2006; Sriskantharajah & Kai, 2007; Caperchione et al., 2013).

Research suggests practical barriers (e.g., lack of time, childcare) are often interwoven with cultural barriers, such as religious modesty, avoidance of mixed-sex activity, and fear of going out alone, and inhibit participation (Lawton et al., 2006; Sriskantharajah & Kai, 2007). For women from this population group at high risk for type 2 diabetes, there is likely much to be gained from engaging in physical activity and much to lose from failure to do so.

IMPLEMENTATION OF A MOSQUE-BASED PHYSICAL ACTIVITY PROGRAM

The growth in the South Asian Muslim population in various areas of Canada (e.g., Metropolitan Toronto) has led to an inevitable growth in their attendance at Islamic places of worship. These places of worship known as mosques and/or *Masjids* promote the identity and security of South Asian Muslim women in a familial-cultural environment. Thus, the provision of women-only exercise sessions in facilities that are culturally safe could serve as a solution to eliminate sex disparity in physical activity participation and empower South Asian Muslim women, especially as the empowerment contributes to their health. Studies indicate health promotion programs in religious institutions (e.g., churches) have demonstrated clinical and psychosocial benefit to women of various ethnic groups (Campbell et al., 2007). Similar to Canadian churches, Figure 30.1 highlights how mosques have key elements identified in the literature to be beneficial in providing physical activity opportunities for Muslim women: partnerships; sex restricted, available, and accessible space; and supportive social relationships (Banerjee et al., 2015).

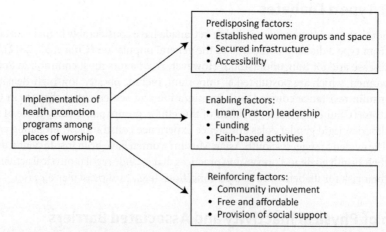

FIGURE 30.1 Factors influencing the implementation of health promotion programs in mosques. (Republished with permission of American Journal of Health Promotion, from Banerjee, A. T., Kin, R., Strachan, P. H., Boyle, M. H., Anand, S. S., & Oremus, M. (2015). Factors facilitating the implementation of church-based heart health promotion programs for older adults: A qualitative study guided by the Precede-Proceed Model. *American Journal of Health Promotion, 29*(6), 365–373; permission conveyed through Copyright Clearance Center, Inc.)

Rationale and Partnership

The South Asian Diabetes Prevention Program (SADPP) at a local health centre conducted a diabetes-screening clinic at a local mosque. The screening team found most women attending the mosque exhibited risk factors for developing diabetes, including a lack of physical activity, and determined there was an immediate need for an integrated and responsive intervention. This led to the successful partnership of our study team composed of the health professionals (e.g., advanced practice nurse, physiotherapist, and kinesiologist) and scientists of the Women's Cardiovascular Health Initiative (Price et al., 2005) at Women's College Hospital, the team (e.g., program coordinator, dietician, and outreach worker) of the SADDP, and council members (e.g., President and Vice-President) of the mosque in the evaluation of the feasibility, acceptability, and effectiveness of a mosque-based exercise intervention for South Asian Muslim women at risk for diabetes.

Exercise Intervention

The intervention included a group exercise program of 24 weeks, offered to South Asian Muslim women in a drop-in format at the mosque location that was accessible by public transit. Participants were able to attend up to three group exercise classes per week. Each class could accommodate up to 30 women.

The exercise program was based on the cardiac rehabilitation program model at Women's College Hospital (Price et al., 2005). Senior female Muslim students in the Faculty of Kinesiology and Physical Education at the University of Toronto who spoke English, Urdu, Gujarati, and Arabic led the exercise sessions. Students of Kinesiology were chosen as they have the expertise to perform physical and functional assessments of women at risk for diabetes and implement group and individual exercise plans to enhance their quality of life.

During each session, women were led through a circuit workout designed to meet Canadian Physical Activity Guidelines (Tremblay et al., 2011), including aerobic, resistance, and flexibility exercises as shown in Figure 30.2. Examples of activities included: walking, resistance band exercises, relaxation exercises, and chair exercises. All exercises required minimal equipment and could be done also in the privacy of their homes. All participants received information about exercise safety.

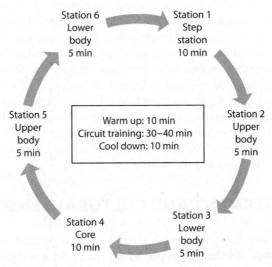

FIGURE 30.2   Exercise Program Model.

Evaluation and Key Findings

Feasibility and acceptability of the program were evaluated in part by numbers of women attending the exercise program. Sixty-two women participated in the mosque-based intervention over a 7-month period. There were no classes offered during the month of Ramadan (the ninth month of the Islamic calendar, and the month in which the Quran was revealed; fasting during the month of Ramadan is one of the Five Pillars of Islam). The exercise participants and research team recognized moderate-to-vigorous exercise was not safe for the women during Ramadan. In addition several classes were cancelled due to unavailability of space and competing demands on the women's time (e.g., weddings). This resulted in a total of 67 exercise sessions held over the 7-month time frame.

Approximately 50% ($n = 28$) of the exercise participants consented to participate in the research evaluation of the intervention. Baseline demographic data were obtained from these research participants. The average age of the women was 51 years (range 23 to 74); most were married (89%); many identified as homemakers (39%); nearly half had less than high school education (46%); and more than half reported a household income of less than $30,000 (54%). In addition, a large number of the research participants described engaging in low levels of physical activity prior to the intervention and had a high readiness to learn how to exercise at moderate-to-vigorous levels.

Of the 28 research participants, 19 completed post questionnaires to determine further measures of feasibility, acceptability, and effectiveness of the intervention. They were asked three questions designed to assess self-efficacy, importance, and readiness toward exercise. Upon completion of the intervention, research participants completed a questionnaire evaluating their overall experience of the 6-month exercise program in the mosque. Most research participants positively rated the exercise classes, indicating that they were convenient, easy to follow, educational, helpful, and supportive. Further, these women increased their exercise and functional capacity as indicated in the measures collected by the Duke Activity Status Index (DASI) (Hlatky et al., 1989) and the International Physical Activity Questionnaire (IPAQ) (Craig et al., 2003).

The 28 research participants had the opportunity to provide qualitative feedback through a questionnaire. Many of the research participants reported that they had been feeling better physically and mentally because of the regular exercise. For example, one woman reported: *"You know, I used to have back pain and was limping but after coming here I am starting to feel better."* The women encouraged each other to be active throughout the intervention. Reinforcing the social support aspect of the program, a woman offered encouragement to her exercise peers who felt reluctant to engage in subsequent classes: *"You will start to feel better after regular exercise, just come to the classes."* The women felt the program was scalable to other Islamic place of worships: *"If you run the classes at another mosque, it would be very successful."*

Overall, the exercise intervention within the mosque was shown to be highly acceptable, feasible, and effective. There were psychosocial and clinical benefits among women in the mosque-based intervention. Apart from these positive outcomes, the most successful and unexpected outcome was achieved at the end of the funding period for this intervention. After careful observation of the emerging health benefits in the women due to the mosque-based exercise program, the mosque council members decided to continue the exercise program. The mosque used their funds to have a female kinesiologist remain and run classes twice per week for an additional 6 months, thus the original intervention translated to a sustainable exercise program for the women at the mosque.

PAR: EMPOWERMENT AND CULTURAL SENSITIVITY

The theoretical framework of PAR is a cyclical process of planning, acting, observing, reflecting, and then re-planning in light of the knowledge gained through the cycle (Choudhry et al., 2002). In this case, it was an ongoing process that used information from the mosque community members (e.g., President, Vice President, and female exercise participants) to shape the intervention. The participation of the mosque community members with the research team was a means to overcome professional dominance, improve strategies (whether they are for practice or research), and show a commitment to democratic principles.

PAR was used to pursue the research objectives with the meaningful involvement of community members of the mosque through all aspects of the exercise intervention research, including identifying the research questions, designing the exercise intervention to be culturally sensitive, and disseminating results. The PAR approach focuses on building community capacity, which leads in turn to consciousness raising and a state of readiness for action (Giachello et al., 2003). The female exercise participants developed the knowledge and skills to take action aiming at changing community conditions for South Asian Muslim women so that a supportive environment existed to sustain exercise behaviour change over time.

Empowerment

As power is an underpinning concept, PAR aims to achieve empowerment of those involved. Empowerment is conceptualized as a shift or dynamic quality of power relations between two or more people or groups, such that the relationship tends toward equity by reducing inequalities and power differences in access to resources (Laverack, 2001). There are subgroups of Muslim women who face forms of male dominance and privilege in their mosque communities, but this male hegemony parallels that experienced by women in various religious and ethnic communities (Trivedi, 1984). Certainly, we find manifestations of social, political, and economic inequality between sexes in Muslim communities. The project team members observed male supremacy in the mosque where the exercise intervention was conducted. Therefore, a goal of the project was to overcome this power imbalance with efforts to change it via physical activity within the mosque culture. The exercise intervention demonstrated the importance of women and brought about gender equity with respect to physical activity opportunities.

In accordance with Reason and Bradbury (2001), PAR was a system for knowledge production in which female participants had the power in setting and conducting the exercise intervention. Class times were set by the women attending the mosque ensuring that the class schedule did not conflict with their family obligations and work responsibilities. Further, women ensured minimal disruption to mosque activities and enabled classes to be adjacent to prayer times. Finally, a female community member from the mosque also assisted the exercise therapists during exercise sessions and learned the structure of the program, reflecting the cross-cultural, community-based, and participatory research.

Commitment to Cultural Sensitivity

Much of PAR is concerned with understanding and creating health promotion programs that are responsive and more reflective of program participant needs (Choudhry et al., 2002). The exercise intervention for the South Asian Muslim women was embedded within specific social, cultural, and historical contexts that impacted program development, implementation, and outcomes. Cultural sensitivity is considered a standard in PAR when working with ethnically diverse populations (Choudhry et al., 2002). Cultural sensitivity is an approach to value and respect the beliefs, norms, and practices of the people to be served (Guimond & Salman, 2013). This approach includes having flexibility and skill in adapting programs to various cultural contexts and situations. Involving the community members directly in the research process was crucial to ensure the exercise intervention was culturally appropriate in a mosque setting. The research team avoided self-assumptions, biases, and perceptions of the Islamic religion and mosque setting during the planning phase. Cultural sensitivity was reflected by the following characteristics of the exercise intervention:

- The exercise classes were conducted in a sex-restricted space for women at the mosque.
- Classes were scheduled during times when there were no prayers being held at the mosque.
- The classes were held in the evening as preferred by the women, and the time shifted accordingly to the timing of the Islamic evening prayer (Salah), which is based on the sun's movement and occurs 5 to 10 minutes prior to sunset.
- There were no classes held during the month of Ramadan.
- Kinesiology students who led the exercises classes were of the Islamic faith and spoke the languages of the women.
- All written material was in English and the Kinesiology students were available to translate consent forms, demographic, and other data collection forms verbally as required.
- Women were able to take an information letter regarding the exercise intervention and consent process home and make decisions with their significant other and/or children with respect to participation in the program and the research component. The consent forms could also be taken home or signed at the mosque.
- All women who wanted to exercise were invited to participate in exercise classes even if they did not want to participate in the research project.
- All women participating in the program were able to wear their traditional attire, such as saris and salwar kameez. They also had the option of removing their hijab (head covering worn in public by some Muslim women) during the exercise class.
- There was no music or mention of "yoga" during the exercise classes as per the religious guidelines of the mosque.
- Exercises were tailored to be low and mid impact as the women were not able to wear shoes during the exercise sessions as per the mosque guidelines.
- All female research team members who were not Muslim wore a hijab when visiting the mosque to meet with the male council members.

REFLECTION: PAR LEADS TO SUCCESSFUL OUTCOMES

Using PAR aspired to engage all organizations (i.e., Women's College Hospital, the health centre, and the mosque) relevant to the development, implementation, and evaluation of the exercise intervention for South Asian Muslim women in a mosque. We produced a successful intervention by using PAR in strengthening knowledge and building skills that were used by the women experiencing barriers to physical activity in an Islamic community. The PAR process engaged those close to the problem (PAR is "participatory") while also promoting positive change (PAR involves "action"). We involved the council members and women of the mosque, health professionals, and researchers from the Women's College Hospital and the health centre. The use of PAR evolved from and was attentive to the local context of the mosque. PAR was not used as a model but as an approach. All stakeholders were considered experts with important knowledge and perspectives. Power relations between the organizations were kept to a minimum. Researchers aimed to question and learn how the mosque community worked and enabled an exercise intervention. PAR engages practitioners in a process of inquiry that became part of the solution and pointed to avenues of successful change. We used mainstream quantitative methods of evaluation that were sensitive to the religious target group. The exercise intervention was flexible in design allowing individualization as necessary and provided all involved with the ability to respond to what was being learned along the way. These elements were essential to the successful long-term adoption of the exercise intervention in a mosque setting.

*To hear full stories of the women reflecting upon their experiences during their participation in the exercise intervention please visit: https://vimeo.com/125616395 and enter password **wch.***

Summary

In this chapter we have tried to provide an overview of what was entailed in carrying out successful action research targeting a specific ethnic community in Canada. The description of a mosque-based exercise intervention highlights a positive experience facilitated by PAR. This form of action research resulted in a culturally sensitive intervention. Muslim women were empowered to demonstrate their importance and brought about gender equity with respect to physical activity opportunities. A salient feature of this PAR-driven project is engaging the mosque community to the full extent in the research process to better understand and take action on health issues important to them.

Our mosque-based intervention program is scalable and may be adopted successfully among other mosque settings in Canada to reach a greater proportion of the eligible population of Muslim women who experience barriers to being physically active. The program we implemented has been shown to be sustainable in a mosque setting and enable South Asian Muslim women to achieve potential long-term benefits of physical activity.

Acknowledgement

The Exploring the Feasibility, Acceptability and Effectiveness of a Mosque-Based Intervention to Promote Physical Activity in South Asian Muslim Women project was funded by the Women's XChange program at Women's College Hospital.

REFERENCES

Banerjee, A. T., Kin, R., Strachan, P. H., Boyle, M. H., Anand, S. S., & Oremus, M. (2015). Factors facilitating the implementation of church-based heart health promotion programs for older adults: A qualitative study guided by the Precede-Proceed Model. *American Journal of Health Promotion, 29*(6), 365–373.

Banning, M., & Hafeez, H. (2009). Perceptions of breast health practices in Pakistani Muslim women. *Asian Pacific Journal of Cancer Prevention, 10*(5), 841–847.

Bryan, S. N., Tremblay, M. S., Perez, C. E., Ardern, C. I., & Katzmarzyk, P. T. (2006). Physical activity and ethnicity: Evidence from the Canadian Community Health Survey. *Canadian Journal of Public Health, 97*(4), 271–276.

Campbell, M. K., Hudson, M. A., Resnicow, K., Blakeney, N., Paxton, A., & Baskin, M. (2007). Church-based health promotion interventions: Evidence and lessons learned. *Annual Review of Public Health, 28*, 213–234.

Caperchione, C. M., Kolt, G. S., & Mummery, W. K. (2013). Examining physical activity service provision to culturally and linguistically diverse (CALD) communities in Australia: A qualitative evaluation. *PLoS One, 8*(4), e62777.

Carroll, R., Ali, N., & Azam, N. (2002). Promoting physical activity in South Asian Muslim women through "exercise on prescription." *Health Technology Assessment, 6*(8), 1–101.

Chiu, M., Austin, P. C., Manuel, D. G., & Tu, J. V. (2012). Cardiovascular risk factor profiles of recent immigrants vs long-term residents of Ontario: A multi-ethnic study. *Canadian Journal of Cardiology, 28*(1), 20–26.

Choudhry, U. K., Jandu, S., Mahal, J., Singh, R., Sohi-Pabla, H., & Mutta, B. (2002). Health promotion and participatory action research with South Asian women. *Journal of Nursing Scholarship, 34*(1), 75–81.

Chudyk, A., & Petrella, R. J. (2011). Effects of exercise on cardiovascular risk factors in type 2 diabetes: A meta-analysis. *Diabetes Care, 34*(5), 1228–1237.

Craig, C. L., Marshall, A. L., Sjostrom, M., Bauman, A. E., Booth, M. L., Ainsworth, B. E., et al. (2003). International physical activity questionnaire: 12-country reliability and validity. *Medicine & Science in Sports & Exercise, 35*(8), 1381–1395.

Giachello, A. L., Arrom, J. O., Davis, M., Sayad, J. V., Ramirez, D., Nandi, C., et al. (2003). Reducing diabetes health disparities through community-based participatory action research: The Chicago Southeast Diabetes Community Action Coalition. *Public Health Reports, 118*(4), 309–323.

Guimond, M. E., & Salman, K. (2013). Modesty matters: Cultural sensitivity and cervical cancer prevention in muslim women in the United States. *Nursing for Women's Health, 17*(3), 210–216.

Hlatky, M. A., Boineau, R. E., Higginbotham, M. B., Lee, K. L., Mark, D. B., Califf, R. M., et al. (1989). A brief self-administered questionnaire to determine functional capacity (the Duke Activity Status Index). *American Journal of Cardiology, 64*(10), 651–654.

Khan, S., & Watson, J. C. (2005). The Canadian immigration experiences of Pakistani women: Dreams confront reality. *Counselling Psychology Quarterly, 18*(4), 307–317.

Laverack, G. (2001). An identification and interpretation of the oganizational aspects of community empowerment. *Community Development Journal, 36*(2), 134–145.

Lawton, J., Ahmad, N., Hanna, L., Douglas, M., & Hallowell, N. (2006). "I can't do any serious exercise": Barriers to physical activity amongst people of Pakistani and Indian origin with type 2 diabetes. *Health Education Research, 21*(1), 43–54.

Price, J., Landry, M., Rolfe, D., Delos-Reyes, F., Groff, L., & Sternberg, L. (2005). Women's cardiac rehabilitation: Improving access using principles of women's health. *Canadian Journal of Cardiovascular Nursing, 15*(3), 32–41.

Reason, P., & Bradbury, H. (2001). *Handbook of action research.* London: Sage.

Sarri, R. C., & Sarri, C. M. (1992). Organizational and community change through participatory action research. *Administration in Social Work, 16*(3-4), 99–122.

Sriskantharajah, J., & Kai, J. (2007). Promoting physical activity among South Asian women with coronary heart disease and diabetes: What might help? *Family Practice, 24*(1), 71–76.

Statisics Canada. (2006). *Canada's ethnocultural mosiac, 2006 census: Definitions.* URL=http://www12.statcan.ca/census-recensement/2006/as-sa/97–562/note-eng.cfm

Statistics Canada. (2013). *Immigration and ethnocultural diversity in Canada. National Household Survey, 2011.* Ottawa: Author. URL=http://www12.statcan.gc.ca/nhs-enm/2011/as-sa/99–010-x/99–010-x2011001-eng.pdf

Tremblay, M. S., Warburton, D. E., Janssen, I., Paterson, D. H., Latimer, A. E., Rhodes, R. E., et al. (2011). New Canadian physical activity guidelines. *Applied Physiology, Nutrition, and Metabolism, 36*(1), 36–46.

Trivedi, P. (1984). To deny our fullness: Asian women in the making of history. *Feminist Review, 17,* 37–50.

Williams, E. D., Stamatakis, E., Chandola, T., & Hamer, M. (2011). Physical activity behaviour and coronary heart disease mortality among South Asian people in the UK: An observational longitudinal study. *Heart, 97*(8), 655–659.

ONLINE RESOURCES

Please visit the Point at http://thepoint.lww.com/Vollman4e for up-to-date Internet resources and additional learning materials on this topic.

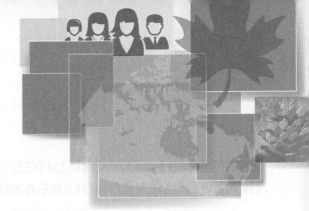

CHAPTER 31

Best Practices in Early Childhood Development Programs in Newcomer Populations

Linda Ogilvie, Anna Kirova, Mahdieh Dastjerdi, and Yvonne Chiu

LEARNING OBJECTIVES

After studying this chapter, you should be able to:

1. Identify early childhood development (ECD) issues specific to newcomer children

2. Comment on the merits of family-focused versus child-focused ECD education in newcomer populations

3. Describe, with examples, what is meant by hybridized parenting, cultural competence, and cultural safety

Introduction

Healthy child development is an important social determinant of health. Health promotion in early childhood is, therefore, a primary health care priority. With an immigrant population of 20% in Canada projected to grow to levels of 25% to 28% by 2031 (Statistics Canada, 2010), immigrant and refugee (newcomer) healthy child development merits significant attention. Newcomer children may be at increased risk of developmental delay related to the stresses of dislocation and resettlement associated with moving to a new country. Refugee children, who may have experienced pre-migration traumatic events or have families who have undergone perilous journeys to safety, may be at particular risk (Beiser, 2005). This multidisciplinary community-based action research project to explore policy-relevant early childhood development (ECD) assessment issues in newcomer children (Ogilvie et al., 2014) also revealed practice-relevant results. As results tended to relate to parenting challenges and adaptations in a new country and the potential for ECD programs to promote positive parenting and integration experiences of newcomer families, the focus of the project, for which ethical clearance was granted and signed informed consent from participants was sought, shifted over time. In collaboration with agency administrators and through interviews with parents and focus groups with front-line staff in ECD programs, issues in ECD assessment identified in the literature were confirmed but the need to create supportive environments for collaboration with families in relation to parenting in a new country took precedence.

ASSESSING EARLY CHILDHOOD DEVELOPMENT IN NEWCOMER TODDLERS AND PRESCHOOLERS

Newcomer ECD and how to assess it is of interest in immigrant-receiving countries worldwide (Hernandez et al., 2008; EACEA, 2009; Fuller et al., 2009; Karoly & Gonzalez, 2011; Bernhard, 2012) and there is recognition that ECD assessment tools grounded in Western developmental norms may lack validity for newcomer children (Greenfield, 1997; Kummerer et al., 2007). Cultural differences in parenting could negatively impact outcomes of standardized ECD testing (Pachter & Dworkin, 1997). In addition, the association between socioeconomic status and health and education outcomes is well established (Bradley & Corwyn, 2002), as is the association of immigration with lower levels of income in Canada (Simich & Jackson, 2010), the USA (Hernandez et al., 2008), and across Europe (EACEA, 2009). Research on ECD and its assessment in newcomer children, therefore, is an important equity issue as newcomer children's knowledge may be devalued and marginalized leading to inappropriate labelling when such children start school without the cultural capital (contextual behaviours and knowledge) needed to succeed (O'Connor, 2011).

While most research on newcomer ECD assessment and programming focuses on the child, there are also advocates of the family-focused approach (Vesely & Ginsberg, 2011; Bernhard, 2012; Bornstein & Cote, 2012). Early childhood development cannot be separated from effective parenting. It is important to recognize that when parents are included, the assessment process itself becomes an intervention. Thus, our most relevant practice recommendations were:

- Initial assessment of recent newcomer children and their families should be flexible and focus on the process of settlement and adjustment, rather than on expectations that they will meet standardized outcome criteria.
- The pace of initial ECD child assessment should be lengthened to allow time for workers to develop trust with families before testing is started and/or completed and to determine if any observed deficits relate more to unfamiliarity with tasks expected than to developmental delay. Front-line workers should exercise discretion in the timing of assessment and funders should provide some leeway.
- Front-line workers need cultural training.
- More culturally relevant family assessment tools for newcomer populations are needed.
- Standardized ECD assessment tools are only one form of assessment and interpretation should be supplemented by observations, parent reports, and systematic collection of artifacts such as artwork.

These practice recommendations, which emerged from focus group and parent interview data, do not negate the need for culturally relevant ECD assessment tools as children do need to be assessed, but without prior engagement with newcomer parents and the creation of a supportive environment, ECD programs for newcomer children are unlikely to yield optimal results.

PERSPECTIVES OF AGENCY STAFF

Issues that were raised in focus groups with 12 front-line workers in ECD programs in three settlement agencies and three government agencies were similar to concerns raised by agency administrators in research team discussions. Emphasis revolved around trust, use of standardized tools, and program characteristics. While policies for funding of ECD programs focused on child assessment and progress, our data overwhelmingly pointed to the importance of accommodating family needs in newcomer ECD assessment and programming. Alleviating family and parental stress emerged as of primary importance in the settlement agency data.

Establishing trust encompassed language considerations that included issues with the use of interpreters; cultural sensitivity both of approaches and questions asked; attention to gender differences; development and maintenance of positive relationships with families and children; optimal timing of standardized testing; and, ethical and conscious awareness of the potential for misuse of information. Solicitation of consents for formal ECD assessment procedures was of particular concern given the negative experiences of some newcomers when signing official forms in their countries of origin. Use of standardized tools incorporated concerns about appropriateness of items in relation to child development norms across cultures, parenting differences, and use of findings that were unlikely to be valid measures of a child's current development or developmental potential. Thus, few front-line staff members administered the tools using recommended or standardized protocols. It was difficult to separate child development issues from family stresses. Staff preferred qualitative assessment methods but funders preferred quantitative measures for both child and program evaluation. Program characteristics were important in two significant ways. Settlement agency programs (all newcomer children) tended to have more cultural and linguistic resources. Front-line staff in government programs (both newcomer and other at risk children) reported fewer issues with the solicitation of consents for ECD assessments. It is possible that the settlement workers, many of whom were also immigrants or refugees, were more conscious of potential parental concerns about signing forms and, therefore, projected their own feelings about signing documents onto clients during the consent process.

PERSPECTIVES OF PARENTS

In our interviews with parents (seven mothers and one father) from Burundi, China, Iraq, Sudan and Vietnam, we found that parents did not necessarily share the perceptions of program staff and administrators. Parents' concerns with language were less about interpretation issues and more related to retention of their heritage language, enhancement of their English language skills in order to become more effective parents in the Canadian context, and the potential for using their child's participation in the ECD program to increase the parents' opportunities to strengthen their communication skills in English. Parents were less concerned about cultural sensitivity and assessment item sensitivity than the research team and front-line staff. One parent mentioned a fear of her child being labelled (misuse of information) and one parent had difficulty with the research consent process, which could translate into a concern about assessment process consent as well. Other issues raised by staff were not introduced by parents. Parents, however, did talk about personal and family issues and the effects of program participation and evaluation on their lives. They perceived participation of a child in an ECD program as an opportunity for the parents to develop personal skills and experience increased social support.

Personal and Family Issues

Personal and family issues included parental concerns about their child's future, parenting in isolation, cultural differences in parenting, and how immigration/settlement processes affect parenting. As with parents everywhere, participants wanted the best for their children: "She wants her kids to be able to, from the beginning, as they are younger to be involved in a good program so that when they grow up they have a great future in this society."

The isolation and loss of an extended family network can make the marital partnership critical as there are fewer people to assume child care responsibilities. Loss of the extended family network, however, was not always perceived negatively.

Here we are only the husband, I, and the children. Now we know ourselves well and the kids. I know they're living in a good place, and eat good food, and they're healthy....But it's back home, like one house you have to see many people and for the food it can become difficult to get money and to get them good education....I'm learning to appreciate the way of life here....One of the things about living here is that I am with my children much more. Whereas before...I could go out, and but, you know do more things more freely, but I was not with my children. So I am really appreciating being here with my children.

Parents spoke of adjusting to life in a new country, with one parent saying that it took 3 years to start believing that life in Canada was better than the life left behind and another parent expressing relief at the safety, including the lack of violence in children's play, experienced in Canada.

Program Participation and Evaluation

Parents had much to say about the effects of the programs on their lives. While not directly related to the ECD assessment process, insights gained from such comments are relevant for planning future ECD programs for newcomer children. Expectations related to enhanced English acquisition were not a surprise but the suggestion that family relationships would improve was interesting. Examples included: "...she want from this program...that her children...respectful to elder and loving brother, sister....Love our people, our culture" and "...you can tell me what going on in Canada, like the rules....Some rules, like giving not beating the children....And child abuse, see and even fighting, husband and wife." In some newcomer populations, child discipline practices and spousal abuse are contentious issues after immigration. These comments reveal awareness and positive attitudes about some Canadian cultural values and practices around family relationships, many of which enhance health.

No negative impacts from involvement in an ECD program were reported but positive outcomes were voiced. For example, in the child, "more confident yea, and maybe friendlier...communicated good with other children"; and, in the mother, "...discipline in a peaceful way...like be calm with the kids...talk to them instead of pushing or physical punishment...a lot of reinforce....Before...always scream at him." For some parents, the home visits were particularly important. One mother commented on the help of a home visitor who reminded her to be a mother to all of her children and not focus all of her attention on the child in the ECD program.

Mothers spoke about increasing their social networks, both across cultures and within their own ethnocultural communities. Such contact not only improved parenting practices but also relieved isolation, built confidence, and increased independence. As one mother said:

I learn many things from the teacher and another person. How, how do I play with children....How do I fix the problem about my children...or become better communication with him....When I came...I just went to do my English....With another person from many country...I learn some more culture...I learn how to teach, prepare the children....When somebody talks to me and they meet me because they feel worried, you know, yeah and now I comfort people....So one of the best things we see is that we feel more comfortable, more confidence...so that we feel more, we don't feel confused or lonely.

Another mother stated:

When I first came it was difficult because the children need to get out, but I wasn't able, I didn't feel able to leave the house. But now, with the program I am more able to leave the house and so we can, which is good for them as well.

An unanticipated finding was the improvement in family relationships and in family expression of emotions. There was change in the marital relationship:

So with my husband we were not that close, we communicating with each other before going to the program. Sometimes we even quarrelled with each other; however, after going to the programs I talked to him about these programs and he also became supportive and he is willing to do a little less hours of work so he could give us a ride to the program. At first my husband wasn't that supportive because he thought it's quite a hassle to go to all these programs with the young children. And also it was just a place that the women will gossip; however, seeing the improvement in the sons and also the happiness in us, he was willing to do that. So in a way, our relationship has become better.

There was also change in the parent-child relationship:

So, the children will be happier. Like, for example, after his activities he would share with me the crafts that he is doing, what he has done during the activities. We kind of have some common topics to talk about. And also, I would learn to play with him. Know how to play with him and our relationship probably would be strengthened more. Here, the westerners, when they love their children, they love their children wholeheartedly, and they show it. For Chinese people, they are usually more reserved. Now we have learned to hug our children, kiss them and also, you know, tell them that we love them. So in a way it is still a bit uneasy for me, say for example when my younger son curls his lip up, he wants to have a kiss. I still kind of feel uneasy but this is good. Expressing our love to them, it is also an important communication to them.

Some participants revealed that the programs enhanced father participation in family outings and recreation time with children, something that was not commonly seen in their countries of origin. Engaging in family activities strengthened family bonds.

While parents were unanimous in their positive assessment of the ECD programs, they did have suggestions for improvement. Parents would like to see more field trips and more program time devoted to helping children with specific learning problems. Mothers would also like to have nonparented activities to allow more personal time. Long wait times between assessment and registration in programs was a source of frustration. There were requests to have resource materials and assessment tests in languages other than English. Better access to interpretation and additional transportation support were also needed.

IMPLICATIONS FOR EARLY CHILDHOOD DEVELOPMENT PROGRAMS IN NEWCOMER POPULATIONS

Three areas for thought and intervention emerged from the information provided by agency front-line workers and parents: hybridized parenting; best practice; and, addressing parents' concerns. What was clear was that focus on ECD assessment tools alone was too limiting and not the appropriate initial step. Much more could be accomplished through advocating a family-centred approach. Enhancing ECD outcomes in newcomer children would enable children to achieve educational success and enhanced employment opportunities in adulthood. Thus, improved ECD assessment and programming for newcomer at risk children is a good example of mediating across sectors to facilitate child and family mental health, school success, and social integration of newcomers.

Hybridized Parenting

The notion of hybridized parenting as a feature of globalization (Sanagavarapu, 2010) is intriguing and a good fit with our parent data. While the term is never clearly defined in Sanagavarapu's paper, the etiology and features of hybridized parenting emerge in her arguments and are well-documented from the literature. Hybridization implies reciprocity in changes in cultural practices with societal change occurring as mutual cultural translation occurs. The parent data suggest that parents were retaining some heritage cultural norms while also embracing what they appreciated as Canadian cultural norms. The inference is that, in the process of integrating into a new society, features of the newcomer's culture collide or interact with features of the host society to lead to new cultural practices that differ from each original practice, and that parenting is one arena in which such new hybridized practices may occur.

For example, parental concern for a child's retention of a heritage language and parents' struggles to master English demonstrate an ideal of bilingualism. It is telling that the needs for interpretation decreased as the process of data collection with parent participants progressed during the interviews in this study. While struggling with English, these parents strove for direct communication with the interviewer even in the presence of an interpreter. They wanted to tell their own story.

In her book, *Stand Together or Fall Apart: Professionals Working with Immigrant Families,* Bernhard (2012) provides critical and well-documented analysis of current programming and professional practices with immigrants. Of particular interest is her differentiation of Type One and Type Two interventions with parents. Type One interventions, characterized by top-down, professionally planned, child-oriented interventions have been unsuccessful in newcomer populations but still form the majority of programs. Conversely, Type Two interventions, which are family-focused, build on parental knowledge and strengths, and involve parents in program design, have led to positive child outcomes. While still rare, Type Two interventions are more likely to result in hybridized parenting and the mutual understanding that would be engendered. The implication is that front-line staff who work with newcomers need to be open and receptive to integrating source country norms into practice settings. Diversity needs to be appreciated for the benefits that Canadian society as a whole can reap through exposure to effective family and parenting differences. Change in a multicultural Canada should not be unidirectional if the true benefits of hybridity are to be realized.

Best Practice

Our recommendations reflect cultural competence and cultural safety best practices. Cultural competence is "an ongoing process of seeking cultural awareness, cultural knowledge, cultural skill, and cultural encounters" (Suh, 2004, p. 96) whereas "cultural safety aims to counter tendencies in health care that create cultural risk (or unsafety)—those situations that arise when people from one ethnocultural group are demeaned, diminished or disempowered by the actions and the delivery systems of people from another culture" (Browne et al., 2009, p. 169). Front-line workers in our study exemplified understanding of best practices congruent with cultural responsiveness to client values, beliefs, experiences, and needs. In addition, the results add to knowledge relevant for services to newcomer families and children. For example, knowing that a newcomer child's participation in an ECD program can influence family relationships, social isolation, and perhaps family integration into the new society could provide sound rationale for innovation in how programs related to issues such as maternal depression or family violence for immigrant and other populations could be conceived and implemented. There is a need to become more creative and inclusive of multiple objectives in program planning if we are to make best use of fiscal and other resources.

Addressing Parents' Concerns

An important feature of action research is the possibility of change. In order to address newcomer parents' desires for their children to both enhance their English proficiency and maintain their heritage language and culture, some of our research team members followed our initial study with a new ECD education initiative. As an example of a Type Two intervention, this new intercultural early learning program employed front-line workers (First Language Facilitators) who were themselves newcomers from countries matched to each child's country of origin. Their role was explicitly to facilitate first language (L1) competency and the preservation of children's cultural heritage (Kirova, 2012). In addition to addressing most of the newcomer parents' concerns identified in the ECD assessment study, the intercultural early learning program fits with Canada's multicultural policies that favour integration with retention of heritage cultural features rather than assimilation into one mainstream culture, and incorporates best practices congruent with suggestions from our collaborative research initiative.

Acculturation, important for integration into the host country, is an ongoing process in which language acquisition plays an important role. There is evidence, however, that school success in newcomer children is related to proficiency in at least one language. While there is consensus among researchers that the maintenance of L1 in immigrant and refugee children is beneficial to their cognitive, educational, and socio-emotional development, the age at which the second language should be introduced is still debated. Bialystok (2007) found that bilingual children who are proficient in both languages have cognitive advantages. Language proficiency is critical to grasping abstract concepts important to educational success, particularly as children progress through the school system.

In addition to academic benefits, maintenance of the L1 at home is the cornerstone of a healthy family life, especially if the parents are not proficient in the majority language. For newcomer children, in particular, maintenance of the L1 is important for the child's self-esteem and for their relationships with their parents in the long term. While both parents and children need capacity in English for integration and everyone recognizes the issue, there are only a few programs that provide examples of best practice in achieving these goals, especially from the parents' point of view, outside of well-known bilingual programs.

In the new initiative, each child's L1 was one of the four languages of classroom instruction. As part of the evaluation of the program at the end of year, three parents were invited to discuss observable changes in the use of the home language. Most parents noticed positive changes in their children's use of their first language, including paying more attention to parents' talk in their home language and showing interest in topics being discussed. Quotes from those who signed consent forms are included here. For example, one mother said, laughingly, "When we say something in our language we don't want him to hear, he now says 'I heard you!'" Younger children were reported as engaging older children in conversation in their mother tongue and teaching their older siblings heritage language words, or bringing new words from school and discussing them with their parents. The parents acknowledged that they too have become a lot more conscious about using their home language with all of their children, as well as encouraging other members of the community whose children who were not part of the program to do the same:

> *Wherever I go I tell my people, "Talk to your children in our language because this will help them learn in school." They don't believe me at first but then I tell them what my child is doing and they listen to me.*

Another noticeable change was the way in which parents understood and were able to accommodate to changes to their child's behaviour that were required by the school, such as approaching adults directly with questions and looking them in the eyes when scolded. One father said, "I don't have a problem with this. We are here in Canada and it is important for our children to learn to stand for themselves and be like the other children." Another father added, "I see her [my daughter] need to blend my culture and this culture in order to fit. So the program has helped a lot. If you live here, you have to be flexible."

The new program, in which not all children are newcomers, is also congruent with the post-colonial concept of hybridity introduced earlier in this paper. Working respectfully together, new programs and ways of being that acknowledge the richness of our diversity can emerge. Most educators, social service providers, and health professionals are unfamiliar with the benefit of heritage language competence in newcomer children for future scholastic achievement, as well as for family cohesion. Many, however, are familiar with education as an important determinant of health and the place of educational success for future employment success.

LESSONS LEARNED

It may be that in work with newcomer populations, deep understanding and enactment of culturally competent and culturally safe care can provide an opportunity for meaningful healthcare and human service system change. Front-line expertise, used wisely, is a powerful tool. The notion of hybridity could guide how we approach human service work and the system change we envision. True respect for differences could lead to new solutions for best practices in health promotion strategies and the provision of enhanced support and care in our culturally diverse societies.

Summary

In this chapter, we presented a community-based multidisciplinary action research project that initially focused on the cultural appropriateness of early childhood development assessment tools and practices for newcomer populations. Results suggested that culturally informed family-focused assessment and intervention were often more critical initially than child-focused programming. Such programs lead to positive changes in parent–child relationships and increased use of the first language and thus enhanced opportunities for hybridized parenting. A follow-up initiative based on the recommendations made by newcomer parents to improve existing ECD programs was described.

Acknowledgements

We appreciate the funding provided by the Prairie Centre of Excellence for Research on Immigration and Integration and by the Canadian Research Institute for Law and the Family, as well as the research team contributions of Elizabeth Burgess-Pinto, Catherine Caufield, Darcy Fleming, Nicole Jarvis, Vivian Lam, Karin Linschoten Lucenia Ortiz, and Sandra Rastin.

REFERENCES

Beiser, M. (2005). The health of immigrants and refugees in Canada. *Canadian Journal of Public Health, 96*(Suppl 2), S30–S44.

Bernhard, J. K. (2012). *Stand together or fall apart: Professionals working with immigrant families.* Halifax: Fernwood.

Bialystok, E. (2007). Cognitive effects of bilingualism: How linguistic experience leads to cognitive change. *International Journal of Bilingual Education and Bilingualism, 10*(3), 210–223.

Bornstein, M. H., & Cote, L. R. (2012). "Who is sitting across from me?" Immigrant mothers' knowledge of parenting and children's development. *Pediatrics, 114*(5), e557–e564.

Bradley, R. H., & Corwyn, R. F. (2002). Socioeconomic status and child development. *Annual Review of Psychology, 53,* 371–399.

Browne, A. J., Varcoe, C., Smye, V., Reimer-Kirkham, S., Lynam, M. J., & Wong, S. (2009). Cultural safety and the challenges of translating critically oriented knowledge in practice. *Nursing Philosophy, 10*(3), 167–179.

EACEA (Educational, Audiovisual and Culture Executive Agency, European Commission). (2009). *Tackling social and cultural inequities through early childhood education and care in Europe.* URL=http://eacea.ec.europa.eu/about/eurydice/documents/098EN.pdf

Fuller, B., Bridges, M., Bein, E., Jang, H., Jung, S., Rabe-Hesketh, S., et al. (2009). The health and cognitive growth of Latino toddlers: At risk or immigrant paradox? *Maternal and Child Health Journal, 13*, 755–768.

Greenfield, P. M. (1997). You can't take it with you: Why ability assessments don't cross cultures. *American Psychologist, 52*(10), 1115–1124.

Hernandez, D. J., Denton, N. A., & Macartney, S. E. (2008). Children in immigrant families: Looking to America's future. *Social Policy Report, 22*(3), 3–23. URL=http://www.srcd.org/sites/default/files/documents//22_3_hernandez_final.pdf

Karoly, L. A., & Gonzalez, G. C. (2011). Early care and education for children in immigrant families. *The Future of Children, 21*(1), 71–101.

Kirova, A. (2012). Creating shared learning spaces: An intercultural, multilingual early learning program for preschool children from refugee families. In F. McCarthy & M. Vickers (Eds.), *Refugee and immigrant student: Achieving equity in education* (pp. 23–44). Charlotte, NC: Information Age Publishing.

Kummerer, S. E., Lopez-Reyna, N. A., & Hughes, M. T. (2007). Mexican immigrant mothers' perceptions of their children's communication disabilities, emergent literacy development, and speech-language therapy program. *American Journal of Speech-Language-Hearing Pathology, 16*, 271–282.

O'Connor, J. (2011). Applying Bourdieu's concepts of social and cultural capital and habitus to early years research. In T. Waller, J. Whitmarsh, & K. Clarke (Eds.), *Making sense of theory and practice in early childhood: The power of ideas* (pp. 115–127). Maidenhead Berkshire: Open University Press.

Ogilvie, L., Fleming, D., Kirova, A., Chiu, Y., Rastin, S., Caufield, C., et al. (2014). Matching policies to needs in early childhood development programs in newcomer populations. In C. Brewer & M. McCabe (Eds.), *Immigrant and refugee students* (pp. 65–88). Toronto: Brush Education.

Pachter, L. M., & Dworkin, P. H. (1997). Maternal expectations about normal child development in 4 cultural groups. *Archives of Pediatric Adolescent Medicine, 151*(11), 1144–1150.

Sanagavarapu, P. (2010). What does cultural globalisation mean for parenting in immigrant families in the 21st century? *Australasian Journal of Early Childhood, 35*(2), 36–42.

Simich, L., & Jackson, B. (2010). What makes some immigrants healthy and others not? *Health Policy Research, 10*, 26–29.

Statistics Canada. (2010). *Projections of the diversity of the Canadian population.* URL=www.statcan.gc.ca/daily-quotidien/100309/dq100309a-eng.htm

Suh, E. E. (2004). The model of cultural competence through an evolutionary concept analysis. *Journal of Transcultural Nursing, 15*(2), 93–102.

Vesely, C. K., & Ginsberg, M. R. (2011). Strategies and practices for working with immigrant families in early education programs. *Young Children, 66*(1), 84–89.

ONLINE RESOURCES

Please visit thePoint at http://thepoint.lww.com/Vollman4e for up-to-date Internet resources and additional learning materials on this topic.

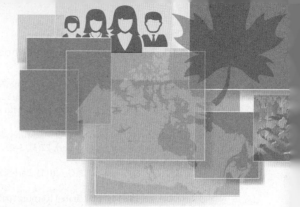

CHAPTER *32*

Influences on Quality of Life of Older Adults in a Remote Dene Community in the Northwest Territories of Canada

Pertice Moffitt and Brianne Timpson

LEARNING OBJECTIVES

After studying this chapter, you should be able to:

1. Understand some of the influences on quality of life of the older adult living in a remote Northwest Territory (NWT) community

2. Identify strategies to create supportive environments for older adults in the NWT

3. Recognize the significance of narrative to knowledge mobilization in Aboriginal communities

4. Appreciate the impact of remoteness and culture on assessment, health promotion, and interventions to create safe communities

Introduction

Older adults' quality of life (QOL) in the Northwest Territories (NWT), as in other parts of Canada, is related to myriad circumstance, environments, belief systems, and personal life stories. Approximately one half of the population of the territory includes Aboriginal people who mostly reside in Dene, Métis, or Inuit communities scattered across the North, while the remaining half are "settlers" from southern Canada and other countries who came to the North for adventure or employment and made the North their home, settling in the larger regional centres. This distinction between where people live and who they are (Aboriginal—mostly in remote and homogeneous communities; settlers—mostly in larger urban centres and heterogeneous communities) can also be stated another way: disparity for the former and prosperity for the latter. Of course, this is a generalization and may appear as polarization but one that bears witness in the health status reports of Aboriginal peoples (Government of the

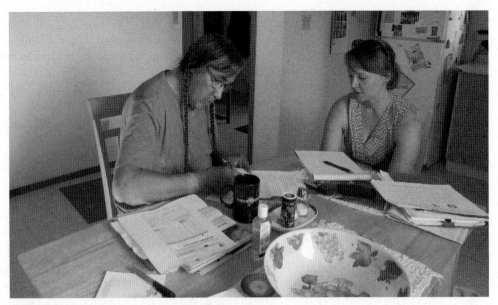

FIGURE 32.1 Interviewing a local older adult.

Northwest Territories [GNWT] Department of Health and Social Services, 2011). It has been found that Aboriginal older adults as a cohort are among the most vulnerable (Health Council of Canada [HCC], 2013).

Between 2013 and 2014, a community-based participatory action research (CBPAR) study exploring the QOL of older adults living in the NWT was conducted by nursing faculty/ researchers at the Aurora Research Institute, a division of Aurora College, and the NWT Seniors' Society (NWTSS). Using focus group meetings, individual interviews (Fig. 32.1), town hall meetings, and sharing circles, influences on the QOL of older adults (i.e., 50 years and older) were explored with 92 older adults from across the territory. In this chapter, we will highlight our results in a case story format about older adults living in a remote Dene community in the North.

THE SETTING

Canada's NWT is located east of Yukon and west of Nunavut. Situated above the provinces of British Columbia, Alberta, Saskatchewan, and the 60th parallel (latitude), the NWT is home to 43,595 residents (GNWT Bureau of Statistics, 2015). This population is dispersed across the Territory in 33 communities; the smallest community, Jean Marie River, is home to 71 people, while 16 communities have fewer than 500 residents (GNWT Bureau of Statistics, 2013). The capital of the NWT, Yellowknife, is home to approximately 20,000 residents, nearly half the total territorial population. Although small in comparison to other Canadian cities, Yellowknife has many of the amenities found in larger urban centres. Stanton Territorial Hospital, the main acute care and out-patient facility for residents across the NWT and Western Nunavut (Kitikmeot Region), is situated in the territorial capital (Stanton Territorial Health Authority, 2015). Inuvik, a town located in the Arctic is home to 3,396 residents, while Hay River, located south of Yellowknife has a population of 3,689 people (GNWT Bureau of Statistics, 2013). The Mackenzie River, 1,738 km long, connects these two towns and many communities along the river, allowing barges to deliver supplies to residents during summer months.

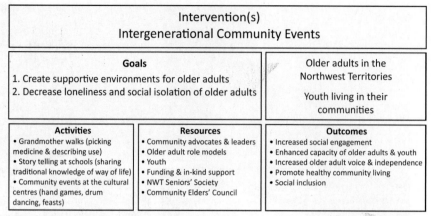

FIGURE 32.2   Logic model.

The landscape of the NWT is remote and rugged. The total land mass of the territory is over 1,000,000 km^2 and consists of many lakes of various sizes (two of which are the largest lakes in the world), rock, Precambrian shield, and tundra (Wonders, 2011). For many residents living in these remote and isolated communities, air travel and ice roads (constructed during the winter months) serve as the means of transportation in the NWT. There are 11 official languages recognized in the NWT, 9 of which are indigenous and broadly categorized in three language families: Dene, Inuit, and Cree (GNWT Education, Culture, & Employment, 2007).

The purpose of this case story is to highlight the influences on QOL of older Dene adults living in a remote NWT community. This is in keeping with the direction document, "Our Elders: Our Community" (GNWT Department of Health and Social Services, 2014) and their policy of supporting of ageing in place. We provide an assessment of a narrative and share a health promotion intervention (see the logic model in Fig. 32.2). The intervention is based on one of the five strategies of the Ottawa Charter—creating supportive environments—through intergenerational health promotion events that enhance social connection between youth and older adults, volunteerism (Hanlon et al., 2014) in their everyday lives, and influences on QOL as described by Moffitt and Timpson (2015).

USING (RE)STORYING FOR KNOWLEDGE MOBILIZATION

Story telling is central to the oral traditions of Aboriginal peoples and also has become salient to scholars as a culturally sensitive way of disseminating research in the Northern territories of Canada (Christensen, 2012; Martin & Gibson, 2012) and elsewhere in Canada within a field of art-based approaches (Bruce et al., 2013). Storytelling, or narrative, is also used as a method of inquiry (Clandinin & Connelly, 2000; Barton, 2004) and as a teaching strategy (Hunter, 2008). Stories resonate with local people, and communicating findings in plain language has been endorsed by our governing bodies. In addition, writing a narrative that is scripted from results of research is particularly relevant for remote communities as a means of protecting anonymity while delivering germane results. Anonymity may be destroyed easily in reporting when details uncover the identities of participants through description even though pseudonyms are used.

The following narrative was constructed from the results of a study conducted in a remote community of the NWT (Moffitt & Timpson, 2015). Pseudonyms have been used for the older adult couple in the narrative and data from several interviews collected have provided depth to establish anonymity.

The Story of Helen and Fred

Helen and Fred live in a remote community on the Mackenzie River in the NWT. They have raised 7 children and have 20 grandchildren. Helen's parents were Adele and Norman from another community on Great Slave Lake and Fred's mother, Sarah, and father, Jacob, along with aunties, uncles, cousins, and grandparents have resided in this community and the surrounding lands for generations. They lived their lives trapping, hunting, and fishing; they travelled in the summer to camps along the river, returning to the settlement during the winter. Helen and Fred maintained that lifestyle in their early years as a couple. Last year, Fred began to wander away from the community and started to forget where he had left his fishing supplies. One day, he almost poured gasoline in the woodstove to start the fire. Helen became concerned and took Fred to the nursing station. After an assessment, it was decided that Fred could no longer stay in the community because of dementia. The only centre for people with dementia is in Yellowknife, so Helen went to Yellowknife with Fred and got him settled in the centre. No one in the centre speaks Fred's Slavey language. Fred is in a room all by himself; Helen went back to the community and has not seen Fred for over 7 months.

Helen is a 75-year-old *Tlicho* woman, the fourth child in a family of 13 children. She loves to tell her grandchildren how it was when she was a girl. She hauled wood for the stove, picked moss in the summer for cleaning the house, cleaned fish, dried meat, and looked after the little ones once they started to walk if she was not doing chores. That was her life until she was 10 years old. Then, her mom and dad thought she should get an education. The only school was 200 km away in Zhati Koe, called the Sacred Heart Mission School. Because her parents led a traditional life in the bush, they had never gone to school. They had friends who went and never wanted to talk about it, but in 1950, they thought it must be much better and a modern education may get their daughter a good job. Helen went to school with her older brother and sister. She stayed for 3 years, from 1950 to 1953. This was before the school closed in the late 50s. She called it a nightmare. She remembers she was not allowed to speak Dogrib; the nuns there spoke English and French, so those were the languages they told her to use. She worked in the kitchen in the winter on the weekends and in the evening. In the summer, she worked in the garden and picked berries. After the first few months, she wanted to go home. She was not allowed. She was not allowed to speak with her brother and sister. If she spoke to them in Dogrib or gave them a hug, she was spanked with the ruler. There were many rules and sometimes children got sick and then she would not see them again. When she was allowed to go home in the summer of 1953, she begged her parents to keep her home and not to send her back. She went with her grandfather to the summer camp and when the plane came to pick her up she was nowhere to be found.

Fred is an 80-year-old *Slavey* man, proud of his knowledge of the land that was passed on to him by his grandfather. He never went to school; he was a traditional hunter and fisher. Up until 2 years ago, he took visitors (educators, nurses, police, and researchers) out on the land. When he passed the waterways and sacred places, he left tobacco and prayed for safe passage. He could run a dog team but he was equally accomplished at repairing a skidoo or fixing a motor. He could predict when a storm was coming and he knew how to survive if stranded in the bush. His mother and grandmother taught him about the medicine that the land provided. He knew where the best fishing and hunting spots were. He noticed he was getting forgetful and told Helen he best stay at home. Things started to go downhill after that.

They have been getting a pension cheque now for 10 years. Fred didn't start to collect his money until a friend in town learned to use the computer in 2004 and learned how to apply for the benefit. The government keeps sending them mail but they just store the letters in the basket. The mail is all written in English and neither one of them can read. They take their cheques to the Northern Store to get them cashed. There is no bank in the community so they store their money in a box in the kitchen. The grandkids all know when it is payday, so they

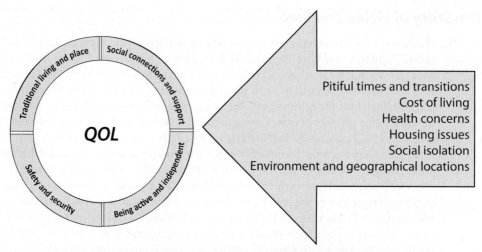

FIGURE 32.3   Influences on quality of life of older adults in the Northwest Territories.

usually come around for a visit and get some cash. That seems to be the only time they see Joe and Frank, their grandsons. They hand out the money until it is gone. Then, they run a credit line at the Northern Store for groceries until the next payday.

Helen and Fred loved to drum dance. Fred had been a drummer for many years and knew all of the prayer songs, wedding songs, and tea dances. When he started forgetting the words a few years back, he stopped drumming and would just go and dance with Helen. Then, that stopped as well because he would wander from the hall; sometimes this was in −40°C temperatures and he would forget his mitts and cap. He was one of the best players on the best hand-games team in the territory. He stopped playing when he started being eliminated early from the game.

Helen cuts the wood for the stove now that Fred is gone. She lives mostly on stew and bannock.[1] Four of her children and their families have moved south. One son is in jail for beating up his wife when he was drunk and another runs a party house in the community. There is such a problem with alcohol and drugs now. Helen was scared last week when her grandson came over demanding money so that he could visit the bootlegger. She gave him all that she had so he would leave. Her daughter comes to visit when she can, but she is working full time in the hamlet office and her evenings are busy in her own home.

ASSESSMENT OF THE NARRATIVE

A strength-based and holistic perspective guides the assessment of the narrative provided (Moffitt & Timpson, 2015). Often, the disparities of Aboriginal peoples in Canada are highlighted in our discourse, particularly where action centres on the fact that Aboriginal people's health lags behind that of other Canadians. Although this is a reality, such discourse that is grounded in risk and despair does nothing to address the resilience of Northern Aboriginal peoples who have lived for centuries amidst harsh climate, geographic isolation, poverty, etc. There is a tendency to describe Aboriginal health through a deficit lens that contributes to a sense of hopelessness for people living in remote Northern communities. An overview of influences on QOL of older adults is presented in Figure 32.3. There are a number of influences on QOL from perceptions of excellence to times of hardship depending on

---

[1]Bannock is unleavened bread like a biscuit and it is usually served with butter and jam. Bannock can be fried, baked, or cooked on a stick over the campfire.

TABLE 32.1   Descriptions of Good Life/Living Well for Older Adults

Themes	Elements
Social Connection and Support	Social interaction
	Supportive networks
	Sense of community
	Love and belonging
	Continuity of generations
	Spirituality
Being Active and Independent	Physically able and mobile
	Good health
	Engaged in community life
	Useful to society
	Volunteer work
	Attend community events
Traditional Living and Place	Connection to the land
	Diverse and hardy people
	Elders' traditional knowledge
	Using your language
	Beliefs, values, and ceremony
	Sharing circles
	Elders and youth together
Safety and Security	Financial security and stability
	Good pensions
	Good health and dental care
	Housing availability and security
	Food security

individual circumstance and context. Descriptors within each influence are further identified in Tables 32.1 and 32.2.

Traditional Living and Place

Dene people have resided for centuries in the NWT. Their relationship to the land can be described as one of reciprocity with all living entities, including plants and animals, which are respected and honoured through traditional practices. Helen's identity as a Dene woman is reinforced when she takes part in the traditional practices of her ancestors. When she gets an opportunity to tan moose hide stretched over poles in her backyard, when she dances at the drum dance, when she provides bannock for the feast, and when she shares stories of Dene women's work with her grandchildren and their friends, she is proud of her heritage. This reinforces her cultural identity. Helen and Fred have led a traditional life in their community. They are respected Elders and up until Fred's deterioration were invited to share their knowledge, direction, and guidance at many local activities. Enabling Helen to continue to attend events and share her knowledge will be supportive for her and others in the community. Older adults contribute to their communities and through their contributions feel validated and self-actualized.

Social Connections and Support

Social connections to friends, family, and community are what make life worth living. Dene people in this community initiate and engage in feasts, drum dances, and hand-games, and older adults are honoured guests at these events. Helen still meets friends at the culture centre

TABLE 32.2 Descriptions of Life's Struggles for Older Adults

Themes	Elements
Pitiful Times and Transitions	Struggle with losses (loved ones, health, choices)
	Colonialism and residential school
	Loss of cultural traditions
	Changing family dynamics
	Leaving community for care
	Lack of land access (fishing/hunting)
	Elder abuse
Cost of Living	Fixed incomes
	Poverty and widening income gap
	Inconsistent application of subsidies
	Expensive airfare
	High fuel costs
	Food availability and cost
Health Concerns	Alcohol and drug addictions
	Chronic disease and disabilities
	Falls and injury
	Pollution of country foods
	Anger, mental anguish, and ageism
	Cognitive failings
	Accessing health care benefits
Housing Issues	Homelessness/squatters
	Affordable accommodation
	Limited seniors' housing
	No home care
	Lack of long-term care beds/home care
	Overcrowding/unsafe housing
	Lack of housing for special needs
	Inconsistent use of subsidies
	Disparity between renting and owning
Social Isolation	Loneliness
	No social network
	Underserviced
	Lack of trust in systems
Environment and Geographical Locations	Cold weather/long winters
	Clean air and water
	Power outages
	Icy streets/uncleared sidewalks
	Unpaved and muddy roads
	No sidewalks
	Lack of wheelchair access
	Transportation concerns

in her community to chat over a cup of tea. In this narrative, Helen has lost an intimate support from Fred, her husband. She grieves the loss of her soul mate because the man she knew is no longer present due to dementia. They are also physically separated from each other as Fred now resides many kilometres distant in care in Yellowknife. It will be important to create connections for the couple, along with community connections for Helen.

Being Active and Independent

Helen and Fred have been active their whole lives. In considering an intervention that creates a supportive environment, Helen must be included in the development of the intervention. Due to her respected position of Elder, she is a key informant about traditional knowledge and will have ideas about cultural events for older adults that lead to community engagement. By engaging Helen and other older adults in the community in creating a proposed intervention that engages older adults with children and youth, they will be valued, cognitively stimulated, and socially included in important community action.

Safety and Security

Helen is not feeling safe in her home since her grandsons have been coming around to get money from her. She is frightened when they have been drinking and show up unexpectedly. In a recent study that surveyed 648 older adults and 57 service providers across the NWT, 70% of participants reported that abuse of older adults[2] occurs in their communities and the most prevalent forms of abuse are neglect and financial (Lutra Associates Ltd., 2015). According to the definition of older adult abuse (Sullivan-Wilson & Jackson, 2014), Helen is experiencing abuse in terms of financial exploitation by her grandsons.

See Table 32.1 for a summary of positive influences on QOL of older adults: descriptions of good life/living well for older adults.

Pitiful Times and Transitions

From this story, we have learned many things about Helen and her family. Helen is a residential school survivor and with this knowledge, it becomes imperative that we consider the legacy of the intergenerational influence of residential schools. Bombay et al. (2014) describe the impact of residential school as historical trauma, identifying that this type of trauma has deleterious effects on the well-being of Aboriginal peoples at personal, family, and community levels. One of the unique ways the territorial governments have chosen to address the legacy of residential school is through the development of a module for inclusion in the high school curriculum in both NWT and Nunavut (GNWT Education, Culture, & Employment et al., 2013). As well, researchers are suggesting that through reconciliation there is hope for community healing (DeGagne, 2007) and supportive interventions (Morrisette & Goodwill, 2013).

Cost of Living

Like many older adults residing in remote NWT communities, Helen lives a modest lifestyle. Her sole income is her pension cheque and the cost of living in her community is formidable. Food is expensive in this small community, since all food is transported there by air. For example, a 2-L carton of 2% milk costs $8.39 in NWT (Canadian Broadcasting Corporation [CBC], 2013) compared to $2.40 to $3.00 in the rest of the country. There are few food subsidies, although most people share meat from the annual caribou hunt. Continuing to use country food is being jeopardized in multiple ways. For example, there is decline in the number and size of caribou herds, changing migration patterns of wildlife, government regulations protecting northern species, lack of traditional hunters in the communities, and rising costs of fuel and for the snow machines that are now in use (GNWT Department of Environment & Natural Resources, 2011).

---

[2]This new term "older adult abuse" replaced the prior language of "elder abuse" in the territory since "Elder" is a respected term used for only some older adults whom are traditional knowledge holders. This was recognized by the NWT Network to Prevent Abuse of Older Adults and changed in 2011 (Lutra Associates Ltd., 2015).

Health Concerns

Fred has been placed in the Dementia Centre; this separation has caused both loneliness and social isolation for Helen. Johansson et al. (2014) describe the difficulties that spouses have to "remain connected" after handing over care of their spouse to an institution. In their research, conducted in Sweden, they describe both facilitators and deterrents to staying connected. Helen does need information about the care of Fred so that she can feel she is partnering in his care even if it is from a distance. One of the challenges that occurs when care is relinquished to an institution is learning to deal with the "separation-individuation" and the accompanying grieving process as you learn to live as a widow (Loboprabhu et al., 2005). Through her social network in the community, Helen needs to redefine herself as an individual and connect with supports that can assist her to keep in touch with others.

Social Isolation

A real problem for Helen is loneliness now that Fred is in care. De Jong Gierveld et al. (2015) have explored the determinants of loneliness. Their findings suggest that personal character-istics, individual social networks and satisfaction with them, and living with socioeconomic challenges are all determinants of loneliness. Helen has experienced a transition within her marriage that sets the stage for her loneliness. She also has limited income, which is just enough to buy her groceries and pay her rent. This affords her little opportunity to pay for airfare to visit her husband in the Dementia Centre.

Environment and Geographical Location

Living in this remote community, there are few amenities. Isolation is a reality. Winters are cold and the harsh weather means that Helen requires transportation to go to community events.

See Table 32.2 for a summary of negative influences on QOL of older adults: descriptions of life's struggles for older adults.

INTERGENERATIONAL SOCIAL CONNECTION

The purpose of the intervention is to create a supportive environment for older adults by pro-moting social inclusion, connection, and engagement with others and diminishing loneliness. Connecting with others through supportive social networks helps to improve the QOL and decrease loneliness of older adults (De Jong Gierveld et al., 2015). Helen participates in Grandmother Walks (NWTSS, 2015), a community-organized event that brings older adults and youth together to spend time with one another. During these walks, Helen and a small group of youth walk around their community looking for traditional plants and berries often used for medicinal purposes. Helen bonds with the youth through storytelling about cultural practices and by sharing her knowledge of each plant's healing properties. In addition to pro-moting social connection and engagement and combating loneliness, Helen and the youth also participate in healthy physical activity.

Another activity in which Helen can participate is modeled after another intergenerational activity that has taken root in the NWT. An elder centre was created within an early childhood educational facility with the purpose to generate connections between older adults and young children (NWTSS, 2015). In this activity, older adults visit daily with preschool children, sharing stories and teaching the children traditional language. Helen could participate in this activity as another way to bond with youth, share her traditional knowledge of her Slavey language and cultural traditions, and improve her social connection with her community.

One way to promote community connections among all community residents is to arrange for a large gathering, such as a community feast. Feasts are a way to get community members together to share stories, participate in cultural activities such as Dene hand-games, beading, drum dancing, or raising a teepee, while feasting on traditional foods. Feasts are often held to celebrate local events such as weddings, band/community meetings, special occasions (e.g., National Aboriginal Day), and national council meetings. These well-attended events promote social connections among community members, reduce loneliness among individuals, and share traditional knowledge between generations.

EVALUATION

Older adults who participated in the various intergenerational projects shared the following: "We want to appreciate one another as a group, family, or individual by recognizing the success of elders and everyone in the community" (NWTSS, 2015, p. 12). Project coordinators commented that the intergenerational activities created a cultural identity with children and reinforced older adult identity through sharing knowledge. In addition, happiness was evident in the smiles and goodwill.

Summary

This case story depicts the context of the lives of older adults who live in remote communities of the NWT. The data collected in the CBPAR study identified various influences on QOL from both beneficial and challenging perspectives. While additional research is needed to more fully explicate QOL for older adults, an understanding of the policy direction, advocacy, and services required to improve social connections and create the supportive environments necessary to age in place in the North is emerging.

Acknowledgements

We appreciate the funding and administrative support of the NWT Seniors' Society (NWTSS) and the many older adults who participated in the study. *Masi Cho!* We are particularly indebted to Barb Hood, Executive Director, and Leon Peterson, President, of the NWTSS. As well, we value the contributions of Gloria Bott, nursing faculty at Aurora College, in the first year of the study, and research assistant Megan Paul, BSN student.

REFERENCES

Barton, S. S. (2004). Narrative inquiry: Locating Aboriginal epistemology in a relational methodology. *Journal of Advanced Nursing, 45*(5), 519–526.

Bombay, A., Matheson, K., & Anisman, H. (2014). The intergenerational effects of Indian residential school: Implications for the concept of historical trauma. *Transcultural Psychiatry, 51*(3), 320–338.

Bruce, A., Makaroff, K. L., Shields, L., Beuthin, R., Molzahn, A., & Shermack, S. (2013). Lessons learned about art-based approaches for disseminating knowledge. *Nurse Res, 21,* 23–28.

Canadian Broadcasting Corporation (CBC). (2013). *Northern food costs remain sky high.* URL=http://www.cbc.ca/news/canada/north/northern-food-costs-remain-sky-high-1.2101753

Christensen, J. (2012). Telling stories: Exploring research storytelling as a meaningful approach to knowledge mobilization with Indigenous research collaborators and diverse audiences in community-based participatory research. *The Canadian Geographer, 56*(2), 231–242.

Clandinin, D. J., & Connelly, F. M. (2000). *Narrative inquiry: Experience and story in qualitative research.* San Francisco: Jossey-Bass.

de Jong Gierveld, J., Keating, N., & Fast, J. E. (2015). Determinants of loneliness among older adults in Canada. *Canadian Journal on Aging, 34*(2), 125–136.

DeGagne, M. (2007). *Toward an Aboriginal paradigm of healing: Addressing the legacy of residential schools.* Ottawa: Aboriginal Healing Foundation.

Government of the Northwest Territories (GNWT) Bureau of Statistics. (2013). *Summary of NWT community statistics.* URL=http://www.statsnwt.ca/community-data/index.html

Government of the Northwest Territories (GNWT) Bureau of Statistics. (2015). *Current indicators.* URL=http://www.statsnwt.ca/

Government of the Northwest Territories (GNWT) Department of Education, Culture and Employment. (2007). *Official languages.* URL=http://www.ece.gov.nt.ca/official-languages

Government of the Northwest Territories (GNWT) Department of Education, Culture and Employment, Government of Nunavut Department of Education, & Legacy of Hope Foundation. (2013). *The residential school system in Canada: Understanding the past-seeking reconciliation-building hope for tomorrow* (2nd ed.,). URL=http://www.ece.gov.nt.ca/files/Early-Childhood/ns_-_residential_schools_resource_-_second_edition.pdf

Government of the Northwest Territories (GNWT) Department of Environment and Natural Resources. (2011). *Caribou forever. Our heritage, our responsibility: A barren-ground caribou management strategy for the Northwest Territories 2011–2015.* URL=http://www.enr.gov.nt.ca/sites/default/files/strategies/2011–2015_barren-ground_caribou_management_strategy.pdf

Government of the Northwest Territories (GNWT) Department of Health and Social Services. (2011). *NWT health status report.* URL=http://www.hss.gov.nt.ca/sites/default/files/nwt_health_status_report.pdf

Government of the Northwest Territories (GNWT) Department of Health and Social Services. (2014). *Our Elders: Our community. Best health, best care, for a better future.* URL=http://www.hss.gov.nt.ca/sites/default/files/our-elders-our-communities.pdf

Hanlon, N., Skinner, M., Joseph, A., Ryser, L., & Halseth, G. (2014). Place integration through efforts to support healthy aging in British Columbia's interior: The role of voluntary sector leadership. *Health and Place, 29,* 132–139.

Health Council of Canada (HCC). (2013). *Canada's most vulnerable: Improving health care for First Nations, Inuit and Métis seniors.* URL=http://www.hhr-rhs.ca/images/stories/Senior_AB_Report_2013_EN_final.pdf

Hunter, L. A. (2008). Stories as integrated patterns of knowing in nursing education. *International Journal of Nursing Education Scholarship, 5*(1), 1–13.

Johansson, A., Ruzin, H. O., Graneheim, U. H., & Lindgren, B. (2014). Remaining connected despite separation – Former family caregivers' experiences of aspects that facilitate and hinder the process of relinquishing the care of a person with dementia to a nursing home. *Aging and Mental Health, 18*(8), 1029–1036.

Loboprabhu, S., Molinari, V., Arlinghaus, K., Barr, E., & Lomax, J. (2005). Spouses of patients with dementia. How do they stay together "till death do us part"? *Journal of Gerontological Social Work, 44*(3–4), 161–174.

Lutra Associates Ltd. (2015). *Networking to prevent older adult abuse: A comparative research study.* URL=http://www.nwtnetwork.com/wp-content/uploads/2013/11/Comparative-Research-Report-Final.pdf

Martin, J., & Gibson, N. (2012). The story that was in danger of being left behind: Re-storying Tlicho culture with land claims and self-government: A conversation with John B. Zoe. *Pimatisiwan: A Journal of Aboriginal and Indigenous Community Health, 10*(2), 147–150.

Moffitt, P., & Timpson, B. (2015). Influences on the quality of life of older adults in the Northwest Territories. Inuvik: Aurora Research Institute. URL=http://www.nwtseniorssociety.ca/wp-content/uploads/2013/11/QOL-Report-Updated-on-Jan-12-2015.pdf

Morrisette, P., & Goodwill, A. (2013). The psychological cost of restitution: Supportive intervention with Canadian Indian residential school survivors. *Journal of Aggression, Maltreatment & Trauma, 22*(5), 541–558.

Northwest Territories Seniors' Society (NWTSS). (2015). *Intergenerational connections handbook. A compilation of stories from intergenerational projects throughout communities in the Northwest Territories.* URL=www.nwtseniorssociety.ca/wp-content/uploads/2013/11/IG-Handbook.pdf

Stanton Territorial Health Authority. (2015). *About us.* URL=http://www.stha.hss.gov.nt.ca/about-us-6

Sullivan-Wilson, J., & Jackson, K. L. (2014). Keeping older adults safe, protected, and healthy by preventing financial exploitation. *Nursing Clinics of North America, 49,* 201–212.

Wonders, W. C. (2011). Northwest Territories. In *The Canadian Encyclopedia (online).* Toronto, ON: Historica Canada. URL=http://www.thecanadianencyclopedia.ca/en/article/northwest-territories/

ONLINE RESOURCES

Please visit the Point at http://thepoint.lww.com/Vollman4e for up-to-date Internet resources and additional learning materials on this topic.

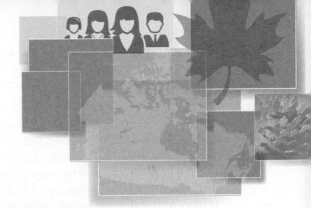

CHAPTER 33

Promoting the Health of Ethnic Women: Cervical Cancer Screening in a Sikh Community

Nelly D. Oelke

LEARNING OBJECTIVES

After studying this chapter, you should be able to:

1. Understand the impacts of ethnicity and immigration on the health of women

2. Appreciate the importance of community engagement in health promotion initiatives

3. Explore approaches to build personal skills and reorient health services for women in ethnocultural communities

Introduction

Canada's population is highly diverse with a mosaic of individuals from a variety of countries representing various ethnocultural communities. Furthermore, Canada has a large population of recent immigrants. The Sikh population, with individuals continuing to emigrate from the Punjab state in India, is one such group of immigrants. These individuals most often settle in large urban centres in Canada. The sociocultural context for individuals in immigrant communities, including the Sikh community, has the potential to impact the health and well-being of its members. Women can be particularly impacted. Given their unique health needs, attention is required to promote the health of women in these ethnocultural communities. This chapter will outline a case story of cervical cancer screening in the Sikh community in a large urban centre in western Canada. Assessment, analysis and planning, intervention, and evaluation sections will focus on community engagement, building personal skills, and reorienting health services. Prior to describing the case in detail, information on Canadian women with a focus on diversity and information on cervical cancer screening will be outlined to provide a background to the case story.

BACKGROUND

In 2011, 21% of Canada's population was born in a country other than Canada. Seventeen percent of these had immigrated to Canada in the last 5 years; 3.5% of Canada's population were new immigrants. Those born in other countries represented over 200 different ethnic groups; 13 of these groups represented more than one million people each. New immigrants to Canada were fairly young, with a median age of 32 years (Statistics Canada, 2013b). South Asians represented the largest visible minority group in Canada (Statistics Canada, 2013b). Statistics Canada (2015) also reported an increase in the number of immigrants settling in the Prairie Provinces.

Research on immigrant health has shown that the health of immigrants deteriorates over time; self-reported health of immigrants that have been in Canada for 10 years or more is poorer than that of newer immigrants (De Maio & Kemp, 2010). Despite Canada's universal health care system and its population being relatively healthy, health inequities persist. Canadian immigrants are considered a vulnerable population by the PHAC (Strategic Initiatives and Innovations Directorate, 2011). Poverty was evident in recent immigrants (Strategic Initiatives and Innovations Directorate, 2011) and 34% reported insufficient funds to address their basic needs (De Maio & Kemp, 2010). Although the gap in low income rates between immigrants and Canadian-born people has decreased, the difference remained 2.6 times greater for those not born in Canada. Immigrants who had lived in Canada for 5 years or less were particularly impacted (Statistics Canada, 2014). Income insecurity and low income had a negative impact on the self-reported health status of immigrants over time (De Maio & Kemp, 2010); women who were not employed outside of the home were more likely to report lower health status (Setia et al., 2011).

Language barriers also affect the health of new Canadians. A total of 39% of Canadians whose first language was neither English nor French stated their health was very good or excellent, but 29% of individuals whose first language was neither English nor French stated their health status was fair or poor (Statistics Canada, 2013a). Women were particularly vulnerable; Setia et al. (2011) found that women whose language abilities were in the lowest quartile were more likely to report poor health than those with greater competency in one or both of Canada's official languages.

Immigrants were also asked about their experiences with discrimination. Over 25% of survey participants stated they had experienced discrimination or had been treated unfairly in subsequent rounds of the Longitudinal Survey of Immigrants to Canada (De Maio & Kemp, 2010). Visible minority status and discrimination were associated with lower levels of self-reported health, particularly mental health (De Maio & Kemp, 2010).

Ethnicity is a complex set of socioeconomic and cultural components (e.g., migration experience, length of time in Canada, social network, socioeconomic status, being a member of a visible minority group) that are known to impact the health of various ethnocultural groups. Using an intersectionality lens may further assist in understanding the complex relationships between the determinants of health and their effect on health inequities (Hankivsky, 2012). Rather than assessing determinants of health as separate categories, intersectionality considers the intersections of characteristics that identify an individual or group and includes social context and inequities in power (Dhamoon & Hankivsky, 2011). For example, how gender intersects with being a new Canadian and socioeconomic status is very different than looking at each of these determinants individually, and better illustrates the greater potential to affect the health of ethnic women.

From 1972 to 2006, cervical cancer decreased in Canada by over 70%, due in large part to relatively high rates of screening (Dickinson et al., 2012). Screening for cervical cancer using the Pap test is an effective measure to decrease the incidence of invasive cervical cancer. The detection and treatment of precancerous lesions prevents cancer of the cervix from developing

(Forte et al., 2012). Not participating in regular screening is a significant risk factor for cervical cancer. Current guidelines for screening vary by age group; screening is recommended for all women aged 25 to 69 every 3 years, while screening for women under the age of 25 is not routinely recommended (Canadian Task Force on Preventive Health Care [CTFPHC], 2013). Although participation in cervical cancer screening in Canada is high, participation rates are lower in those women who speak a language other than English or French, are born in another country, have lower income and education levels, and are older (Lofters et al., 2010; Cancer Care Ontario, 2014).

Health promotion initiatives to prevent cervical cancer and improve participation in screening among women from various ethnocultural communities are essential, given the diversity of our population, the complex intersections between ethnocultural determinants of health, and the lower rates of cervical cancer screening among ethnic women.

THE PROJECT

The aim of this case story is to describe health promotion activities to increase participation in cervical cancer screening for ethnic women. The target population for this project was the Sikh community in a large urban centre in western Canada. Adult women of all ages were included in the project, even though screening is recommended only for those 25 years of age and over. Using the Ottawa Charter as a framework for health promotion initiatives, the intervention emphasized community engagement as a foundation for building personal skills and reorienting health services. More specifically, the intervention involved awareness and education strategies to reach women in this community as well as creating screening services to better meet their needs.

At the beginning of the project, a plan for engaging women in the community was developed. Data were collected through individual interviews with women. Women were recruited in a variety of ways (Box 33.1). In recruiting women to participate in interviews, maximum variation was sought in those interviewed to gather a variety of perspectives from women with different demographic characteristics (e.g., age, length of time in Canada, language[s]). Interviews were informal and conversational in nature, promoting trust and rapport with the women. We facilitated conversations to obtain information from women about their personal experiences with cervical cancer screening as well as their perceptions of women in the community as a whole. Interviews began by asking women to talk a bit about themselves (e.g., when they came to Canada, their family, age). Following some general conversation, we asked about the Pap test, what it meant to them, benefits of screening, barriers to screening, and family and community influences on screening. Finally, we asked women about their own participation in screening. Some interviews were conducted in English and others were conducted in Punjabi with a skilled interpreter present.

Once interviews were completed and the data analyzed, three focus groups were conducted with more women to validate the results and gather additional information. Unlike the interviews, participants for the focus groups were recruited through community champions who

---

Box 33.1 Recruiting Women

- Posters in Punjabi and English in various locations where women visited (e.g., *Gurdwara*, community service agencies, public health clinics, breast cancer screening event)
- Information provided to key community contacts
- Advertisements with Punjabi media
- Informal network within the community (e.g., word of mouth)

TABLE 33.1 Summary of Assessment Results

Theme	Detailed Description
Inside our bodies	• The cervix is a hidden part of the body and often not discussed
Lack of awareness	• Many women were unaware of the Pap test • Women lacked knowledge of cervical cancer and anatomy of their bodies • Others were not aware of the need for regular screening • <50% of women interviewed had been screened regularly; one had never had a Pap test • Older women and newer immigrants were less aware • Pap tests were often associated with contraception, postnatal check-ups, and STD screening rather than cervical cancer screening
Lack of focus on prevention	• Seeking care with no symptoms was unnecessary/inappropriate • Regular pregnancy care had become an acceptable practice • Cost may have prohibited regular check-ups in India
Influence of the family	• Traditional practices (e.g., arranged marriages, living with extended family) may impact health practices • Domination by male and elderly community members; mother-in-law tended to control the house • Obligations in the family, cultural obligations in the community, and outside work took precedence over a woman's needs • Sikh women did not put a priority on their own health • Permission for medical appointments may be required • Some women spoke of the support from families for obtaining screening, including cervical cancer screening
Cultural honour and morals	• Cervical cancer screening is a very private topic decreasing overall knowledge among women in the community • Topic can be offensive as related to sexuality • Protection of family honour; physician visit can have negative impact • Maintaining the family's socioeconomic status in the community; lack of time and available resources to cover potential health care costs
Provider issues	• Family physicians not providing information to women • Preferred a female provider • Language of the provider and issues using a family member to translate for private issues • Tension between seeing a provider from the community and confidentiality in a close knit community • Access to a family physician

worked with women. Questions used with women in the focus groups were similar to those used in the interviews with one additional question: "What advice do you have for us about how cervical cancer screening resources and services can best be delivered to you and the women in your community?" Focus groups were conducted in the *Gurdwara,* the temple for Sikh religious communities, and another community organization. Guiding principles for the focus groups, especially related to privacy and confidentiality, were emphasized at the beginning and end of each session. This tactic was of particular importance, given the relatively small size of the Sikh community.

Large amounts of data were collected during interviews and focus groups; a summary of the results is located in Table 33.1.

During focus groups, women shared many thoughts on strategies to reach women with information about cervical cancer screening as well as strategies to increase participation in screening. These suggestions identified by women from the community are presented in Table 33.2.

Information gathered from women in interviews and focus groups provided comprehensive information to assist in developing a plan of action to promote cervical cancer screening.

TABLE 33.2 Strategies to Reach Women

Education and Awareness

Approach	Actions
Media	• Ethno-specific media such as Punjabi television, radio, newspapers, and magazines • Should include both advertising and educational information
Educational Sessions	• Presentations at community-based organizations/gathering places • "Education Camps" held at the *Gurdwara* accompanied with screening
Word of Mouth	• Utilize the informal social networks to spread information in the community
First Language Resources Materials	• Written materials in both Punjabi and English placed in physicians' offices, *Gurdwara,* beauty salons, and Indian stores • Development of a video in Punjabi
Other	• Announcements at the *Gurdwara*

Screening Strategies

Approach	Actions
Provider Strategies	• Access to female providers • Screening by nurses would be an acceptable option
Strategies to Increase Participation	• Same-day screening (educational session with screening available) • Address barriers to promote screening (e.g., transportation, translation services)

Community Engagement

Community engagement is key to successful implementation of health promotion initiatives (South & Phillips, 2014; West, 2014). In this case story, engagement occurred over time. Components of the intervention to engage women are outlined in Table 33.3. The importance of building trust and rapport with women and within the community as a

TABLE 33.3 Intervention—Community Engagement

Component	Actions
Establishing trust and rapport	• Building on previous work in the community (i.e., Project Leader had completed a previous health promotion initiative in the community) • Spending time at the *Gurdwara* talking to community members (men and women) • Sharing some information about one's self (e.g., family, work) • Participating in the day to day activities (e.g., peeling vegetables for the daily meal at the *Gurdwara,* which was also the community gathering place) • Trying to learn a few Punjabi words • Attending social celebrations to build relationships and rapport among women
Connecting with key community contacts	• Working with those women known to the Project Leader • Connecting with other women/community members they recommended via phone/email • Contacting community organizations via phone/email • Contacting religious leaders at the *Gurdwara* by phone
Seeking permission from community leaders	• Women recommended community leader(s) be contacted to address health promotion issues, particularly if a sensitive issue such as cervical cancer screening
Community champion	• Working with a highly respected/well-connected woman in the community
Interpreter	• Using a trained/skilled interpreter • Engaging an interpreter respected by the target group • Interpreters require more than just language skills, they need to be cultural brokers
Using print and media	• Distributing posters to community organizations and other places women frequented • Making announcements at the *Gurdwara* and on Punjabi radio and TV

whole cannot be underestimated; they are the foundation on which all project strategies and activities were developed. Specific activities and time were required to support these efforts, particularly given the privacy concerns and sensitivity of the topic of women's reproductive health.

Regular and continuous efforts were required to involve women in the Sikh community around this topic area. To this end, an engagement plan is essential to facilitate and sustain engagement over time for such an initiative. Involving key stakeholders in the development of plans assisted in community engagement.

Connecting with women we knew provided a starting point to link with the community. Soliciting ideas for further contacts and using their networks assisted in connecting with other key community contacts. The importance of working with a champion was evident in the number of women recruited for the focus groups. Connections made with community contacts often required several follow-up phone calls and emails; most community organization leaders did not respond the first time. One approach that worked very well was connecting with the large faith-based organization to then link with women attending services.

Seeking permission from a community leader or leaders was not specifically required for our small and time-limited project; however, the Project Leader had a conversation with the religious leader in the community and learned that for the development of a full-scale health promotion initiative to promote cervical cancer screening, explicit permissions should be pursued. Given the dominance of males and the elderly in this ethnocultural community, approval would need to be sought from the male leader(s) of the community and likely a well-respected older woman seen as a formal or informal leader in the community.

To evaluate community engagement, it is important to consider the number of women reached, the quantity and quality of the data, and whether the results resonated with community members. For the assessment and planning processes, 13 women were interviewed and 40 women participated in three focus groups. Recruitment initially was slow. Engagement strategies were re-evaluated and a presentation was conducted for a group of senior women to get them involved in the project.

One of the most important lessons learned is that relationship building and community engagement require time. Contacts need to be made regularly and in a timely manner. Furthermore, spending time in the community at social events and community gathering places was most beneficial in establishing trust and rapport with the women and the community as a whole. Another important realization is that community engagement efforts never end; the process is ongoing. It should be woven throughout the project, ensuring that women and other community members are engaged throughout the health promotion process.

Building Personal Skills

Building personal skills refers to the sharing of information and education to enhance the health of individuals and communities (see Chapter 6). Building both individual and community capacities facilitates empowerment and self-care. Many women in this Sikh community lacked knowledge about cervical cancer and associated screening. The sensitivity of the issue and preservation of family honour are imperative considerations in the types of activities being considered and the content of the materials and educational sessions. English literacy was mixed, with many Sikh women not comfortable in speaking or reading English. Materials prepared in consultation with Sikh women and in Punjabi language would be needed to reach all women in the community, particularly newer immigrants and older women.

Educational sessions were recommended by women in our focus groups as an important strategy to raise awareness regarding cervical cancer and screening. A variety of education sessions were recommended—from small groups to larger, more organized "Education Camps"— that should occur in community locations (e.g., the *Gurdwara*). Also recommended was to develop comprehensive advertising campaigns, such as posters and advertisements in Punjabi media venues. Cultural media such as TV, radio, and print, particularly those specific to the Sikh community were strongly recommended as appropriate avenues to target community women.

Women in the project discussed the strength of informal social networks among friends and families. These networks are often very strong and an important means of information sharing. Despite women stating that the topics of cervical cancer and Pap testing were not often shared among friends and family, they felt that social media could be an essential strategy to initiate discussions about such an important issue.

Evaluation of the success of the project should consider outputs such as the number of presentations completed, the number of women who attended, and the type and number of advertisements distributed and where. To measure whether women's knowledge increased, evaluations could be conducted at presentations. Evaluations could also provide feedback on the quality of the education session, its time, and location. Ultimately, the goal of raising awareness and education about cervical cancer screening would be increased screening rates. Pre- and post-intervention screening rates should be measured as a primary outcome for this initiative.

Reorienting Health Services

The Ottawa Charter (World Health Organization [WHO], 1986) identified the reorientation of health services as one component for health promotion action. Key components of changing health service delivery include a focus on health promotion as opposed to treatment, and ensuring that health services address the whole person and their various health needs. In this case story, prevention and promotion were not a high priority for women in the Sikh community. They tended not to participate in screening when no symptoms were present, instead focusing more on seeking health care when there was an actual problem that needed attention. Furthermore, busy work schedules, family commitments and obligations, and community activities prevented them from focusing on their own health.

A number of challenges were identified that prevented women in the Sikh community from obtaining Pap tests from their family physicians. Issues included, but were not limited to, the lack of information, transportation to attend appointments, and appropriate translation services. Male family members often drove and accompanied women to their medical appointments. Males acting as interpreters, though, resulted in very uncomfortable situations and were generally avoided. Hence, information about screening and the actual procedure would likely not have been completed. Discomfort with male providers was also a barrier. Providing creative options for cervical cancer screening for women in this Sikh community are essential to ensure better uptake of screening for this largely preventable disease. Organizing same-day screening clinics to accompany education sessions would assist in addressing transportation issues. Having a trained female interpreter available at the screening clinic/event would ensure that women understand the procedure and feel more comfortable. Exploring options of nurses doing Pap tests will assist with addressing the issue of a nonfemale provider conducting the procedure.

Finally, the need to address the overall health of women in the community was evident in their comments about other health issues. For example, mental health and well-being were key issues raised by some of the women interviewed. Employing a more comprehensive, holistic approach to health and well-being and being attentive to other concerns and issues beyond cervical cancer screening will be essential to promote the health of women in this Sikh community (e.g., breast cancer, hypertension, and diabetes screening).

From an evaluation perspective, outputs to be measured would include the number of educational events and screening clinics, and the number of women attending. Outcomes to be measured should include the acceptability of services (gathered through evaluation forms at clinics and events and/or conducting focus groups with women in the community during and after the screening), and the number of women screened. As noted in the previous section, pre- and post-intervention screening rates should be measured.

Summary

The primary purpose of this project was to engage Sikh women in this community to assess their perspectives on cervical cancer and screening. Information on their preferences for cervical cancer screening resources and services was also obtained and shared with stakeholders in the community, community members, and with Cancer Prevention Services staff.

REFERENCES

Canadian Task Force on Preventative Health Care [CTFPHC]. (2013). Recommendations on screening for cervical cancer. *CMAJ, 185*(1), 35–45.

Cancer Care Ontario. (2014). *Cancer Fact: Cervical cancer screening rates below provincial target and vary with neighbourhood income.* URL=https://www.cancercare.on.ca/common/pages/UserFile.aspx?fileId=296664

De Maio, F. G., & Kemp, E. (2010). The deterioration of health status among immigrants to Canada. *Global Public Health, 5*(5), 462–478.

Dhamoon, R. K., & Hankivsky, O. (2011). Why the theory and practice of intersectionality matter to health research and policy. In O. Hankivsky (Ed.), *Health inequities in Canada: Intersectional frameworks and practices* (pp. 16–50). Vancouver: UBC Press.

Dickinson, J. A., Stankiewicz, A., Popadiuk, C., Pogany, L., Onysko, J., & Miller, A. B. (2012). Reduced cervical cancer incidence and mortality in Canada: National data from 1932 to 2006. *BMC Public Health, 12*, 992.

Forte, T., Decker, K., Lockwood, G. A., McLachlin, C. M., Fekete, S., & Bryant, H. E; Pan-Canadian Cervical Cancer Screening Initiative: Monitoring Program Performance Working Group. (2012). A first look at participation rates in cervical cancer screening programs in Canada. *Current Oncology, 19*(5), 269–271.

Hankivsky, O. (2012). Women's health, men's health, and gender and health: Implications of intersectionality. *Social Science & Medicine, 74*(11), 1712–1720.

Lofters, A. K., Moineddin, R., Hwang, S. W., & Glazier, R. H. (2010). Low rates of cervical cancer screening among urban immigrants: A population-based study in Ontario, Canada. *Medical Care, 48*(7), 611–618.

Setia, M. S., Lynch, J., Abrahamowicz, M., Tousignant, P, & Quesnel-Vallee, A. (2011). Self-rated health in Canadian immigrants: Analysis of the Longitudinal Survey of Immigrants to Canada. *Health & Place, 17*(2), 658–670.

South, J., & Phillips, G. (2014). Evaluating community engagement as part of the public health system. *Journal of Epidemiology and Community Health, 68*(7), 692–696.

Statistics Canada. (2013a). *Table 105–0504—Health indicator profile, by linguistic characteristic (mother tongue, first official language spoken), two year period estimates, by sex, Canada, provinces and territories, occasional, CANSIM (database).* URL=http://www5.statcan.gc.ca/cansim/a26?lang=eng&etrLang=eng&id=1050504&paSer=&pattern=&stByVal=1&p1=1&p2=31&tabMode=dataTable&csid=

Statistics Canada. (2013b). *Immigration and ethnocultural diversity in Canada. National Household Survey, 2011.* Ottawa: Author. URL=http://www12.statcan.gc.ca/nhs-enm/2011/as-sa/99–010-x/99–010-x2011001-eng.pdf

Statistics Canada. (2014). *Study: Immigration, low income and income inequality in Canada: What's new in the 2000s?* URL=http://www.statcan.gc.ca/daily-quotidien/141215/dq141215c-eng.pdf

Statistics Canada. (2015). *Study: Changes in the regional distribution of new immigrants to Canada.* URL=http://www.statcan.gc.ca/daily-quotidien/150318/dq150318b-eng.pdf

Strategic Initiatives and Innovations Directorate, Public Health Agency of Canada. (2011). *Canadian Reference Group on social determinants of health.* URL=http://www.who.int/sdhconference/resources/BackgroundCanada_PHAC.pdf

West, J. F. (2014). Public health program planning logic model for community engaged Type 2 diabetes management and prevention. *Evaluation and Program Planning, 42*, 43–49.

World Health Organization (WHO). (1986). *The Ottawa Charter for Health Promotion.* Geneva: Author.

ONLINE RESOURCES

Please visit thePoint at http://thepoint.lww.com/Vollman4e for up-to-date Internet resources and additional learning materials on this topic.

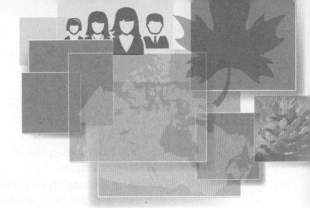

CHAPTER 34

A Community College Dental Hygiene Program Supports Victoria's Underserved Population

Cynthia Smith, Melissa Schaefer, and Shirley Bassett

LEARNING OBJECTIVES

After studying this chapter, you should be able to:

1. Identify barriers to dental care experienced by vulnerable and underserved populations

2. Discuss the benefits of low-cost community-based oral health services

Introduction

> *"Health workers have an obligation to address the issue of poverty directly rather than remain content to deal with its effects" (Raphael, 2002).*

Compared to the rest of the Canadian population, certain population groups (e.g., the elderly, working poor, children and adults living in poverty, and new immigrants) are less likely to have access to oral care services and dental professionals. People living in poverty are particularly disadvantaged with respect to access to dental care, and the oral health needs of people who are experiencing homelessness are often ignored (Wallace et al., 2014). When dental care is obtained it is more likely to be emergency in nature, often tooth extractions, and rarely preventive or restorative (Wallace, 2000).

With most oral disease concentrated among populations with low incomes, those who need the most dental care receive the least; this has been described as a market failure (Ramraj et al., 2014) (see Chapter 9). Of the approximately $14 billion spent on dental care in Canada annually, only 5.5% comes from public funds (Ramraj et al., 2014), with the remainder paid for through private sources (e.g., direct out-of-pocket payment and private insurance plans).

Barriers to dental services such as affordability, availability, and acceptability prevent low-income people from accessing dental care. There is a poor fit between private practice dentistry, public dental benefits, and the oral health needs of people living on low incomes. Many private dental practices are inhospitable to people living on low or fixed incomes and to those who have difficulty keeping appointments and paying their bills (Wallace & MacEntee, 2012). Wallace et al. (2014) identified that "there is a wide gulf of distrust between people living in poverty and the system of dental care around them" (p. 198). Further, they report that dental practitioners often have inaccurate and negative perceptions of people on social assistance: "Dentists cite financial risks, low reimbursement rates, excessive and complicated paperwork, broken appointments, unpredictably disruptive behaviour and a general disregard for oral health as reasons for refusing to accept patients with public dental benefits" (p. 198). Although private sector dentistry provides good quality oral care for most Canadians, it is not a good model of oral health care provision for vulnerable groups who have the highest levels of oral health problems (Canadian Academy of Health Sciences [CAHS], 2014). Clearly, alternatives to the private practice model of oral health care delivery are necessary to address the needs of vulnerable and underserved populations.

Oral health is an essential component of overall health and is necessary for active and productive participation in society. Poor oral health has been linked to cardiovascular disease, respiratory disease, diabetes, premature birth, and low–birth-weight babies (Cullinan et al., 2009). People with poor oral health also suffer from reduced dignity, self-respect, social connectedness, and employability (CAHS, 2014).

THE SETTING

Camosun College is a community college in the city of Victoria, British Columbia, on south Vancouver Island, which offers a variety of health programs including a 3-year Diploma in Dental Hygiene. As part of the curriculum, the dental hygiene students provide preventive and therapeutic services in the College clinic to over 800 public clients annually. Clients of the College clinic include immigrants, refugees, the elderly, low-income families, and Aboriginal people; many of these groups face challenges with health literacy, income, culture, and education. The goal of the College clinic is to provide services that are accessible, sensitive to clients' needs, and caring. Only nominal fees are charged, making care more affordable; further, good public transportation facilitates access to this centrally located service. While the College clinic is the primary practice site for students, a variety of community initiatives are undertaken in an additional effort to improve the oral health of the vulnerable and underserved people within the Greater Victoria community.

In both the on-site College clinic and in the community, dental hygiene students have developed a reputation for gentle, professional, and personalized care for clients of all ages and from all walks of life. Faculty and students employ a combination of health promotion strategies to facilitate access to oral health information and care for people at high risk for oral disease.

In greater Victoria, 26% of the population are identified as financially insecure (Victoria Foundation, 2014) and about 24% of seniors are considered low income (Vancouver Island Health Authority, 2010). Almost 1,800 people used shelters in 2013/2014 (Elliott, 2014) and almost 1,800 people were living in facilities including temporary emergency beds during the same period (Rabinovitch et al., 2014). Currently, there is a 6-month wait list at the only other low-cost dental health clinic in Victoria besides the Camosun College's clinic.

Client demand for service at the College clinic is greater than can be accommodated. In order to help meet community need, the College's dental hygiene program partners with community agencies to increase access to services and support the needs of the population by providing dental outreach to members of the community where they live. One initiative involves providing care at an inner-city community centre in Victoria. The centre, called Our Place, which opened a new facility in 2007, provides services to the working poor, impoverished elderly, mentally and physically challenged people, people with addictions, and those who are homeless. Our Place serves over 1,200 meals per day, provides hot showers and free clothing, and offers a variety of health-related services (e.g., mental health, spiritual wellness, counselling, foot care, acupuncture, acupressure, and chiropractic care) as well as outreach services. The facility also has 45 transitional housing units. People who use the services are referred to by the staff and other clients as "family members."

INTERVENTION

A faculty member from the University of Victoria School of Nursing made the initial introduction of Camosun College to Our Place; nursing students were doing practicum placements at Our Place and had assessed the need for dental care for clients there. Important contacts were made that ultimately led to the invitation to partner with Our Place.

The overall intent of the dental hygiene outreach program is to involve students in activities that reinforce what they are learning in the classroom, namely the Ottawa Charter (World Health Organization [WHO], 1986) strategies of developing personal skills, strengthening community action, creating a supportive environment, and, to some degree, reorienting health services. In partnership with Our Place staff and family members (i.e., clients), the following five project goals were established:

1. Creating a supportive environment conducive to building the trust of Our Place family members in oral health professionals through the practice of cultural attunement (Hoskins, 1999). (See Chapter 11.)
2. Promoting oral and overall health through the provision of dental hygiene services.
3. Strengthening community action and reorienting health services by reducing barriers to dental hygiene care for Our Place family members (i.e., clients) through the provision of on-site dental hygiene services and referrals. (See Chapters 5 and 8.)
4. Increasing student awareness and understanding of the determinants of health in an underserved population. (See Chapter 1.)
5. Providing an opportunity for students to better understand the role of the dental hygienist as an advocate in order to reduce inequities in oral health and increase access to dental services in their community.

A logic model (Table 34.1) is provided that summarizes the key elements of the project.

TABLE 34.1 Logic Model for the Dental Hygiene Outreach Project

Resources	Activities	Outputs	Outcomes
Our Place staff Our Place facility Dental hygiene students Dental hygiene instructor Mobile dental equipment and supplies	Student tour of Our Place prior to rotations Student rotations through Our Place clinic: • Clinic operates 1 day a week throughout the Winter semester • Third year dental hygiene students rotate in pairs providing services to 2 of Our Place members, accompanied by a dental hygiene instructor	Services provided to Our Place members: • Oral cancer screening • Dental hygiene assessments • Individualized oral hygiene education • Scaling and debridement • Fluoride application • Dentist consultations at no cost through referrals to the Camosun College's dental hygiene clinic	Our Place members receive culturally safe, high-quality dental hygiene services Our Place members are more knowledgeable about their oral health status and the need for any necessary referrals Students are more knowledgeable about the diversity of this underserved population Students gain increased awareness of the social determinants of health and their role as advocates Students gain experience in an alternative practice setting, delivering mobile dental hygiene services

Student Practicum

The oral health needs of the population in Victoria had been well documented through a number of community action research projects that emerged from the Capital Urban Poverty Project (Wallace, 2001). Camosun College's dental hygiene program was part of the collaborative advocacy group that supported the development of the only other low-cost dental health clinic in Victoria besides the Camosun College's clinic.

Third-year dental hygiene students in their final semester were identified as being at the right stage of learning as they have had sufficient academic preparation and clinical experience to carry out the services required. With limited time available in the dental hygiene program curriculum and timetable, adjustments were made to substitute practicum time within the College's on-site clinic for practicum time in the community.

Take Note

One of Camosun College's pillars is community engagement, and all programs in the School of Health and Human Services have a community-based service component; therefore, support was readily provided for the necessary resources and faculty to supervise students.

This service learning opportunity (see Box 34.1) allows students to connect with a vulnerable and underserved population in their community and witness first-hand the impacts of poverty, mental illness, addiction, and social isolation. Community-based practicum experiences provide an opportunity to increase students' knowledge of oral health disparities, as well as increasing confidence in working with individuals facing a variety of challenges. As well, learning experiences that take place outside of traditional dental clinics may increase the likelihood that students will choose a career in community settings following graduation (Piskorowski et al., 2012).

Dental health services need to be accessible, sensitive, caring, and aware of the special needs of different populations. As well as teaching preventive and curative clinical services, the dental hygiene program curriculum includes a focus on community health by addressing topics such as literacy, community development, advocacy, and cultural safety. In these ways, Camosun College is reorienting health services by providing needed services in the community where people live and, at the same time, changing professional education and training.

At Our Place, a dental hygiene clinic is set up using portable equipment and runs once a week during the winter semester, from January to April, each year. Due to space limitations, the clinic is held in a large shower stall; this provides a sanitary environment that also affords privacy for clients receiving care (Fig. 34.1). Clients are booked on a first-come, first-served basis. Staff at Our Place strongly support the project and advertise the clinic in the community,

Box 34.1 Service Learning

Service learning is a structured learning experience that combines community service with preparation and reflection. Students engaged in service learning provide community service in response to community-identified concerns and learn about the context in which service is provided, the connection between their service and their academic coursework, and their roles as citizens.

(Seifer, 1998, as cited by Community-Campus Partnerships for Health [CCPH], n.d.)

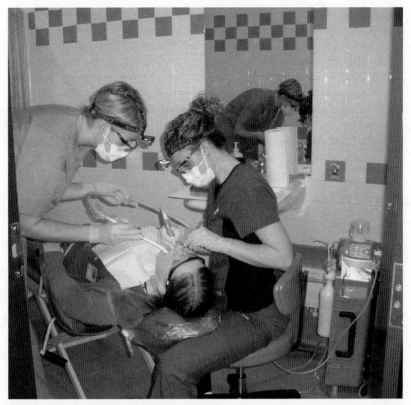

FIGURE 34.1 Camosun College dental hygiene students providing care at Our Place.

helping to recruit clients. The Our Place website, under the banner of "Dental Hygiene," states that "In co-operation with the Camosun College's dental hygiene program, dental hygiene students provide health advocacy...and direct patient care to the Our Place family" (Our Place Society, 2014).

Under the supervision of an instructor (present at all times), students provide oral cancer screening, oral health assessment, and when necessary, referrals to a dentist for further consultation on issues beyond the scope of practice of the dental hygienist. Additional services include scaling (i.e., removal of hard deposits from the teeth), application of fluoride, and oral health education. Counselling usually focuses on improving oral hygiene, preventing disease, and helping clients understand the connections between oral health and general health. Since the project's inception in 2010, 130 dental hygiene students have completed this community rotation providing care to approximately 100 people at Our Place.

Awareness of the diversity of needs of different populations is integral to professional dental hygiene practice. The dental hygiene program educates students on the principles and strategies of health promotion, which supports their understanding of the value of personal and social development for positive health outcomes. They are educated not only to enhance clients' life skills by playing a role in providing information and education to clients but also going further upstream to create a supportive environment by advocating for community supports for clients to experience positive health. In doing so, they can increase the options available to people to be able to make choices conducive to health.

In their classes at the College prior to the community practicum, students are introduced to both psychological and emerging social theories that help to explain health and health-related behaviours, in order that they may better treat clients in a holistic manner, in an atmosphere of nonjudgement, and with dignity, respect, and empathy. Specifically, students are expected to apply the Transtheoretical Model of Change (Prochaska & DiClemente, 1982), which respects the client's readiness to take on certain health behaviours (see Chapter 18). However, the Life Course Analysis theory (Watt, 2002) helps students understand that the determinants of health, namely social, cultural, and historical conditions, are at the roots of, and influence, individual health behaviours and must be taken into account.

Students provide care that is client-centred and begins where clients are with respect to their values and ways of being, understanding that many factors, over many years, have influenced clients' current circumstances. Through these understandings, students can develop trusting relationships with clients. In addition, they are encouraged to advocate for the broader social, political, economic, and physical environments affecting health.

Evaluation

As mentioned earlier, approximately 100 people have received dental hygiene services from the dental hygiene students at Our Place since the project's inception. There is ongoing evaluation of the students' performance with clients. At the end of the treatment session, clients are asked for their voluntary feedback, both verbal and, if they are willing, via written questionnaire, on their experience. In general, the responses indicated a high level of satisfaction.

All of the clients who completed the questionnaire ($n = 20$) responded "yes" to the question, "Are you more aware of your level of oral health?" Client responses to the question "Are you satisfied with the services you received?" were all positive.

"Despite being just students with [instructor] assistance, these guys give excellent dental hygiene services. Very thorough, professional, give good explanation of what they are doing. And also giving very valuable advice on how to continue to floss, brush teeth and keep healthy."

Clients were asked for suggestions for service improvements; no specific suggestions were received, except requests to continue providing dental hygiene services at Our Place.

"The best way to improve is simply continue to be here at Our Place. Your services are very much appreciated and valued by everyone in the community—especially by those who are vulnerable and are not able to afford high-quality dental hygiene. Thank you very, very much!"

To add another perspective to the evaluation of dental hygiene services by students, Our Place staff members were asked to provide input and feedback on what they believed to be the value of the service. The Community Engagement Program Coordinator expressed that she had observed an increase in confidence of some of the family members (clients) as a result of receiving dental hygiene care, stating: "it helped them feel more secure within themselves and feel more 'normal.'" Family members (clients) reported to her that the dental hygiene students "put them at ease" and were "very caring and professional." She believed the students and the services they provided "have a huge and positive impact on their [family members (clients)] self-esteem." An outreach staff member reported that family members (clients) "feel honoured and grateful for the treatment they received."

This evaluation feedback indicates the development of an increasingly trusting relationship between the clients and the students. In addition, it is clear that this client group values oral health and is interested and willing to access dental hygiene services if they are made available. This feedback supports earlier research results by Wallace (2000), who surveyed low-income, homeless, and other individuals living in disadvantaged circumstances in the Victoria area and found that 99% believed oral health was important (72% thought it was very important and 27% felt it was somewhat important) and 82% would seek service if it was available and affordable.

In addition to the evaluation of the service from the clients and staff, discussions of student experiences occur immediately after client appointments and are followed up with discussions in class. Students are also required to submit a reflective assignment based on their experience to their instructor. The reflections are guided by the following questions:

1. What was the most valuable thing you learned from this experience?
2. How will this experience inform your future practice as a dental hygienist?
3. What recommendations do you suggest for future practicum experiences?

The majority of the responses to the first question included the importance of providing "nonjudgemental care" as well as "challenged assumptions" students held regarding this population. The following two examples describe this:

> *"The most valuable thing that I learned at Our Place was the value of acceptance and not passing judgement on others. As a health care professional, I believe that it is in our nature to want the best for our clients. Sometimes, the desire to help achieve optimal health forces our beliefs on to our patients. It is important for us to accept that what we think individuals "should" do may not be in their best interest. While it is important to present clients with findings, facts, and all of the treatment options, it is also critical to accept their choice."*

> *"The clients we saw displayed a sense of inner strength I was not expecting, and were very self-aware."*

Another theme emerging from student reflections is the increased awareness of the extent of oral health disparities and the impacts of the broader social determinants of health on people in their community. This awareness is illustrated by the following student comments:

> *"I believe the most valuable thing I learned from my experience at Our Place was a concrete realization that health disparities do exist, even in a city like Victoria. We are taught in the dental hygiene program about the various health disparities that exist in marginalized populations, but to witness it firsthand is of incredible importance. I think to some extent I have turned a blind eye to the crisis that exists in my own city. My experience at Our Place really put into perspective the extreme need for health services for people facing challenging financial and personal situations, to read about it and to discuss it is one thing, to experience it is a completely eye-opening experience ... it has made me really want to make a difference in my own community, to advocate for these people and be part of the change."*

Overwhelmingly, the feedback from the students who participated in a practicum at Our Place suggests that it provides fertile ground for dispelling the myths and stereotypes many students held regarding low-income and vulnerable populations. The experience challenged assumptions and gave rise to a desire to do more community-based work after graduation.

Their feedback supports the conclusion that the project has resulted in students having an increased awareness of the determinants of health and the dental hygienist role as advocate, as stated in the intended outcomes. Many students indicated that they would have benefited from more than a 1-day community experience and recommended expanding the number of days for future classes.

Impact of the Dental Hygiene Outreach Program

As a result of this experience, we conclude that a shift to community-based delivery of oral health care is necessary in order to reduce oral health disparities and improve the health of all Canadians. By developing interest, knowledge, and skills of graduates to work in the community, programs such as Camosun College's dental hygiene outreach may lead to the expansion of community practice settings (Wallace et al., 2014). Blue (2013) suggests that "community-based, service-learning experiences facilitate the personal and professional development of dental and dental hygiene students" (p. 1044). Specifically, these educational strategies have been found to increase students' awareness of underserved populations, positively influence their attitudes about an individual's right to access dental care, increase their self-efficacy in providing care for diverse populations, and increase their empathy. Increasing the availability and accessibility of oral health care and working to ensure that those who most need oral health services receive them is the responsibility of all dental professionals. Developing personal skills through oral health education is a key component of dental hygiene education; providing people with the knowledge and skills necessary to maintain their oral health is integral to dental hygiene practice.

Blue (2013) asserts that "the future of the dental workforce...will need to supply society with dental hygienists who are willing to provide service to all human beings equitably and work to address health disparities in their communities" (p. 1050). It is heartening that so many students have expressed a passionate intent to do just that—advocate for the changes needed for improving health, reducing health disparities, and improving access to dental services to underserved populations. Whether or not this desire will turn into a reality is yet to be determined. At the present time in British Columbia, new graduates must complete at least 3,500 hours of private practice experience before being eligible to work without the supervision of a dentist, preventing the provision of direct services immediately following graduation.

For over 20 years, the Camosun College's dental hygiene program has been providing service to the Greater Victoria community. The dental hygiene outreach program at Our Place contributes to increasing the health status of the community by reorienting health services from curative care to preventive, culturally sensitive, and accessible care that focuses on developing personal skills for those who could not otherwise access dental care in a supportive environment.

Summary

Camosun College's community-based, service-learning experience at Our Place contributes to the personal and professional development of its dental hygiene students. Each year, since the inception of this practicum into the dental hygiene program at the College, there has been class consensus that this experience is valuable to student learning and should be continued in the future.

As the promotion of social responsibility for the common good is a core responsibility of the profession of dental hygiene, dental hygiene education should include opportunities for students to provide services in the community, better preparing them for future alternative practice settings. Camosun College's dental hygiene program will continue to work towards expanding community treatment alternatives by supporting the development of graduates and encouraging their interest to work in these new settings.

REFERENCES

Blue, C. M. (2013). Cultivating professional responsibility in a dental hygiene curriculum. *Journal of Dental Education,* *77*(8), 1042–1051.

Canadian Academy of Health Sciences (CAHS). (2014). *Improving access to oral health care for vulnerable people living in Canada.* Ottawa: Author.

Community-Campus Partnerships for Health (CCPH). (n.d.). *Focus areas – service-learning.* URL=https://ccph. memberclicks.net/service-learning

Cullinan, M., Ford, P., & Seymour, G. (2009). Periodontal disease and systemic health: Current status. *Australian Dental Journal, 54*(Suppl 1), S62–S69.

Elliott, D. (2014). *Creating homes, enhancing communities.* Victoria: Greater Victoria Coalition to End Homelessness.

Hoskins, M. L. (1999). Worlds apart and lives together: Developing cultural attunement. *Child and Youth Care Forum, 28*(2), 73–85.

Our Place Society. (2014). *Our place.* URL=https://www.ourplacesociety.com/about-us

Piskorowski, W. A., Stefanac, S. J., Fitzgerald, M., Green, T. G., & Krell, R. E. (2012). Influence of community-based dental education on dental students' preparation and intent to treat underserved populations. *Journal of Dental Education, 76*(5), 534–539.

Prochaska, J. O., & DiClemente, C. C. (1982). Transtheoretical therapy: Toward a more integrative model of change. *Psychotherapy: Theory, Research & Practice, 19*(3), 276–288.

Rabinovitch, H., Pauly, B., & Zhao, J. (2014). *Patterns of homelessness in Greater Victoria.* Victoria: Greater Victoria Coalition to End Homelessness. URL=http://victoriahomelessness.ca/get-informed%20/coalition-reports/

Ramraj, C., Weitzner, E., Figueiredo, R., & Quiñonez, C. (2014). A macroeconomic review of dentistry in Canada in the 2000s. *Journal Canadian Dental Association, 80,* e55.

Raphael, D. (2002). Addressing health inequalities in Canada. *Leadership in Health Services, 15*(2), 1–8.

Vancouver Island Health Authority. (2010). *Report of the chief medical health officer on the health status of Vancouver Island residents.* Victoria: Author.

Victoria Foundation. (2014). *Vital signs.* Victoria: Author.

Wallace, B. (2000). *Brushed aside: Poverty and dental care in Victoria.* Vancouver: Vancouver Island Public Interest Research Group.

Wallace, B. (2001). *Towards a downtown community dental clinic in Victoria.* Vancouver: Vancouver Island Public Interest Research Group.

Wallace, B., Figueiredo, R., MacEntee, M., & Quiñonez, C. (2014). Homelessness and oral health. In M. Guirguis-Younger, R. McNeil, & S. W. Hwang, (Eds.), *Homelessness and Health in Canada* (pp. 189–210). Ottawa: University of Ottawa Press.

Wallace, B. B., & MacEntee, M. I. (2012). Access to dental care for low-income adults: Perceptions of affordability, availability and acceptability. *Journal of Community Health, 37*(1), 32–39.

Watt, R. G. (2002). Emerging theories into the social determinants of health: Implications for oral health promotion. *Community Dentistry and Oral Epidemiology, 30*(4), 241–247.

World Health Organization (WHO). (1986). *The Ottawa Charter for Health Promotion.* Geneva: Author.

ONLINE RESOURCES

Please visit the Point at http://thepoint.lww.com/Vollman4e for up-to-date Internet resources and additional learning materials on this topic.

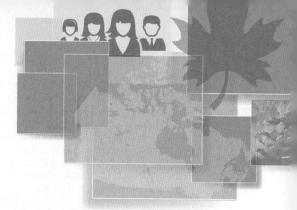

CHAPTER 35

Influencing Food Security Through Mediating Public Policies: How It Works in Brazil

Melody Mendonça and Cecilia Rocha

LEARNING OBJECTIVES

After studying this chapter, you should be able to:

1. Understand how public policies and processes can influence food security

2. Appreciate how multiple public policies from various levels can work together to achieve a common goal

3. Identify the aspects of the public policies that put the Ottawa Health Promotion Strategies in action

Introduction

Food security exists "when all people at all times have physical and economic access to sufficient, safe and nutritious food to meet their dietary needs and food preferences for an active and healthy lifestyle" (World Food Summit, 1996). Based on this definition, the dimensions of accessibility, availability, adequacy, and acceptability of food for all are key requirements to maintain an active and healthy lifestyle. When any of these dimensions are compromised, whether it is at the individual, household, regional, or national level, food security is compromised. The Centre for Studies in Food Security at Ryerson University further expands on the definition of food security by adding the dimension of "agency" (Table 35.1). Agency refers to the policies and processes required to enable food security. It addresses *how* we ensure food security. It is this aspect of food security that we focus and elaborate on in this chapter.

Food security is a growing issue in Canada. According to the 2007–2008 Canadian Community Health Survey (CCHS), nearly 2.2 million Canadians were food insecure, which is approximately 8% of the population. Furthermore, 228,500 children between the ages of 12 and 17 lived in food insecure households, nearly one third of which were severely food insecure (Health Canada, 2010). The situation continues to decline. Data tabulated from the 2012 CCHS estimates that 4 million Canadians including 1.15 million children experienced some level

TABLE 35.1   The Five As of Food Security

Concept	Description	Questions
Availability	Sufficient food for all people at all times	Is there enough food? For everyone? All the time?
Accessibility	Physical and economic access to food for all at all times	Can you get to the food? Can the food get to you? Can you afford it?
Adequacy	Access to food that is nutritious and safe, and produced in environmentally sustainable ways	Is the food adequately nutritious? Is it safe to eat? How sustainable is the food supply?
Acceptability	Access to culturally acceptable food, which is produced and obtained in ways that do not compromise people's dignity, self-respect or human rights	Is the food and the system of delivery culturally acceptable and appropriate?
Agency	Policies and processes that enable the achievement of food security	Is there a way to take action to change unfavourable situations?

From Centre for Studies in Food Security. (n.d.).

of food insecurity (Tarasuk et al., 2014). In other words, about 13% of Canadians are food insecure. Certain segments of society such as Aboriginal peoples, immigrants, and single parents showed higher rates of food insecurity. The prevalence of food insecurity in Aboriginal households was 28.2%, about double the rate reported in Canadian households (Tarasuk et al., 2014).

Food insecurity is a major public health concern. Adults in food insecure households have higher rates of diabetes, heart disease, and obesity, and experience poor physical and mental health (Tarasuk et al., 2014). Good nutrition in children is especially important as they go through phases of immense growth and cognitive development. Research has shown that hunger adversely impacts the physical as well as mental health of Canadian children and manifests itself in disorders such as asthma or depression that persist into adulthood (Tarasuk et al., 2014). Public policies that support increased access to nutritious food, particularly among vulnerable segments of society, can reduce food insecurity.

Brazil has been particularly successful at influencing food security through public policies that prioritize food access for vulnerable populations and strengthen family farming as a strategy to increase availability of food and support sustainable livelihoods (United Nations Standing Committee on Nutrition [UNSCN], 2013). (See Box 35.1.) We examine two policies that are part of the country's Food and Nutrition Security Plan: the Food Acquisition Program (*Programa de Aquisição de Alimentos* [PAA]) and the National School Meals Program (*Programa Nacional de Alimentação Escolar* [PNAE]). The federal government funds the PAA

Box 35.1   Circle of Food

Food security is everyone's business. Food security includes the circle of:

- Planting
- Growing
- Harvesting
- Transporting
- Shopping
- Preparing
- Eating
- And preserving our environment
  Food security means equity and choice at every point.
  (Avenue Food Security Network. (n.d.).

and PNAE but requires the cooperation of state and municipal governments to implement the programs (UNSCN, 2013). In this case story, we focus on the Municipality of Belo Horizonte to explain how local programs mediate the implementation of PAA and PNAE to influence food security based on the five As of Food Security and discuss how the strategies of the Ottawa Charter have been applied.

PROJECT DESCRIPTION

Belo Horizonte, a large urban centre in Brazil, has been a leader in reducing food insecurity by launching a comprehensive set of programs dating as far back as 1993 (Rocha et al., 2012). With a population of almost 2.5 million, it is Brazil's sixth largest city and the capital of the second most populous state, Minas Gerais (*Instituto Brasileiro de Geografia e Estatística* [IBGE], 2014). Together with 34 other municipalities, Belo Horizonte forms the greater metropolitan region that has a population of almost 5.2 million and a large geographic spread of 9,460 km² (IBGE, 2014). The municipal department of Food and Nutrition Security of Belo Horizonte (*Secretaria Municipal Adjunta de Segurança Alimentar e Nutricional* [SMASAN]) is responsible for implementing the national and local food policies.

Take Note

The population size and spread of the Belo Horizonte Metropolitan Region are similar to large metropolitan cities in Canada surrounded by agricultural lands. For example, the Toronto census metropolitan area has a population of 5,583,064 in a land area of 5,905.71 km² (Statistics Canada, 2015).

We conducted an exploratory, ethnographic study with the primary aim of describing the local implementation process of PAA and PNAE from the viewpoint and perspectives of local administrators, family farmers, and other stakeholders (Mendonça & Rocha, 2015) (see Box 35.2). The local municipal food security programs were also visited and documented (see Box 35.3). It should be noted that the policies and programs described here are only the ones visited during the study. At both the national and local level there are many more policies that influence food security in a variety of ways, directly and indirectly.

Qualitative data were collected over 2 weeks in May 2013 through chain (snowball) sampling, site visit observations, and conversations with key stakeholders, including farmers participating in the programs, program administrators from SMASAN, nutritionists, agronomists, public school principals, and a president of a community garden. All informants were made aware of the intentions of the researcher, gave verbal consent, and openly provided information for study use.

Box 35.2 A SnapShot of National Programs Influencing Food Security in Belo Horizonte

National Food Security and Nutrition Policies

National School Meals Program (Programa Nacional de Alimentação Escolar [PNAE])

The National School Meals Program dates as far back as 1955. It provides federal funds for school meals to children in daycare centres, preschools, and primary schools in the public school system. The program reaches 53 million elementary school children on a daily basis (Peraci & Bittencourt, 2011).

PNAE Minimal 30% Local Procurement Law

In 2009, the Brazilian government passed a national law requiring schools to spend at least 30% of their school meals budget on fresh foods from local family farms (Peraci & Bittencourt, 2011). The requirement of at least 30% local procurement of fresh produce by PNAE positively affects family farmers and increases access to fresh fruits and vegetables for schoolchildren, thus further supporting their academic and physiological development (Sidaner et al., 2013).

Food Acquisition Program (Programa de Aquisição de Alimentos [PAA])

PAA strives to foster local family agriculture including actions related to the storage of foods and purchase and distribution of agricultural products for people in conditions of food and nutritional insecurity (MDS, n.d.). Its function is to support the commercialization of products grown on family farms through direct state purchases at near market prices. These purchases are redistributed to government food programmes such as schools, daycare centres, popular restaurants, and food banks (Rocha et al., 2012).

Box 35.3   A SnapShot of Local Programs Influencing Food Security in Belo Horizontea

Local Municipal Programs

Popular Restaurants

Popular Restaurants are government subsidized cafeteria-style restaurants that serve nutritious balanced meals at breakfast, lunch, and dinner, and follow a universal, unrestricted access policy (Rocha & Lessa, 2009). They serve the broader public and also capture the most vulnerable segments of society. A meal costs 2 reais [BRL] ($1 CAD) but is half price for families on social assistance and free for homeless people.

Food Bank

Belo Horizonte has one food bank. It coordinates the donation of food and household items to 46 community-based organizations on a weekly basis (Mendonça & Rocha, 2015). The food bank works in partnership with the Sanitation Department to collect daily the unsold fresh fruits and vegetables from stores around the city (Rocha & Lessa, 2009).

Sacolões ("Large Bags") are commercial outlets that sell fresh fruits and vegetables by the kilo at a set price that is about 20 to 50% below market prices (Rocha & Lessa, 2009). The city licenses private operators (21 in 2012) to set up sacolões in key locations (Prefeitura Municipal de Belo Horizonte [PBH], 2013). Since prices of other items sold in these outlets are not regulated, operators are able to make a profit.

Straight from the Country (Direto da Roça) facilitates direct interaction between small rural producers and urban consumers by eliminating wholesale intermediaries. Its main goal is to help rural families establish themselves in the countryside and reduce the rural–urban migration that has inflated Belo Horizonte's population in poorer neighbourhoods (Rocha & Lessa, 2009). Rural producers obtain a licence from the municipality and are assigned fixed sale points throughout the city.

Community Gardens are communal spaces where fruits, vegetables, and medicinal plants are produced using participatory community involvement and promotion of sustainable agro-ecological methods (Rocha & Lessa, 2009).

School Gardens are small plots located at municipal schools used to engage students, teachers, and school administrators on how to grow and care for plants. Vegetables and herbs produced in the gardens are used in preparing school meals onsite (Rocha & Lessa, 2009).

Workshops for Planting in Alternative Spaces teach techniques for planting herbs and medicinal plants in alternative areas such as pop bottles, wooden boxes, rubber tires, etc. (Rocha & Lessa, 2009).

In 2012, Belo Horizonte had 48 community gardens, 108 school gardens, and offered 91 workshops on gardening in alternative spaces (PBH, 2013).

Based on analysis of the primary data, we mapped the causal mechanisms involved in implementing the two national programs, PAA and PNAE, in Belo Horizonte to identify contextual factors impacting local implementation (Mendonça & Rocha, 2015). We further analyzed the primary data collected from stakeholders at the different local sites using the 5 As to Food Security, supplemented with secondary data acquired through literature reviews and municipal documents provided by program implementers.

MEDIATING PUBLIC POLICY TO INFLUENCE FOOD SECURITY

In Belo Horizonte, local programs mediate the implementation of PAA and PNAE. Together, the national and local programs work as agents to influence food security. PAA focuses on improving food availability and food access (Chmielewska & Souza, 2010). It targets the most vulnerable as it is aimed at food insecure people, social assistance and government program recipients, and small-scale family farmers who, despite contributing to a large proportion of the domestic food supply, face difficulty accessing markets and overcoming poverty (UNSCN, 2013).

PAA guarantees a minimal market price and participating farmers can receive up to 4,500 reais [BRL] (equivalent to $2,250 Canadian dollars [CAD]) per year. The income generated by supplying fresh produce through PAA helps farmers cover the costs of food production, while continuous access to local markets encourages them to grow more and to diversify production, thus increasing the regional availability of food (Peraci & Bittencourt, 2011).

The municipality of Belo Horizonte purchases food from family farmers through PAA to simultaneously donate to the Food Bank and Popular Restaurants. PAA is beneficial to family farmers and vulnerable segments of society in Belo Horizonte as it has the capacity to promote regional food security, better access to nutritious food, social inclusion, and income generation (Mendonça & Rocha, 2015).

Food Accessibility Programs

The *Food Bank's* main aim is to provide food to people who cannot afford (or access) food. In contrast to food banks in Canada, the Food Bank is run by the municipality and does not serve people directly. Instead, community-based organizations receive food weekly from the food bank to prepare community meals for their beneficiaries (e.g., the homeless, people living with AIDS, seniors, etc.). In this manner, some degree of food acceptability is maintained by lowering the extent to which food assistance compromises human dignity.

The Food Bank ensures food adequacy with respect to nutrition and safety. Despite relying on donations, the majority of food received was fruits and vegetables. In addition to the produce obtained from local farmers through PAA, the Food Bank also obtained perishable food donations from the *Sacalões* and nonperishable food products donated by large supermarket chains. The supermarkets also provided products like detergents, soaps, diapers, etc. Usually, the donated items were within the expiry date but had some packaging defects (e.g., damage to outer packaging or label misprint). All donated food items undergo a quality control check by the nutritionist at the Food Bank. The Food Bank also employs workers trained in food safety to separate out the consumable produce from that which is past the point acceptable for human consumption.

At the same location of the Food Bank is the municipality's Reference Centre for Nutrition and Food Security (*Centro de Referencia de Nutricion & Seguranca Alimentar*). The Centre delivers workshops for running school gardens, tests and standardizes recipes for school menus, and provides nutrition education to children and School Meals program supervisors.

At the time of our site visit, there were four *Popular Restaurants* operating in Belo Horizonte, each serving 3,000 to 8,000 meals daily for up to 700 people at a time (Göpel, 2009, p. 11). The federal government funds the construction of the restaurants after which the municipal government is responsible for their administration and maintenance. The Popular Restaurants follow a semi-private management model; the municipality outsources the labour to private contractors who run the restaurants. Municipal program operators and public health nutritionists oversee administration, food security, and nutrition aspects.

The Popular Restaurants' affordable pricing and locations in high-foot traffic areas support economic and physical access to food. They also directly support consumption of adequate amounts of nutritious food and indirectly support food availability as the nutritionists on site develop weekly balanced menus taking into account seasonal produce. Only 1% of food was purchased through PAA. Although program operators would have preferred to purchase more food through PAA, participating family farmers found it difficult to supply the large volumes required daily to run the Popular Restaurants (Mendonça & Rocha, 2015). The remaining 99% of food is supplied through a private contractor.

The Popular Restaurants policy of universal unrestricted access also supports the acceptability of food. Program operators stated that the high quality of the meals at low prices served in well-maintained establishments also attracts the working middle class and student population. As a result, the Popular Restaurants are able to overcome some social class barriers while making food accessible to poorer segments of society.

The federal Ministry of Education transfers PNAE funds directly to states and municipalities responsible for its implementation (Rocha & Lessa, 2009). Municipal schools provide public education for children between 1 and 14 years of age. The School Meals (*Merenda Escolar*) Program for municipal public schools is coordinated centrally. High schools are state run and provide secondary education for students over age 14. In contrast to the municipal School Meals Program, the programs in high schools are decentralized; each high school is responsible for administering its own meal program to its students.

The School Meals Program increases food security in school children through food access. It supports the social and cultural acceptability of food by serving hot meals, in keeping with regional food habits, to all students irrespective of whether they are food insecure. Breakfast, lunch, and an afternoon meal are served daily, and together must provide at least 70% of the student's daily caloric needs according to current legislation (Sidaner et al., 2013).

In Belo Horizonte, 250 municipal schools are served by the School Meals Program, which has been integrated into the school day. All schools have a fully equipped kitchen and service area on site and a standardized menu is followed to ensure equal access in terms of food amount and quality to all students across the city. The municipality supplies a variety of perishable and nonperishable food and the schools have a budget to purchase bread and leafy greens.

As part of implementing the School Meals Program in Belo Horizonte, groups of family farmers are contracted to supply perishable foods directly to the schools. Family farmers can earn up to 20,000 reais [BRL] ($10,000 CAD) annually and are paid through PNAE. In 2012, family agriculture supplied only 7.5% of procured food (far below the minimum 30% procurement) in Belo Horizonte. Factors such as transportation costs, the task of supplying large volumes of food daily and in meeting the quality standards required by municipal schools create challenges to family farmers that need to be addressed (Mendonça & Rocha, 2015). Similar to PAA, supplying the School Meals Program not only generates a steady income for family farmers but also improves their standard of living, social inclusion, and the incentive to increase food production thus improving the availability of nutritious foods to those in need (Mendonça & Rocha, 2015).

School principals and nutritionists from SMASAN describe multiple benefits of the program in their local schools. They found that students were less anxious about food access because they could depend on quality meals being served at school. Many nutrition education components are also incorporated into the program: skill-building workshops (e.g., planting and gardening), drama and theatre activities, and video shows.

The school day is designed so that it is mandatory for students to attend in the morning while the afternoon component is optional. However, by offering an afternoon meal, the School Meals Program provides an incentive for students to stay for the full day. Further, nutrition education workshops are held in the afternoon. We learned that students would ask their parents to prepare meals similar to those served at school, thus promoting healthy food choices at home.

A number of challenges face the administrators of the School Meals Program. Local vendors selling sweets just outside the school enabled children to access junk food. In turn, children who brought junk food to school resisted eating the healthy hot meals offered. Another difficulty was getting students to accept the dish prepared in the afternoon; the children found the meal too heavy or unappealing in taste. A societal challenge faced by administrators was that parents who earned more than others in low-income neighbourhoods would often send their children to school with processed food and unhealthy snacks. Program operators found that education on healthy eating and nutritious food, although helpful, was more effective with students than with parents.

Food Availability Programs

The *Sacolões* support physical and economic access to adequate food. At the time of the study, the designated 20 fresh food items cost 0.92 reais [BRL]/kg (approximately 50 cents/kg). To obtain a licence to run a *Sacolão*, vendors must participate in a public bidding process. Once they obtain a licence, they hold a 5-year contract to run their businesses. If the retailer has to build a new facility to run the business, the contracts are for 10 years. Whether the vendor builds the facility or occupies an already established space, all vendors pay rent to the municipality for use of the space. Program administrators state that the contracts are in high demand as the prime locations in the city generate large revenues to the vendor. Furthermore, the location of *Sacolões* in high traffic areas and sale of other products in addition to the low-priced fresh food attracted people from all segments of society to shop there. Thus, it supports food access in a socially acceptable manner.

The municipality makes 40 *Straight from the Country* licences available that allow local farm producers to sell their produce in neighbourhoods across the city, thus promoting physical access to adequate nutritious food. Farmers with small areas of land and limited access to labour find this program optimal as it gives them the opportunity to sell directly to the consumer, does not require them to supply large volumes, and eliminates the need for a middleman. Through the program, small farmers increase food availability while maximizing their income and sustaining their food production capacity. During a site visit to a participating farmer's stall, the farmer said she enjoys the direct relationship she has established with her clients. The farmer operates her stall 2 days a week and is usually sold out within 4 hours.

We visited a *Community Garden Program* plot located in one of the poorer neighbourhoods of Belo Horizonte. The garden was one hectare (100 m × 100 m) in size with 16 plots (6.25 m²). The municipality initially provided the land, seeds, and irrigation; over time, the municipality's main role has become the provision of technical assistance. A municipal agronomist supports and advises community garden participants on growing techniques.

The Community Garden Program promotes access and acceptability of adequate food by gardening for self-consumption. Most of the produce goes home with the gardeners. Participants also make food available to the community by supplying three local School Meals Programs and offering produce to their neighbours.

As the growers were mostly experienced farmers who gave up their livelihoods in the countryside, the Community Garden Program helps them maintain the skills they left behind when they moved to the city. The community garden also had laying hens, so eggs were also available. Community garden participants prepare a meal and eat together on the weekends.

THE OTTAWA CHARTER IN ACTION

Belo Horizonte has developed *healthy public policy* through its multisectoral and complementary approach to food security, demonstrating how joint action across different sectors can contribute to healthier public services, better access to quality food, and increased feasibility in making the healthier choice the easier choice. Public policy for food security has moved beyond health care to health promotion by supporting income generation amongst local farmers; reducing inequality through universal access policies that encourage people from all strata of society to eat together; and involving the nonhealth sector in the implementation of these policies.

PAA and PNAE create a *supportive environment for health* at the local level through their legislated program objectives, structure, and provision of funds mediated through the several local programs in Belo Horizonte that work together to promote food security. Universal food access programs support healthy child development and health equity in vulnerable groups.

Brazil's National Law for Food and Nutrition Security supports *strengthening community action* by mandating the participation of civil society in policy formulation. Such participation has the potential to empower communities to take ownership of their health, livelihoods, and well-being. In recent years, civil society campaigns have led to important results, such as making the Right to Adequate Food a fundamental right in 2010 (*Ministério do Desenvolvimento Social Ministério do Desenvolvimento Social* [MDS], n.d.).

Personal skills development is supported by information and education for health and life skills provided by the various programs. For example, training and support by nutritionists and agronomists teach novice gardeners techniques in gardening and help farmers who migrated from the countryside to maintain their skills. Sustainable livelihoods are promoted by the School Meals and Straight from the Country Programs, whereby farmers are incentivized to build capacity that improves their income while improving the availability and access to food. Universal programs allow food to be accessed in ways that preserve dignity and promote social inclusion.

Brazil's reformed health care system (the Unified Health System) was designed with the principles in the Ottawa Charter in mind (Wallerstein et al., 2011). Decision makers included health in other public policies as it *reoriented the health system* toward prevention. Recognizing the cross-cutting nature of food insecurity, the federal government created the Ministry of Social Development and Fight Against Hunger in 2003 to oversee its comprehensive food security strategy that has evolved into the current National Food and Nutrition Security Plan (MDS, n.d.). In Belo Horizonte, the municipality created SMASAN to implement national and local programs to promote food security. The diversity in policies and programs aimed at influencing local food security demonstrate SMASAN's motivation to support individuals and communities to access health.

THE CANADIAN CONTEXT

To influence food security in Canadian communities and successfully apply the lessons learned from Belo Horizonte, we must understand the barriers and enablers that exist in Canada. The autonomous nature of the provinces with regard to health makes it difficult for the Canadian government to institute national food and nutrition policies. Yet, there is a history of successful health-promoting public policies in Canada that originated at the municipal level. Local, regional, and provincial/territorial public health departments across Canada are actively engaged in influencing food security as a means of supporting population health, addressing the determinants of health and reducing health inequities (see Chapter 1). Nevertheless, additional collaborative efforts outside the health sector are needed. Building one's own capacity to engage in policy and influence decision makers is a good starting point.

Summary

This case story illustrates how Belo Horizonte was able to influence food security by mediating national public policies through local program implementation. The diverse approaches used to tackle food insecurity and the multisectoral and collaborative nature of the public policies demonstrates how the strategies outlined in the Ottawa Charter have been applied. For such complex policies to be designed and applied in Canadian settings, it is important to consider local political contexts and identify current strengths and weaknesses in the policy process.

REFERENCES

Avenue Food Security Network (n.d.). *Circle of food.* URL=http://avefsn.weebly,com/circle-of-food.html

Centre for Studies in Food Security, Ryerson University. (n.d.). *Food security defined.* URL=http://www.ryerson.ca/foodsecurity/our-approach.html

Chmielewska, D., & Souza, D. (2010). *Market alternatives for smallholder farmers in food security initiatives: Lessons from the Brazilian Food Acquisition Programme (Working Paper No. 64).* Brasilia: International Policy Centre for Inclusive Growth, United Nations Development Programme.

Göpel, M. (2009). *Celebrating the Belo Horizonte Food Security Programme. Future Policy Award 2009: Solutions for the food crisis.* Hamburg: World Future Council.

Health Canada. (2010). *Household food insecurity in Canada in 2007–2008: Key statistics and graphics.* URL=http://www.hc-sc.gc.ca/fn-an/surveill/nutrition/commun/insecurit/key-stats-cles-2007–2008-eng.php

Instituto Brasileiro de Geografia e Estatística (IBGE). (2014). *Belo Horizonte, Minas Gerais: Censo demographico 2010.* URL=http://www.ibge.gov.br/cidadesat/xtras/perfil.php?codmun=310620

Mendonça, M., & Rocha, C. (2015). Implementing national food policies to promote local family agriculture: Belo Horizonte's story. *Development in Practice, 25*(2), 160–173.

Ministério do Desenvolvimento Social (MDS) e Combate à Fome. (n.d.) *Programa de Aquisição de Alimentos – PAA [Food Acquisition Programme].* URL=http://www.mds.gov.br/segurancaalimentar/aquisicao-e-comercial-izacao-da-agricultura-familiar

Peraci, A. S., & Bittencourt, G. A. (2011). Family farming and price guarantee programmes in Brazil: The Food Acquisition Program. In J. G. Da Silva, M. E. Del Grossi, & C. G. De Franco (Eds.), *The Fome Zero (Zero Hunger) Program: The Brazilian experience* (pp. 193–223). Brasilia: FAO.

Prefeitura Municipal de Belo Horizonte (PBH). (2013). *Promovendo a segurança alimentar e nutricional.Relatório de prestação de contas 2012, Secretaria Municipal Adjunta de Segurança Alimentar e Nutricional (SMASAN).* Belo Horizonte: Secretaria Municipal de Políticas Sociais.

Rocha, C., & Lessa, I. (2009). Urban governance for food security: The alternative food system in Belo Horizonte, Brazil. *International Planning Studies, 14*(4), 389–400.

Rocha, C., Burlandy, L., & Maluf, R. (2012). Small farms and sustainable rural development for food security: The Brazilian experience. *Development Southern Africa, 29*(4), 519–529.

Sidaner, E., Balaban, D., & Burlandy, L. (2013). The Brazilian school feeding programme: An example of an integrated programme in support of food and nutrition security. *Public Health Nutrition, 16*(6), 989–994.

Statistics Canada. (2015). *Population and dwelling counts, for census metropolitan areas, 2011 and 2006 censuses.* URL=http://www12.statcan.gc.ca/census-recensement/2011/dp-pd/hlt-fst/pd-pl/Table-Tableau.cfm?T=205&S=3&RPP=50

Tarasuk, V., Mitchell, A., & Dachner, N. (2014). *Household food insecurity in Canada 2012.* Toronto: Research to Identify Policy Options to Reduce Food Insecurity (PROOF). URL=http://nutritionalsciences.lamp.utoronto.ca/resources/proof-annual-reports/annual-report-2012/

United Nations Standing Committee on Nutrition (UNSCN). (2013). *Country policy analysis: Nutrition impact of agriculture and food systems: Brazil.* UN System Standing Committee on Nutrition country study for the second International Conference on Nutrition. URL=http://unscn.org/files/Publications/Country_Case_Studies/UNSCN-country-case-study-Brazil-FINAL.pdf

Wallerstein, N., Mendes, R., Minkler, M., & Akerman, M. (2011). Reclaiming the social in community movements: Perspectives from the USA and Brazil/South America: 25 years after Ottawa. *Health Promotion International, 26* (Suppl 2), ii226–ii236.

World Food Summit. (1996). *Rome declaration on world food security.* URL=http://www.fao.org/docrep/003/w3613e/w3613e00.htm

ONLINE RESOURCES

Please visit thePoint at http://thepoint.lww.com/Vollman4e for up-to-date Internet resources and additional learning materials on this topic.

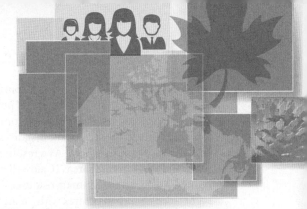

CHAPTER 36

Creating Healthy, Active Rural Communities Through Active Transportation

Kate Hall and Sue Shikaze

LEARNING OBJECTIVES

After studying this chapter, you should be able to:

1. Explain how active transportation planning can be used as a health promotion strategy in small rural communities

2. Describe a community development process for building capacity to improve conditions for active transportation

3. Discuss strategies for implementation and evaluation of active transportation initiatives

Introduction

A gap exists between the health of rural and urban residents in Canada; those living in rural areas have overall poorer health. In a national study, researchers examined various health risks and mortality rates between rural and urban populations and found that in rural Canada, health-related lifestyle factors such as smoking and obesity rates were higher, while leisure time and physical activity rates were lower (DesMeules & Pong, 2006; Noxon Associates Limited, 2009). Lack of physical activity (i.e., a sedentary lifestyle) is one factor associated with the development of several chronic diseases.

Compared to residents of urban settings, people living in rural communities are generally more dependent on their cars and are more likely to have health problems associated with being overweight (Heart and Stroke Foundation, 2005). They are also less likely to have access to sustainable transportation options such as public transit, bicycles, and walking paths (Transport Canada, 2006). Small and rural communities across Canada are facing a greater and faster-growing proportion of older adults than urban areas (Noxon Associates Limited, 2009), which makes independent mobility options like walking and cycling important in rural parts of Canada. Building active transportation capacity is an important consideration because there is often no (or limited) access to public transit in rural small towns.

Transportation planning in rural communities is usually focused on infrastructure for automobiles due to the significant distances between homes and destinations and a low-density land use base (Young, 2008). As a result, there are fewer multiuse trails, sidewalks, and bicycle paths and lanes in rural areas (Caldwell et al., 2015). Rural municipalities typically have more limited financial and human resources to plan transportation infrastructure compared to higher-density urban centres with greater tax bases (Noxon Associates Limited, 2009).

People in rural communities often live far from where they work, shop, worship, or go to school. However, the towns and villages that they drive to are usually compact, with most services and businesses located in close proximity to one another and to public parking. The scale of rural communities is an asset, and people are able to walk to do their errands.

There is a correlation between the sedentary act of driving and an increased risk of obesity. The risk of obesity has been shown to increase by 6% for each hour spent in a car per day (Frank et al., 2006). People can reduce their risk for obesity by building physical activity into their daily lives. Health promotion, encouragement, and better community design and infrastructure make it easier for people to be physically active. Walk-friendly neighbourhoods are associated with more active transportation, and pedestrian-friendly streetscapes encourage physical activity and support the local economy. Both are associated with lower body weights, fewer traffic accidents, and less crime (Canadian Institute of Planners [CIP], 2010).

Take Note

Walkable retail areas with unique visual, cultural, social, and environmental qualities have a "place-making dividend" that attracts people to visit often, stay longer, and spend more money (McMahon, 2010). Patrons of retail businesses that come by foot and bicycle visited more often and spent more money per month than those who came by car (Ryerson Planning and Consulting, 2014).

Public health departments are responsible for addressing health at the population level; they accomplish public health goals through prevention, promotion, and protection activities. As evidence of the association between health and the built environment has grown, it has become increasingly important for the public health sector to work collaboratively with municipal governments and others (e.g., urban planners and transportation engineers) whose work affects community design and the built environment. There are many examples of public health departments and local municipalities working together to improve health through community design (Perrotta, 2011).

Transportation networks and rural/urban design play significant roles in shaping how residents move around a community. A motor vehicle–centric road network encourages residents to drive—even for short distances. By accommodating active modes of transportation, many of the physical and psychological barriers to physical activity can be overcome.

HEALTH AND ACTIVE TRANSPORTATION

Active transportation refers to any form of human-powered transportation. It is any trip made for the purpose of getting to a particular destination (e.g., work, school, recreation facility, shop, etc.). Active transportation most commonly refers to walking and cycling, but might also include the use of mobility devices such as wheelchairs, in-line skates, skateboards, and boats (Noxon Associates Limited, 2009). Communities across Canada and North America are taking steps to improve conditions that support active transportation, recognizing the many benefits of using vehicles less in favour of more physical activity (Transportation Association of Canada [TAC], 2012).

A good active transportation network is safe, connected, and integrated. Safety is important because active transportation users can be vulnerable while on the sidewalks, pathways, roads, and waterways. Engineering strategies and design elements that increase road, path, and water safety include signs and signals, pavement markings, and physical barriers or separation between active transportation users and motor vehicles. Road design (e.g., paved shoulders) can also improve safety for vehicles and motorcycles (Hallmark et al., 2010). A well-connected network provides efficient links among multiple destinations; integrating active transportation networks into the overall community transportation plan facilitates transitions between different modes of transport (e.g., sidewalks between parking lots and business districts, bicycle parking at transit stops).

Regardless of whether people live in urban or rural communities, access to transportation can present a barrier to employment, education, health and social services, and social interaction. Approximately 20% of Canadian households do not own a motor vehicle, another 10% are not able to drive because of a disability, and 10% do not have the income to support car ownership (Litman, 2003); active transportation networks therefore contribute to equity by allowing more economical modes of transport to be safe and convenient.

Planning for active transportation is an ideal way for urban planners and public health departments to implement a number of health promotion strategies as outlined in the Ottawa Charter. Much effort on active transportation involves working with municipal governments to advocate for public policy that supports active transportation and healthy community design, and to build awareness among decision makers that health is an important lens to consider when making policy decisions. Creating supportive community environments that encourage active transportation makes the healthy choice (i.e., physical activity) an easy choice. Planning for active transportation should include public participation and community engagement; residents are able to provide insight into what is working well, what is not working, and suggest improvements. Taking the opportunity to be more active when moving around the community presents opportunities to build personal skills and knowledge (e.g., cycling skill, safe road/water conduct, knowledge about community pathways to a variety of destinations).

Active transportation initiatives support priorities of particular relevance to rural communities in addition to addressing the present and future needs of an aging population—economic development, tourism, and community pride. Walking and cycling are important quality-of-life activities that can attract and retain residents and businesses. Creating safe and attractive streets increases the vibrancy of a community, making it more attractive to retirees and a variety of professionals who prefer a rural lifestyle (Caldwell et al., 2015). Walk Score ratings (www.walkscore.ca) from "Car Dependent" (0 to 24) to "Walker's Paradise" (90 to 100) are often found in real estate listings, and communities are rated for their livability.

Take Note

Livability is the sum of the factors that add up to a community's quality of life—including the built and natural environments, economic prosperity, social stability and equity, educational opportunity, and cultural, entertainment, and recreation possibilities.

(Partners for Livable Communities, 2016)

In summary, active transportation plays an important role in improving economic vitality, public safety, and population health, particularly in rural communities. It is "a creative, cost-effective, simple solution that addresses multiple challenges in a single step: affordable transportation, changing demographics, obesity and economic development" (Rails-to-Trails Conservancy, 2011, p. 22).

ACTIVE TRANSPORTATION IN HALIBURTON COUNTY

Haliburton County is a rural region located in central eastern Ontario, approximately 200 km north of Toronto. Covering an area of approximately 4,500 km^2, the county has a year-round population of approximately 17,000 people and a population density of about 4 people/km^2 (Statistics Canada, 2012). Tourism is one of the main economic drivers with a large number of seasonal residents that increases the population by approximately 45,000 in the summer. The seasonal nature of the economy has a significant impact on employment rates. As of April 2011, the unemployment rate for the county was 9.5%, which was higher than the provincial rate of 7.7% (Hirstwood, 2011). The county also has a large number of seniors, with the county's median age of 54 years considerably higher than that of the province of Ontario (40.4 years) (Statistics Canada, 2012).

In terms of overall health, county residents have higher rates of hospitalization due to cardiovascular disease, cancer, hypertension, and respiratory disease than those of Ontario as a whole (Prime Time Strategies Inc., 2011). The most recent journey to work data from the 2006 census showed that 6% of workers in Haliburton County walked or bicycled to work, similar to the provincial rate of 6.8% (Statistics Canada, 2007).

The Communities in Action (CIA) Committee is a coalition formed in 2004 to plan for active transportation as a way to increase physical activity and create a healthier, more active population. It is a community-based coalition that includes representatives from the public health department, community economic development, business organizations, and groups interested in seniors, trails, and cycling. Prior to 2004, there was little in the way of policy or initiatives in Haliburton County that focused on active transportation or healthy built environments; most Official Plans (policy documents in Ontario that direct land use planning at the local municipal level) did not include policies addressing active transportation or healthy active communities. There was also limited community awareness about active transportation and its benefits, and there were no community groups to plan or promote active transportation activities.

In 2004, work being done elsewhere on active transportation was in an urban context, meaning that best practices could not be simply reproduced for a rural setting. The CIA Committee had to adapt and, in many cases innovate, in order to identify practices appropriate for a rural setting.

The CIA Committee initiatives targeted both municipal government decision makers and the general community. With regard to municipal government, the CIA Committee work focused on advocacy for policy changes and investments in infrastructure. At a community level, the CIA Committee's focus was on increasing active transportation by promoting it as an affordable, accessible, and enjoyable way to incorporate physical activity into daily living. Bringing about policy change and commitment to invest in infrastructure requires building community-level interest. In this way, the CIA Committee worked from both the "top down" and "bottom up" in order to accomplish active transportation initiatives.

Municipalities in Haliburton County do not have staff dedicated to cycling, walking, or active transportation; therefore, having an interest group to advocate, raise awareness, and educate was critical for bridging the knowledge gap for both the public and municipal government decision makers. The CIA Committee was supported by funds from federal, provincial, and local sources and chaired by a health promoter from the public health department, providing staff capacity during periods between grants.

The CIA Committee used the following approaches: advocacy for healthy public policies, collaboration with multiple stakeholders, community education and promotion, and research and planning. The CIA Committee also conducted evaluations to assess the contribution and impact that efforts have had on active transportation in Haliburton County.

Advocacy for Healthy Public Policy

As a community-based group, the CIA Committee itself did not build infrastructure. Its role was to advocate to local municipalities for supportive policy and investments in active transportation. The World Health Organization [WHO] (1988) states: "The main aim of health[y] public policy is to create a supportive environment to enable people to lead healthy lives. Such a policy makes health[y] choices possible or easier for citizens. It makes social and physical environments health-enhancing" (p. 1). (See Chapter 1.)

Policy instruments include municipal by-laws, zoning regulations, and roadway design standards. The CIA Committee participated in and contributed to local Official Plan reviews. The group communicated regularly with municipal government through delegations, information briefs, letters, and phone conversations. Advocacy efforts included making the case for investment in infrastructure, communicating the benefits of cycling and road life/maintenance, safety, and tourism. The CIA Committee endeavoured to "connect the dots" by providing information and evidence that illustrated the links between active transportation and these priorities.

Public education efforts focused on raising awareness of the "why," "where," and "how" of active transportation. The CIA Committee chose the message "Park the Car and Get Moving" to encourage people who drive to town to park and walk to do their business.

Collaboration and Partnership

Collaboration is key to addressing capacity issues that exist in rural communities. A primary focus of the CIA Committee was to build positive relationships with several sectors, and its partners included municipal government, schools, police, seniors groups, businesses, and tourism stakeholders. The public health department was a key partner in the CIA Committee from its inception. This intersectoral relationship benefited both the CIA Committee and the public health department, with each helping the other to achieve its mandate and objectives.

Municipal government was also a key partner, as it was responsible for public policy and community infrastructure. (See Box 36.1.) The CIA Committee sought local champions and hosted a variety of workshops and events for its partners, often bringing in outside experts to demonstrate that progressive communities elsewhere were embracing active transportation policies. Activities such as community walk audits were opportunities to engage municipal government staff and politicians in an analysis of the county's walking environment.

Box 36.1 Share the Road: An Example of Partnership

In 2009, a comprehensive Share the Road project was undertaken by municipal government, public health department, the CIA Committee, and Ontario Provincial Police (OPP). The project installed road signs across the county and developed and distributed educational material to the public. The partnership capitalized on the strengths of each partner. The municipal government administered the funds and ordered and installed "Share the Road" signs on local roads. The public health department and the CIA Committee took the lead on implementing a social marketing campaign with input from the OPP. This project received a Sustainable Communities Award in 2010 from the Federation of Canadian Municipalities.

Community Education and Promotion

The CIA Committee undertook a variety of projects to educate and raise awareness about active transportation. These initiatives were important in building community support and also served to demonstrate community interest in and demand for active transportation. Early on, the CIA Committee decided to focus its social marketing messages on the villages of Haliburton and Minden rather than on the whole county, advertising a feasible goal—for people to use active transportation in town.

Numerous resources were developed to encourage and promote active transportation. "Walk, Bike and Be Active" maps were developed for downtown Haliburton and Minden showing walking and cycling routes, and large maps were located in public parking areas to help people navigate from where they parked into and around town. The CIA Committee led or supported a number of events and activities including guided walks, a commuter challenge, bike/walk to school promotion, and a cycling festival. The CIA Committee promoted active transportation through multiple media: public service announcements, radio and television interviews, and articles in local newspapers.

Research and Planning

The CIA Committee built a strong evidence-based case to support active transportation, developed tools and resources, and conducted community-based research. Community-based research methods such as focus groups and surveys provided important information on active transportation activity and community assets and problems, and served to raise awareness. In a rural community where the time and resources of municipal government staff are limited, community groups and volunteers enhanced local capacity to collect data. The CIA Committee enhanced its own capacity by accessing the time and skills of university students from Trent University in Peterborough, Ontario working with the coalition through a local community-based research centre on various research projects.

The CIA Committee developed active transportation plans for both Haliburton and Minden (Young, 2008); these plans included concept illustrations or digitally altered images of problem areas that helped provide a vision of what could be improved. These illustrations laid the foundation for further advocacy for supportive policies and infrastructure investment, and helped establish the CIA Committee as a credible resource.

EVALUATION AND ACHIEVEMENTS

In 2011/2012, the CIA Committee undertook a comprehensive evaluation to measure changes in active transportation since 2005 and to assess its contribution to these changes as detailed in a logic model (Fig. 36.1). The evaluation comprised a variety of approaches to collect quantitative and qualitative information: an inventory of policy and infrastructure changes; a survey that asked residents to self-report their active transportation awareness and behaviour; an observational study that produced manual counts of people walking and cycling at several locations in the villages of Haliburton and Minden; and key informant interviews with government decision makers.

Noxon Associates Limited (2009) stated "non-governmental organizations in smaller communities can play critical roles as champions that create awareness, shape public opinion, instill a sense of ownership, and harness community energy" (p. 5). By the evaluation results, the CIA Committee was identified as playing an important role in these ways. The outcomes that emerged in the evaluation included changes to policies, improvements to infrastructure, and increased awareness of active transportation. Broader impacts included a change in culture in support of active transportation and an overall increase in active transportation activity.

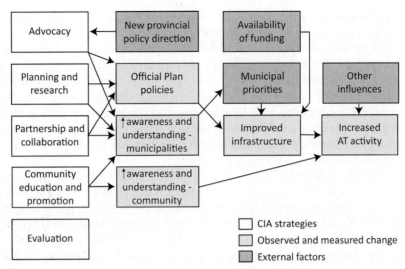

FIGURE 36.1 Activities and impacts of the Communities In Action Committee.

The CIA Committee's actions helped to establish it as a credible partner and resource to municipal government and communities. Municipal government key informants viewed the CIA Committee as expanding their capacity and making an important contribution to the changes that had taken place.

"...to have [the CIA Committee] as an independent body to provide the municipal and county levels with direction and to highlight best practices and bring resources to the table is very effective." (Municipal Key Informant; Hall & Shikaze, 2013, p. 22)

In 2004, active transportation was not part of the conversation at either a community or local government level. Noxon Associates Limited (2009) identified the challenges of overcoming this "car-first" culture that exists in many small, rural communities: "Efforts to improve travel options in small and rural communities must first overcome a culture of decision making that favours cars and people that have access to them, while it disadvantages residents who cannot use cars, such as children, the elderly and persons with disabilities" (p. 4). A cultural shift began to occur in Haliburton County, with increased recognition among the public and municipal decision makers of the benefits of active transportation and significant investments in infrastructure.

As of 2014, all Official Plans at the lower and upper tier in Haliburton County have policies specific to cycling, active transportation, healthy communities, and walking. The successful advocacy efforts of the CIA Committee are reflected in new policies. The village of Minden created a Downtown Improvement Plan (a long range planning and visioning document) that reflected several of the recommendations advocated by the CIA Committee.

"Land use patterns and development should promote energy efficiency, improved air quality, and allow for compact development that is designed in such a way to support and encourage active transportation." (County of Haliburton Official Plan, 2010, 2.3.5.3)

The physical landscape for active transportation has changed since 2004. In downtown Minden, the road width was reduced and sidewalks were widened. Overall aesthetics were improved with coloured concrete, new planters, and street furniture. Crosswalks were painted at intersections where previously there were none. In addition, the downtown Riverwalk trail was completed, including installation of a pedestrian bridge and boardwalk connecting downtown with the cultural centre, arena, and recreation centre. Riverwalk has become a well-used trail for both recreation and transportation.

In the Village of Haliburton, a two-phase project to improve two downtown streets was completed in 2013. These were large-scale projects that included digging up and repaving the existing streets and rebuilding and reconfiguring the roadway and surrounding environment. Earlier community consultations conducted by the CIA Committee helped build community support for this project by raising awareness of the benefits of making the downtown more walkable. The transformation was dramatic with the installation of new curbs, sidewalks, paving stones, plantings, crosswalks, bicycle racks, benches, and lighting, which resulted in great improvements to the walking environment.

The CIA Committee and its partners played a critical role in advocating that paved shoulders be included in road projects. The county began adding 1- to 1.2 m wide paved shoulders to major road projects in 2008, with approximately 30.5 km of paved shoulders completed as of 2014. A marker of the CIA Committee success was that Haliburton County's 2014 Four-year Capital Works Plan included paved shoulders as a standard in major road projects.

At a community level, responses to surveys provided qualitative evidence indicating increased awareness of active transportation.

"People are becoming more physically active as there is more public education around things like obesity and diabetes. Parents and kids are using them more for a healthy lifestyle." (Community Survey Respondent; Hall & Shikaze, 2013, p. 21)

The public appreciated the changes that supported their active transportation, and they enjoyed the benefits of villages that were more walking and cycling friendly. Observational studies indicated that there were more people walking. Since the work of the CIA Committee was about improving health through active transportation, the increased level of active transportation activity was an important indicator of potential health impact (Table 36.1).

As a result of its efforts, other rural communities have looked to the CIA Committee and its accomplishments and have modeled their initiatives from the lessons learned in Haliburton County.

TABLE 36.1 Increase in Active Transportation Activity in Selected Locations[a]

Location	Year	Number[a]
Haliburton		
Highland Street	2005	146
	2012	277
York Street	2005	106
	2012	135
Courtesy Crossing	2005	55
	2012	56
Minden		
Invergordon Avenue	2007	10
	2012	21
Pritchard Lane	2007	7
	2012	24
Water Street	2007	5
	2012	75

[a]Average number of people walking or cycling per hour based on 3 h of observation.

LESSONS LEARNED

Through the work of the CIA Committee, there are lessons learned that may be applied in other communities that wish to undertake active transportation initiatives.

1. Identify a manageable message and focus when encouraging active transportation. In a rural community, messages that people feel are realistic will assist in acceptance and uptake. Active transportation has many benefits, so it is helpful to integrate those benefits with messages and initiatives wherever possible. While active transportation is a health promotion strategy, the health message may not be sufficient to capture the attention of municipal decision makers.
2. Build partnerships and collaborate with different sectors. Collaboration makes the most of human and financial resources, increases and builds capacity, taps into community expertise, and helps achieve multiple goals and outcomes.
3. Articulate how active transportation supports municipal priorities and link active transportation to provincial priorities and direction. It helps to show that higher levels of government see value in planning for and promoting active transportation.
4. Use community engagement strategies to demonstrate demand and develop an active transportation plan. The planning process presents an opportunity to acquire community input, engage stakeholders, create a vision, and identify solutions. Plans can also be a starting point for policies that will have longer-term impacts.

Summary

Implementation of active transportation initiatives is achievable in small, rural communities and is a valuable health promotion strategy to encourage physical activity. There are unique opportunities for partnerships. While the overall geography can be vast, typically there is a concentration of services around key hubs, which can be the focus for active transportation promotion and planning.

Community organizations, especially public health departments, play an important leadership role in initiating active transportation in small, rural communities where resources may be limited. Active transportation addresses many public health priorities such as increasing physical activity, preventing injuries, improving safety and accessibility, and promoting mental health. Public health departments can use a range of health promotion strategies to encourage more active transportation.

Measurement, monitoring, and evaluation are required to make the case for investment. Community-based research is a valuable and effective approach to evaluation; it is a legitimate and accessible methodology that community groups can use to measure and evaluate the effectiveness of their work. Using multiple methods of data collection, both quantitative and qualitative, is useful in order to triangulate results and validate what has been observed.

Influencing change takes time; having and articulating a consistent vision is important. There are many factors at work when it comes to changing active transportation behaviour. The CIA Committee's experiences indicate that taking a variety of approaches and targeting a range of audiences are effective ways to convey the messages that effect change and impact health.

REFERENCES

Caldwell, W. J., Kraehling, P., Kaptur, S., & Huff, J. (2015). *Healthy rural communities tool kit – A guide for rural municipalities.* Guelph: University of Guelph. URL=http://www.ruralhealthycommunities.ca/Rural_Healthy_Communities/Toolkit.html

Canadian Institute of Planners (CIP). (2010). *Healthy communities practice guide.* URL=https://www.cip-icu.ca/Resources/Resources/Healthy-Communities-Practice-Guide

County of Haliburton. (2010). *Official plan.* URL=https://haliburtoncounty.ca/wp-content/uploads/2013/08/OfficialPlan.pdf

DesMeules, M., & Pong, R. (2006). *How healthy are rural Canadians? An assessment of their health status and health determinants.* Ottawa: Canadian Institute for Health Information. URL=https://secure.cihi.ca/free_products/rural_canadians_2006_report_e.pdf

Frank, L. D., Sallis, J. F., Conway, T. L., Chapman, J. E., Saelens, B. E., & Bachman, W. (2006). Many pathways from land use to health: Associations between neighbourhood walkability and active transportation, body mass index and air quality. *Journal of the American Planning Association, 72*(1), 75–87.

Hall, K., & Shikaze, S. (2013). *Seven years later: Evaluating impact on active transportation in Haliburton county.* URL=http://www.haliburtoncooperative.on.ca/CIA/images/stories/pdfs/final%20report%20-%20communities%20in%20action_new%20logos.pdf

Hallmark, S. L., McDonald, T. J., Hsu, Y., Tian, Y., & Andersen, D. J. (2010). *Safety benefits of paved shoulders.* Ames: Iowa State University, Center for Transportation Research and Education.

Heart and Stroke Foundation. (2005). *Report card on Canadians' health: Has the suburban dream gone sour?* URL = http://www.heartandstroke.com/site/apps/nlnet/content2.aspx?c=ikIQLcMWJtE&b=4955951&ct=4512815

Hirstwood, S. (2011). *Haliburton County business retention and expansion report.* Prepared for the Haliburton Highlands Chamber of Commerce. URL=http://haliburtonchamber.com/articles.php?id=13927

Litman, T. (2003). *Social inclusion as a transport planning issue in Canada.* Contribution to the FIA Foundation G7 Comparison Paper, presented at the European Transport Conference, Strasbourg. URL=http://www.researchgate.net/publication/37183839_Social_Inclusion_as_a_transport_planning_issue_in_Canada

McMahon, E. T. (2010). The placemaking dividend. *Urban Land Magazine.* URL=http://urbanland.uli.org/economy-markets-trends/the-place-making-dividend/

Noxon Associates Limited. (2009). *Improving travel options in small and rural communities.* Prepared for Transport Canada. URL=http://data.tc.gc.ca/archive/eng/programs/environment-urban-guidelines-practitioners-improvingtravelsrcomms2009-menu-1656.htm

Partners for Livable Communities (2016). URL=http://livable.org/about-us/what-is-livability

Perrotta, K. (2011) *Public health and land use planning: How ten public health units are working to create healthy and sustainable communities.* Prepared for the Clean Air Partnership and the Ontario Public Health Association. URL =http://www.cleanairpartnership.org/files/CAP%20PHLUP%20Background%20Report%20April%202011.pdf

Prime Time Strategies Inc. (2011). *Haliburton County community picture 2011.* Prepared for the Haliburton Kawartha Pine Ridge District Health Unit. URL=http://www.hkpr.on.ca/Portals/0/PDF%20Files%20-%20CDIP/Haliburton%20County%20Community%20Picture.pdf

Rails-to-Trails Conservancy. (2011). *Active transportation beyond urban centers: Walking and bicycling in small towns and rural America.* Washington: Author. URL=http://www.railstotrails.org/resource-library/resources/active-transportation-beyond-urban-centers-report/

Ryerson Planning and Consulting. (2014). *Bike lanes, on-street parking, and business: A study of Danforth Avenue in Toronto Danforth neighbourhood.* Toronto: Ryerson University, Urban and Regional Planning. URL=http://www.tcat.ca/knowledge-centre/bike-lanes-on-street-parking-and-business-a-study-of-danforth-avenue-in-toronto-danforth-neighbourhood/

Statistics Canada. (2007). *Haliburton, Ontario (Code3546) (table). 2006 Community Profiles. 2006 Census. Catalogue no. 92–591-XWE.* Ottawa. URL=http://www12.statcan.ca/census-recensement/2006/dp-pd/prof/92–591/index.cfm?Lang=E

Statistics Canada. (2012). *Haliburton, Ontario (Code 3546) and Ontario (Code 35) (table). Census Profile. 2011 Census. Catalogue no. 98–316-XWE.* Ottawa. URL=http://www12.statcan.gc.ca/census-recensement/2011/dp-pd/prof/index.cfm?Lang=E

Transport Canada. (2006). Sustainable transportation in small and rural communities. Urban Transportation Showcase Program, Issue Paper 61. Ottawa: Author.

Transportation Association of Canada (TAC). (2012). *Primer on active transportation: Making it work in Canadian communities.* URL=http://tac-atc.ca/sites/tac-atc.ca/files/site/doc/resources/primer-active-trans2012.pdf

Young, P. (2008). An active transportation plan for Minden. Report produced for The Communities in Action Committee. URL=http://lin.ca/sites/default/files/attachments/AT%20PLAN%20MINDEN%20JULY%202008%20-%20web.pdf

World Health Organization (WHO). (1988). *Adelaide recommendations on healthy public policy.* Geneva: Author.

ONLINE RESOURCES

Please visit the Point at http://thepoint.lww.com/Vollman4e for up-to-date Internet resources and additional learning materials on this topic.

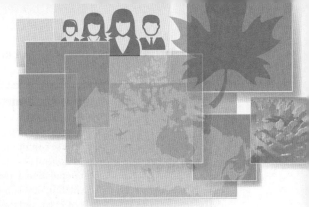

CHAPTER 37

Empowering Mothers of Murdered Children: A Community-Based Approach

Annette Bailey and Sky Starr

LEARNING OBJECTIVES

After studying this chapter, you should be able to:

1. Identify the impact of the death of a child from gun homicide on mothers, families, and the community

2. Describe the grief process that bereaved mothers experience after the death of a child to gun homicide

3. Describe how the Out Of Bounds Forgotten Mothers program reflects a health promotion approach

Introduction

Mothers are unduly affected by the loss of children to gun homicide (Bailey et al., 2015); there are very few experiences that can be compared to the pain of losing a child. Research has highlighted that more than 5 years after the violent loss of their children, bereaved mothers still struggle with complicated grief and posttraumatic stress disorder (PTSD) (Murphy et al., 2003). Persisting social difficulties that contribute to a complex, prolonged, and complicated grief process commonly accompany their loss experiences (McDevitt-Murphy et al., 2012; Bailey et al., 2015). Bereaved mothers living in marginalized communities suffer debilitating psychological and social consequences of grief accompanied by social isolation, social stigma, discrimination, and resource depletion (Bailey et al., 2013; Hannays-King et al., 2015). Despite these mothers' propensity for resiliency and meaning making, loss of a child to gun homicide has serious mental health implications for them, their families, and their communities (Bailey et al., 2013; Burke & Neimeyer, 2014; Sharpe et al., 2014).

Grief and grief-associated PTSD have a very long lifespan. Yet, practical strategies to address the needs of survivors of gun homicide are not in place. One-time debriefs and short-term counselling (Salloum et al., 2001; Ziegler et al., 2004), while well intentioned, have been ineffectual for managing long-term grief and trauma responses (Currier et al., 2008). Meeting the unique traumatic grief needs of gun homicide survivors requires sustainable health

> ## Box 37.1 The Jane-Finch Community
>
> Jane-Finch, located at the centre of Toronto's Black Creek neighbourhood, is one of the most linguistic and ethnically diverse communities in the world. In comparison to Toronto's 140 neighbourhoods, Black Creek is rated as the least livable. With a population of 22,057, the neighbourhood has the highest population density ($6,356/km^2$), the highest concentration of immigrants, the largest representation of youth ages 15–24, the highest female-headed lone parent families (41% vs. city rate of 21%), and the lowest average after-tax household income ($47,362 vs. city average of $70,945) (City of Toronto, 2014).
>
> The area of Jane-Finch has become synonymous with poverty and social dysfunction. Ranked as having the highest rates of poverty in Toronto, this marginalized community has been the focus of nation-wide media and public attention, often framed in negative discourses about violence, urban decline, and social unrest. Criminal activities and violent crimes shape the stigmatized reputation of the community and are often used to frame the area as a social/political problem in need of reform (Nangwaya, 2014). Jane-Finch continues to be one of the top five communities in Toronto affected by homicide, particularly gun homicide. In 2010, 50% of homicides in Toronto were committed with guns. With majority of these gun homicides occurring within blocks of the intersection of Jane-Finch, this community continues to rank high in gun-related deaths (Charron, 2011).

promotion strategies (Bailey & Velasco, 2014). The Ottawa Charter (World Health Organization [WHO], 1986) acknowledges the centrality of the community in supporting and enabling individuals and families to improve their health and well-being. For grieving mothers at great risk for marginalization, alienation, and psychological collapse, health promotion strategies should involve approaches that cultivate their capacities for healing and empowerment. Community-based agencies, however, are often challenged by the lack of available resources and strategies to bolster the capacities of this unique population.

Out Of Bounds (OOB) provides pragmatic grief support for bereaved mothers and their families in the marginalized community of Jane-Finch in Toronto. It is situated in the Jane-Finch community, one of 13 priority (socioeconomically disadvantaged) neighbourhoods in Toronto, Ontario (United Way, 2012) (see Box 37.1).

An empowerment model (Fig. 37.1) has been developed for OOB's Forgotten Mothers program and a multiple-part narrative of two mothers is used to illustrate its application. Woven throughout are the experiences of bereaved mothers and grief therapist, Rev. Sky Starr. Quotes presented in this case story have been accumulated from OOB's work with bereaved mothers during group sessions and years of crisis response in the community. Pseudonyms have been used to protect privacy.

GUN HOMICIDE AND MOTHERS' TRAUMATIC GRIEF

I think my heart came out. I mean it came right out of my body. It was racing so fast that I thought I saw it jump right out of my chest. I think it wanted to go with him. I lost my heart that day.

For over 15 years, OOB has witnessed mothers' devastating experiences of traumatic grief. The above statement represents the debilitating emotional responses that shape the realities of mothers who have experienced gun homicide loss and are in the stage of fresh grief. These responses are often followed by dissociation, flashbacks, nightmares, panic disorders, hypervigilance, and depression (Allen et al., 1999; Margolin & Gordis, 2000). Understanding that these psychological consequences are further perpetuated by poverty, lack of support, self-blame, and feelings of helplessness, OOB's initial work with bereaved mothers is focused on regaining basic equilibrium by building stabilization skills, also termed mental health first-aid.

Deep-breathing exercises, positive affirmations of personal strength, mindfulness-based cognitive therapy, and accompaniment are among the services provided by OOB's grief therapist, who also becomes a "stabilizing agent" for mothers for the duration of the grief journey.

During the grief process, mothers continuously encounter re-traumatization. Their re-traumatization is activated by the stigma of gun homicide, fear of judgement, silence, and emotional warfare that intersect and persist to create layers of subjugation, powerlessness, and social isolation (Bailey et al., 2015; Hannays-King et al., 2015). For mothers, especially single mothers with other children, working through the interplay of these complex factors and the social burden that comes with this loss seems impossible. Without ongoing support, complicated grief is inevitable, with consequences to family structures and community capacity. To ease mental health impairment, OOB also addresses mothers' social needs; most often, this includes providing guidance with funeral arrangements, assisting with victim service processes, preparing mothers for interaction with the police and the legal system, and facilitating access to various social services.

Overcoming the pervasive influence of loss necessitates resilience in coping with the social factors that reinforce the victimization of gun homicide survivors. Becoming resilient is no easy feat, but some mothers recognize that resilience is not an option—it is a necessity (Bailey et al., 2015). Maintaining family structures provides an impetus for working through social chaos. Mothers' resilience, demonstrated through altruism, social change actions, and community intervention, is often fuelled by spirituality, cultural fortitude, and meaning making (Bailey et al., 2013; Bailey et al., 2015). OOB recognizes this resilience as strength and models the Ottawa Charter by fostering a supportive environment and providing access to information and life skills to ignite bereaved mothers' innate capacity for resilience. Mothers who are unable to channel their capacity and transform pain into resilience often remain mentally and physically incapacitated. This incapacitation represents a major health service need for survivors of gun homicide. Therefore, health promotion efforts for survivors should go well beyond personal coping; promoting collective empowerment for sustained healing and social change is also important. OOB functions with a clear understanding that the disempowerment and disconnection experienced by bereaved mothers should be addressed from a health promotion perspective.

The experiences of many bereaved mothers dealing with traumatic grief are represented in the OOB Model of Empowerment (Fig. 37.1). The approach works in tandem with other tactics used by OOB to help mothers find their way out of fresh grief and move toward resilience. At

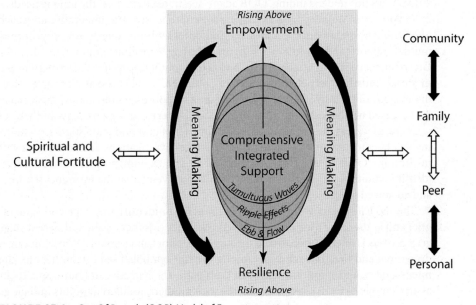

FIGURE 37.1   Out Of Bounds (OOB) Model of Empowerment.

the onset of fresh loss, there is intense grief and trauma in the form of extreme psychological pain that gives the effects of strong wave-like emotions. These emotions occur at the inner circle where *tumultuous waves* are strongly felt. Lines emanating out from the centre represent *rippling effects,* or emotions felt on the personal level that extend out to the family and community. Spaces between the ripples symbolize the intervals of reprieve and/or steady growth over time; these are termed the *ebb and flow.* Getting mothers to this point requires *comprehensive integrated support* in the forms of social support, education, and spiritual encouragement, which are provided simultaneously to create interlocking, revolving, and reciprocating processes of care with mutual peer support as its nucleus.

The Ottawa Charter provides guidance for creating supportive environments, developing coping skills, and enhancing mothers' personal health. The activities of the OOB Forgotten Mothers program strengthen mothers and allow to them to develop *empowerment* and *resilience. Rising above the waves* is indicative of mothers who, following active involvement in the program, are able to make meaning in their loss. *Meaning making* combines support, skill building, and mothers' spiritual and cultural fortitude. These processes, congruent with grief, are not linear, but fluid and interchanging.

TRAUMATIC GRIEF SUPPORT FOR MOTHERS

OOB is a not-for-profit, community-based organization aimed at empowering mothers and other survivors of violence. The program began in the summer of 2005 under the direction of a grief therapist who initiated the program after an upsurge in the incidence of gun homicide left youth, families, and the community debilitated by grief. A subsidiary program called Forgotten Mothers was created specifically to address the traumatic grief and isolation of mothers following the gun homicide of their children.

OOB's mandate is to strengthen the resilience of these mothers. As shown in Figure 37.1, OOB provides individual and community support to mothers dealing with trauma and grief-related PTSD. Research has shown that a complex interplay between pre-existing social challenges and the stigma of gun homicide can significantly increase mothers' social and psychological struggles. This interplay creates emotional chaos in the lives of bereaved mothers and sparks readiness to engage them in capacity-building and transformation (Bailey et al., 2015). With this understanding, OOB adapts its strategies to meet the unique needs of mothers in its Forgotten Mothers program. Using a comprehensive and integrative approach, services offered incorporate education and training interventions, one-to-one psychotherapy, peer mutual support, and community support to enhance healing, empowerment, and resilience. Given the social stigma attached to gun violence, mothers' psychosocial experiences are rooted in social injustice, perpetual oppression, and stereotypical social discourses that affect all dimensions of their lives. Grief-related trauma responses are often a psychosocial experience for bereaved mothers. An integrative approach is therefore responsive to mothers' psychological care, as well as the personal and social impact of gun homicide stigma, including preparing mothers to respond to the media and police investigations and to interact within social institutions. OOB offers a 10-week grief and trauma training program that educates people to identify symptoms of grief-related PTSD and bereavement at the introductory, intermediary, and advanced levels.

The model of empowerment (Fig. 37.1) helps to identify the stage and state of mothers' grief and at the same time envisages their resilience. Mothers' pain at different stages in their grief process is often demonstrated through metaphors and symbols. Waves, ocean, sea, water, drowning, and breathlessness are among the top symbols used by mothers to illustrate the intense, deep, and emotional nature of their pain. The narrative of Louise and Thelma is used as an example of OOB's use of the model with mothers at different points in their grief.

Lives of Two Mothers Turned Upside Down

> *Look at what they did to my son. He is a good child. He wanted to be an RN [Registered Nurse] to help people. Oh God, look at what they did to my son.*

Thelma wailed in dismay and fresh traumatic grief as she learned the dreadful news that her 16-year-old son and his 15-year-old friend were gunned down at the door of the friend's home. They were returning home from a summer program when they were both shot multiple times by three male youth on bicycles.

Amid continuous wailing Thelma lamented on things that could have been and pleaded with police officers and others at the scene, "Help me understand. Please help me understand. How could this happen? My son was a good kid. He looked after his younger brother. He always walked him to school and to his programs. He's never in any trouble. Somebody help me understand."

There were howling screams as Louise, the second mother, arrived at the scene. "Where's my son? I want to see my son. Show me my son. This is not happening. Where is my son? It can't be my son." Her ordinarily reserved nature was replaced with hysteria to the amplified traumatic scene. Her son had been taken to a trauma centre where he was pronounced dead on arrival. A female police officer approached her and said, "I'm so sorry madam. I'm so sorry madam. He didn't make it." After what seemed like ages of frenzied bemoaning, this mother fainted and had to be lifted off to a neighbouring community health centre for intense trauma-focused care. When she eventually regained her composure, she repeatedly stated, "I can't go back there. I can't go back there. I feel sick. I can't go back there." The shooting happened at the front door of her house. She was taken to her brother's home outside of the community.

Within the two-week period of awaiting release of the bodies from the coroner's office, the first mother busied herself in preparing. "I want to do the best funeral I can do for my son. It has to be the perfect send-off," she stated. Her grieving was placed on hold as she busied herself. The second mother became intensely incapacitated, leaving her brother and other family members to arrange final rites.

These mothers' lives were irrevocably altered. This double homicide is particularly painful for Louise and Thelma who are not allowed to see, touch, or be close to their children during the police investigation. The burden of pain, suffering, and eventual PTSD on these mothers involves a long, arduous road of deep-rooted agony that alters their lives, livelihood, and functioning. The psychological impact on family members, friends, neighbours, and community life are intense and long-lasting.

Tumultuous Waves

At the peak of their sorrow, mothers most often liken their grief and trauma emotions to tumultuous waves. Like waves on a shoreline, grief-related emotions smash these bereaved mothers with irresistible force, volatility, and unnerving conflicting highs and lows. A mother in fresh grief described her experience:

> *This huge wave of pain picked me up like a rag doll and tossed me so far and so deep that I could literally feel sea water stinging my nose; I could taste it in my mouth, burning my throat and filling my lungs till I couldn't breathe.*

Recognizing that waves are the forward motion of the ocean's water (Briney, n.d.), OOB sees traumatic pain, even at the most tumultuous stage, as indicative of forward motion in the grieving process. Therefore, OOB works with mothers to help them understand that the tumultuous emotions will eventually recede like a wave. With support and repetitive reminders mothers gradually shift in the grief process such that they are able to manage and accept each wave because they realize the wave-like emotion will recede. Understanding what triggers these emotions and gaining awareness of their pain are incremental transformations in their grief process that begins the process of their empowerment. OOB recognizes that empowerment is achievable for these mothers. However, the intensity of fresh grief, which is compounded by their social circumstances, is a key deterrent to mothers' ability to set and achieve self-determined goals, with some measure of control over their grief and recovery. A strong structure of support is required to modify the impact of tumultuous grief. Heightened relational support from interactions with OOB's therapist and other grieving mothers is critical at this time.

Lives of Two Mothers Turned Upside Down (cont'd)

Like waves moving back and forth, Thelma rocked back and forth as she sat on the concrete surface just across from where her son was killed. With both hands clasped beneath her belly, she repeated, "My stomach is ripping, my stomach is ripping. It [wave] keeps coming. It keeps coming." Arriving at the scene, the grief therapist's familiarity with Thelma facilitated an immediate connection. She sat next to Thelma with careful body alignment ensuring that her body was touching Thelma's. This "body-touching" made Thelma aware that she was not alone, but that someone familiar was also helping to share her grief. At this tumultuous stage, the grief therapist uses few words, but makes herself present and supports the mother through validation, acknowledgement, consolation, and empathy. To address the bodily sensations, mothers are reminded that these symptoms are the body's indicators of the intense trauma they are facing. Establishing safety techniques serve to orient mothers, like Thelma, that they are on dry land, without the ocean waves that threaten to drown them. Thelma was encouraged to concentrate on what was happening in her body. While allowing her lament, cognitive approaches were applied to redirect thought patterns and reassure her that she was not alone. These initial actions are critical to mothers' awareness that they are the experts of their grieving process, establishing a platform to build on their innate capacity for personal healing and resilience.

Ripple Effects

Death's impact is never compartmentalized or isolated. Like the proverbial "pebble in a pond," the sudden traumatic death of a loved one from gun homicide ushers in ripple effects that expand beyond time, space, and imagination. These deaths erode equilibrium and create challenges for family functioning. In cases where the lost member contributed to emotional, social, spiritual, and financial functioning, family disintegration is predictable. Family members become more vulnerable, easily overwhelmed by the intensity of unshared emotions. Families that once enjoyed emotional stability may find themselves isolated, dejected, and often torn apart. Extended families, communities, and institutions (e.g., schools) also feel the ripple effect, creating domino consequences of anger, retaliation, and re-traumatization. In communities like Jane-Finch, already challenged by frequent occurrences of gun homicide, re-traumatization is inevitable (West, 2014). Facilitating resilience for mothers requires a comprehensive integrative approach that is deliberately focused on addressing the ripple effects on families, peers, and communities. The WHO makes it clear that "no one survives without community and no community thrives without the individual" (Friedli, 2009, p. iv). Therefore, it is necessary to create supportive environments that are conducive to healing and empowerment in response to the effects of gun homicide on individuals, families, and communities.

Lives of Two Mothers Turned Upside Down (cont'd)

The double homicide of two stellar young men was the first of its kind in the community, igniting an outcry within the entire community. OOB reacted promptly by organizing a community vigil in collaboration with the Jane-Finch Crisis Response Network, which consists of social service agencies and community members. Over 200 youth attended the vigil. The vigil offered solace to Thelma and Louise, provided a safe space for people to voice their concerns, and helped youth to curb thoughts of retaliation. During the vigil, Thelma and Louise were physically encircled by about 12 mothers and heard from them about how they had become resilient in the face of loss.

Mutual support among bereaved mothers is an essential component in OOB's model of traumatic grief care for building mothers' resilience and empowerment. In the context of health promotion, mutual support is an important mechanism to enhancing individual and community coping (Epp, 1986). OOB facilitates mutual support for mothers through community gatherings such as community vigils to create a healing space for expression and remembrance. Mothers are encouraged and consoled by other mothers and community members in these vigils. Now in her second year of bereavement, Thelma shared with OOB's grief therapist that the vigil contributed to her sense of self and provided the encouragement and hope needed to promote her resilience and current level of empowerment.

Ebb and Flow Tide

During the active grieving stage, mothers grapple with emotional ebb and flow. Contrasting emotions similar to the ocean's tide stirs large-scale, overpowering torrents of successive pain. Irrational thought patterns often evoke suicidal tendencies when overwhelming and large-scale emotions seem intolerable. Once these heightened emotions have ebbed, mothers flow into a dull numbing that threatens their survival. Thoughts become irrational, evasive, and suicidal. However, it is during this time that they have a desperate urge to seek help. One mother gave insights to the ebb and flow:

I decided that I didn't want to live. I knew how to end it. The pain, my life. Suicide was always at the back of my mind. Sometimes it rushed forward when I was very low but then there were times when it wasn't so bad.

In this phase, mothers demonstrate knowledge, awareness, and an acceptance of triggers that shape their survival. Although mothers may feel that they are drowning in emotion, they actively participate in pushing against the tide of active grief, thus building their resilience and empowerment. Key to building mothers' resilience is that they are encouraged to control the rate and method of their grieving. The therapist's work with mothers at this stage depends on each mother's shifting needs. While the therapist maintains the role of stabilizer, she also provides social support and therapy to build coping skills so that mothers understand and manage their grief-related responses.

Lives of Two Mothers Turned Upside Down (cont'd)

Six months following the shooting, Louise shared her story with 22 participants in one of OOB's trauma-focused training sessions. She agreed to share her story, being aware that it might trigger extreme emotion. Sharing experiences is a crucial part of group activities where survivors listen to each other in a contained, safe, and caring environment. Louise received validation and empathic understanding from the group. Mothers gain confidence, acquire coping strategies, and achieve incremental healing towards resilience and empowerment as they remember and share their grief journey.

Rising Above the Waves

"Rising above the waves" is a signal that the mothers are healing and growing as they move towards resilience. The time it takes for each mother to rise above the waves hinges on the level of intimacy and emotional connection with the deceased child; the deeper the intimacy with the child, the longer the time it takes. Meaning making begins with a steady acceptance of loss, where mothers transform the meaninglessness of their children's deaths to gain a new sense of purpose for their lives. Mothers' resilience emerges as activism and altruism in realizing the meaning they created (Bailey et al., 2013).

Within this phase, OOB's strategy concentrates on building mothers' capacity by bolstering their strengths, as observed throughout the grieving process. Validation of a mother's ability to bounce back and her willingness to live, along with the identification of previous coping methods, are emphasized. To support this approach, mothers are paired in a buddy system with women of similar circumstances. Buddies listen, encourage, and validate each other's experiences during tumultuous waves, ebb, and flow, and celebrate each other rising above the waves.

Lives of Two Mothers Turned Upside Down (cont'd)

To celebrate the first anniversary of their sons' death, Thelma and Louise initiated, planned, and participated in the implementation of a community event to honour their sons. This event attracted a wide range of community interest and participation. Although very emotional, the mothers spoke to over 600 attendees about their journey, declared their gratitude to the community, and proclaimed the event as an annual celebration in their sons' honour. This was a visible testament of their strength and ability to shift to a healthier stage of grieving and empowerment.

Thelma and Louise established an annual OKAY Tournament to honour their sons—this event is now well recognized, with meaningful sponsorship and collaboration from community organizations, law enforcement, and local media.

DISCUSSION

The body of literature on the devastating mental health impact of gun homicide on survivors and communities continues to grow (e.g., Currier et al., 2006; McDevitt-Murphy et al., 2012; Bailey & Velasco, 2014). An understanding of this impact on parents, families, youth, and the overall community is crucial for reorienting community services. Community-based trauma interventions are necessary to ensure that the mental and social impacts of gun homicide do not go unnoticed (Buchanan, 2014). Because of the social stigma of gun homicide, mothers and other survivors of gun violence require services that are comprehensive, integrated, and well situated in health promotion perspectives (Buchanan, 2014; Bailey et al., 2015). Currently, services tend to be provided as reactive solutions to community crisis, and not as integrated and sustained approaches. Traumatic grief support services, especially for mothers who are often the main family caregivers, should be responsive to approaches that recognize and build the coping skills and resilience of gun violence survivors.

Lack of funding continues to be a barrier to the types, duration, and sustainability of programs to support grieving families of violent crimes. Due to the scarcity of resources in marginalized communities such as Jane-Finch, there is limited sharing of resources to support families. Competition for available funding sometimes deters partnerships between community agencies, whose combined efforts could broaden the structure of support needed for mothers. Although agencies come together at the onset of a crisis, partnerships are not sustained over the long haul. Funding decisions should consider groups and communities affected by violence in order to break the cycle of violence.

Summary

The level of trauma experienced by gun homicide survivors affects their daily lives and family function. Existing services may be reoriented to address survivors' trauma; however, specialized care for traumatic grief is needed because unless trauma is addressed, survivors' mental health care remains inadequate. OOB offers hands-on, realistic support that forms the backbone of crisis and trauma services in the Jane-Finch community. Traumatic grief services are focused at the individual, family, group, and community levels and incorporate educational interventions, individual and group psychotherapy, peer mutual support, and community support to enhance healing and resilience for mothers who are survivors of gun homicide. Inadequacies in grief care after gun homicide can be attributed to a lack of recognition of traumatic grief as a mental health issue, as well as lack of funding for programs and services. Mental health system reform needs to recognize and address these gaps to create lasting support for families and communities affected by gun homicide.

Acknowledgements

The authors wish to acknowledge Levar Bailey and Jay Starr for their contribution to the development of the Out Of Bounds Model of Empowerment.

REFERENCES

Allen, J. G., Huntoon, J., & Evans, R. B. (1999). Complexities in complex posttraumatic stress disorder in inpatient women: Evidence from cluster analysis of MCMI-III personality disorder scales. *Journal of Personality Assessment, 73*(3), 449–471.

Bailey, A., Akhtar, M., Clarke, J., & Starr, S. (2015). Intersecting individual, social and cultural factors in Black mothers' resilience building following loss to gun violence. In N. Khanlou & B. Pilkington (Eds.), *Women's mental health: Resistance and resilience in community and society* (pp. 311–326). New York, NY: Springer.

Bailey, A., Clarke, J., & Salami, B. (2015). Race-based stigma as a determinant of access and support in Black mothers' experience of loss to gun violence. In S. Pashang & S. Gruner (Eds.), *Roots and routes of displacement and trauma: From analysis to advocacy & policy to practice* (pp. 262–276). Oakville, ON: Rock's Mills Press.

Bailey, A., Hannays-King, C., Clarke, J., Lester, E., & Velasco, D. (2013). Black mothers' cognitive process of finding meaning and building resilience after loss of a child to gun violence. *British Journal of Social Work, 43*(2), 336–354.

Bailey, A., & Velasco, D. (2014). Gun violence in Canada. In C. Buchanan (Ed.), *Gun violence, disability and recovery* (pp. 207–221). Freshwater, NSW: Surviving Gun Violence Project.

Briney, A. (n.d). *Waves: Ocean waves.* URL= http://geography.about.com/od/physicalgeography/a/waves.htm

Buchanan, C. (2014). *Gun violence, disability and recovery.* Freshwater, NSW: Surviving Gun Violence Project.

Burke, L. A., & Neimeyer, R. A. (2014). Complicated spiritual grief I: Relation to complicated grief symptomatology following violent death bereavement. *Death Studies, 38*(4), 259–267.

Charron, M. (2011). *Neighbourhood characteristics and the distribution of crime in Toronto: Additional analysis on youth crime.* (Crime and justice research paper series). Ottawa: Statistics Canada, Canadian Centre for Justice Statistics. URL= http://www.statcan.gc.ca/pub/85-561-m/85-561-m2011022-eng.pdf

City of Toronto. (2014). *2011 Neighbourhood Census/NHS Profile: Black Creek.* URL=http://www1.toronto.ca/City%20Of%20Toronto/Social%20Development,%20Finance%20&%20Administration/Neighbourhood%20Profiles/pdf/2011/pdf4/cpa24.pdf

Currier, J. M., Holland, J. M., & Neimeyer, R. A. (2006). Sense-making, grief, and the experience of violent loss: Toward a meditational model. *Death Studies, 30,* 403–428.

Currier, J. M., Neimeyer, R. A., & Berman, J. S. (2008). The effectiveness of psychotherapeutic interventions for bereaved persons: A comprehensive quantitative review. *Psychological Bulletin, 134*(5), 648–661.

Epp, J. (1986). *Achieving health for all: A framework for health promotion.* Ottawa: Health and Welfare Canada.

Friedli, L. (2009). *Mental health, resilience and inequalities.* Copenhagen: World Health Organization, Regional Office for Europe. URL= http://www.euro.who.int/_data/assets/pdf_file/0012/100821/E92227.pdf

Hannays-King, C., Bailey, A., & Akhtar, M. (2015). Social support and Black mothers' bereavement experience of losing a child to gun homicide. *Bereavement Care, 34*(1), 10–16.

Margolin, G., & Gordis, E. B. (2000). The effects of family and community violence on children. *Annual Review of Psychology, 51*, 445–479.

McDevitt-Murphy, M., Neimeyer, R. A., Burke, L. A., Williams, J. L., & Lawson, K. (2012). The toll of traumatic loss in African Americans bereaved by homicide. *Psychological Trauma: Theory, Research, Practice, and Policy, 4*(3), 303–311.

Murphy, S. A., Johnson, L. C., Chung, I. J., & Beaton, R. D. (2003). The prevalence of PTSD following the violent death of a child and predictors of change 5 years later. *Journal of Traumatic Stress, 16*(1), 17–25.

Nangwaya, A. (2014). Police violence in Toronto's Jane and Finch Community: Cops act like "military police in occupied territories" [Blog post]. URL=http://toronto.mediacoop.ca/blog/ajamu-nangwaya/32229

Salloum, A., Avery, L., & McClain, R. P. (2001). Group psychotherapy for adolescent survivors of homicide victims: A pilot study. *Journal of the American Academy of Child & Adolescent Psychiatry, 40*(11), 1261–1267.

Sharpe, T. L., Osteen, P., Frey, J. J., & Michalopoulos, L. M. (2014). Coping with grief responses among African American family members of homicide victims. *Violence and Victims, 29*(2), 332–347.

United Way. (2012). *Strong neighbourhoods: Responding to a call to action.* Toronto: United Way Toronto and City of Toronto, Social Development, Finance and Administration Division. URL=http://www.toronto.ca/legdocs/mmis/2012/cd/bgrd/backgroundfile-45145.pdf

West, C. (2014). *Violence in the lives of Black women: Battered, black, and blue.* New York, NY: Routledge.

World Health Organization (WHO). (1986). *The Ottawa charter for health promotion.* Geneva: Author.

Ziegler, R. G., Howe, J., & Pasternak, G. (2004). Psychotherapeutic debriefing of children and adolescents after exposure to violence in home or community: Integrating narrative techniques. *Journal of Infant, Child, and Adolescent Psychotherapy, 3*(2), 163–184.

ONLINE RESOURCES

Please visit the Point at http://thepoint.lww.com/Vollman4e for up-to-date Internet resources and additional learning materials on this topic.

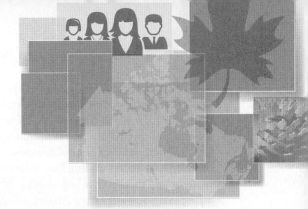

CHAPTER 38

Cultural Continuity: Re-storying Identity of Indigenous Youth

Brigette Krieg

LEARNING OBJECTIVES

After studying this chapter, you should be able to:

1. Describe the colonial policies that disrupted the cultural continuity in Aboriginal families and communities

2. Appreciate the challenges faced by urban Aboriginal youth

3. Describe some options for cultural programming that can support the development of positive self-esteem and identity of urban Aboriginal youth

Introduction

Statistical representation of Aboriginal youth in Canada presents an alarming picture of adversity characterized by substance abuse, suicide, teen pregnancy, and academic underachievement. Using Photovoice as a vehicle for community dialogue and education, the goal of this research project was to examine the strengths and resilience of the youth. The project, entitled "*I want you to know: Understanding Indigenous youth in Canada,*" documented the lived experiences of Aboriginal youth residing in urban centres and identified issues and responses to the challenges they experience.

Research indicates that colonial policies have created a loss of cohesion and identity in Aboriginal communities that have impacted families, eroded language and cultural traditions, and led to cultural discontinuity (MacNeil, 2008). Recognizing the devastating effects of colonization on their ancestors, Aboriginal youth across Canada identified culture and identity as a sense of loss and an important factor for healing in a special committee for the Royal Commission on Aboriginal People (Thira, 2000). Literature identifies the devastating effects of cultural loss on Aboriginal youth, and there is consensus among Aboriginal youth that they are "suffering from a loss of culture and a loss of family" (Morris, 2007, p. 137). Aboriginal youth believe that reconnecting with their culture would benefit them on individual, familial, and community levels (MacNeil, 2008).

Cultural continuity is the ability to preserve the historical traditions of a culture and carry that culture forward into the future, and is closely linked to the concept of cultural identity (Brown, 2003), which has a major influence on confidence and self-esteem. Due to years of colonial policies, Aboriginal communities feel disconnected from cultural values and traditions (Morris, 2007). Cultural disconnection and lack of cultural continuity create a loss of confidence in understanding how to live life and make decisions (MacNeil, 2008). Oritz (2011) spoke of how these people feel "confused…ambiguous and uncertain" (p. 285), and many who do try to acknowledge their Aboriginal identity feel invalidated.

This loss of cultural continuity and identity has taken a particularly devastating toll on Aboriginal youth. Chandler et al. (2003) and MacNeil (2008) have connected cultural continuity as a protective factor in addressing suicide among Aboriginal youth. They attribute this to the loss of cultural continuity that leads to a loss of self-continuity or self-identity, and a loss of self-confidence in understanding how to live life and make decisions. Chandler et al. (2003) identified adolescence as a time of heightened risk to suicide because it is a transitional developmental time and is also a critical time to develop strategies for promoting cultural continuity and for preserving confidence and identity at the individual level. Specifically, Chandler et al. (2003) found that "First Nations communities that succeed in taking steps to preserve their heritage culture and to recover some measure of control over [their] institutions…are also dramatically more successful in insulating their own children against the risks of suicide" (p. 115).

One of the strategies to promote cultural continuity is to provide youth with access to the arts that are important in their culture. Aboriginal youth have identified returning to traditional values, reconnecting with cultural teaching, and relearning Aboriginal languages as beneficial (Morris, 2007). They have also identified the importance of having positive Aboriginal role models from their family and community (Brown et al., 2007). Not just limited to youth, many Aboriginal people consider contemporary art practices to be a process of decolonization, re-appropriation, reclaiming, and healing (Trépanier, 2008).

The literature clearly demonstrates that Aboriginal youth have a vision for their future; they understand what is needed to create success for their future. Youth feel they have something valuable to contribute and feel it beneficial that their contributions be valued and included in responses designed to address their needs (Thira, 2000; Brown et al., 2007; Morris, 2007).

PHOTOVOICE AND DIGITAL STORYTELLING

Photovoice, a method in action research, is a grassroots community assessment tool enabling local people to identify, represent, and enhance their community through the use of photography as a medium for communication (Strack et al., 2004). Photovoice enables local people to actively participate in the research process, using cameras to record their views on their own communities. By using photography as the catalyst for both individual and community change, Photovoice allows participants to document their own worlds, discuss issues with policy makers, and become active agents in social action. Photovoice enhances the empowerment process by allowing marginalized peoples a central role in the mutual sharing of expertise and knowledge-building (Wang & Burris, 1997).

Digital storytelling is a multimedia art form combining both visual and auditory elements. Authors write a brief autobiographical script, which they then narrate as voiceover paired with a series of still images to relate a personal story (Gubrium, 2009). Though each story is unique to the individual, the process of creating a digital story also emphasizes connection to community through the workshops where participants learn to use the necessary technology and that function as the site of group bonding and growth as individuals share their stories (Gubrium, 2009). Digital stories are both a catharsis for the individual and also a vehicle to deliver a message to an audience—fellow participants or society at large. Distinctive aspects of digital storytelling include the importance of the story, narration in the unique rhythm of the author's voice that allows for authoritative self-representation, and the author's choice in images, which function as a connection point between an individual's story and cultural context (Benmayor, 2008). The process of constructing a digital story facilitates the author's self-reflection, while the performance allows for personal reconstruction and growth with the power to envision and direct the author's own identity and life story (Hull & Katz, 2006).

In the research project presented here, participants were Aboriginal youth between ages 14 and 18 years who were accessing youth programs offered through a local grassroots organization called *P A Women of the Earth Inc.* Through key informant and snowball sampling, 10 Aboriginal youth from Prince Albert, Saskatchewan, were invited to join the project. Over a 6-month period, the youth participated in 20 to 30 2-hour meetings (approximately once weekly) to identify the relevant issues and develop ways in which they could use their experiences to promote change. They were asked to create digital stories based on personal experience around identity to educate the community about identity for Aboriginal youth.

Data Collection

When the youth photographer group was established, the researcher/facilitator presented an initial theme for the photography "*I want you to know: Understanding Indigenous youth in Canada.*" The group discussed the initial theme to identify key issues and stimulate ideas about potential photos and how they could be represented on film. The group decided to make a photo book and combine their stories to create a narrative that identified and dispelled the various stereotypes and assumptions they felt society made about them and helped people understand how these stereotypes and assumptions impacted the way youth interacted with society. While they chose several photos to be showcased in the book, all photos were used as research data. As a group, everyone was assigned a role to play in the project, based on their strengths (e.g., photographers with strong organizational skills assisted with setting up group meetings and those who demonstrated strengths in public speaking presented at peer reviewed conferences).

Data Analysis

When the group felt they had exhausted their photographic possibilities, they met to discuss the photos. Using an analysis technique typically employed in the Photovoice process, the group was involved throughout the three-stage process that provided the foundation for analysis: selecting the photos they felt best represented their community's needs and assets; contextualizing or telling stories about what the pictures meant to them; and codifying or identifying issues, themes, and stories that emerged (Wang & Burris, 1997).

First, the group selected their favourite photos and discussed why they felt those were most significant. The person that took a particular photo then told the story represented in that photo to the group that also included the researcher. It included an explanation of why the photo was taken, and stories told by the person in the photo were shared. McIntyre (2003) recommends that photographers rely on instinct when choosing photos and analyze them according to the following questions: "What does the photo mean to you? What was the relationship between the content of the photo and how the youth perceived the community? How did the youth see the photo as reflecting issues that are salient to them?" (p. 53).

In the second round of analysis, the group organized two to four photographs into topic groups. Together, the group collected their ideas, identified similarities across photos, and constructed holistic analysis of the clusters of photographs through open dialogue (Lykes, 2001). The group then codified the issues, themes, and theories emerging in the discussions that arose from the photographs (Wang & Burris, 1997).

With the permission of the group, all discussions were audio-recorded and later transcribed. The written transcriptions were taken back to the group to ensure the transcriber had accurately captured the information shared. When the transcripts were accepted as accurate, the researcher then analyzed the data using a computer-assisted analysis program, which was then compared to the manual analysis completed during the group discussions.

YOUTH NARRATIVES

One of the biggest challenges the group identified in trying to understand their social position as Aboriginal youth was a combination of loss of cultural and community connection that taught them what it meant to be an Aboriginal person and the external definitions they received through stereotypes and assumptions that people made about them because of their appearance. The group described that many of the lifestyle choices they made because of their background were reflected in the stereotypes and assumptions made by society about Aboriginal youth. They thought these stereotypes existed because of racist attitudes that lowered societal expectations for the futures of Aboriginal youth. The group felt that stereotypes and assumptions influenced how people interacted with them and how they, in turn, viewed their place in society. This perception was articulated clearly in the narrative of a 16-year-old Aboriginal youth:

I want people to know that we aren't all bad people who cause problems. We don't drop out of school voluntarily and we aren't all gang members. We are diverse, some gifted with art, music, culture, math, and other such talents. We are capable of being great leaders within the city but with all the alienation, how can we thrive? Young kids seem to be dropping out of school because they want to. Most reasons for failure are from the feeling of being unwanted and pushed out and the effects of alienation. As an Aboriginal youth, I experience "the look". "The look" is the stare you receive when you enter a store, when you enter a class, or when you are giving your future employer your resume. Did you know that most native youth are poor because of the effect of racism, poverty, and colonialism? We are caught between two worlds and both parties have a strong will. When I say strong will it is both ways of life. It is the being in the mainstream culture with the wants and needs to nourish the Aboriginal identities. We just want to belong.

Negative stereotypes and assumptions limited the ability and desire of Aboriginal youth to succeed; it is difficult to make positive changes when "other people don't think [we] can really do this." It took incredible strength and resilience for the group to balance how they felt society defined them with their understanding of what it meant to be an Aboriginal youth.

The group felt that a part of knowing who you are is being proud of what you are (see Fig. 38.1):

We are members of Treaty Six and we are Cree people. Our culture is very beautiful; we honour the earth and treat every child to the oldest elder with respect. I am writing this to tell you what it means to be an Aboriginal youth. As a native youth you are considered a double whammy due to the idea that natives are gangsters and drunks. And then there is the presumption that youth are shoplifters and uncontrollable. Put those together and you have a bad stereotype of two misjudged people. Have you heard this quite often? This is true. You as an Aboriginal youth stay true to who you are. Keep yourself balanced within the medicine wheel. You will be young and full of knowledge. My advice is to take advantage to a lot of opportunities to travel, dance, sing, and expand your "to do" list. See what the Creator has made to discover. Experience all the beautiful cultures. Don't cut yourself short because society doesn't think you are worth it. So, stand tall and embrace your culture because we are worth standing up for.

The group admitted that they struggled to maintain the motivation to improve their situations because the doubt and expectation to fail they received from external sources

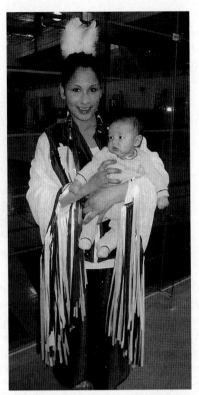

FIGURE 38.1   "I am sacred; I am Cree and I am proud." (Photo by project participant.)

superseded their internal belief in their ability. The group felt that recognition of their ac-complishments and external belief in their ability was essential to their personal growth and development. They believed society needed to be challenged to think critically about the reality of the lives of Aboriginal youth to inform their understanding through dialogue with Aboriginal youth:

Not every Aboriginal kid is bad or dangerous. You need to take time to realize that we all have potential. Spend some time with us so that you know that we are almost the same as other kids our age. Learn a thing about our beautiful culture and understand that we're all human and we deserve to be treated like it.

The group shared their experiences of racism in society, from other youth, at school, and in their workplaces. Exposure to stereotypes and racism had a detrimental effect on their identity as Aboriginal youth. The group identified feelings of shame about their Aboriginal culture, stat-ing that many Aboriginal youth try to dismiss their heritage in order to free themselves from stereotypes and racist attitudes in society, which had detrimental effects on their self-esteem and confidence. The photo in Figure 38.2 exemplifies this emotion.

It's a young girl with moccasins on but her pants are basically hiding them, and that's because some are ashamed of their culture and some don't want to be Aboriginal—that's why you see blonde hair and blue eyed natives with light brown skin, it's because they dyed their hair blonde put in blue contacts.

The group identified the delicate balance of defining and redefining who they are as Ab-original youth as a daily struggle. For urban youth, this struggle was compounded by the lack of opportunity to become engaged in cultural activities. Having the opportunity to engage in Aboriginal culture, learning the language and engaging in ceremonies, offered opportunity to redefine who they are as Aboriginal youth.

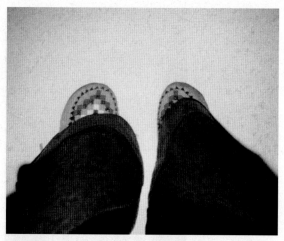

FIGURE 38.2 Feelings about Aboriginal culture. (Photo by project participant.)

The group shared concerns of losing cultural teachings and were concerned about the lack of available cultural programming in urban centres. They felt that it would be beneficial for Aboriginal youth, especially females, to have a traditional understanding of women in society. The group felt that traditional teachings emphasizing women's strength and importance in society, as well as respecting their power as women, would be valuable lessons for Aboriginal youth. Locating trusted and respected elders to provide these teachings in urban centres was a challenge (see Fig. 38.3).

I don't think, without Elders, I don't think . . . our culture can survive. Let's face it, there are very few young people who are interested in culture now a days. And with Elders, no matter of how bad of a kid you are, almost all native kids looked up to their Kokum or their Mushum.

To be an Aboriginal youth is to be the descendants of past Aboriginal generations that are the original in-habitants of our land. When I was younger I never really got any teachings or lessons that I needed. . . . Take

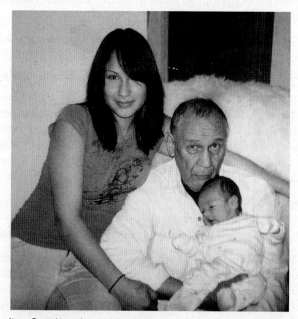

FIGURE 38.3 Feelings flow through generations. (Photo by project participant.)

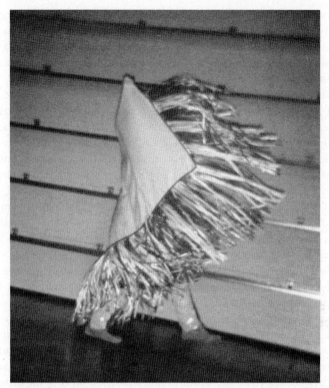

FIGURE 38.4   Feeling connected through cultural teachings. (Photo by project participant.)

every opportunity you can to go to camp with Mushum and Kokum. (They) can teach you things about the
wilderness and let them tell you stories about our past. Listen to them and ask them questions so you can
pass on these stories to your grandchildren. Keep the stories flowing through the generations.

Cultural programming was seen as essential. The group felt that cultural teachings specific to Aboriginal youth was key in their social, emotional, and spiritual development. They felt that cultural teachings specific to youth infused respect for their culture that had eroded over the years. The group shared stories of involvement in cultural activities that gave them a clearer sense of identity and importance (see Fig. 38.4). Protocols maintain that those taking part in ceremonies and cultural activities need to be drug and alcohol free and therefore participation would promote healthy lifestyle choices, as well as increasing confidence and self-esteem.

It gives them a reason to not do things, like, if you're making a dress then you have a reason not to drink,
if you're going to a sweat lodge or going to a traditional dance or a wake or something you know not to
do drugs or to abstain from doing harm to yourself.

DISCUSSION

Community issues were seen as generational. The legacy of residential schools had begun the process of stripping away not only Aboriginal identity but also the importance of women in society. The group felt that the consequences of residential school could still be seen today in the struggles of Aboriginal families, their experiences in the foster care system, and the lack of recognition of female Aboriginal role models. The combination of these issues could be explained by the loss of culture in the family and community. The group viewed their identity as a constant struggle against negative societal perceptions of Aboriginal youth. Reclaiming identity was seen as especially important in challenging current perceptions for their own success and for the success of future generations. Raising children and youth to understand and value the role of family, culture, and community provides a basis for individual strength in identity and respect for Aboriginal culture.

Given the importance of cultural programming in developing and strengthening the identity of Aboriginal youth, the group expressed disappointment that community programs that genuinely promoted Aboriginal teachings were not readily available in urban settings. Programming specific to the needs of Aboriginal youth would offer an opportunity to promote identity development through cultural activities, teachings, and access to role models and mentors. The group recommended that such programs should be gender specific to help develop a positive sense of identity for both female and male youth. The group spoke to the importance of instilling a sense of pride in being Aboriginal and the importance that pride held for family and community. They noted that youth involved in cultural activities had a sense of responsibility to live their lives mindful of the impact their decisions had on themselves, their families, and their communities.

During this project, the group was able to derive a holistic picture that included reflection into the emotional, social, and cultural issues of Aboriginal youth living in urban centres. These issues were viewed as iterative cycles with limited support in one area feeding into lack of success in another. These cycles were characterized by a struggle to create a sense of identity in which to situate themselves within their culture, families, and communities. The tone of the discussion and the images caught on film were described by the counterpoints of desperation and hope. The group was able to articulate their struggles, and they were also able to identify what they needed to be successful in life. Reflecting on this, the group recognized that what they sought was a connection to someone or something.

By engaging with the project and each other, the group began to think of themselves less as victims and more as teachers. They felt that they had experienced and overcome many hardships in the course of their lives, and their survival left them with important lessons to share with other youth experiencing similar adversity. They believed that Aboriginal youth need the opportunity to talk openly about the reality of their lives in order to ease their feelings of isolation.

The Aboriginal youth in the project were able to speak thoughtfully and concretely about their circumstances and needs. The group found that healing began with acknowledging the adversity in the lives of urban Aboriginal youth and then emphasizing the importance of family and community support. Recognizing their own potential as role models highlighted the importance of having role models to guide and support them.

Summary

The voices and perspective of Aboriginal youth in this project supported the results of earlier studies in which youth suggested that they clearly understood what was necessary to make positive and lasting changes (Thira, 2000; Brown et al., 2007; Morris, 2007). A common theme throughout the project's Photovoice and digital storytelling processes supported current literature on the importance of cultural continuity in creating positive and lasting change for Aboriginal people, families, and communities. As the group reflected on the issues and needs of urban Aboriginal youth, they recognized the importance of regaining cultural knowledge and ties to recapture their lost identity. Reconnecting with their Aboriginal culture and identity was key to addressing many of the current socioeconomic concerns; incorporating these teachings into their everyday lives generated respect for their minds, bodies, and spirits and challenged them to live their lives in a way that respected each of these.

The level of insight and maturity demonstrated by the group was astounding; these Aboriginal youth were able to consider their personal circumstances within the broader context of family, community, and culture. In so doing, the group did not get trapped in a cycle of negativity by reminiscing about past wrongs but instead created prospects for positive change and hope for their generation.

REFERENCES

Benmayor, R. (2008). Digital storytelling as a signature pedagogy in the new humanities. *Arts and Humanities in Higher Education, 7*(2), 188–204.

Brown, I. (2003). Aboriginal health and wellness. In *Touch Magazine, Vol. 26.* Ottawa: National Indian & Inuit Community Health Representatives Organization (NIICHRO).

Brown, J., Knol, D., Prevost-Derbecker, S., & Andrushko, K. (2007). Housing for Aboriginal youth in the inner city of Winnipeg. *First Peoples Child and Family Review, 3*(2), 56–64.

Chandler, M. J., Lalonde, C. E., Sokol, B. W., & Hallett, D. (2003). Personal persistence, identity development, and suicide: A study of native and non-Native North American adolescents. *Monographs of the Society for Research in Child Development, 68*(2), 1–138.

Gubrium, A. (2009). Digital storytelling: An emergent method for health promotion research and practice. *Health Promotion Practice, 10*(2), 186–191.

Hull, G. A., & Katz, M. L. (2006). Crafting an agentive self: Case studies of digital storytelling. *Research in the Teaching of English, 41*(1), 43–81.

Lykes, M. B. (2001). Creative arts and photography in participatory action research in Guatemala. In P. Reason & H. Bradbury (Eds.), *Handbook of action research: Participative inquiry and practice* (pp. 1–14). Thousand Oaks: Sage Publications.

MacNeil, M. (2008). An epidemiologic study of Aboriginal adolescent risk in Canada: The meaning of suicide. *Journal of Child and Adolescent Psychiatric Nursing, 21*(1), 3–12.

McIntyre, A. (2003). Through the eyes of women: Photovoice and participatory research as tools for reimagining place. *Gender, Place and Culture, 10*(1), 47–66.

Morris, K. (2007). Re-examining issues behind the loss of family and cultural and the impact on Aboriginal youth suicide rates. *First Peoples Child and Family Review, 3*(1), 133–142.

Oritz, S. (2011). Aboriginal continuance: Collaboration and syncretism. *The American Indian Quarterly, 35*(3), 285–293.

Strack, R. W., Magill, C., & McDonagh, K. (2004). Engaging youth through photovoice. *Health Promotion Practice, 5*(1), 49–58.

Thira, D. (2000). What are the contributing factors to Aboriginal youth suicide? In *Through the pain: Suicide prevention handbook.* Vancouver: Thira Consulting.

Trépanier, F. (2008). *Aboriginal arts research initiative: Report on consultations.* Ottawa: Canada Council for the Arts, Strategic Initiatives Division URL=http://canadacouncil.ca/~/media/files/research%20-%20en/aboriginal%20arts%20initiative%20aari/aarifinalreport.pdf.

Wang, C., & Burris, M. A. (1997). Photovoice: Concept, methodology, and use for participatory needs assessment. *Health Education and Behavior, 24*(3), 369–387.

ONLINE RESOURCES

Please visit thePoint. at http://thepoint.lww.com/Vollman4e for up-to-date Internet resources and additional learning materials on this topic.

Index

Note: Page numbers followed by f, t, and b indicate figures, tables, and boxed material, respectively.

RRS1605